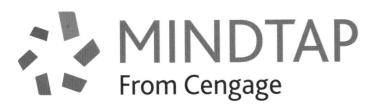

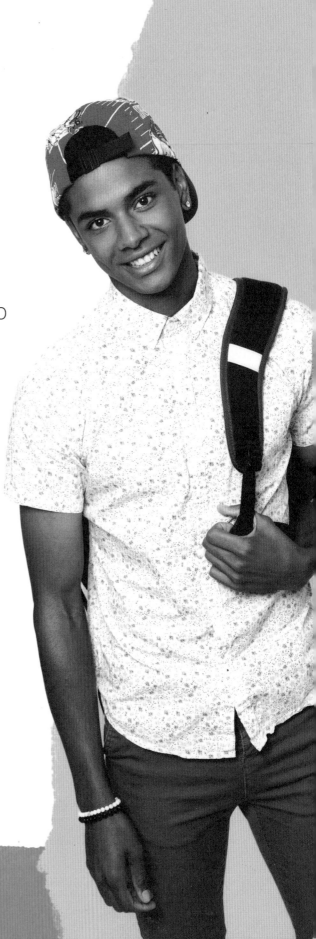

DRUGS
ACROSS THE
SPECTRUM

8th EDITION

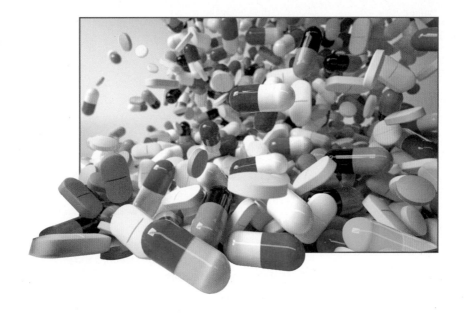

Raymond Goldberg, Ph.D.

Pardess Mitchell

Associate Professor, William Rainey Harper College

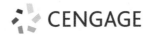 **CENGAGE**

Australia • Brazil • Mexico • Singapore • United Kingdom • United States

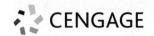

Drugs Across the Spectrum, **8th Edition**
Raymond Goldberg, Pardess Mitchell

Product Director: Dawn Giovanniello

Product Manager: Krista Mastroianni

Project Manager: Tyler Sally

Content Developer: Laura Lawrie

Product Assistant: Marina Starkey

Marketing Manager: Ana Albinson

Manufacturing Planner: Karen Hunt

Image Researcher: Lumina Datamatics Ltd.

Text Researcher: Lumina Datamatics Ltd.

Production Management and Composition:
  MPS Limited

Art and Cover Direction: MPS Limited

Text Designer: MPS Limited

Cover Image: iStockPhoto.com/Artfoliophoto

For product information and technology assistance, contact us at
Cengage Customer & Sales Support, 1-800-354-9706

For permission to use material from this text or product,
submit all requests online at **www.cengage.com/permissions.**
Further permissions questions can be emailed to
permissionrequest@cengage.com.

Library of Congress Control Number: 2017951369

Student Edition:
ISBN: 978-1-337-55736-8

Loose-leaf Edition:
ISBN: 978-1-337-55753-5

Cengage
20 Channel Center Street
Boston, MA 02210
USA

Cengage is a leading provider of customized learning solutions with employees residing in nearly 40 different countries and sales in more than 125 countries around the world. Find your local representative at **www.cengage.com.**

To learn more about Cengage platforms and services, visit **www.cengage.com.**

To register or access your online learning solution or purchase materials for your course, visit **www.cengagebrain.com.**

Printed in the United States of America
Print Number: 01   Print Year: 2017

CONTENTS

PREFACE

Mind-altering substances have had a profound effect on society ever since humans first roamed the planet. The goal of this book is to impart an understanding of drugs and their impact on individuals, families, communities, and society. In addition to providing a thorough review of illicit drugs, the book devotes much attention to licit, or legal, drugs. This focus is pertinent because drugs such as tobacco and alcohol account for far more deaths and disabilities than do illicit drugs. Also, millions of people use prescribed and over-the-counter drugs that are potentially harmful. This book also covers performance-enhancing drugs such as anabolic steroids because of their increased use in the past decade.

Unlike some texts, *Drugs Across the Spectrum* goes beyond the presentation of abstract concepts and impersonal information to examine issues that warrant personal reflection. One goal of *Drugs Across the Spectrum* is to make the information relevant to the reader. It is understood that no one is immune from the effects of drug use. People face decisions about their own drug use and drug use by family members and friends. Societal effects and public policy are also areas that require knowledge on which to base responsible decisions.

Organization

Drugs Across the Spectrum is divided into three parts. The first five chapters, Chapters 1 to 5, provide an overall view, including a historical perspective, the motivations for drug use, social implications of drug use, legal ramifications, and factors affecting how drugs interact with the human body. Chapters 6 through 14 focus on specific categories of drugs, exploring their psychological and physiological effects. The final chapters, Chapters 15 and 16, critically examine treatment and prevention, including various modes of drug treatment, the effectiveness of drug treatment, and the impact of education and prevention in addressing problems caused by drug use, misuse, and abuse.

Notable Changes in This Edition

The science of drugs continues to evolve, as new ways to study addiction help us understand the impact of drugs and drug dependence. Designer drugs continue to arise in society of which their popularity continues to change as new drugs replace older ones on the market. This edition includes updated information on designer drugs such as kratom and flakka.

Moreover, as the landscape regarding drug use continues to change, this edition contains current references regarding drug use and includes recent studies of drug use.

Furthermore, this edition contains updated case studies with including high profile media profiles. New figures and tables were added with questions to help students think about the data presented and encourage students to interpret data (quantitative literacy).

For all chapters and highlights, we have:

- Added a "Consider this" for each chapter
- Added relevant case studies in each chapter
- Created several new figures and tables and revised others to enhance learning
- Revised chapter objectives to reflect different levels of learning based on Bloom's Taxonomy
- Expanded on 'Cultural Considerations' using Gloria Ladson-Billing's (2009) principles of culturally relevant pedagogy to enhance students' development of cultural competence
- Added questions throughout the text to promote critical thinking skills among students

Chapter 1
- Took out short histories for each drug and placed them in the chapter pertaining to that drug
- Added section about motivations for drug use
- Added section on theories of addiction
- Updated text on biological risk factors for drug dependence

Chapter 2
- Updated all data from Monitoring the Future and National Survey on Drug Use and Health
- Presented new figures from National Survey on Drug Use and Health
- Added more information on the impact of drugs on the family using updated references
- Added a section on the online drug trade
- Expanded section on public assistance and drug testing
- Added figures with questions to promote interpretations of graphical data
- Took out section on designer drugs and the drug business (added in chapter 3)

Chapter 3
- This chapter discusses drug laws (previously in chapter 4)
- Added section on the business of drugs (previously in chapter 2)
- Added relevant case study on marijuana with questions to ponder
- Expanded and updated section on drug paraphernalia including major cases portrayed in the media
- Expanded and added relevant information on racial considerations

Chapter 4
- Updated information on neurotransmitters
- Added case studies relevant to the study of neurotransmission
- Discussed how pleasure derived from drugs and pleasure derived from food are different
- Updated statistics on age and drug use
- Updated and added information on the different ways drugs are metabolized by gender and race/ethnicity
- Added a case study on ethnicity and in the effects of drugs

Chapter 5
- Chapter on designer, synthetic and performance enhancing drugs
- Included a history of designer drugs
- Added section on designer drugs with updated references including media headlines regarding its use
- Expanded information on performance enhancing drugs with updated statistics and trends
- Added drug business section with updated trends including high profile cases (i.e. El Chapo, Rodrigo Duterte (Philippine's President)

Chapter 6
- Updates all statistics regarding alcohol consumption trends
- Added section on the consequences of prohibition
- Updated and included information on the impact of heavy alcohol use on the brain
- Updated and included additional information regarding the factors that contribute to alcoholism
- Included new DSM V criteria for alcohol use disorder

Chapter 7
- Updated all statistics regarding tobacco use
- Updated new cultural considerations with questions for students to ponder

- Updated new on Campus box regarding smoke-free campus policies
- Added section on electronic cigarettes
- Added section on using tobacco from a hookah

Chapter 8
- Updated statistics on narcotic use
- Updated section on the use of naloxone
- Updated section on NEPs
- Added relevant case studies

Chapter 9
- Added section on Ketamine
- Added case study on date rape drugs on campus
- Changed classification of inhalants to gases, nitrites, volatile solvents, and aerosols
- Added case study on the use of sleeping aids
- Updated statistics on use of sedative hypnotics

Chapter 10
- Added section on mental disorders and substance abuse
- Expanded on comorbidity and dual diagnoses

Chapter 11
- Added section on cocaine's impact on neurotransmitters
- Updated cocaine treatment section

Chapter 12
- Updated State laws regarding medical and recreation marijuana use
- Updated current research regarding therapeutic benefits of marijuana
- Expanded on current conditions that may benefit from marijuana use
- Updated guidelines from National Academies of Science, Engineering, and Medicine

Chapter 13
- Expanded on research regarding the therapeutic benefits of psilocybin and LSD.
- Added case studies and historical contexts for hallucinogenic drugs

Chapter 14
- Expanded section on cold and cough medicine abuse on college campuses
- Presented arguments for and against changing RX medications to OTC
- Expanded section on herbal supplements including research regarding the actual contents of these medicines

Chapter 15

- New tables were created highlighting similarities between substance abuse treatment and chronic disease treatment
- Presented an argument how relapse is a natural progression of treatment, using examples from chronic disease models
- Expanded on types of outpatient therapies used for treatment including benefits of each type.
- Added a case student regarding the arrest of a drug using pregnant women

Chapter 16

- Added principles of an effective substance abuse prevention program
- Added information on Red Ribbon Certified Schools

Features

- Chapter objectives at the beginning of each chapter put the content into a meaningful framework.
- Color photos, illustrations, and tables reflect the latest drug statistics and trends.
- "Thinking Critically" questions at the end of each chapter promote critical thinking and stimulate classroom discussion.
- "Cultural Considerations" boxes in each chapter provide key information about how drug use, drug abuse, and legal penalties vary between ethnic groups, age groups, and nations.
- "On Campus" boxes in each chapter focus on facts and statistics that are relevant to college students.
- Each chapter includes "Fact or Fiction?" questions that enable readers to examine their beliefs and possible misconceptions about various drugs.
- Key terms are highlighted and defined as they are discussed in the text to give readers easy access to the meaning of vocabulary essential to their understanding.
- A brief summary concludes each chapter.
- Web resources at the end of each chapter have been thoroughly updated and include brief descriptions to direct readers to specific information related to chapter topics.

Ancillaries

The following ancillaries have been developed to support the printed textbook:

- **Instructor's Manual:** Contains chapter outlines, discussion questions, lecture outlines and select activities.

- **Test Bank:** Powered by Cognero, the test Bank is a flexible, online system that allows instructors to author, edit, and manage test bank content from multiple Cengage Learning solutions; create multiple test versions in an instant; and deliver tests from your Learning Management System (LMS), your classroom, or anywhere you want.
- **PowerPoint Presentation: Includes materials from** each chapter that can be customized for use in the classroom.
- **Drugs Across the Spectrum MindTap:** Drugs Across the Spectrum MindTap brings course concepts to life with interactive learning, study, and exam preparation tools that support the printed textbook. The MindTap includes an interactive eReader, and interactive teaching and learning tools including quizzes, flashcards, and more. It also contains built in metrics tools that monitors student engagement in the course.

Acknowledgments

This book has benefited from the assistance of many people. The individuals who were instrumental in seeing this project come to fruition include Dawn Giovanniello, Product Director; Krista Mastroianni, Product Manager; Laura Lawrie, Content Project Manager (Lumina); Tyler Sally, Associate Project Manager; Jim Zayicek, Project Manager; Manoj Kumar, Senior Project Manager (MPS); Tom Griffin, Senior Media Producer; and Marina Starkey, Product Assistant. Their expertise and support throughout this endeavour are greatly appreciated.

I would like to give special thanks to the reviewers, whose input has been very valuable for this revision:

Dr. Deborah M. Wilson, Bethune-Cookman University
James W. Brenner, West Chester University
Joaquin Fenollar Bataller, University of Kentucky
Kathleen Phillips, PhD, Eastern Illinois University
Mark Plonsky, PhD, University of Wisconsin
Pardess Mitchell, EdD, Harper College
Shannon Norman, Bemidji State University

I would like to thank my wife, Barbara, and my daughters, Tara and Greta, for their continuing love and support.

I would like to thank my husband Jack, my sons, Devin and Jase, and my daughter Arieanne for their support.

—Raymond Goldberg and Pardess Mitchell

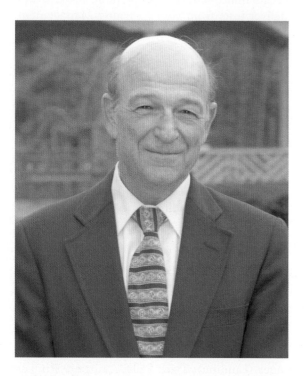

Raymond Goldberg is a professor emeritus of health education and associate dean at the State University of New York at Cortland. He recently retired from Vance-Granville Community College, where he served as the Dean of Health Sciences. Over the course of his professional life, Ray has taught a variety of drug-related courses, authored numerous articles on health- and drug-related topics, and received several significant research grants for his work in health and drug education. Ray is also the author of *Taking Sides: Clashing Views on Controversial Issues in Drugs and Society* (McGraw-Hill). He received his undergraduate degree from the University of North Carolina at Pembroke, his master's degree from the University of South Carolina, and his Ph.D. from the University of Toledo.

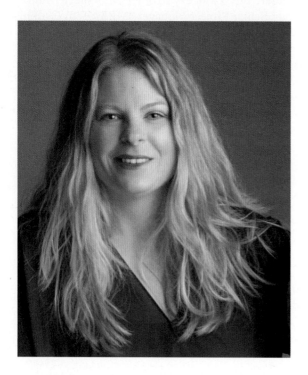

Pardess Mitchell is an Assistant Professor at Harper College in Illinois where she is the Department Co-Chair for the Kinesiology and Health Education Department. She has previously held positions at the College of Lake County. She teaches in the areas of Health Education. Professor Mitchell received her Bachelor of Science for University of Maryland College Park, her Masters of Science, Health Education, from Southern Illinois University, Carbondale, and her Doctor of Education from Northern Illinois University.

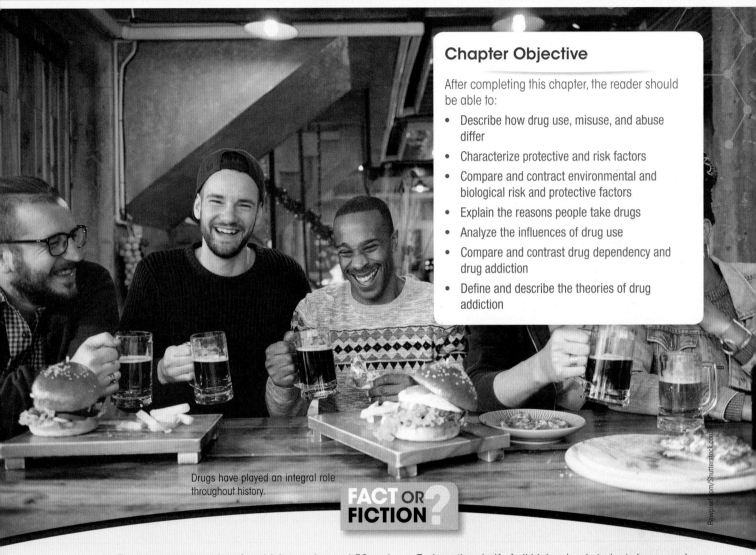

Drugs have played an integral role throughout history.

Rawpixel.com/Shutterstock.com

Chapter Objective

After completing this chapter, the reader should be able to:

- Describe how drug use, misuse, and abuse differ
- Characterize protective and risk factors
- Compare and contract environmental and biological risk and protective factors
- Explain the reasons people take drugs
- Analyze the influences of drug use
- Compare and contrast drug dependency and drug addiction
- Define and describe the theories of drug addiction

FACT OR FICTION?

1. The most common drug for which people aged 50 and older receive treatment is alcohol.

2. The use and abuse of drugs is a recent phenomenon.

3. The elderly are less likely to misuse drugs compared to younger adults.

4. Drug abuse can cause one to develop a mental illness.

5. One-third of all emergency room visits were attributed to pharmaceutical drugs.

6. Drug awareness programs at schools (such as D.A.R.E.) raise a child's curiosity regarding drug use.

7. Less than half of all high school students have used alcohol in the past year.

8. Adolescents that use alcohol before the age of 15 are more likely to become alcohol dependent as an adult.

9. European, American, and Chinese adolescents are more likely to be influenced by peers in their drug use behaviors compared to African American adolescents.

10. Religious groups in the United States are not permitted to use illicit drugs for religious ceremonies.

Turn the page to check your answers ➔

The use and abuse of drugs have always played a role in society. Archaeological evidence suggests that as early as the fourth millennium BC, people were consuming alcohol. People coming together to drink alcohol is an activity that has remained constant throughout history. Images of drinking scenes, from the fourth millennium BC, have been uncovered and imply the use of alcohol has been around almost as long as people have.[1] The use of **drugs** in prehistoric times is not limited to alcohol. Societies have been using mind-altering substances (i.e., hallucinogens) for spiritual and healing purposes.[2]

Drug use and **drug abuse** continue to impact society. It is estimated that illicit drugs cost the United States more than $700 billion annually.[3] The cost of crime, lost work productivity, and healthcare are taken into account when determining the cost of **illicit drug use** in the United States. Drug use impacts everyone in society, not just users, but nonusers as well.

A historical perspective on drugs provides insight into the role that drugs have played over time. We also can benefit from a common understanding of what the terms **drug, drug misuse**, and **drug abuse** mean. Many factors affect how these words are defined. Is a substance defined as a drug according to its behavioral effects, pharmacological effects, effects on society, or chemical makeup? If drugs are viewed as only illegal or menacing substances, we may not acknowledge substances such as caffeine and tobacco as drugs. If caffeine and tobacco are not considered drugs, one may think they cannot be misused or abused because only illegal drugs are misused or abused. Or a person may grow up thinking that any drug use, from aspirin to nasal decongestants, is unacceptable. If someone takes three aspirins a day, is he or she misusing or abusing drugs? What if a person has a glass of beer with dinner and a glass of wine each night before going to bed? What about the use of hallucinogenic drugs to enhance a person's spirituality? The Native American Church uses the hallucinogen peyote in a spiritual context but not recreationally.[4] Our attitudes regarding drug use are shaped not only by our own experiences with drugs, but also by our motivations for taking drugs.

Although definitions for the word drug are numerous, there is no legal definition. **Drugs** therefore can be defined as any substance when taken in the body that alters the structure and function of the body. This definition excludes food substances. Could foods be included as drugs? If you have ever seen a small child hyped up on sugar, you may come

CONSIDER This

Drug abuse impacts nonusers. Think of ways drug abuse would impact the following people:

- A mother to a college-age person who is abusing alcohol
- An older sibling to a high school age person who is smoking marijuana
- A spouse to a person who is abusing pain medication
- A child to an alcoholic parent

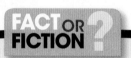

1. **FACT** Among people aged 50 and older, almost 60% receive treatment for alcohol abuse.

2. **FICTION** The fact is—Images of drinking scenes have been discovered from the fourth millennium BC.

3. **FICTION** The fact is—Almost 20% of the elderly combine alcohol with prescription medication

4. **FICTION** The fact is—while there is a relationship between drug abuse and mental illness, it is unclear whether drug abuse can cause a mental illness.

5. **FACT** Pharmaceutical drugs were attributed to one-third of all of emergency room visits.

6. **FICTION** The fact is—Many of the drug awareness programs that include ex-drug addicts and police officers raise children's curiosity about drugs and may result in increased experimentation.

7. **FICTION** The fact is—Over half of all high school student reported using alcohol in the past year.

8. **FACT** The younger a person is when they use alcohol, the more likely they will develop alcohol dependency as an adult.

9. **FACT** Studies have shown African American adolescents are less influenced by their peer drug use compared with European, American, and Chinese adolescents.

10. **FICTION** The fact is—Some religious groups are given special permission to use psychedelic drugs in their religious ceremonies. The Native American Church has been permitted to use peyote as part of their religious ceremony.

IS SUGAR A DRUG?

Almost two decades ago, researchers looked at the impact of sugar on babies (aged 9–12 weeks). Do babies have a preference for sugary substances and how can one measure these preferences? It may surprise you to discover that babies are impacted by sugary substances and develop a preference for those people who deliver that sugary substance (think sugar dealer). Researchers gave babies a sugary substance while staring into their eyes. They discovered that babies then developed a preference for the people who supplied their sugary substance. This became clear when a group of strangers and the sugar-dealing researcher entered the room while the mom was holding the baby. The babies' gaze was analyzed and it was found that the babies had a preference for the sugar-dealing researcher over the stranger.[1]

Almost a decade later, researchers conducted a study on rats to determine if they have a preference for sugary substances. The researchers used Oreos as their sugary substance. They discovered that rats formed equal preferences for eating Oreos as they did for cocaine or morphine. To make matters more interesting, they also found that eating Oreos activated more neurons in the brain's pleasure center than the drugs heroin and cocaine. [2,3]

HOW WOULD YOU MAKE THE ARGUMENT THAT SUGAR IS A DRUG?

Think back on the definition of a drug. How would you make the argument that sugar is not a drug?

1. Elliot M. Blass, Carole A. Camp, "The Ontogeny of Face Recognition: Eye Contact and Sweet Taste Induce Face Preference in 9 and 12 week-old Human Infants," *Developmental Psychology* 37, no 6 (2001), 762–774.

2. Simon McCormack, "Oreos more Addictive than Cocaine? Study shows Cookies might produce more Pleasure than Coke in Rats." *Huffington Post.* October 18, 2013. Available at: http://www.huffingtonpost.com/2013/10/17/oreos-more-addictive-than-cocaine_n_4118194.html.

3. Connecticut College, "Student-faculty research suggests Oreos can be compared to Drugs of Abuse." *Connecticut College News Archive.* Available at: 2016, https://www.conncoll.edu/news/news-archive/2013/student-faculty-research-suggests-oreos-can-be-compared-to-drugs-of-abuse-in-lab-rats.html#.V-UL-iTA24o

to believe sugar is a drug. There are many parents who take actions to limit the amount of sugar given to their children to avoid such behavior. Many people crave ice cream and chocolate to cope with unpleasant experiences or simply to raise their spirits. Should these be considered drugs? Are they used differently from many substances identified as drugs?

One definition of **psychoactive drugs** is "substances that act to alter mood, thought processes, or behavior, or that are used to manage neuropsychological illness."[5] These substances can be used recreationally, medically, illegally, or legally. The legality of drug use depends on many factors that change over time and can change situationally. Consider a person who is over 21 who drinks a glass of wine with dinner. Compare this to a person who is under 21 who drink a glass of wine with dinner. In the first instance, this would be considered a legal recreational behavior, whereas in the second instance it would be considered an illegal recreational behavior. The only difference in the two examples is age, which in the United States, is a factor that defines when a person

can legally consume alcohol. What about a person who occasionally uses illicit drugs without major detriment to one's health? Is it possible for a person to be a responsible illicit drug user? Can one use a drug in a way to minimize risk? Imagine a successful business person who uses cocaine occasionally when out with friends. Could this be considered responsible use?

drug Any substance that alters one's ability to function emotionally, physically, intellectually, financially, or socially

drug misuse The unintentional or inappropriate use of prescribed or over-the-counter drugs

drug abuse The intentional and inappropriate use of a drug resulting in physical, emotional, financial, intellectual, or social consequences for the user

illicit drugs use Illegal drug use

psychoactive drug Any substance that has the capability of altering mood, perception, or behavior

Drug Misuse

Drug misuse refers to the unintentional or inappropriate use of prescribed or over-the-counter drugs. More information regarding the abuse of prescription drugs is elaborated on later in the text. One group especially vulnerable to drug misuse is the elderly.[6] Although individuals aged 65 and older represent 13% of the population, this age group accounts for one-third of all medications prescribed.[7] The elderly are more likely to be prescribed long-term medication and multiple prescriptions.[8] The elderly population experiences higher rates of sleep disorders, pain, and anxiety, which results in higher use of medications. In fact, prescription drug misuse among the elderly is increasing.[9] Almost 20% of older Americans combine the use of alcohol with medication.[10] Alcohol can cause adverse effects when combined with either prescription or over-the-counter medication. This coupled with a declining cognitive function may result in improperly using the prescribed medication. Additionally, many of the elderly are on a fixed income and struggle to find ways to pay for their medication. As a result, they may not take the prescribed amount as a way to reduce costs.[11] Furthermore, this does not take into account the impact over-the-counter medicines many elderly take and how these impact drug interactions between the prescribed and nonprescribed medication. These older adults are more likely to experience negative effects of these drug interactions due to increased drug sensitivity and slower metabolisms.[12]

Drug misuse may result from not understanding a drug's effects. For example, if a student studies for a test and drinks alcohol to improve his or her study skills, the student is misusing alcohol because it does not improve learning. Misuse may arise from deluding oneself about one's purpose for using drugs. This is illustrated by a person who consumes five glasses of wine daily and says it is for spiritual purposes. Examples of drug misuse are the following:

- Discontinuing prescribed medicines against the physician's recommendation (discontinuing antibiotics once the symptoms of an illness disappear)
- Mixing drugs (some drugs, particularly depressants, can be fatal when consumed together)
- Consuming more of a drug than prescribed (if one pill or tablespoon is good, five is not five times as good!)
- Using more than one prescription at a time without informing the physician who wrote the prescription
- Saving or using old medications (the properties of drugs and their effectiveness change over time)

- Not following the directions for a drug; some drugs are ineffective when taken at certain times, such as after eating

Drug misuse has been a concern since the 1990s. There are several conditions present that make addressing issues of drug misuse particularly challenging, particularly in regards to treatment. Take, for example, the idea that prescription and over-the-counter medication have health benefits as well as risks for the user. How does one go about countering the impact of the negative consequences while maintaining the benefits received from these medications? Since many of the medications are over-the-counter and do not require a prescription, how does one go about gathering information to determine to what extent these medications are used and how misuse occurs? Lastly, there are few studies that have been done to characterize the factors that contribute to medication misuse.[13]

Drug Abuse

Drug abuse is the intentional and inappropriate use of a drug resulting in physical, emotional, financial, social, or intellectual consequences.[14] In other words, harm caused from using drugs would be considered drug abuse. Drug use and drug abuse are not the same. Consider a person who drinks beer when going out with friends. If the person drinks responsibly, less than two drinks in a 3-hour period, the behavior would not be considered abuse. Take the same situation, but this time, the person overdrinks and has four

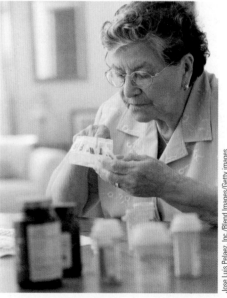

Jose Luis Pelaez, Inc./Blend Images/Getty images

The elderly use more prescription and over-the-counter drugs than people in other age groups.

Case Study-Protective and Risk Factors - adapted from: http://school.discoveryeducation.com /teachersguides/pdf/health/ds/rm_deadly_highs .pdf

SCENARIO 1

Allison is having a bad year. After years of not getting along, her parents had finally decided to get a divorce. While there was a lot of tension in the house, her parents were trying hard to be polite to each other and to be considerate of Allison's and her younger brother's feelings. Always a good student, Allison continued to find comfort in studying hard and getting good grades in school. Her best friend, Susie, had really been there for her, too. Every weekend Susie planned something fun for them to do by themselves or with other friends. Over the past several months, Allison and Susie have gone ice-skating on a regular basis, seen many movies, and gone bowling. Allison has also continued to play soccer on her school's team. Throughout the year, Allison has been able to talk to her parents about the pending divorce. Allison's parents have been willing to listen to her concerns and discuss her anger about this big change in her life. Allison feels really sad, but she knows she's going to be alright.

SCENARIO 2

Laura feels as if her life is falling apart. Her parents have just told her that they are getting a divorce. Although her parents haven't gotten along for years, Laura has always hoped that they would find a way to stay together so they could continue to be a family. Instead, her parents don't seem to have any time to talk to her about her feelings. Laura always thought she had a few good friends, but she isn't feeling like she can turn to them now. Her friend Katy has a boyfriend, and she doesn't get a chance to see her soccer teammates much outside of games and practices. Laura has always been a good student, and she continues to complete her assignments on time. But she has noticed that it is becoming increasingly difficult to concentrate on her schoolwork. Because she is feeling lonely and isolated, Laura is considering going to a party with Katy. She has heard that some kids bring drugs to these parties. For that reason, she has always stayed away. Now, however, she thinks it might be a way to get out of the house and forget about her problems for a little while. It might be fun. Laura is thinking that unless something else happens so that her social life improves, she might just go.

Questions

1. Which girl do you think is more likely to use drugs? Why?
2. List Allison's protective and risk factors.
3. List Laura's protective and risk factors.
4. Based on the above scenarios, which protective factors do you feel are strongest and why?

drinks in 3 hours. This amount of alcohol in a short period of time would be considered binge drinking and thus be characterized as drug abuse.

Where does the line exist between drug use and drug abuse and what factors impact whether a person crosses that line? **Protective** and **risk factors** play a role in whether an individual is more or less likely to abuse a drug. Protective factors reduce a person's risk for drug use behavior. On the other hand, risk factors increase a person's risk for drug use behavior.[15]

Environmental and biological factors make up protective and risk factors. Environmental factors include family, peers, school, and neighborhood conditions. Biological factors include a person's stage of development when first taking a drug and other conditions (i.e., mental disorders).[16] Some drug use and abuse results from conditions related to mental disorders. One study reported that adolescents with prior mental disorders had higher rates of alcohol and illicit drug abuse.[17] Furthermore, anxiety disorders were a factor related to the transition from nonuse to first use and from use to problematic use.[18]

Almost 2.5 million emergency room visits were associated with drug use or misuse.[19] Less than 5% of these visits were attributed to alcohol alone, while

protective factors Reduce a person's risk for drug use behavior

risk factors Increase a person's risk for drug use behavior

Table of Risk and Protective Environmental Factors

Risk Factors	Protective Factors
Lack of parental supervision	Parental monitoring and support
Poor social skills	Positive relationships
Availability of drugs at school	School antidrug policies
Community poverty	Neighborhood pride
Parental abuse of drugs	Parents reinforce nonuse of drugs

National Institute on Drug Abuse, "Drugs, Brains, and Behavior" The Science of Addiction, Revised July 2014. Available at: https://www.drugabuse.gov/publications/drugs-brains-behavior-science-addiction/drug-abuse-addiction.

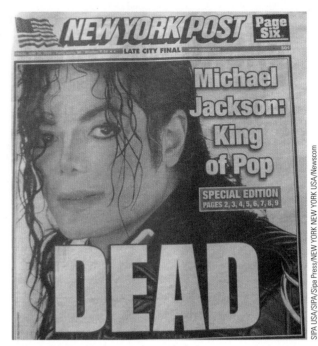

Michael Jackson is dead!

one-third of these visits were attributed to pharmaceutical drugs.[20] Hospital visits resulting in serious outcomes were associated with alcohol and other drug combination use.[21]

Drug addiction is pervasive in society. As indicated, addictions are not limited to substances. The following list identifies substances and behaviors to which people are addicted along with the number of people in the United States for whom these substances or behaviors are a problem.[22]

- Alcohol—6.6 million people over the age of 12 report alcohol dependence or abuse. Males have higher rates of abuse compared to females.
- Drugs—persons aged 18 to 25 have the highest rate of illicit drug dependence and abuse at 7.4% of the population.
- Gambling addiction—5.7 million people have a gambling disorder.[23]

Drug use and abuse is a problem in society. Why do people start using drugs in the first place? We live in a society where information is at our fingertips; a person only has to ask the question about the dangers of drug use in order to view thousands of webpages with that information. Media headlines about famous people dying from drug overdoses cover the front pages of magazines and newspapers. One would imagine these would positively influence a person's decision to try drugs. In the following section, motivations for drug use will be described with a focus on the factors that influence a person's motivation for taking drugs.

In many ways, drug use mirrors the broader society. Reasons for drug use and the needs that drugs fulfill are affected by societal changes. In our scientifically advanced, technological world change occurs so rapidly that our ability to adapt cannot keep pace. Many inventions of the 20th century provide

instant or immediate feedback: Computers offer instant access to information; banks with automatic teller machines dispense money at any time of the day or night; fast-food restaurants and microwave ovens satisfy hunger speedily; communication with friends is instantaneous through our cell phones. People adapt to a changing society by learning to cope, by withdrawing, or by escaping. Drugs are one means to that end.

Alternatives to using drugs include exercise programs, support groups, Internet games, watching television, listening to music, talking to friends, taking walks, and reading. In view of these alternatives, and others, why are drugs so popular?

Reasons for Drug Use

Drugs are easy to use, and they work quickly. If a person desires to alter consciousness, drugs can accomplish this relatively easily; little effort is required to inhale marijuana, swallow a pill, snort cocaine, or drink alcohol. Drugs are a quick fix. To overcome illness or to experience pleasure quickly, some people look to drugs because they fulfill immediate needs. This feature of modern society is called *immediacy*, the desire and expectation that things should be handled rapidly. It could well be the main reason that people use drugs.

People use drugs for many other reasons, too. The family structure and society have changed dramatically. Both parents working outside the home, the rising cost of living, the emphasis on immediate gratification, mass media, and the high degree of mobility all have contributed to stresses on the family. The 1990s recession placed additional stress on the family due to financial hardships and unemployment.[24] To deal with these stresses, some people experiment with drugs, others use drugs occasionally, and still others take drugs frequently or compulsively.

Experimentation

Curiosity is a common reason to try drugs. Especially among young people, curiosity is a natural phenomenon that easily leads to experimentation. Infants continually place objects in their mouths. Children cannot wait to open a package to find out its contents. Many schools inadvertently arouse interest and curiosity in drugs through "drug awareness programs," in which former addicts, police officers, pharmacists, judges, physicians, clergy, or drug therapists talk to students about the dangers of drugs. Newspapers and popular magazines contain articles about drugs, particularly drug use by well-known athletes, politicians,

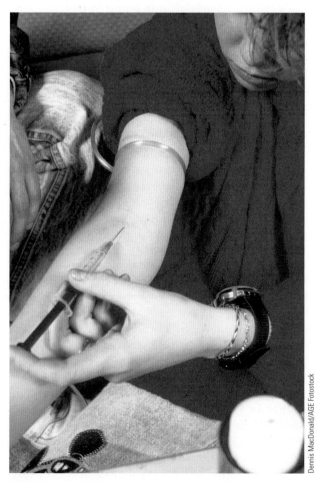

■ People who inject drugs are more likely to be compulsive drug users.

musicians, and actors. While drug-use trends showed lower rates in 2015 compared to previous years, there are some areas of concern regarding drug-taking behaviors of high school students. About 58% of high school students reported having drank alcohol and roughly 35% report having used marijuana/hashish.[24] Almost 15% of high school students reported using a narcotic (other than heroin) over the past year.[25]

The age by which alcohol is consumed is reflected in alcohol problems as an adult. The longer one waits before drinking alcohol, the less likely one will have alcohol problems as an adult.[26] Adolescents that drink alcohol before the age of 15 are four times more likely to meet the criteria for alcohol dependence at some point in their lives.[27] Similarly, the earlier children experiment with cigarettes, the more likely they are to become regular smokers. Other factors affecting the initiation of smoking include social and media influence, having friends who smoke, and living with a smoker.[28]

Some adolescents experiment with drugs due to poor impulse control or simply due to the undeveloped brain. In adolescents, the affective areas of the brain (those areas in control of rewarding aspects of alcohol use) are more dominant, while the prefrontal cortex (the area that controls the inhibitory response or "just say no") is less dominant.[29] Also, the use of one type of drug may lead to experimentation with another drug. For example, marijuana users who do not view marijuana use as having adverse effects are more likely to experiment with ecstasy.[30]

Pleasure/Escape from Boredom

Another reason for using drugs is pleasure. Many people simply like the feelings they receive from drugs. If drugs did not provide some type of perceived benefit, their use would be discontinued. Pleasure is the antithesis of boredom, and an individual who is bored will engage in something pleasurable to relieve the boredom. Drugs become a source of reward.

The adolescent brain is underdeveloped. Research in the area of adolescent brain development suggests the rewards for alcohol use are highly sensitive and provide a stronger positive reaction to alcohol use compared to adults.[31] Thus the pleasure received from alcohol (and drug use) can be seen as more rewarding for adolescents than adults. In a study of high school seniors that was conducted 30 years ago, 49% indicated that they used drugs "to feel good or get high," 41% "because it tastes good," and 23% "because of boredom, nothing else to do."[32] Perhaps reasons for drug use have not changed greatly over time. It has been argued that the desire to get high may be genetically programmed into some people.[33] One study found that 18-year-olds used marijuana

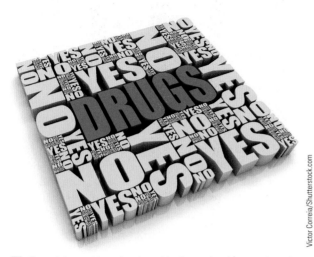

The adolescent's undeveloped brain can lead to poor impulse control.

and alcohol to regulate emotions and for the experience.[34] Substance use among older people is not uncommon; many older people take drugs to escape from the psychological, social, and health problems they incur.[35]

Drugs that are used to increase pleasure or to reduce boredom are reinforcing, especially if the drugs are effective. The accompanying euphoria provides **positive reinforcement**, which encourages continued drug use. Conversely, drugs taken to alleviate discomfort can provide **negative reinforcement**. Distinguishing whether reinforcement for drug use arises from the urge for euphoria or the desire to eliminate dysphoria is sometimes difficult. Nevertheless, the drug user achieves some type of physical or social reward.

An interesting question pertains to whether drug use for the purpose of achieving pleasure should be viewed as acceptable. Some argue that drugs are part of society, most people can moderate their drug use, and drug use for pleasure should be accepted.[36] Many people use drugs to increase their happiness levels. Some argue the government protects this right in the Declaration of Independence, specifically the statement "Life, Liberty and the pursuit of Happiness."[37]

Others disagree, saying that people cannot easily control their drug use and that pleasure can turn into pain over time.[38]

Peer Influence

Many young people use drugs to gain peer acceptance or approval. Commonly referred to as peer pressure, it is defined as feeling pressured or urged by peers and is subjective.[39] While all age groups are susceptible to peer pressure, young people tend to place more value on their peers' opinions compared to adults. Erik Erikson, a psychologist who is well known for his theory on stages of psychosocial development, described adolescence as a time period that is focused on how one appears to others. During this time, a sense of belonging to a peer group is highly sought after.[40]

For adolescents, the greatest influence in their lives is their peers' perception of them. Starting in early adolescence, the influence of peers begins to exert a relatively greater role than the family as a socializing agent. Thus peers have more influence than parents on adolescent drinking behavior. Parents tend to have very little influence on their adolescent children regarding drug use (they do have a much stronger influence during earlier years). In a study done on adolescents who use cannabis, users reported their parents' opinions on drugs and specially, marijuana use, did not influence their use of the drug.[41] Thus the strongest predictor for adolescent drug use is peer substance use.[42]

Adolescents attribute marijuana and alcohol use with increased popularity rates.[43] Schools plays a role in perceived popularity among these users. For example, in schools that reported high connectivity rates among their students (smaller class sizes, emphasis on scholastic success, students feel happy and secure at school), the extent to which popularity is associated with marijuana use is decreased.[44] Schools in communities that have higher levels of socioeconomic statuses tend to have higher rates of school connectedness among their students. Conversely, schools located in areas with lower of socioeconomic statuses tend to have lower rates of school connectedness.[45] Adolescents at highest risks for drug use are from areas that have fewer educational opportunities and are generally made up of underrepresented racial and ethnic groups.

This point is illustrated in research on alcohol use by fraternity and sorority members. Rates of alcohol consumption by fraternity and sorority members were found to be significantly higher than those of non-Greek-affiliated college students.[46] Fraternity members had higher rates of alcohol use than sorority members. In a study conducted on dry (alcohol-free housing) and wet (alcohol allowed in the house), it was discovered that fraternity members had no difference in alcohol consumption behavior while for dry sorority houses, there was a significant decline in alcohol use.[47] Students, especially those in fraternities and sororities, consistently overestimate how much others drink.[48] Not confined to the Greeks at colleges, adolescents often overestimate drug and alcohol use among their peers. They rate their peers as using more drugs and alcohol than what is reported.[49]

Just as drug use can be attributed to peer approval, drug abstinence can be associated with peer disapproval. The relationship between peer group affiliation and drug use is reciprocal.[50] It has been shown that teachers can set a climate in the school that promotes respect and healthy norms among students. Nondrug use becomes acceptable behavior.[51] Groups implicitly reinforce behaviors by showing acceptance and affection toward others who share their behaviors.[52] Parents, however, who explicitly tell their children that they do not tolerate drug use affect their children's use of drugs.[53]

Peer influence is affected by one's culture. European, American, and Chinese adolescents were found to be more affected by peers in their drug use than were African American adolescents.[54] Among South Korean youths, peer influence was critical to drug use.[55] Similarly, French adolescents are more likely to use drugs if peers do.[56] In a recent study, US teens were shown to have higher rates of illicit drug use compared to European teens. Conversely, US teens have lower rates of cigarette and alcohol use compared to European teens.[57]

At the same time, basic values, life goals, and aspirations still are influenced more by parents. Parents who communicate well with their children are able to pass on values, discouraging drug use.[58] Positive family relationships deter drug use. Positive parent communication with their children serves as a deterrent to alcohol and drug use.[59] Living in neighborhoods that have greater rates of crime and violence may contribute to drug use.[60] A recent study looking at the impact of disadvantaged neighborhoods and alcohol use among adolescents showed that neighborhood disadvantage is a significant predictor of adolescent alcohol use.[61]

Parents indirectly alter their children's drug use by influencing their choice of friends and by emphasizing education.[62] Also, parental attitudes and reactions to the use of tobacco seem to have a greater effect on adolescent smoking than whether parents actually smoke. In addition, children of mothers who smoked during pregnancy are more likely to be dependent on nicotine compared with children whose mothers did not smoke.[63]

The most likely common denominator within an adolescent's peer group, after age and sex, is drug use. Rather than peers exerting an influence on drug-taking behavior, those who use drugs could well seek out others who consume drugs. Young people choose to associate with those who share the same interests. If you are a parent or thinking of becoming a parent, what is the message? Either choose your child's friends carefully or make sure your child chooses friends who hold values similar to yours. One encouraging finding is that parents are becoming more aware of their children's use of drugs, especially cigarettes.[64]

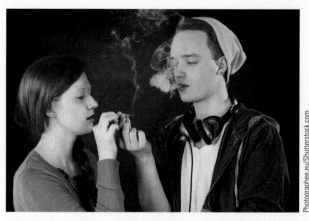
Peer pressure is of the main reasons why adolescents use drugs.

Spiritual Purposes

Throughout history, people have used drugs to seek out or communicate with something or someone greater than themselves. Drugs have played a role

CULTURAL Considerations

■ Ethnic and cultural identity may significantly influence drug use and abuse.

■ Among adolescents, those who are Puerto Rican, African American, and Asian, who have strong ties with their ethnic groups and communities, have lower levels of drug use and abuse.

■ Strong ethnic identification serves as a protective factor against drug use and abuse.

■ Prevention programs aimed at adolescents should take into consideration the ethnic background of the participants and incorporate cultural and ethnic content into the curriculum.

Source: P. Zickler, "Ethnic Identification and Cultural ties may help prevent drug use," *National Institute on Drug Abuse: NIDA NOTES*, 14, no.3 (1999). Available at: http://archives.drugabuse.gov/NIDA_Notes/NNVol14N3/Ethnic.html.

positive reinforcement Rewarding a positive behavior
negative reinforcement Removing negative stimulus after a behavior

in this discovery process by being used to enhance spirituality and the search for the spiritual self.[65] Ironically, spirituality plays a protective and facilitating role in substance use. Studies suggest involvement in an organized religion serves as a protective factor against alcohol and drug use and abuse.[66] Religion and spirituality also serve as a recovery aid for substance abusers. Consider the 12-step program associated with Alcoholics Anonymous. This program includes a spirituality component that asks its members to give in to a higher power to aid in the recovery process.[67] On the other hand, spirituality plays a role in the consumption of alcohol and drugs by their inclusion in certain spiritual rituals. In Judaeo-Christian ceremonies wine is used as part of the religious ritual. In other religions, psychedelic substances are used as part of ceremonies to enhance spirituality. A concept common to some world religions is that animals and plants acquire their special characteristics from a spirit contained within them. By consuming a plant with such a spirit, the person becomes endowed with the spirit. Hence, psychoactive plants have played a meaningful role in the religious and spiritual practices of many societies around the world.

The Aztec, Toltec, and Navajo cultures use psychedelic substances to aid in achieving an altered state for the purpose of its spiritual effects.[68] Many American Indian cultures use hallucinogens in a religious context. The Native American Church uses the hallucinogen peyote during religious ceremonies to treat alcoholism. Another drug used for spiritual purposes is bhang. Derived from cannabis, bhang is incorporated into Hindu religious rites. Holy men consume it to "center their thoughts on the eternal."[69] Moreover, it is used during Hindu festivals, marriages, and family celebrations. In the 1920s

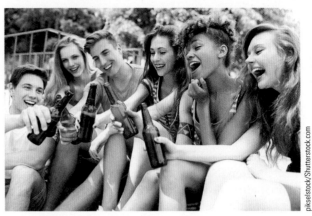

Being a member of a fraternity increases the chance of drinking.

and 1930s, the religion Rastafarianism was formed in Jamaica. This religion uses marijuana as part of its rituals and condemns the use of alcohol.[70] Subscribers to this religion believe the Tree of Life mentioned in the Bible was a marijuana plant, and while they condemn using marijuana solely for the purpose of getting "high," it is seen as a way to enhance feelings of unity. Timothy Leary promoted LSD in his religion, the League of Spiritual Discovery. Its motto was "Turn On, Tune In, and Drop Out." Unlike the Native American Church, which had been permitted to use peyote legally, members of the League of Spiritual Discovery were not legally sanctioned to use LSD. More recently, the First Church of Cannabis Inc. was approved in Indiana in 2015. Cannabis is listed as the church's sacrament in its doctrine and is used to promote health among the followers.[71, 72]

Spirituality in the context of personal growth, development, and life change has had an influence on drug use among young adults. In a study of college students, 81% claimed that they had a spiritual experience while using a hallucinogen.[73] Scholars have connected the use of ecstasy at dance music/rave scenes with Generations' X and Y desire to enhance spirituality.[74] Abuse is unlikely if drugs are restricted to religious rituals.

Social Interaction

As social beings, humans have a great need for interaction. These interactions range from working and dining together to being in the same organization to simply talking together. Drugs are used sometimes to facilitate interactions with others. In his research, Skager notes that young people use drugs because they feel that drug use is the social thing to do.[75] Young adults use alcohol because they feel it helps them socialize with their peers. People who view alcohol consumption positively with social interactions are

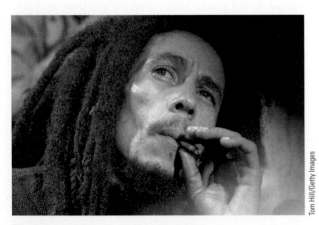

"Glory be to the father and to the maker of creation. As it was in the beginning, is now and ever shall be world without end." The prayer recited before a pipe is smoked in the Rastafari religion.

more likely to use a moderate amount of alcohol in social settings.[76] One social ritual in the United States is drinking at football games. High levels of alcohol consumption occur during college football games.[77] In the United States, alcohol-related arrests are three times higher on game days compared to nongame days.[78] One study of 18- to 24-year-olds found that prior to the game 16% of students engaged in heavy drinking, which was defined as ten or more drinks for males and eight or more drinks for females.[79]

Illegal drugs are also used in a social context. Some people consider marijuana to be a drug that binds people together. As a sign of friendship, heroin addicts share drugs as well as hypodermic needles. For others, cocaine is a social lubricant, included as part of a romantic evening and to attract a sexual partner.

Rules and norms govern drug use in a social context. Even as alcohol use in a college dormitory might abound, there may be rules regarding when and where to drink. Parents who smoke marijuana might wait until their children go to bed. Certain social groups determine *how* a drug is used. For instance, it was found that social milieu of street life leads many young people to escalate their drug use, resulting in their injecting drugs.[80] Furthermore, having a sexual minority status (LGBTQ) places people at a higher risk for alcohol and drug abuse.[81] Many gay men, and to a lesser extent lesbians, use drugs to deal with homophobia.[82]

Drug use by soldiers in Vietnam provides an example of the moderating effect of social environment. At least 35% of enlisted men used heroin, and more than half of them became addicted while in Vietnam.[83] Contrary to dire expectations and warnings of government officials, only 10% of the addicts remained addicted after returning to the United States. One reason is that the social sanctions revolving around heroin use while in Vietnam were quite different from those found in the United States.

Rebelliousness

Another reason why some people take drugs is that they are told not to. Rebelliousness is one of the best predictors of increased drug use among adolescents. A strong relationship has been found between drug use and recklessness and predelinquent behaviors such as aggression and poor emotional control. Young people rebel against the conventions of society, including warnings about drugs' dangers. Institutions such as religious groups, schools, and government identify rules by which people should behave. The more affiliated one is with these institutions, the less likely one is to use drugs. Similarly, participating on

ON CAMPUS

A study conducted on college students showed stress and neuroticism as significant predictors of drug use. This study analyzed two types of drug users: minor drug users were defined as marijuana and alcohol users and major drug users, which included narcotic use. Results from this study indicate higher levels of neuroticism (characterized by anxiety, fear, jealousy, envy). Similarly, stress scores were high among minor and major drug users. Furthermore, high levels of stress and neuroticism indicate the greatest risk factor for drug use.

Source: Jennifer Coleman and Joseph Trunzo, "Personality, Social Stress, and Drug use among College Students," *The International Honor Society in Psychology*, 20, no.1 (2015):52–58.

sports teams reduces the use of cigarettes and illicit drugs, although alcohol use is not reduced.[84] On the other hand, antisocial behavior is a good predictor of drug abuse.[85]

From a young age, children are taught to conform. Parents and other adults impose rules when we visit relatives, attend school, walk through a shopping mall, get a haircut, pick out clothing, and so forth. Among the many ways to rebel against these proscriptions is to engage in behaviors that are deemed inappropriate. A recent study that analyzed externalizing behaviors (oppositional defiant, conduct problems, etc.) and internalizing factors (stress, depression, anxiety, etc.) found that externalizing behaviors were related to increased and problematic cannabis use as an adult. The same association was not found for internalizing factors.[86] Adolescents who demonstrate oppositional behavior are more likely to engage in health risk behaviors including drug use.[87]

Other motivations for drug use range from relieving anger and tension to staying awake to feeling more energetic. Figure 1.1 highlights environmental factors, interpersonal and social factors, and individual factors contributing to the use of alcohol and other drugs.

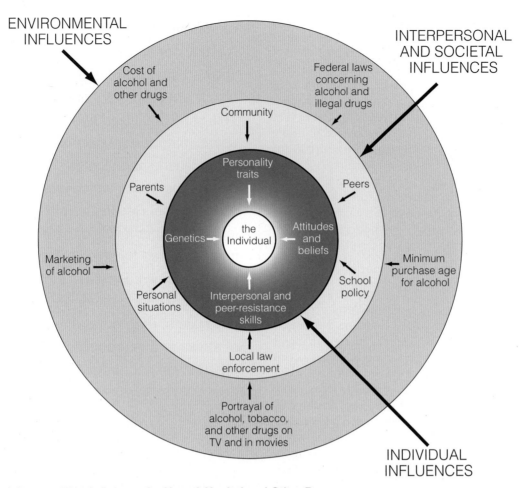

Figure 1.1 Factors That Influence the Use of Alcohol and Other Drugs

Source: Prevention Plus II Office for Substance Abuse Prevention, 1989.

Drug Dependency Versus Drug Addiction

Drug dependency can be physical or psychological. Before elaborating on the differences, we have to differentiate between the terms **drug dependency** and **drug addiction**. Both connote a compulsive need to use a drug and an inability to cease using it even if serious consequences ensue. Similarly, both *dependency* and *addiction* mean that drug use takes precedence over many other behaviors in one's life.

Before the terms *addiction* and *physical dependence* were used, the term *habit* was used to describe people who could not stop using drugs. As early as 1914, the *American Journal of Public Health* included articles about the habit of drug abuse and how detrimental this habit was. This 1914 article advocated that habitual drug abusers receive treatment rather than incarceration.[88]

So how do these terms differ? Physical dependence occurs when the body adjusts to the drug's

presence and will exhibit withdrawal symptoms if the drug is discontinued.[89] Stereotypically, the term *drug dependent* conjures up an image of someone who is ill and in need of treatment and compassion. Addiction, on the other hand, includes a physical dependence to a drug, but also encompasses characteristics associated with drug abuse such as the inability to stop using a drug, failure to meet work, social, and family obligations, and tolerance and withdrawal.[90] A *drug addict* might be perceived as a criminal and a degenerate who is best served by incarceration, not hospitalization. The terms *dependency* and *addiction* are applied to different drugs as well. For example, heavy smokers seldom are called nicotine addicts, whereas heroin users typically are called addicts. Because the notion of dependence evokes less condemnation than addiction does, the World Health Organization (WHO), four decades ago, proposed substituting the word *dependence* for *addiction*.[91] Similarly, the committee members who worked on the DSM-V replaced the word addiction with dependence.[92] O'Brien argues for this distinction by stating the word dependence is associated with the physical dependence of the drug while addiction encompasses the compulsive desire to continue drug use.[93] The compulsive use of some drugs can be based on the psychic or perceived need for the drug, not only on the physical need. Furthermore, it is important to consider that drug dependence can occur without addiction. Think about a person who is prescribed a narcotic to deal with chronic pain. After a period of time, that person will become physically dependent on the drug, but if he or she follows protocol for drug administration, addiction may not occur. Similarly, a person can exhibit signs of addiction, but not be physically dependent. Consider a person who is addicted to gambling; there is no physical dependence on gambling but rather a compulsive need to continue the behavior.[94] In a nutshell, then, addiction is "an ingrained habit that undermines your health, your work, your relationships, your self-respect, but that you feel you cannot change."[95] To stay consistent with current terminology, the term drug dependence will be used in this text to refer to drug dependence and addiction. Regardless of how compulsive drug use is defined, the National Institute on Drug Abuse views compulsive drug use as a treatable illness.[96]

1. *Physical dependency* is marked by **withdrawal symptoms**—the physical symptoms that appear after drug use ceases. People who are physically dependent on a drug need to take the drug to ward off withdrawal symptoms.
2. *Psychological dependency* refers to one's perceived need for a drug.

Some symptoms that show up after drug use ceases may be psychological rather than physical, and some drugs have more potential to cause addiction than others. Important factors in determining whether a drug results in addiction are how quickly it gets to the brain and its potency. Even though many withdrawal symptoms are psychological, they are quite real. Moreover, psychological dependency is harder to overcome than physical dependency, as illustrated in Figure 1.2. This lends credence to the idea that dependency reflects the inability to adapt to one's environment, or at least the inability to adapt in the absence of drugs.

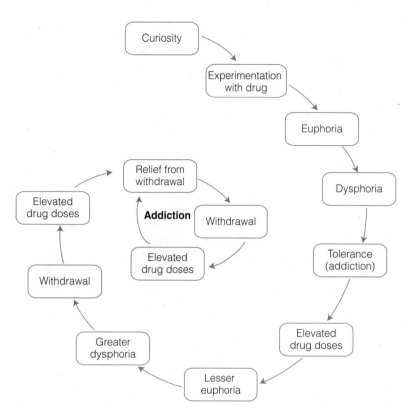

Figure 1.2 Downward Spiral of Psychological Addiction

From TURNER/SIZER/WHITNEY/WILKS. Life Choices, 2E. © 1992 Brooks/Cole, a part of Cengage Learning, Inc. Reproduced by permission. www.cengage.com/permissions

Addiction is classified as a complex disease that affects the brain.[97] Drug addiction changes the brain's functioning and physical structure, which can be long-lasting.[98]

Many people question using the term disease to describe drug dependence as some believe drug dependence is a choice. While it is true that the initial decision to take drugs in a choice, it becomes a compulsion that takes the notion of choice out of the equation. The brain changes from drug use in a way that impairs the areas of the brain that impact judgement, decision making, learning, and memory.[99] If these areas of the brain are damaged from drug use and can be measured, then one must question whether drug dependence is truly a choice.

Another question pertaining to drug dependence is why some people are able to use a drug sparingly

drug dependency The body adjusts to the presence of a substance and will exhibit withdrawal symptoms if the drug is discontinued

drug addiction A complex disease that impacts the brain

withdrawal symptoms Physical symptoms that appear after a drug is discontinued

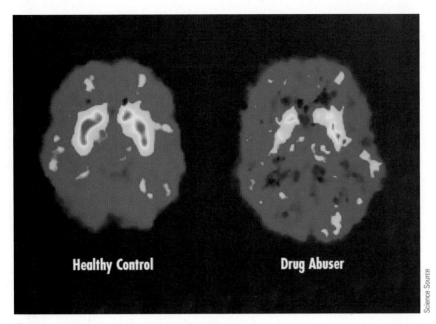

Drugs change the brain's ability to function.

and seemingly responsibly while others become drug dependent. Just like any disease, some people are more prone to getting a disease while others have less risk. Consider heart disease. There are some measures that can be taken to reduce the risk of getting this disease such as eating a healthy diet, regularly exercising, and controlling hypertension. These are considered controllable risk factors. On the other hand, there are also risk factors that are uncontrollable such as family history and genetic predisposition, which can increase the risk of getting heart disease. Drug dependence is similar but there are controllable and uncontrollable risk factors. Scientists estimate that genetic factors account for about 50% of a person's susceptibility to drug dependence.[100] Biological risk factors include family history, genetics, and mental disorders with mental disorders being one of the greatest risk factors.[101]

Is dependency a valid reason for legally prohibiting drugs? Scribner argues that antidrug laws do not protect against addiction and are counterproductive.[102] Volkow and others maintain that many addicts have no choice but to take drugs; however, she asserts that addicts are accountable for their behavior while on drugs and that they should be treated medically rather than criminally.[103]

Theories of Drug Addiction

The US Department of Health and Human Services states that addiction is a "chronic, life-threatening condition that has roots in genetic susceptibility, social circumstance, and personal behavior."[104] Many theories attempt to explain addiction. It has been attributed to poor self-control, ignorance, personality traits, bad genes, poverty, disease, and the absence of family values. When addicts were asked what caused their addiction, most attributed it to psychological factors such as fear, anxiety, and sorrow.[105]

When laypeople were surveyed to determine what they thought was the basis for heroin addiction, their political beliefs were a factor. Conservative voters tended to attribute addiction to low moral standards, and liberal voters attributed addiction to psychological and social reasons.[106] Although no single theory adequately covers every aspect of drug addiction, elements of various theories provide insight into drug addiction. A number of theories regarding drug abuse are examined here.

Personality Theories

Some specific personality traits have been related to drug dependence. Personality refers to "a dynamic set of traits acquired by a person that influences his or her perceptions, motivations, and behaviors in various occasions."[107] What is difficult to know is whether certain personality traits lead to drug dependency or if drug dependency alters personality. It has been noted that substance abusers have lower reasoning skills compared to nondrug users.[108] Persons with high reasoning skills are good abstract thinkers and have the ability to consider the consequences of a decision and make appropriate decisions based on foreseeing the outcomes of the decision. Drug-dependent people tend to be negative, self-deprecating, depressed, and tense and have a sense of helplessness.[109] Learned helplessness is the idea that one's actions do not impact outcomes.[110] Thus one feels powerless to control the outcomes of his life. The learned helplessness trait has been associated with poorer levels of self-control and internal motivations among drug-dependent people.[111] Low levels of self-esteem have also been implicated in increased risk for drug abuse. In a study that looked at almost 4,000 participants, it was found that low levels of self-esteem were related to lifetime substance use.[112] To deal with low self-esteem and accompanying tension, some people rely on drugs. A New Zealand study found methamphetamine use is linked to poor self-esteem and feelings of aggression.[113] Among adolescents, delayed behavioral or emotional development may be a factor in their substance abuse.[114]

Personality characteristics associated with drug abuse include the following:

- Low self-esteem
- Poor interpersonal skills
- Need for immediate gratification
- Defiant feelings toward authority
- Little tolerance for anxiety, frustration, and depression
- Impulsivity
- Risk taking
- Low regard for personal health

The problem with identifying personality characteristics is that drug abuse may have led to a change in personality rather than personality causing drug abuse.

Drug use can be a means of coping with anxiety. In reality, though, the person is probably exchanging one set of problems for another. "Addicts have problems with self-regulation and impulse control and tend to use drugs as a substitute for coping strategies."[115] Coping with feelings of anxiety and arousal by using drugs is one way to reduce negative aspects of one's life. Some people use narcotics to deal with internal feelings of aggression and rage. Traumatic events in a person's life often trigger substance abuse.[116] Figure 1.3 illustrates the cycle of psychological addiction.

Some people point to an addictive personality trait as reasoning for increased susceptibility to drug use and abuse. To say that one has an addictive personality would imply that certain personality traits place a person more at risk for drug abuse. As discussed earlier in this section, research has shown relationships between low self-esteem, learned helplessness, and impulse control with an increases risk for drug use. However, there are some scientists who do not believe an addictive personality trait exists. Thornburg states "there does not seem to be a personality type or set of characteristics that predictably fit either addicts or alcoholics."[117] In her study, she found much variability between drug addicts' and alcoholics' personality traits. Supporting this idea, Mayberg conducted a study on people who abuse alcohol and methamphetamines and concluded there was no specific personality type in either group that would predict drug use.[118]

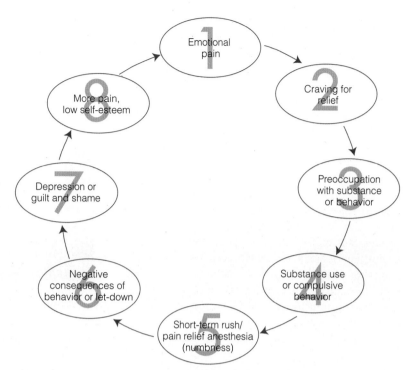

Figure 1.3 Cycle of Psychological Addiction

From TURNER/SIZER/WHITNEY/WILKS. Life Choices, 2E. © 1992 Brooks/Cole, a part of Cengage Learning, Inc. Reproduced by permission. www.cengage.com/permissions

Reinforcement Theory

All animals are believed to have pleasure and reward circuits in the brain that turn on when they are stimulated by addictive substances. The basis for craving drugs may lie within our genes.[119] A behavior that results in stimulation of these circuits is reinforced—the animal is motivated to repeat that behavior. In some humans, addiction may arise from the reward system of the brain not functioning properly.[120]

Reinforcers are stimuli or events that increase the likelihood of a particular behavior. Reinforcers can be primary or secondary. **Primary reinforcers** reduce physiological needs or are inherently pleasurable (e.g., food, water, and sex). **Secondary reinforcers** act as signals for the increased probability of obtaining primary reinforcers; money, for instance, is a secondary reinforcer because it does not provide immediate pleasure, but it can be used to secure a primary reinforcer.

reinforcers Stimuli or events that increase the likelihood of a particular behavior

primary reinforcers Reduce physiological needs or are inherently pleasurable

secondary reinforcers Act as signals for the increased probability of obtaining primary reinforcers

Drugs can be primary or secondary reinforcers. People take drugs because of a payoff or benefit. The payoff might be acceptance from people with whom one wants to be associated, the pleasure derived from altering one's consciousness, or the relief accompanying elimination of withdrawal symptoms.

Reinforcement can be positive or negative. When a person is motivated to repeat behaviors because of the pleasurable sensations they bring, he or she is receiving positive reinforcement. Drugs produce a euphoria that many people seek to repeat. If behaviors provide relief from or avoidance of pain, the desire to repeat those behaviors is motivated by negative reinforcement. Examples of negative reinforcement are use of drugs to avoid the effects of withdrawal and the fear of losing status or approval among peers. A drug-dependent individual falls into one of two camps: the maintainers or the euphoria seekers. The maintainers seek to avoid pain. The euphoria seekers want to feel high.

Biological Theories

Theories focusing on the biological aspects of addiction deal primarily with genetic determination and metabolic imbalances.

Genetic Theory

The genetic theory postulates that a person is predisposed to drug addiction, including addiction to alcohol, by hereditary influence. Studies involving families, twins, and adoptees offer persuasive evidence that addiction is partly genetic and runs in families.[121] There is also research showing a link between compulsive eating and drug abuse, suggesting that both behaviors have a similar genetic component.[122]

Recent research places much emphasis on genetics. In a study on people who underwent weight loss surgery, it was discovered that many people replaced their eating addiction with another addiction.[123] There has been a rise in alcohol and narcotic dependence among those who underwent surgery to treat an eating addiction.[124] What is known as an addiction transfer has been linked to the dopamine receptors in the brain, specifically the D2 receptor. The fewer D2 receptors present in the brain, the more likely one is to become addicted. To illustrate this case, in a study on chronic drug users and overeaters, it was discovered that both types of individuals had fewer D2 receptors in the brain.[125] This suggests a genetic link between addiction and genetic makeup.

Because of biological differences, people become intoxicated at differing levels of consumption and metabolize drugs at different rates. Isolating bio-

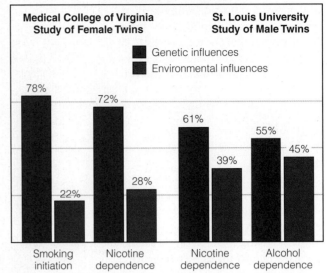

Figure 1.4 **A Medical College of Virginia study involving 949 female twin pairs found genetic factors to be more influential than environmental factors in smoking initiation and nicotine dependence. Likewise, a St. Louis University study of 3,356 male twin pairs found genetic factors to be more influential for dependence on nicotine and alcohol.**

Source: P. Zickler, "Evidence Builds That Genes Influence Cigarette Smoking," NIDA Notes, 15 (June 2000): 1–5.

logical or genetic factors from personality and environment is difficult, and most of the research linking genetics and drugs is limited to alcohol. Determining whether addiction is a result of heredity or environmental influences is also difficult. Nonetheless, Figure 1.4 assesses the genetic and environmental effects on twins.[126]

Metabolic Imbalance

Addiction to narcotics sometimes is attributable to a metabolic disorder.[127] Just as the diabetic person needs insulin, the narcotic user covets narcotics. Narcotics help addicts stabilize the metabolic deficiency caused by absence of the drug. Although this theory can be applied to narcotics users who take methadone to stabilize their desire for narcotics, little evidence is available to support the metabolic deficiency theory. Many people receiving methadone for heroin dependence continue to crave heroin.[128]

Social Theories

According to social theories, cultural and social influences contribute to drug abuse.[129] If individuals are rewarded for their behaviors, such as drug use, the risk of continuing those behaviors becomes greater. Rewards are derived from groups and others with whom we associate. Based on this premise, drug abuse is socially learned and benefits the individual by group acceptance. Moreover, those with a substance abuse disorder tend to overestimate the extent of drug use by their peers.[130] Drug abuse arises from antisocial behavior,[131] although no one theory adequately determines drug addiction.[132]

Whether a behavior is categorized as a problem is a function of how society labels the behavior. In some instances, behaviors outside of social norms actually are considered desirable and are reinforced. In a convoluted way, "bad" is "good," and vice versa. In some social groups, drug abstinence is not valued, whereas drug use, although condemned by many people, is considered good.

Mass Media and Drugs

The impact of the media on drug use is hard to determine because it is only one factor in the total picture of parents, friends, siblings, religion, and schools. In 2012, the Surgeon General stated that exposure to cigarette use in movies may cause young people to start smoking.[133] One encouraging sign is that scenes of smoking in movies has declined significantly. In 2005, there were 4,000 scenes involving smoking, and in 2009, there were 1,935 scenes.[134]

Unfortunately, after the year 2010, tobacco incidences in movies increased to 2,500 incidents in 2014. Incident levels in 2015 have reduced closer to the levels seen in 2009.[135]

Highlighted here are some forms of mass media that feature drugs—advertisements, billboards, television, music, and celebrities.

Advertisements

An estimated $25 billion is spent on advertising for tobacco, alcohol, and prescription drugs. The American Academy of Pediatrics recommends banning tobacco advertising in all media as a way to dissuade young people from smoking.[136] Advertising for prescription drugs amounted to $4.2 billion.[137] The overriding message of advertisements for drugs is that drug-taking is acceptable and, in fact, the norm.

In 2014, the Federal Drug Administration launched a public campaign called "The Real Cost." The purpose of this campaign was to reduce tobacco use among 12- to 17- year-olds in the United States. This national campaign aired on television, online, radio, and other media channels and achieved an 80% rate of youth awareness of the campaign. The perceived effectiveness of the campaign was rated highly among nonsmoking teens.

Summary

Definitions related to drugs frequently reflect the biases of those who come up with the definition. What one person classifies as drug use, another may classify as misuse or abuse. Generally, misuse involves the unintentional or inappropriate use of a drug, whereas drug abuse typically entails chronic use of a drug that results in physical, intellectual, financial, social, or emotional problems. Even the word *drug* is subject to interpretation. One could argue that sugar and chocolate are forms of drugs.

Drug dependency and drug addiction have been used to describe drug use behavior interchangeably. However, these terms are not synonymous. Drug dependency refers to a physical dependence on the drug, and when that drug is discontinued, a person will experience withdrawal symptoms. Drug addiction, on the other hand, refers to the compulsive use of a drug, regardless of the negative consequences that occur from taking the drug.

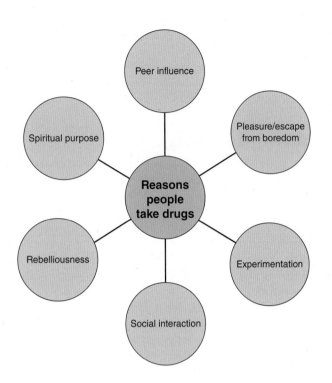

Theories of Drug Addiction

Personality Theories

- Specific personality traits related to addiction
- Traits include learned helplessness, low self-esteem, poor interpersonal skills, etc.

Reinforcement Theory

- Reward system in the brain not functioning properly
- Reinforcers—stimuli that increase the likelihood of a particular behavior
    - Primary reinforcers—reduce physiological needs or are pleasurable
    - Secondary reinforcers—increase probability of obtaining a primary enforcer

Biological Theories

- Genetic theory—a person is predisposed to addiction by hereditary influence
- Metabolic Imbalance—drugs helps stabilize a metabolic imbalance

Social Theories

- Culture and social influences contribute to drug addiction

Thinking Critically

1. Religion and spirituality play a protective and facilitating role in drug use. Many religions incorporate the use of drugs as part of their religious ceremonies. Wine is used in Judaeo-Christian ceremonies and psychedelic substances have been part of other religious ceremonies to enhance spirituality. While some religious sects have received special provisions to use psychedelic substances as part of their ceremonies, others have not. Do you believe all religious sects should be allowed to use drugs as part of their ceremonies? How would you determine which religions should be granted special permissions to do so?

2. Addiction is considered a complex disease that affects the brain. The brain of a drug-addicted person is different in structure and function compared to a person who is not addicted to drugs. In light of this, society often doesn't view addiction in the same way that it views diseases such as cancer. For the most part, cancer is viewed as a disease that one must fight and battle with in hopes of a victory. Addiction, on the other hand, is viewed as a personal weakness that one must learn to control. If addiction is considered a disease, do you think more help should be available to those suffering from it? Do you think society's views on addiction would change to be more sympathetic toward individuals suffering from addiction?

3. Look at the most popular songs for the past month. How many refer to drugs? Are drugs portrayed positively or negatively? Do the lyrics have any effect on your behavior or the behavior of those around you?

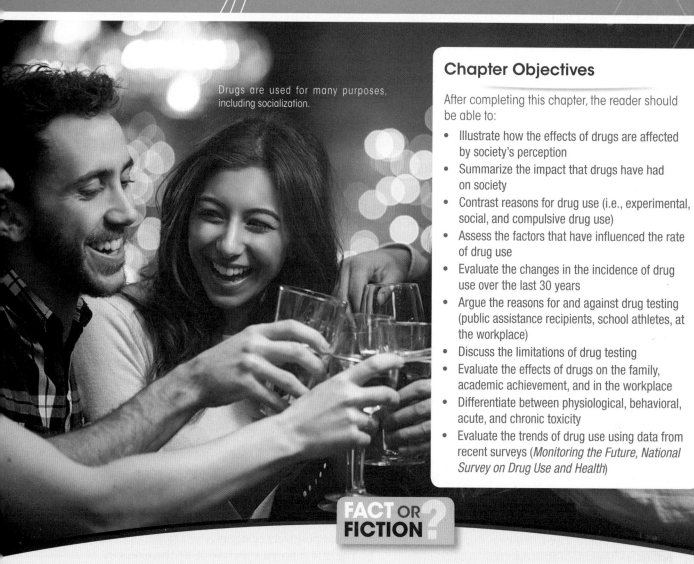

Drugs are used for many purposes, including socialization.

Chapter Objectives

After completing this chapter, the reader should be able to:

- Illustrate how the effects of drugs are affected by society's perception
- Summarize the impact that drugs have had on society
- Contrast reasons for drug use (i.e., experimental, social, and compulsive drug use)
- Assess the factors that have influenced the rate of drug use
- Evaluate the changes in the incidence of drug use over the last 30 years
- Argue the reasons for and against drug testing (public assistance recipients, school athletes, at the workplace)
- Discuss the limitations of drug testing
- Evaluate the effects of drugs on the family, academic achievement, and in the workplace
- Differentiate between physiological, behavioral, acute, and chronic toxicity
- Evaluate the trends of drug use using data from recent surveys (*Monitoring the Future, National Survey on Drug Use and Health*)

FACT OR FICTION?

1. The federal government spends more money on preventing drug use than on prosecuting drug users.
2. About three out of every four US voters feel that the war on drugs has been a failure.
3. Parents who use drugs are more likely to have children who use drugs.
4. Most adolescents aged 12 to 17 who are in substance abuse treatment were referred there by their schools.
5. Individuals in the 12 to 17 age group are more likely to use illegal drugs on a monthly basis than individuals between ages 18 and 25.

6. The United States has one of the highest incarceration rates in the world.
7. All hospitals drug test women who have given birth to determine whether their babies may have drugs in their bloodstreams.
8. People who were abused as children have higher rates of alcoholism during adulthood compared with those people who were not abused as children.
9. The most commonly used illicit drug is cocaine.
10. E-cigarettes have the highest use rate among all tobacco products.

Turn the page to check your answers

Drugs pervade every facet of life. A fetus is affected by the mother's use of caffeine, tobacco, sedatives, and alcohol. Children are given stimulants to help them function more effectively in school. Adolescents use drugs to cope with daily stresses and to fit in with others. College students ingest amphetamines to stay awake and study late into the night. Club drugs such as ecstasy and GHB are taken at nightclubs and rave parties to enhance the user's mood. Homemakers rely on tranquilizers such as Xanax to deal with life's problems. People living in poverty take drugs to mask the situations in which they find themselves. Affluent individuals use drugs out of boredom. Elderly people rely on drugs to manage ailments that accompany aging. Deeply imbedded in the human psyche is the tendency to use drugs to deal with pains, problems, frustrations, disappointments, and social interactions.

The Prevalence of Drug Use

Nearly every American has used a mind-altering substance by having a glass of wine, a cigarette, a cup of coffee, a soft drink, or a cup of hot chocolate. In the United States, sales of prescription drugs totaled $309 billion in 2015.[1] American children consume 90% of all Ritalin produced worldwide.[2] In 2011, the number of people who visited emergency rooms that involved drug misuse abuse in 2011 was 2,460,000 which includes nonmedical use of pharmaceutical drugs.[3] Of these nonmedical pharmaceutical drugs, prescription stimulants (Adderall, Ritalin, etc.) are the mostly widely abused among college students.[4] Nine out of ten pharmaceutical companies, meanwhile, are spending more money on marketing prescription drugs than on research and development of these drugs.[5] Not surprisingly, these companies contribute a large amount of money to the US Food and Drug Administration (FDA).[6]

Among persons aged 12 or older, an estimated 27.1 million reported to using an illicit drug in the past month.[7] This is about 1 out of every 10 Americans. Of illicit drug use, marijuana is the most commonly used drug.[8] A little over 20 million people aged 12 and older had a substance use disorder in 2015. Of these, the most commonly reported substance use disorder was attributed to alcohol (15.7 million).[9]

Drug abuse is an expensive problem. The use and abuse of tobacco, alcohol, and illicit drug use is estimated to cost the United States $700 billion dollars annually, which includes costs related to crime, lost work productivity, and healthcare.[10,11,12] Only 11% of those who need treatment for drug dependence receive services. Thus out of 22.7 million people who could benefit from treatment, only 2.5 million actually receive treatment.[13] The economic cost of alcohol misuse in the United States is estimated to be about $249 billion annually.[14]

Over half of all state and federal prison inmates are in jail on drug offense charges.[15] To address problems associated with drugs, the US government is increasing its funding. By way of comparison, in 1980, the figure for combating drug abuse was $1 billion; in 2017, the US government requested $31.1 billion for drug control.[16,17] About half of the money earmarked in 2017 is for the prevention and treatment of drugs. Figure 2.1 shows the drug control budget for the 2017 fiscal year.[18]

FACT OR FICTION?

1. **FICTION** The fact is—Far more money is allocated for prosecuting drug offenses than for preventing drug use.

2. **FACT** According to Zogby International, 76% of US voters feel that the war on drugs has been unsuccessful.

3. **FACT** Children who grow up in drug-dependent families are more likely to use drugs.

4. **FICTION** The fact is—Adolescents in substance abuse treatment are more likely to be referred by the criminal justice system than by their schools.

5. **FICTION** The fact is—Individuals between the ages of 18 and 25 are almost twice as likely to have used an illegal drug in the previous month.

6. **FACT** A little over 1% of the US's population is in jail.

7. **FICTION** The fact is—Some hospitals have tested pregnant women whom they suspected of having used drugs; however, most hospitals do not routinely test for drugs.

8. **FACT** More people who were abused as children are likely to be alcoholics as adults, although most abused children do not become alcoholics.

9. **FICTION** The fact is—Marijuana is the commonly used illicit drug.

10. **FACT** A little over 15% of 8th and 12th graders have reported to using e-cigarettes.

Budget Authority in Millions of Dollars.
Source: ONDCP, February 2016

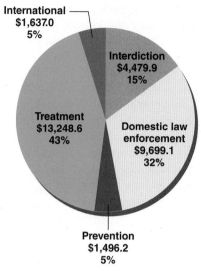

International
$1,637.0
5%

Interdiction
$4,479.9
15%

Treatment
$13,248.6
43%

Domestic law
enforcement
$9,699.1
32%

Prevention
$1,496.2
5%

Figure 2.1 United States Budget for Drug Control 2016

Source: "National Drug Control Budget: FY 2017 Funding Highlights" (Washington, DC: Executive Office of the President, Office of National Drug Control Policy), February 2016, Table 1,p. 16, and Table 3, p.19. https://www.whitehouse.gov/sites/default/files/ondcp/press-release/fy_2...

The Impact of Drug Use and Abuse

Alcohol use is prevalent in the United States with almost 90% of adults aged 18 or older report to using alcohol at some point in their lifetime.[19] Furthermore, almost one-fourth of all adults aged 18 or older reported they engaged in binge drinking during the past month and almost 7% reported they engaged in heavy drinking over the past month.[20] It is not surprising then that alcohol use disorder the United States is cause for concern. Of adults aged 18 and older, almost 7% have an alcohol use disorder.[21] It is not surprising then to discover that almost 90,000 people die per year due to alcohol, making alcohol-related deaths the fourth preventable cause of death in the United States.[22, 23]

The use of alcohol by college students is particularly concerning. College students use alcohol at rates that are higher than their noncollege attending peers.[24] College students report heavy drinking and binge drinking at rates that are higher than their noncollege-attending peers.[25, 26] Not only has binge drinking at American colleges been linked to student deaths, but it has also been associated with weak academic performance, injuries, vandalism, and property damage.[27] About 25% of students reported academic problems

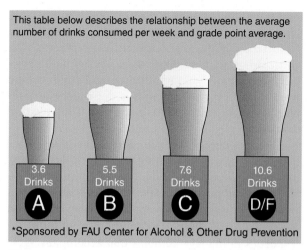

This table below describes the relationship between the average number of drinks consumed per week and grade point average.

3.6 Drinks **A**
5.5 Drinks **B**
7.6 Drinks **C**
10.6 Drinks **D/F**

*Sponsored by FAU Center for Alcohol & Other Drug Prevention

The more one drinks the less likely he will be successful in school.

as a result of their drinking alcohol.[28] Female college students who drink alcohol are perceived as being more sexually interested.[29] Similarly, college women are more likely to experience verbal, sexual, and physical aggression on days they drink heavily.[30]

In 2010, among college students aged 18 to 24, 1,825 died from alcohol-related unintentional injuries, 599,000 were unintentionally injured while under the influence of alcohol, 690,000 were assaulted by another student who had been drinking, and 97,000 were victims of alcohol-related sexual abuse.[31] Moreover, 100,000 reported being too intoxicated to know if they consented to having sex.[32]

Some people are concerned that drug use is destroying the fabric of society, that families and communities are undermined by drug use, and that moral decay will fester. In many instances, however, family and community problems might be the precursors to, rather than the effects of, drug abuse.[33] When addressing drug-related problems, there is a sense of frustration that something must be done. A public opinion poll indicated that 32% of Americans consider drug abuse a crisis across the country and 55% see it as a serious problem. However, only 12% reported feel drug abuse is a crisis in their own community.[34]

Impact of Drug Use and Abuse on the Family

Parental drug abuse has a detrimental impact on children. Children who are raised by parents who abuse drugs experience much instability during their childhood. The needs of the child become secondary to the drug dependence needs of the parent. In families with one parent abusing drugs, the financial needs of the children become second to the drug needs of the parent.[35] Thus monies that should be used for food, clothing, etc., are being misappropriated and used for drugs. Children who are raised by parents who abuse drugs are more likely to be abused both physically and mentally.[36] One study found children who were raised by a parent who is dependent on opioids were more likely to have nutritional and medical disorders.[37]

Parents/caregivers who abuse drugs are more likely to have poor parenting skills (includes abuse), inadequate coping skills, a lack of basic resources, limited social support, and experience high employment rates and housing instability.[38] Drugs can be seen as a way to escape these circumstances, even though it is detrimental to their children. It should come as no surprise to discover that more than half of all welfare cases and at least two-thirds of all cases where children are taken out of the home are due to parental substance abuse.[39]

Children raised in homes with parental substance abuse problems suffer from emotional trauma, which results in lower academic achievement, truancy, suicidal involvement, teenage pregnancy, eating disorders, and substance use and abuse.[40] Furthermore, in a recent study, it was discovered that children who are raised by a mother who abuses alcohol experience emotional neglect, physical abuse, emotional abuse, and sexual abuse.[41] Parental substance use and abuse is a risk factor for child substance use and abuse. This becomes a cycle where the children raised in drug-dependent families use drugs to escape their reality grow up and raise their children in households where substance abuse is taking place.

In families with no parental substance abuse, substance dependency by a child negatively impacts the family's ability to function. The addiction becomes the family's focus, often to the detriment of other children in the family. Families describe feeling torn between wanting to deal with the child who is suffering from addiction and the desire to maintain a stable environment for the other children in the family.[42] Mothers, in particular, are especially vulnerable in the family and carry the heaviest burden while trying to be a successful caregiver to those outside of the family.[43] The relationship between the parents also becomes strained and the anger and frustration that is felt toward the child with the substance abuse problem begins to manifest itself as anger between the parents.[44] Siblings of the substance-dependent child also suffer with direct and indirect consequences. Direct consequences include being assaulted or stolen from, while indirect consequences include feeling neglected because all the attention is going to the child with the substance abuse problem.[45]

Although drug use has not been *proved* to increase marital separation and divorce, an association exists between drug use and the likelihood that a couple will separate or divorce. Women with alcohol-dependent partners have significantly more family and marital problems. Also, women subjected to violence have higher rates of alcohol dependence and other drug abuse problems.[46] Family life may reduce drug involvement. Family interventions into adolescent alcohol use reduce the initiation and frequency of alcohol use.[47] Teaching adults how to improve their parenting skills has been shown to reduce the use of alcohol and other drugs among children and adolescents.[48]

It has been shown that marijuana use by young Black males is significantly reduced when both parents are present.[49] Parental divorce, however, increases the likelihood that children will be prescribed Ritalin.[50] In a study of Finnish twins, intoxication by the father was shown to increase the likelihood of marijuana smoking, although cigarette use was a stronger predictor of marijuana use.[51]

In a study of marriage, it was found that individuals' illicit drug use declined after they married. Both husband and wife reduced their illicit drug use, but husbands were slightly more likely than wives to use drugs.[52] When couples cohabitate, licit and illicit drug use declines, although marriage produces a greater decline.[53] In a study of divorced couples, researchers noted that frequent alcohol intoxication was strongly related to divorce. Frequency of marijuana use was not a strong predictor of divorce.[54]

Substance abuse is a prominent factor in many cases of child abuse and domestic abuse. For instance, in a study of US soldiers, it was noted that 13% of those involved in child maltreatment were under the influence of alcohol or an illicit drug at the time of the incident.[55] Moreover, many of those individuals who were abused as children or abused by their intimate partners end up in substance abuse

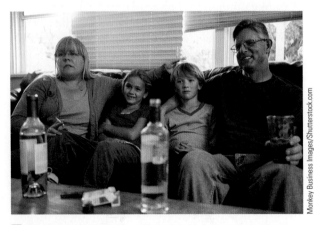

One in ten children live with a parent who has a substance abuse problem.

Monkey Business Images/Shutterstock.com

treatment. It was found that women in treatment who were abused as children are about 2.5 times more likely to be victims of intimate partner violence.[56] Although alcohol is implicated with child and domestic abuse, alcohol is also linked to other drugs. For example, it has been shown that there is a strong relationship between binge drinking and cocaine use.[57]

A study in Brazil reported that alcohol use or abuse was associated with the perpetration of sexual aggression, especially toward boys.[58] Adolescents who were sexually abusive and engaged in criminal sexual conduct were more likely to have caregivers who had histories of substance use and abuse.[59] Conversely, women who were sexually abused by age 13 have a greater incidence of alcohol dependence and abuse. Children who are neglected are at greater risk for being arrested on drug and alcohol violations.[60] Children who were sexually abused are more likely to develop drug-related problems as adults.[61] Substance abuse does not figure into every incident of maltreatment; however, caseworkers often cite it as a major factor. One study found that individuals who were abused or neglected as children do not necessarily grow up abusing alcohol, but have a greater risk of abusing alcohol.[62]

Impact of Drug Use and Abuse on Society

Currently, the United States has one of the highest incarceration rates in the world.[63] Since the 1970s incarceration rates have grown 700%.[64] This amounts to over 1 per 100 Americans in jail.[65] Half of all people in state and federal prisons are serving sentences for drug-related offenses.[66] This places a large burden on the taxpayers, as the budget for state prisons has quadrupled over the past two decades.[67] It costs taxpayers about $30,000 to house an inmate for one year.[68] While prisons serve a necessary role in society, it is easy to question the justification of whether it is a good use of taxpayers' money to place nonviolent offenders, and in particular drug offenders, in prison.

In contrast, there is an association between illegal drug use and violent crime.[69] In 2010, among people arrested for committing a crime, those who tested positive for drugs ranged from 52% in Washington, DC to 83% in Chicago.[70] Since 1972, the number of people incarcerated for drug-related crimes has increased fivefold, but despite this increase, drug use and crime have not declined.[71] Alcohol, more than any other drug, is a factor in violent crimes such as murder, rape, and assault.[72] Driving while intoxicated in the third most commonly reported crime in the United States and is the number one cause of death,

injury, and disability in people under the age of 21.[73] Furthermore, it is estimated that four out of five juveniles in state institutions were under the influence of alcohol or drugs while committing their crimes.[74] Alcohol accounts for twice as many violent incidents in bars, nightclubs, and restaurants.[75]

Newspaper headlines recount disturbing stories of drug-crazed people perpetrating crimes on others. In August 2016 a 19-year-old Florida State University student was suspected of a double homicide and one attempted murder. In this bizarre story, he found stabbing a man while biting the man's face.[76] What is called the "zombie drug" Flakka has been implicated as a contributor in this incident. Flakka is a synthetic cathinone related to bath salts. It causes the user to experience hyperstimulation, paranoia, and hallucinations.[77] More on bath salts will be discussed in a later chapter.

Prenatal exposure to drugs and alcohol can have devastating effects for the baby. Although rates for pregnant women (~5%) are lower than for nonpregnant women (~10%), there is still cause for concern.[78] Alcohol use during pregnancy follows the same trend, with fewer pregnant women consuming alcohol (10%) compared with nonpregnant women (55%).[79] Of particular concern are teens who are pregnant, as they have the highest rate of drug use among pregnant women. Pregnant teens (22%) have higher rates of tobacco use compared with nonpregnant teens (13%).[80] Additionally, of young mothers aged 15 to 19, 11.7% used marijuana in the previous 30 days.[81] In self-reported surveys, roughly

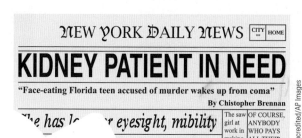

5% of pregnant women admitted to using marijuana during pregnancy.[82] More research is being done to determine the impact of marijuana on a fetus. This, along with the impact on other drugs and alcohol on the fetus, will be presented in later chapters. In 2010, the Child Abuse Prevention and Treatment Act, including the Keeping Children and Families Safe Act, was reauthorized by Congress and states that physicians must notify child and protective services if an infant is affected by illegal substances at birth. This poses ethical, legal, and social concerns. Some states authorize either civil commitment or detention of women to protect a fetus from substance exposure while others consider maternal substance use child abuse and will remove the infant from maternal custody when born.[83] Furthermore, in many states there is no clear distinction on whether maternal substance use constitutes child abuse. This also presents a problem when considering the privacy rights of pregnant women. The 14th amendment protects personal privacy rights including the rights of a woman to decide whether or not to bear a child. Some would say that maternal substance abuse would fall under these privacy rights, while others believe a fetus' rights cannot be separated from the women's rights.[84] One must consider the purpose of these laws and how to best implement them to protect the mother's rights and the fetus' rights. If infants are taken away immediately from substance abusing mothers, does this serve as a deterrent for mothers taking substances while pregnant or does it punish mothers who use drugs?

In 2012, there were approximately 1.2 million persons aged 13 and older living with HIV infection.[85] HIV is the virus that causes AIDS. In 2014, there were almost 45,000 newly diagnosed HIV cases.[86] The impact of HIV and AIDS disproportionally impacts underrepresented persons. Black/African Americans account for almost half of newly diagnosed cases.[87] Furthermore, Hispanics/Latino represent 17% of the population, but account for 23% of HIV diagnoses.[88] Injection drug use accounts for approximately 6% of all newly diagnoses HIV cases, which is down 63%.[89] Needle-exchange programs have been shown to reduce the transmission of HIV.[90]

Drugs are widely available, especially in the largest metropolitan areas where illegal drug use is more common. In the United States, 9.4% of people aged 12 and older used an illicit drug in the past month.[91] Marijuana was the most commonly used illicit drug representing 7.5% of users.[92] In New York City, marijuana can be obtained at newsstands, record shops, video rental outlets, and so on. In 2011, a large Internet site called the Silk Road popped up and became a place where illegal drugs (and other items) could be purchased on the Internet and delivered right to someone's door.[93] Much like eBay, the website was a virtual place that connected dealers to buyers. It is an anonymous black market website that had an estimated 30,000 to 150,000 active buyers.[94] While not the only black market website, it gained notoriety after an article in Gawker was posted highlighting the services and goods that could be purchased through this website.[95] It is estimated that there were around 340 different types of illicit drugs for sale on the website.[96] The site was closed down in 2013, followed by Silk Road 2.0 being relaunched by some of the initial administrators from Silk Road. This site was also shut down and three of the administrators were arrested.[97]

To curb drug availability, billions of dollars are allocated for drug enforcement, prevention, and treatment. In 2017, it was predicted that the federal government's requested expenditures to interdict drugs would total $4.1 billion.[98] High schools and colleges conduct drug tests, especially with athletes. Passing a drug test is a condition of employment for some companies.

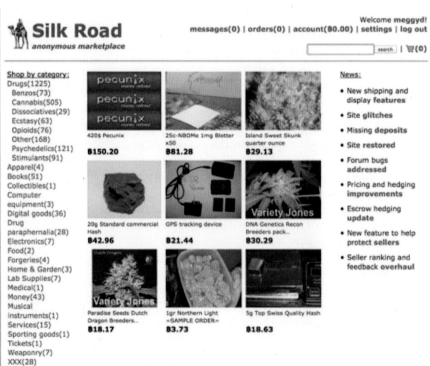

Silk Road: An illicit website that sold drugs

Drugs unquestionably can lead to violent behavior; dependency; mental and physical maladies; strained relationships among siblings, children, parents, and spouses; work-related problems; legal dilemmas; problems in school; financial difficulties; accidents and injuries; and death. Over the last several decades, the United States has become much less tolerant of drug use. The sentiment of zero tolerance extends to other countries as well. For example, in Australia, there is a movement away from minimizing the harm of drugs to zero tolerance.[99]

A report from the Brookings Institute suggested that the debate over how to address the drug problem is based on speculation, not on fact.[100] It is unclear how much of a drug a person has to take before problems arise and how often one has to use drugs before becoming dependent or developing a psychological or medical problem. No hard-and-fast rules are available for determining when drugs become a problem for an individual.[101]

Drugs from a Social Perspective

The effects that drugs produce are influenced greatly by society's perception of them.[102] For example, illegal drugs are condemned much more than legal drugs. Consequently, people who use legal drugs are not viewed in the same negative light as those who use illegal drugs. Tobacco use, in the form of cigarettes, was perceived more negatively in the 2010s than in the 1980s. However, perceptions of e-cigarettes have not shown the same trajectory. In a study conducted on young adults, of those who were aware of e-cigarettes, 44% agreed they can help a person quit smoking, 52% agreed they were less harmful than cigarettes, and 26% felt they were less addictive than cigarettes.[103] Society's reaction to an injection of morphine in a hospital is very different from that to an injection in one's home after obtaining morphine illegally. In addition to the pharmacological effects of drugs, social and psychological factors surrounding drug use play an important role.

Whether a given drug is defined as good or bad, socially acceptable or undesirable, conventional or "deviant" is not a simple outgrowth of the properties or objective characteristics of the drug itself, but is in no small measure a result of the history of its use, what social strata of society use it, for what purposes, the publicity surrounding its use, and so on. Whether the effects are experienced as pleasurable (euphoric) or unpleasant (dysphoric), weak or intense, hedonistic or depressing, hallucinatory or mundane,

serene or exciting is largely a function of sociological factors.[104]

Risk factors that increase the potential for young people to use drugs include growing up in a chaotic household, having parents who abuse drugs, and lacking mutual attachment and nurturing. Parental drug use and poor family relations increase the likelihood of children using drugs[105] (see Figure 2.2).

Other risk factors include school failure, extreme shyness or aggressiveness in the classroom, poor coping skills, the perception that drug use is acceptable, and associating with peers who engage in drug use and other deviant behaviors.[106] In contrast, protective factors that reduce the likelihood of drug use are strong bonds with families, parents who take an active role in their children's lives, academic success, parents who monitor their children and provide clear rules for them, and children who adopt conventional norms regarding drug use.[107] The simple act of eating meals together reduces the likelihood of children using drugs.[108]

Patterns of Drug Taking

In the 1970s, the National Commission on Marihuana and Drug Abuse devised a typology of five general patterns of drug-taking behavior: experimental, social-recreational, circumstantial-situational, intensified, and compulsive.[109] Despite when these typologies were developed, they remain appropriate.

Experimental Use

Individuals who use drugs infrequently and out of curiosity typify **experimental use**. This pattern involves short-term drug use. Experimental use is limited to ten or fewer experiences with a given drug. Drug use usually does not go beyond the experimental phase, because the experimenter no longer has access to the drugs or simply does not find the drug experience enjoyable. If the person continues to use drugs, the drug use no longer is a matter of curiosity or experimentation.

Social-Recreational Use

Social-recreational use, the most common pattern, refers to taking drugs in a social environment to

experimental drug use Infrequent drug use usually motivated by curiosity

social-recreational drug use Taking drugs in a social environment to share pleasurable experiences among friends

share pleasurable experiences among friends. Social-recreational users do not tend to escalate their drug taking to the point of abuse. Women are more likely to be introduced to drug use by a sexual partner.[110] Adolescent females, in particular, are influenced more by romantic partners as compared to men.[111] These situations could be classified as a social-recreational situations.

Circumstantial-Situational Use

Taking a drug on a short-term basis to contend with immediate distress or pressure characterizes **circumstantial-situational use**. Adolescents are more likely to use drugs when they are under stress. Several studies on multiple stressors have found a significant relationship between stress and substance use and abuse among adolescents. In two recent studies regarding Latino and Hispanic adolescents, stress related to culture and minority status was identified as being a risk factor for substance use and abuse.[112,113] It seems that holding a minority status in itself is a risk factor for substance use and abuse. For instance, gay, lesbian, bisexual, and transgender youths, who are often under much stress, have significantly higher rates of substance use. In a large study conducted on adolescents, the identification with being a gender minority was associated with increased use of alcohol, marijuana, and illicit drugs. This same study identified this group as experiencing more episodes of bullying, which also placed them at an increased risk for substance use and abuse.[114] Moreover, there are few intervention programs tailored to these youths.[115] Also, easy access to drugs increases the likelihood of teenagers using drugs.[116] Likewise, easy accessibility for healthcare professionals can lead to drug abuse. Physicians have been found to abuse alcohol and drugs at similar rates to the general population.[117] A study done in 2004 found that physicians abused prescription drugs at higher rates compared to the general population.[118] This could be attributed to the availability of prescription drugs for physicians. In another study done in 2015, the researchers found illicit and prescription drug use to be uncommon among physicians. Using self-reported surveys, roughly 12% of male and 21% of female doctors met the criteria for alcohol abuse or dependence. Risk factors for the physicians in this study included burnout, depression, suicidal ideation, lower quality of life, lower career satisfaction, and recent medical errors.[119] In New York State, 2% of all practicing doctors must be monitored for problems of substance abuse or mental health concerns.[120] Joyous occasions such as weddings and holidays sometimes stimulate people to drink alcohol excessively. A student who has to write a 10-page paper that is due the next day might take amphetamines to stay up all night.

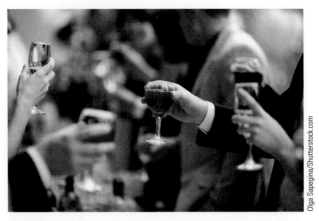

Holiday gatherings can prompt people to drink more alcohol than they had originally intended.

This type of use can become a problem if the need to rely on drugs to cope with problems increases or if stressful events lead to consuming alcohol. Holiday times are stressful as well. There is a higher rate of drug-related suicides of 12- to 17-year-olds and those over age 50 in December.[121]

Intensified Use

A person's drug-taking behavior is **intensified use** if he or she uses drugs on a steady, long-term basis to "achieve relief from a persistent problem or stressful situation or his [or her] desire to maintain a certain self-prescribed level of performance."[122] **Chronic drug use** indicates some extent of physical or psychological dependence. Unlike compulsive drug users, who tend to be alienated from society, chronic drug users maintain their place in society.

Compulsive Use

The person who consumes drugs compulsively and obsessively is not integrated into society. Acquiring and consuming drugs is the compulsive user's main focus. To a large extent, the media emphasize drug use by teenagers. A major problem, however, is compulsive drug use by hardcore users. In 2014, an estimated 435,000 people aged 12 or older were current heroin users.[123] Although heroin use by individuals aged 12 or older represents only 0.3% of the population, its

circumstantial-situational drug use Short-term drug use to contend with immediate distress or pressure

intensified drug use Taking drugs on a steady, long-term basis to relieve a persistent problem or stressful situation

chronic drug use The habitual use of drugs

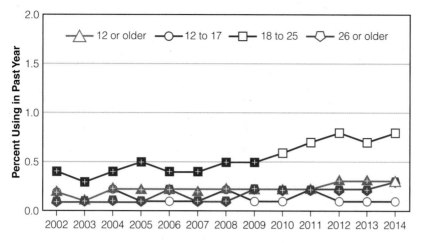

⁺Difference between this estimate and the 2014 estimate is statistically significant at the .05 level.

Figure 2.2 Heroin Use by Persons Aged 12 And Older Has Been on the Rise

Source: https://nsduhweb.rti.org/respweb/homepage.cfm##

use continues to increase.[124] Cocaine use estimates have remained steady since 2002, with an estimated 1.5 million users.[125] These hardcore users also are responsible for most of the crime, child abuse, and fatal overdoses in the United States.

The compulsive user's lifestyle revolves around drugs. The compulsive user takes drugs to avoid discomfort, not to achieve pleasure. Unlike with other patterns of use, the social environment surrounding drug use does not dictate how and why drugs are used. In fact, the individual takes drugs despite the social situation. Society is justified in worrying about **compulsive drug use** because this pattern is destructive to the user and others. Compulsive drug

users are likely to underestimate the extent of their drug use. Most people who use drugs, however, do not become compulsive users.

Extent of Drug Use

To determine precisely the extent of drug use is not easy because people might not answer questions about their personal behavior honestly, especially when illegal drugs are involved. Although obtaining information about the use of legal drugs, such as tobacco, alcohol, and prescription medicines, is easier, even that information may not be entirely accurate.

Even so, surveys repeated over time provide good data with respect to trends in drug use. Two comprehensive, large-scale studies are the *National Survey on Drug Use and Health* and the *Monitoring the Future: National Results on Adolescent Drug Use* survey, which looks at drug use by 8th-grade, 10th-grade, and 12th-grade students.

National Survey on Drug Use and Health

Data regarding drug use have been collected periodically from US households since 1971.[126] Those who participate represent a random cross-section of people. The data received are grouped by respondents' ages (12–17, 18–25, and 26 or older). Table 2.1 shows monthly use of various drugs based on age groups.

Respondents were asked if they ever used drugs, if they had used them in the past year, and if they had used them in the past month. In 2014, an estimated 27 million Americans aged 12 or older were current illicit drug users and 6.5 million reported using nonmedical use of psychotherapeutic drugs.[127] The group with the highest rate illegal drug use during the past month was the 18 to 25 age group at 22%, and those 26 and older had the lowest monthly rates at 8.3%. The most commonly used illicit drug was marijuana. It is used by approximately 8.4% of the population, which reflects an increase over previous

compulsive drug use Obsessive drug use without regard for society

TABLE 2.1 Types of Illicit Drug Use in Lifetime, Past Year, and Past Month Among Persons aged 12–17

Drug	Lifetime (2014)	Lifetime (2015)	Past Year (2014)	Past Year (2015)	Past Mouth (2014)	Past Month (2015)
Illicit Drugs[1,2]	nc	25.3	nc	17.5	nc	8.8
Marijuana	16.4	15.7	13.1	12.6	7.4	7.0
Cocaine	0.9	0.8	0.7	0.6	0.2	0.2
Crack	0.1[a]	0.1	0.1[a]	0.0	0.0	0.0
Heroin	0.1	0.1	0.1	0.1	0.1	0.0
Hallucinogens	nc	3.1	nc	2.1	nc	0.5
LSD	1.2	1.3	0.9	1.0	0.3	0.2
PCP	0.2	0.2	0.1	0.1	0.0	0.0
Ecstasy	nc	1.4	nc	0.8	nc	0.1
Inhalants	nc	9.1	nc	2.7	nc	0.7
Methamphetamine	nc	0.3	nc	0.2	nc	0.1
Misuse of Psychotherapeutics[3]	nc	nr	nc	5.9	nc	2.0
Pain Relievers	nc	nr	nc	3.9	nc	1.1
Tranquilizers	nc	nr	nc	1.6	nc	0.7
Stimulants	nc	nr	nc	2.0	nc	0.5
Sedatives	nc	nr	nc	0.4	nc	0.1
Illicit Drugs Other Than Marijuana[1,2]	nc	15.9	nc	9.1	nc	3.0

Reference: Center for Behavioral Health Statistics and Quality. (2016). *2015 National Survey on Drug Use and Health: Detailed Tables*. Substance Abuse and Mental Health Services Administration, Rockville, MD.

years. Key facts regarding this dataset from 2014 are presented below:[128]

- 27 million Americans use illicit drugs. This represents 10% of the population. These estimates are higher compared to previous years. Figure 2.3 highlights past month illicit drug use.
- 66.9 million Americans are tobacco users. This represents a decrease in tobacco use, especially among adolescents. In 2002 13% of adolescents were cigarette smokers compared to 4.9% in 2014.
- 139.7 million Americans drank alcohol in the past month.
- 60.9 million Americans report to binge drinking while 16.3 million report to using alcohol heavily. These rates are similar to those of past years.
- Around 21 million Americans had a substance use disorder and 3.3% had both a mental illness and a substance use disorder.
- Marijuana is the most used illicit drug with an estimated 22.2 million Americans reported being current users. This represents a higher number of users compared to previous years.
- 2.5% of the population reported nonmedical use of psychotherapeutic drugs. This includes the use of pain relievers, tranquilizers, stimulants, and sedatives. Two-thirds of nonmedical use of psychotherapeutics are pain relievers.

- 0.1% reported to using LSD in the past month and 0.2% reported to using ecstasy (MDMA). These are similar rates to previous years.
- Almost a half a million users reported to using inhalants, comprising mostly young adolescents.

Monitoring the Future: National Results on Adolescent Drug Use—Overview of Key Findings, 2014[129]

Beginning in 1975, the National Institute on Drug Abuse funded research examining the extent of legal and illegal drug use by high school seniors throughout the United States. The research, titled "Monitoring the Future," expanded in 1991 to include 8th- and 10th-grade students. Besides drug usage, data were collected regarding attitudes about drugs, age at which drug use was initiated, and the availability of drugs. Although this annual survey excludes students who drop out of school and those who are absent from school on the day the survey is administered (suggesting that actual figures are underreported), it provides an excellent barometer of trends concerning drug use by 8th-, 10th-, and 12th-grade students.

The year 2014 data, which included about 42,000 students nationwide, showed a mixed picture

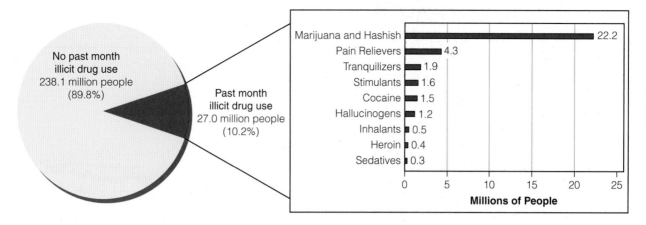

Note: Estimated numbers of people refer to people aged 12 or older in the civilian, noninstitutionalized population in the United States. The numbers do not sum to the total population of the United States because the population for NSDUH does not include people aged 11 years old or younger, people with no fixed household address (e.g., homeless or transient people not in shelters), active-duty military personnel, and residents of institutional group quarters, such as correctional facilities, nursing homes, mental institutions, and long-term hospitals.

Note: The estimated numbers of current users of different illicit drugs are not mutually exclusive because people could have used more than one type of illicit drug in the past month.

Figure 2.3 Numbers of Past Month Illicit Drug Users among People Aged 12 or Older: 2014

Source: Substance Abuse and Mental Health Services Administration (SAMHSA). 2014 National Survey on Drug Use and Health (NSDUH)

in illicit drug use among 8th-, 10th-, and 12th-grade students since the mid-1990s. One of the purposes of this study is to analyze cohort effects as they pertain to differences in substance use attitudes and behaviors. Cohort effects look at attitudes regarding substances at over time. Individuals who grow up at a certain time in history share certain ideas and attitudes regarding drugs. These cohort effects impact drug use. For example, as cigarette use among adolescents declines, one also sees a decline in cigarette use among adults as these adolescents grow up resisting cigarettes and grow into adults who resist cigarette use. Thus, over time, cigarette use will continue to decrease. On the other hand, these cohort effects can predict increased use of certain drugs. Consider the use of e-cigarettes, which has been observed to be on the increase in young adolescents. This trend may then continue to adulthood with as the adolescents grow up and continue to use e-cigarettes.[130]

Results from this survey show a decline in the use of licit (legal) and illicit drugs. Unlike the results from the *Monitoring the Future National Survey Results on Drug Use*, this survey showed a decrease in marijuana use among by young adolescents. Conversely, while marijuana use has declined, attitudes regarding acceptance of marijuana use has increased while perceived risk for marijuana decreased. Other drugs that have a decreased prevalence include: synthetic marijuana, bath salts, narcotics other than heroin, ecstasy (MDMA), hallucinogens other than LSD, salvia, over-the-counter cough and cold medicines, amphetamines use without doctor's orders, Ritalin, Adderall, "crack" cocaine, and

any prescription psychotherapeutic drug.[131] Drug use that remained steady were inhalants, tranquilizers, and the club drugs GHB, cocaine, heroin, methamphetamine and crystal methamphetamine, sedatives, rohypnol, ketamine, and anabolic steroids. Other data revealed in the survey include the following:[132]

- Cigarette smoking continues to be on the decline. Rates between 1996 and 2014 have declined by 81% for 8th graders and 77% for 10th graders. Increased risk and disapproval rates have increased steadily since 1996 and seem to have halted in 2013.
- Smokeless tobacco rates decreased from the mid-1990s to the early 2000s. These levels rebounded from the 2000s to the 2010s. Since 2010, the levels have declined but remained steady in 2014. Since 2010, there has been a decline in the use of smokeless tobacco, some of which may be attributed to the increase use of e-cigarettes.
- Alcohol is the most widely used substance among today's teenagers, with 66% having reported to have consumed alcohol. In 2014, half of all 12th graders and 11% of 8th graders reported being drunk at least once in their life. See Figure 2.4 for alcohol trends among these grade levels.
- E-cigarettes have the highest 30-day prevalence use compared to all tobacco products. Use was 8.7% of 8th graders, 16.2% of 10th graders, and 17.1% of 12th graders. E-cigarettes is being perceived as less risky compared to cigarettes with about 14% of respondents perceiving a "great risk" associated with e-cigarettes compared to on

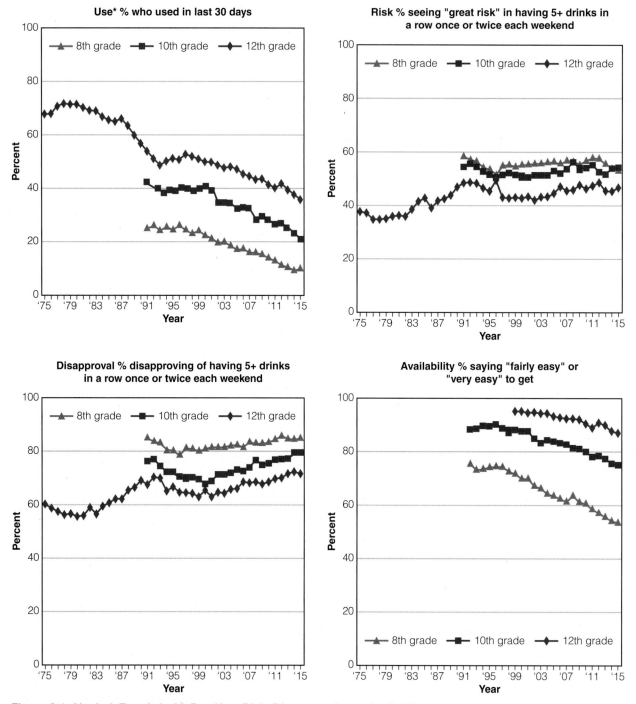

Figure 2.4 Alcohol: Trends in 30-Day Use, Risk, Disapproval, and Availability

*Beginning in 1993, a revised set of questions on alcohol use was introduced, in which a drink was defined as "more than just a few sips."

Source. The Monitoring the Future study, the University of Michigan.

average about 73% perceiving a "great risk" with smoking one or more packs of cigarettes a day.

- Daily prevalence rates of marijuana use have declined with about 1% of 8th graders, 3.4% of 10th graders, and 5.8% of 12th graders reporting daily use. For 12th graders, the availability of marijuana has remained steady since 1975, with between 81% and 90% of 12th graders saying

they could get marijuana easily compared to 81% in 2014. The availability of marijuana for 8th graders is much lower at 37%.

- Synthetic marijuana was first monitored in 2011 among 12th graders. Prevalence at this time was 11.4%, making it the second most used illicit drug after marijuana. Rates did not begin to decline until 2012 and continued to decline into 2014.

- LSD was the most commonly used hallucinogenic drug until 1996. From 1996 to 2006 use declined and has remained at low levels. Since 2000, perceived risk has been declining, suggesting a phenomenon called "generation forgetting." Young teens are less knowledgable about the drug with more participants responding "can't say, drug unfamiliar" to questions about LSD.
- Cocaine use among 8th, 10th, and 12th graders has been sporadic. Over the past 15 years, however, use has declined, with only an annual use of 2.6% among 12th graders and lower numbers for 8th and 10th graders. Perceived risk among all grade levels rose from 1992 to 2000 and continues to rise slightly each year.
- Crack cocaine is a separate item on the "Monitoring the Future" survey. Use rose rapidly in the early 1980s with the highest levels recorded in 1986 with a 4% prevalence rate among 12th graders. In 2014, historic lows were recorded among 8th and 10th grades (prevalence rates dropped 80%) and near historic lows among 12th grades (prevalence rates dropped 60%). Perceived risk of trying crack rose slightly in 2014 among 8th and 10th graders and leveled off among 12th graders. Perceived risk of regular use of crack dropped significantly in 2014 among all grade levels.
- Heroin use fell significantly between the years 1975 and 1979 and held at a low rate until 1994. Use rose in the mid-to-late 1990s (along with other drugs). Use of heroin reached its peak in the late 1990s and early 2000s among 8th, 10th, and 12th graders. Use then began to decline until 2013 with only 0.6% of students reporting heroin use. In 2014, there has been no further change in prevalence.
- The prevalence rates for ecstasy was high in 1996 among 10th and 12th graders with 4.6% reporting ecstasy use; this was higher than college students and young adult use. Since that time, use has declined slightly. In 2014, use was reported at 0.9% for 8th graders, 2.3% for 10th graders, and 3.6% for 12th graders. The term "molly" was added to the survey in 2014 because there were some questions about whether students included it in their answers. In the 2014 survey, which included the term, there seems to be no difference in prevalence rates.

CULTURAL Considerations

Rave parties have been associated with the use of club drugs. A study was conducted to determine if there is an association between attending rave parties and drug use. This study was conducted in 2015 among a nationally represented population of US high school seniors. The results are below:

- One out of five high school seniors attended a rave in their lifetime
- A little over 7% reported attending raves monthly
- Females and religious students were less likely to attend raves
- Hispanics, those who live in cities, and those with higher incomes were more likely to attend raves
- Students who attend raves were more likely to use illicit drugs compared to those students who did not attend raves (35.5% vs. 15.6%)
- Frequent attendance of raves was the highest variable associated with illicit drug use

Source: J.J. Palamar, J.Griffin-Tomas, and D.C. Ompad, "Illicit drug use among rave attendees in a nationally representative sample of US high school seniors", *Drug and Alcohol Dependence*, 152 (2015): 24-31.

Drug Abuse by Older Adults

Drug abuse by Americans 60 years of age and older is an invisible epidemic. In the United States in 2008 more than 49,000 people aged 55 and older went to an emergency room as a result of an adverse reaction to an illicit drug, and more than 151,000 went to an emergency room due to the nonmedical use of a pharmaceutical drug.[133] Another 39,000 people aged 55 and older went to an emergency room after experiencing an adverse reaction from alcohol in combination with another drug.[134] Approximately 2.5 million older Americans have problems related to alcohol. It is estimated that 6% to 11% of elderly patients admitted to hospitals exhibit symptoms of alcoholism, as do 20% of elderly patients in psychiatric wards. Some older adults misuse over-the-counter drugs that have high alcohol content, such as cough suppressants. The majority of older people engaging in substance misuse are men, even though women outnumber men. The small percentage of older adults who abuse illicit drugs usually are aging criminals and long-term heroin addicts.

Substance abuse by older adults accelerates the normal decline in physiological functioning that accompanies aging. Also, because older people are more affected by drugs, they are at higher risk for accidents and illness. Further, the percentage of older adults in the general population is projected to increase, so substance abuse problems are expected to become more apparent. A clear relationship exists between alcohol problems early in life and alcohol problems later in life. Also, there is an association between separated, divorced, and widowed adults and alcohol abuse.

Close to 30% of older adults have a prescription to take 5 or more medications.[135] This places older adults at a higher risk for drug misuse as the number of medications that are prescribed is higher and thus the likelihood of adverse drug interactions increased.[136] Risks for an adverse drug interaction is at 13% for two drugs, 58% for five drugs, and 82% for seven drugs.[137] Thus as the number of prescriptions for older populations increase the number of adverse effects also increase. Older people are more likely to be noncompliant in their medication adherence due to poor communication skills with their physician, using multiple pharmacies (who may not be aware of other prescriptions), and the decline in cognitive functioning.[138] Couple this with the increasing amount of over-the-counter (OTC) medications, the use of which is often not shared with physicians and/or pharmacists. It is estimated that older adults take four OTC medications along with four prescribed medications.[139] Almost one-fourth of older adults take a combined total of 10 or more OTC and prescription medications.[140] As previously mentioned, many people do not inform their doctors and/or pharmacists of the OTC medications they are taking, many of which can adversely interact among each other. For example, Wafarin is a drug that is prescribed to reduce the risk of stroke and heart attacks. When mixed with Ginkgo Biloba, a popular herbal drug in the United States taken to improve memory and brain functioning, may result in an increased risk of bleeding.[141] If Warafin is taken with St. John's Wort, another popular herbal medicine believed to help with depression, it can result in a moderate reduction in the effects of Warafin.[142]

Problems with substance abuse by elderly people may be more common than believed, because healthcare providers underestimate, underidentify, underdiagnose, and undertreat the problem. However, diagnosing symptoms of substance abuse in older adults is difficult because many symptoms mimic symptoms of medical and behavioral disorders common to this population. Older adults also experience more noncancer-related pain compared to younger populations.

A survey conducted indicates that almost 60% of older people experience noncancer related pain lasting at least one year.[143] It has also been reported that 40% of older people experience daily pain.[144] In a study that was conducted on older people who admitted to misusing drugs a little over 70%

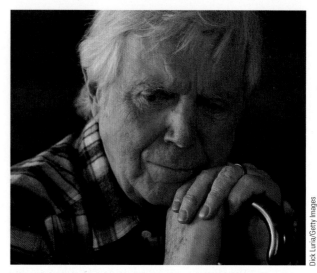

Many older people use drugs to deal with loneliness.

reported to being in fair or poor health and almost 87% reported to having severe physical pain over the past year. Additionally, almost 45% reported severe depression. When asked about their drug-misusing behavior, almost 81% reported misusing the drug to alleviate severe pain followed by almost 15% using the drug as a replacement for another drug and another 15% reported using the drug to get "high."[145] Thus when looking at opioid misuse among the older population one must consider the motivations for misusing the drug and identify ways to better manage pain.

Contributing to substance abuse problems of older adults are shame and *ageism*. Many older adults feel shamed if they have a substance abuse problem; consequently, they are reluctant to seek treatment. Moreover, adult children of older individuals feel shamed if their parents have a substance abuse problem and therefore choose not to address the problem.

Too often, substance abuse by older adults is ignored because of the unspoken but pervasive attitude that treating older adults is not worth the trouble. Some people think that older people will not be around that much longer anyway, so why interfere with their lives if they are enjoying themselves?[146] Unfortunately, older adults who self-medicate with alcohol or prescription drugs are more likely to characterize themselves as lonely, and they report lower life satisfaction.

Drugs in the Workplace

Substance abuse has a profoundly negative effect in the workplace, resulting in lessened productivity and increased accidents, absenteeism, and healthcare costs. According to the American Council for Drug Education, over 70% of substance users hold jobs. It is estimated that employee drug abuse costs the workplace $25.6 billion.[147] People who are unemployed are more likely to use drugs than people who are employed; however, most substance users and those with substance abuse disorders work full time.[148] Part-time workers also have higher rates of drug use than full-time workers. The industries with the highest rates of drug use are food service workers and construction workers.[149] The latter have the highest rates of occupational injuries among the major industries.[150]

In recent years, "the percent of American workers testing positive for illicit drugs such as marijuana, cocaine, and methamphetamine has increased" (p. 58).[151] Rates of drug users identified in the workplace through urine tests have increased in 2014 with about 4.7% testing positive for drugs.[152] In 2007, the number of workers testing positive for cocaine and methamphetamines declined significantly from the previous year.[153] Most surveys figured that fewer than 10% of workers used alcohol or other drugs—excluding tobacco and caffeine—on the job. Nonetheless, alcoholism results in 500 million lost workdays each year. The majority of employees who use drugs are men. However, almost one in five women who are employed full time engaged in binge drinking within the previous month and 6.4% used an illicit drug.[154]

Workplace drug use is not consistent throughout the country. The number of workers testing positive for methamphetamine use is greater in the Western states.[155] Workers in Hawaii had the highest rate of methamphetamine use.[156] Among active duty military personnel, 11.9% tested positive illicit drugs, including nonmedical use of prescription drugs.[157] Drug use in the workplace is not limited to the United States. An Australian study revealed that 8.7% of workers drank alcohol at work and almost 1% used drugs at work. Hospitality workers had higher rates of drug use than other professions.[158] In Norway, nearly one-fourth of workers reported to work with a hangover, and 6% were absent from work due to alcohol.[159]

Identifying drug problems in top-level managers is more of a dilemma than recognizing drug problems in other workers, because upper-level managers have less supervision, and corporations often deny that their executives abuse drugs. To address drug abuse, most Fortune 500 companies use some type of drug testing and undercover surveillance. It is believed that drug testing has greatly reduced drug use among American workers. The percentage of individuals testing positive for drugs has declined since the 1980s.[160]

An interesting question involves whether employers can fire workers who test positive for marijuana even though marijuana was used for medical purposes. The California State Supreme Court ruled by a margin of 5 to 2 that employers do have the right to fire workers who test positive for marijuana.[161] Other states (Colorado, Michigan, Oregon, Washington, and New Mexico) have had similar decisions

---

CASE STUDY: Marijuana

"Rojerio Garcia disclosed during his job interview with Tractor Supply Company that he had been diagnosed with HIV/AIDS, and was participating in New Mexico's medical cannabis program under the state's Compassionate Use Act (CUA). Garcia was required to undergo a drug test as a condition of hire and was terminated after his drug test showed positive for cannabis metabolites. He sued Tractor Supply, alleging that the company terminated him based on his serious medical condition and his physicians' recommendation to use medical marijuana." "[Judge] Johnson explained that New Mexico's medical marijuana law does not include affirmative requirements mandating that employers accommodate medical marijuana cardholders, as some states—like Connecticut and Delaware—do. "The court finds that the CUA, combined with the New Mexico Human Rights Act, does not provide a cause of action for Mr. Garcia, as medical marijuana is not an accommodation that must be provided for by the employer," he said. The court also dismissed Garcia's claims that Tractor Supply fired him because of his serious medical condition, "as marijuana use is not a manifestation of HIV/AIDS, nor is testing positive for marijuana conduct."

In addition, the court ruled that requiring Tractor Supply to accommodate Garcia's use of a drug that is still illegal under federal law would require it to permit conduct that is prohibited under the federal Controlled Substances Act (CSA)."

Source: R. Maurer, "Court rules medical marijuana users can be fired," Society for Human Resource Management, (January 29, 2016). Available at: https://www.shrm.org/resourcesandtools/hr-topics/talent-acquisition/pages/medical-marijuana-users-can-be-fired.aspx.

regarding marijuana use on the job. In a recent federal court case in New Mexico, the court rules that a company may not permit conduct that allows use of a substance that is prohibited under the federal Controlled Substance Act.[162] Thus, because marijuana still is categorized as a schedule I drug, its use is prohibited under the federal Controlled Substance Act, which supersedes state law.

The Department of Labor ended the drug-free workplace program in 2010.[163] Workplace alcohol and drug policies have been shown to reduce the impact of substance use and abuse. For example, in a study conducted in Australia regarding workplace alcohol and drug policies, researchers found that having these policies significantly decreased the odds of high risk drinking and drug use.[164]

Employee Assistance Programs

Many corporations have devised employee assistance programs (EAPs) to help workers deal with legal, family, health, or other problems that affect job performance.[165] Some EAPs are offered on a voluntary basis, and others require that employees attend. Many workers benefit from EAPs, especially those who are given the choice of attending a program or being fired. Employers benefit because absenteeism declines, productivity increases, job-related problems decrease, and employee morale improves. In a literature review regarding the return of investing on health-promotion programs, a positive relationship was found between workplace health promotion and a return on investment. Thus costs associated with EAPs have been found to have a greater return on investment due to the benefits mentioned above.[166]

Managers rely on EAPs to help identify employees who would benefit from an alcohol and drug treatment through brief screenings with employees. Employees benefit from EAPs by having a support service to engage in rehabilitation services while being able to maintain employment.[167] "EAPS are the principal invention mechanism for dealing with alcohol and other health and behavioral problems in the workplace" (p. 56).[168] A worksite program designed to prevent alcohol misuse by working adults found that alcohol consumption and problems related to alcohol use can be reduced.[169] It was reported that among workers who went to an EAP for alcohol or drug problems, mental health improved in 66%, physical health improved in 56%, and absenteeism showed an 80% improvement.[170] The Hazelden Foundation indicated that alcohol addiction improved in 89% of people treated through their employers.[171]

Employees who are in recovering from substance abuse treatment are protected under several laws regarding discrimination. These laws include the American with Disabilities Act (ADA), Rehabilitation Act of 1973, Fair Housing Act (FHA), and the Workforce Investment Act (WLA).[172] These do not cover those employees who are using and abusing alcohol and other drugs at the workplace or if the abuse of alcohol and other drugs impacts their job performance.[173]

Drug Testing

In the 1986 classic, *America's Habit: Drug Abuse, Drug Trafficking, and Organized Crime,* the President's Commission on Organized Crime advocated that all federal workers be drug tested and that federal contracts be withheld from private employers who do not initiate drug testing programs. In 2011, the federal government earmarked $283.1 million for drug-related activities in schools.[174] Random workplace drug testing has effectively identified frequent users of illicit drugs.[175] It is important to note that 40% of industrial accidents are attributed to alcohol use and alcoholism.[176] Drug-using employees are five times more likely to file for workers' compensation.[177] Drugs inevitably affect an individual's ability to work. Companies that test employees for performance, however, found that fatigue, stress, and illness are the most common factors leading to poor job performance.[178] In 2007, a study was conducted to determine the extent of drug testing in the United States. The researchers found that 46% of workers and 90% of Fortune 200 companies have some sort of drug testing at the company.[179]

Some employers maintain that there are numerous benefits to drug testing employees. One benefit is that employee morale is improved because employers are committed to providing a safe work environment. Low-performing employees are weeded out and workers that have been identified as being a drug user during screening may not be hired in the first place.[180] Drug testing may lead to a worker seeking out treatment whereas they would not have been motivated to do so before being asked to submit to drug testing.[181]

An interesting dilemma is that 14 states and the District of Columbia allow individuals to receive marijuana for medical purposes. Yet, because of how long marijuana stays in the body (see Table 2.2), an individual who has used marijuana for medicinal purposes may test positive at work even weeks later. So

employee assistance programs (EAPs) A confidential workplace assistance program designed to help employees and their families with personal problems.

TABLE 2.2 Detectability of Drugs

Drug	Urine Detection Period	Hair Detection Period
Alcohol	6–12 hours	Not detectable
Amphetamines/methamphetamines	4–5 days	Up to 90 days
Barbiturates	2–12 days	Not assayed
Cocaine	4–5 days	Up to 90 days
Marijuana	3–30 days	Up to 90 days
PCP	2–10 days	Up to 90 days

far, the courts have ruled in favor of employers who dismiss employees testing positive for marijuana even if the employees have a doctor's note.[182]

Not all critics support drug testing, some arguing that it represents a billion-dollar business for the private sector. In one study, drug testing was associated with a reduced rate of minor injuries (with no lost work), but had no impact on injuries that resulted in lost work.[183] In another study that conducted a literature review on the efficacy of drug testing, it was found that studies that showed significant reductions in occupational accidents associated with drug testing had weaker methodology practices. Researchers of this study felt that there is a need for better research studies, specifically in regards to methodology, to show a relationship, or lack thereof, between drug testing at the workplace and reduced accidents.[184]

Who should be drug tested? For example, should teachers be drug tested? When school superintendents were asked about drug testing teachers, the majority felt they had the right to drug test teachers but most would not because they felt the problem of drug use by teachers is too small to warrant testing. The superintendents were more comfortable drug testing as a condition for hiring teachers.[185] The previous governor of Hawaii proposed drug testing all teachers but that effort was thwarted by the Hawaii Teachers Association.[186] In 2015, The Hawaii Teachers Association and the Department of Education reached an agreement regarding drug testing of teachers; drug testing was implemented in exchange for an 11% pay increase for teachers.[187] While drug testing teachers is lawful, it is an expensive endeavor.

Most Americans view drug testing as degrading and dehumanizing.[188] A group especially subjected to drug testing is pregnant women. In addition, Black women are 1.5 times more likely to be tested for illicit drugs than non-Black women.[189] In many jurisdictions, physicians are required to report women who use drugs during pregnancy or infants who test positive for drug use by their mothers. However, the Supreme Court indicated that pregnant patients cannot be tested for illegal drugs if the purpose is to alert police to crime. Rather, drug testing is permissible if the purpose is to help the pregnant

woman receive better health care.[190] Drug testing with the intent of punishing the pregnant woman is opposed by the American Medical Association, the American Congress of Obstetricians and Gynecologists, and the American Academy of Pediatrics.[191]

Women whose babies test positive for drugs such as cocaine are subject to losing custody of their children because they are viewed as unfit parents. As a result, women may not receive adequate prenatal care for fear of losing their children. And, even though cocaine use during pregnancy is unhealthy, alcohol use and cigarette smoking during pregnancy have been shown to cause worse problems.

Testing of Public Assistance Recipients

In recent years, there has been much discussion about the need to require people who seek public assistance to be drug free. In 1996, President Clinton passed the Personal Responsibility and Work Opportunity Reconciliation Act of 1996 that allowed states to take control of their welfare systems.[192] Additionally, it made it more difficult for individuals to apply for and receive assistance.[193] States have been trying to pass legislative requiring welfare recipients and applicants to submit to nonsuspicious drug testing.

Proponents for drug testing public assistance recipients believe that monies given to recipients would be used for drugs rather than items such as food, housing, etc. They believe reducing the amount of people who receive assistance would save the state money by reducing the amount of assistance provided. Furthermore, they believe drug testing could identify people who could benefit from treatment.[194] Opponents believe drug testing places additional stigma regarding public assistance and drug use suggesting to the public that public aid recipients use and abuse drugs at higher rates than the general public. Furthermore, these programs are expensive and money is being diverted from public assistance programs to pay for drug testing.[195] In 2011, when Florida enacted drug testing for public assistance recipients, 98% of the tests came back as negative.[196] One must consider the purpose of drug testing public assistance recipi-

VALLEY & STATE

Welfare recipients face drug tests

'Reasonable cause' now triggers screening

By Amy B Wang
THE ARIZONA REPUBLIC

What is the purpose of drug testing those on public aid? Is it to identify those who could benefit from treatment or to exclude people from receiving benefits?

ents. Is it to identify those that are drug users to provide them with help in the form of treatment, or to identify people to exclude from the program?

Testing of Athletes

Drug testing is a concern in many professional and amateur athletic programs. To increase alertness, competitiveness, and aggression, some competitors use stimulants. Others use beta-blockers to reduce anxiety. Still others use steroids to augment muscle development.[197] Beta-blockers are especially beneficial in sports requiring steadiness, such as putting in golf.[198] One unfortunate side effect is that they interfere with sexual performance.

Almost all high schools randomly drug test athletes, while 65% randomly drug test students participating in extracurricular activities and 14% randomly drug test all students.[199] Court rulings have been mixed as to whether drug testing violates the privacy of high school and college athletes. Random drug testing of students, not just student-athletes, has been shown to reduce drug use. One large study found that 16% of students in schools with mandatory random drug testing used drugs compared to 22% of students in schools without random drug testing.[200]

The US Supreme Court said that drug testing does not violate a student-athlete's right to privacy[201] and confirmed a school district's decision to drug test all students involved in extracurricular activities. In a 2001 ruling, the Supreme Court upheld lower court rulings that prevent school districts from drug testing nonatheletes.[202] However, steroids are used by non-athletes because friends use them, to enhance physical appearance, and to improve physical performance.[203]

The effectiveness of drug testing is questionable. In Texas, $6 million was allocated for testing student-athletes for steroids. Of 10,000 students, only two tested positive.[204]

Some people argue that drug testing of athletes should be abandoned for several reasons, among them questions regarding the validity of the tests and whether the levels that are considered inappropriate are arbitrary.[205] The American Academy of Pediatrics opposes the random drug testing of athletes. They believe initiating a random drug testing program could have adverse effects such as decreased participation in sports and an increase in substance use that is not tested by drug panels.[206] Another concern is that drug testing has not kept up with new ways to avoid detection; thus, there is inconsistency in which athletes are caught doping.[207]

Some athletes use performance-enhancing drugs to keep up with the competition. Despite this point, many athletes support drug testing. One study of 240 elite track and field athletes found that the majority supported the antidrug movement.[208] Elite athletes in Australia favor drug testing for performance-enhancing drugs, although they are not in favor of penalizing athletes who use illicit, recreational drugs.[209]

Methods of Drug Testing

Testing for drugs can be done by examining urine, saliva, hair, blood, or breath. The ability to detect drugs depends on the type of test, the dose, and the sensitivity of the test. A new test for detecting drugs developed by University of Illinois researchers involves a litmus-like paper strip that examines molecules in saliva, urine, or blood.[210] Urine testing is the most common method and has been shown to be accurate and reliable. The methods used to test urine for drugs are immunoassay, gas chromatography, thin-layer chromatography, and gas chromatography/mass spectrometry.

1. **Immunoassay** is fast and less expensive than other methods but may give false-positive readings.
2. **Gas chromatography** is more expensive and time-consuming than other methods.
3. **Thin-layer chromatography** is simple and inexpensive, but it requires expert interpretation, and is less sensitive than the immunoassay procedure.
4. **Gas chromatography/mass spectrometry** is highly sophisticated and sensitive but is time-consuming and expensive.

The detectability of drugs in urine or hair varies with the drug. Although amphetamines and methamphetamines are detectable in urine 4 to 5 days after use, a hair test can detect their presence up to 90 days after use. Phencyclidine (PCP) is detectable in urine 2 to 10 days after use and is detectable through hair analysis up to 90 days after use. Urine tests can detect cocaine 4 to 5 days after use, and hair tests can detect cocaine 90 days after use. A person can test positive for heroin 1 to 2 days after use via urine and 90 days after use via a hair sample. Marijuana can be detected from 3 to 30 days after use by a urine test and up to 90 days later through a hair test. In one county in Iowa, Child Protective Services is hair-testing children soon after they are born to determine whether they have been exposed to smoked drugs, especially crack.[211] Table 2.2 compares the detectability of drugs through urine and through hair.

Two problems with drug testing are false positives and false negatives:

1. A **false positive** means that a person tests positive for a drug even though no drug is present in the person's urine. For example, ibuprofen, the active ingredient in Motrin and Advil, may cause a false-positive test for marijuana. A person may test positive for opiates after consuming poppy seeds or cough syrups containing codeine. It has been shown that individuals who lack the enzyme UGT2B17 may test positive for excessive testosterone.[212]
2. A **false negative** means that a person tests negative even though drugs are present in the person's urine.

Some people employ inventive ways to test negative: by obtaining someone else's urine, by drinking vast amounts of water before testing, or by placing salt and detergent in the urine sample. Another potential problem with drug testing is that one's medical condition may be revealed to the employer. For example, a drug test may indicate whether a person is taking certain medications for certain medical conditions or is genetically predisposed to other conditions such as heart disease or cancer. It may cause an

immunoassay A drug-testing procedure that tests for metabolites of drugs

gas chromatography A drug-testing procedure that is more specific, sensitive, and expensive than the immunologic assay

thin-layer chromatography A simple, inexpensive, urine-based drug test

gas chromatography/mass spectrometry A type of drug test, highly sophisticated and sensitive, but time-consuming and expensive

false positive A test that is positive for drugs even though no drugs are present in the urine

false negative A test that is negative for drugs even though drugs are present in the urine

employer to forgo hiring a prospective employee to avoid potential health insurance costs.

Legality of Drug Testing

The legality of drug testing was debated in two cases that came before the US Supreme Court: *Skinner* v. *Railway Labor Executive Association* and *National Treasury Employees Union* v. *von Raab*. The *Skinner* case dealt with the constitutionality of random drug testing of employees and applicants of private railways. In 1985, the Federal Railroad Administration (FRA) adopted regulations that prohibited employees from possessing or using alcohol or any controlled substance while at work or from reporting to work while under the influence of alcohol or a controlled substance. These regulations were implemented because a number of employees had come to work impaired by alcohol or had become drunk while at work.

In 21 or more railway accidents between 1972 and 1983 that involved fatalities, serious injuries, and millions of dollars of damage to property, alcohol or other drugs were the probable or contributing cause.[213] By a 7–2 vote, the Supreme Court upheld the FRA's plan to test railway workers. While recognizing the need to protect individuals' rights, the Supreme Court noted that the safety considerations of certain jobs override those rights. Because the impairment of railway workers posed a considerable threat to the public, the Supreme Court ruled that drug testing is warranted.

The second case before the Supreme Court, *National Treasury Employees Union* v. *von Raab*, dealt with whether applicants for the US Customs Service must pass a drug test. Individuals testing positive would not have to turn over the results for prosecution. The purpose was to prevent individuals from getting the jobs in the first place. The Customs Service argued that drug users were subject to bribery and blackmail, that drug users may be unsympathetic to their task of interdicting narcotics, and that drugs might impair employees who carry firearms.

Even though only 5 employees of 3,600 had tested positive for drugs, the Supreme Court narrowly (5–4) agreed with the Customs Service. Because the testing program was designed to prevent drug use and the integrity of the Customs Service had to be maintained, the Court ruled that the testing program was justified.

In a study of commercial aviation employees, it was found that employees who tested positive for drugs were three times more likely to be involved in an accident. Marijuana accounted for two-thirds of employees testing positive for drugs. Nonetheless, drug violations contributed to a very small percentage of aviation accidents.[214]

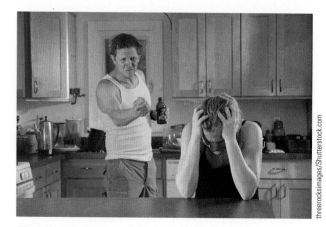

Drug use increases the risk of domestic violence.

Consequences of Drug Use

Drug use is a factor in family stability, social behavior, education and career aspirations, and personal and social maturation. A relationship has been reported between adolescents' substance use, depression, and suicidal thoughts and attempts. It could be argued that drugs are not *the* problem, but just one piece of a much larger puzzle in which drug use is simply another component. An important question is whether drugs are a problem or whether they are symptomatic of other problems.

Drugs and Deviant Behavior

Drug use and deviant attitudes and behavior are closely associated.[215] The most important distinction between drug users and nonusers is their extent of *conventionality*.[216] Deviant social childhood and adolescent behavior are related to an increased in vulnerability for drug use.[217] Whether drug use provokes deviant attitudes and behaviors or whether deviant behaviors and attitudes provoke drug use is unclear. Humans are social animals where much time is spent interacting with others. Positive social interaction stimulates the reward system in the brain, which reinforces social interaction. Some believe that positive social play and the rewards system for drugs of abuse work on the same neural systems in the brain and the same neurotransmitters (i.e., endogenous opioids, dopamine). Thus positive social play produces a rewarding sensation much in the same way drugs do. In small doses, most drugs of abuse will enhance social play behavior in rats but in larger doses will reduce social play.[220] Drug users display more independence, rebelliousness, acceptance of deviant behavior, and rejection of moral and social norms than nonusers.[221] Children of parents who use drugs are more likely to engage in delinquent behaviors than their peers whose parents do not use drugs.[222] The significance of this association is revealed by one study reporting that almost 7.5 million alcohol-dependent or alcohol-abusing parents have at least one child living with them.[223]

Some drugs are more likely to produce violent behavior whereas others, such as marijuana and heroin, are more likely to produce a passive response. (Heroin is linked to criminal behavior but not to violent behavior.) Stimulants such as methamphetamines and cocaine are associated with violence. The combination of hyperactivity and increased suspiciousness may cause sudden, unwarranted aggressiveness. The factor relating to violence may not be the amphetamine but, rather, the paranoia the drug causes.

The drug involved with the most violent incidents is alcohol. The level of aggression associated with alcohol was found to be dose related. The more one drank, the more aggressive one became. This applied to both males and females.[224] Binge drinking is associated with unsafe sex and violence as well as with nonconsensual sex.[225] Combining alcohol and caffeine, which is popular among some groups of people, exacerbates the potential for violence.[226]

The person using alcohol may perpetrate the violence or be the victim of another alcohol user. Among many victims of violence, it was believed that the perpetrator was under the influence of alcohol at the time; for example, of individuals who were victimized at work, 35% believe that the offender was under the influence of alcohol or other drugs.[227] In a study of 20,274 adolescents, 16% reported being victims of dating violence. Most cases of dating violence occurred in the South, and in many instances, alcohol was implicated.[228]

Drugs, Education, and Employment

There is a higher dropout rate from school for those who used alcohol, illicit drugs, and cigarettes.[229] In a study of African American students, it was found that the desire to do well academically was related to less marijuana use, parental substance use norms, and family financial concerns.[230] There is a relationship between academic performance and drug use. It is not always clear whether drug use causes poor academic performance or whether one uses drugs because one is doing poorly in school. A study was conducted on marijuana users who attended college. The college students were divided into five categories based on their marijuana use: non-users, infrequent users, decreasing users, increasing users, and frequent users. Results from this study discovered higher rates of dropping out of college and delayed gradation among decreasing and frequent users. Additionally, all marijuana users reported lower GPAs.[231] Feeling connected to school serves as a deterrent to drug use.[149] One study of college students found that males who perceive themselves to be under much stress are more likely to consume energy drinks, which negatively affects academic performance.[232]

Drug use is assumed to be a predictor of welfare dependency. In 1997, the federal government passed a law stipulating that all welfare recipients be denied Social Security income and disability insurance if alcohol and drug addiction were exclusively responsible for their disabilities. In 2011, Florida Governor Rick Scott proposed that all welfare recipients be drug tested and those who fail will not receive welfare for a year. A second failed drug test would disallow a person from receiving welfare for three years.[233]

The relationship between drug use and welfare dependency is not limited to the United States. In New Zealand, marijuana use among adolescents and young adults negatively affected educational achievement, reduced employment, and increased welfare dependency.[234] Similarly, Norwegians who use marijuana are more likely to receive welfare assistance in that country.[235]

The Higher Education Act of 1965 stipulates that college students who are convicted of a drug offense are denied federal financial aid. Legislation has been introduced to have federal financial aid restored to college students if they enroll in treatment and pass two drug tests.[236] Since 2000, more than 180,000 students have been denied federal financial aid due to a drug conviction.[237]

Employed drug users have less stable job histories than nonusers. Whether job instability results in drug use or drug use causes job instability is unclear. Alcohol abusers earn significantly less money than moderate drinkers and abstainers.[238] Finally, drug use is associated with higher accident rates on the job and lower productivity.

Drug Toxicity

At a certain dose, many drugs are beneficial. At higher doses, the same drugs may be poisonous, or *toxic*. The difference between a safe level and a dangerous level, the **margin of safety**, can be slight. Even if one does not overdose, drug use can be fatal. In a study of US veterans, it was found that substance use increased the risk of premature death significantly.[239] An Australian study reported that substance use was highly correlated to suicide attempts.[240]

Toxicity can be physiological, behavioral, acute, or chronic:

1. *Physiological toxicity* refers to the danger to the body as a result of taking the drug. An example is taking an excessive amount of barbiturates, causing breathing to cease.
2. *Behavioral toxicity* means that a drug interferes with one's ability to function. Behavioral toxicity is illustrated by drowning or getting into an automobile accident after consuming alcohol.
3. *Acute toxicity* alludes to the danger from a single experience with a drug, such as getting drunk.
4. *Chronic toxicity* is the danger posed by repeated exposure to a drug. An example is cardiac or pulmonary damage resulting from long-term cigarette use.

Toxicity does not reflect the legal status of a drug. The drug causing the highest death rate in the United States is tobacco, which is responsible for more than 400,000 deaths per year even though its production is subsidized by the federal government! The notion that if a drug is legal, it is safe—or at least safer than illegal drugs—must be dispelled.

Drug Abuse Warning Network

To get a better grasp of the magnitude of drug-related problems, the federal government monitors emergency room visits in many metropolitan areas through a system called the Drug Abuse Warning Network (DAWN). DAWN collects information on the number of times drugs are implicated in nonlethal visits to emergency rooms and in fatalities.

From 2005 to 2009, the number of drug-related suicide attempts by males resulting in visits to emergency rooms increased from 58,775 to 77,971.[241] For women, the number of drug-related suicide attempts went from 92,682 to 120,418.[242] The type of drug that was most implicated with suicide attempts was nonmedicinal pharmaceutical drugs.

Emergency room visits arise from adverse emotional or physical reactions to drugs. The user may hallucinate or become irrational, overly anxious, or suicidal. The medical examiner determines whether death is caused by drugs. When a person visits an emergency room or has a fatal overdose, more than one drug is usually involved.

Many factors play a role in drug overdoses. Injected drugs pose a greater health threat than ingested drugs, and mixing drugs augments their potency significantly. Also, drug dosage, drug purity, and frequency of use figure into the potential risks. Adverse effects increase when larger amounts are consumed or when the drugs are taken at more frequent intervals. The DAWN data reflect **acute** drug-related problems, not chronic drug use.

In 2011, DAWN was discontinued and integrated with the National Hospital Care Survey (NHCS). This allowed for an expansion on the type of information collected, which includes the reporting of mental disorders.

If it were categorized by itself, alcohol would head the lists for both lethal and nonlethal incidents. One study found that among individuals reporting an emergency room visit, 245 had engaged in "risky drinking," which was defined as 14 or more drinks per week for men and 7 or more drinks per week for women. Eight percent reported being problem drinkers and 3% were alcohol dependent.[243]

It should be noted that drug mortality figures only represent a small percentage of drug overdoses. It is estimated that only 20% of all deaths are reviewed by a medical examiner or coroner. In 2009, there were 19,551 deaths attributed to prescribed and over-the-counter medicines.[244]

margin of safety Difference between an effective dose and a lethal dose

toxicity A drug's ability to disturb or nullify homeostasis

acute Describes a condition that arises abruptly and is not long lasting

Summary

Drugs affect people throughout life, from the fetus to the elderly. Drug-use patterns vary considerably—from experimental use motivated by curiosity, to social-recreational use, to circumstantial-situational use, to intensified use, or to compulsive use dictated by a psychic or physical need for drugs. The age group most likely to use illegal drugs is 18 to 25. National surveys pointed to an upward trend in the early 1990s, although modest declines are now occurring. As people perceive drugs to be harmful, the rate of use tends to go down.

The impact of drug abuse is considerable for families. Children raised in homes where drug abuse occurs are more likely to experience instability, less financial support, experience nutritional deficiencies, and emotional trauma. Unfortunately, these may result in lifelong consequences including performing poorly academically, which leads to poorer job outcomes, higher stress, and increased risk for substance use and abuse.

In regards to the impact on society, drug use and abuse accounts for nearly 50% of all people in prison. Furthermore, drug use and abuse contributes to cases of violent crime.

Prenatal exposure to drugs and alcohol can have devastating and long-lasting effects for the baby. Pregnant teens have higher rates of alcohol use compared to pregnant adults, along with tobacco and marijuana use. While physicians must notify child protective services if an infant is affected by illegal substances at birth, one must consider the ethical, legal, and social consequences of this.

To address drug use in the workplace, many companies have developed employee assistance programs (EAPs) designed to help employees deal with personal problems including those that are drug related. The purpose of these drug programs is to help employees, not to punish them. Companies benefit from EAPs because they are able to retain already trained employees rather than having to replace them. As a condition of employment, many companies require applicants to take drug tests. The constitutionality of drug testing remains to be answered definitively.

One danger posed by drugs is their toxicity. Although many illegal drugs are toxic, the chronic use of cigarettes is the leading drug-related cause of death.

Thinking Critically

1. The purpose of the Child Abuse Prevention and Treatment Act is to protect children and now includes language prenatal exposure to drugs and alcohol. If infants are taken away immediately from substance abusing mothers, does this serve as a deterrent for mothers taking substances while pregnant or does it punish mothers who use drugs? If pregnant women perceive a risk of having their baby taken away if they admit to using drugs and alcohol, do you think they would actively seek help? If the focus is on treatment, how would you encourage pregnant women to seek help?

2. The cohort effect can indicate social tolerance and acceptance for certain drugs. These effects change over time. In the 1980s cocaine was one of the most used and abused recreational drug. It was depicted in films, television, and many celebrities used the drug. Think about your personal cohort effect. What drugs do you feel were discouraged? Encouraged? Which drugs were popularized by the media? How did growing up in your time period impact your thoughts about certain drugs?

3. Are drugs really a problem in society, or is the concern excessive? The drawbacks to using drugs are numerous. In the attempt to reduce drug use and abuse, what is the best approach? Should drug policy focus on reducing the supply of drugs or the demand for drugs? Which approach would result in the least harm?

4. Drug testing, many argue, invades an individual's right to privacy. But employers contend that drugs cost their businesses, and therefore consumers, a great deal of money. How can the rights of the individual be balanced against the rights of the employer? Should regulations regarding testing be determined by the type of job—for example, airline pilot, sales clerk, nurse, carpenter? If so, which jobs would you include?

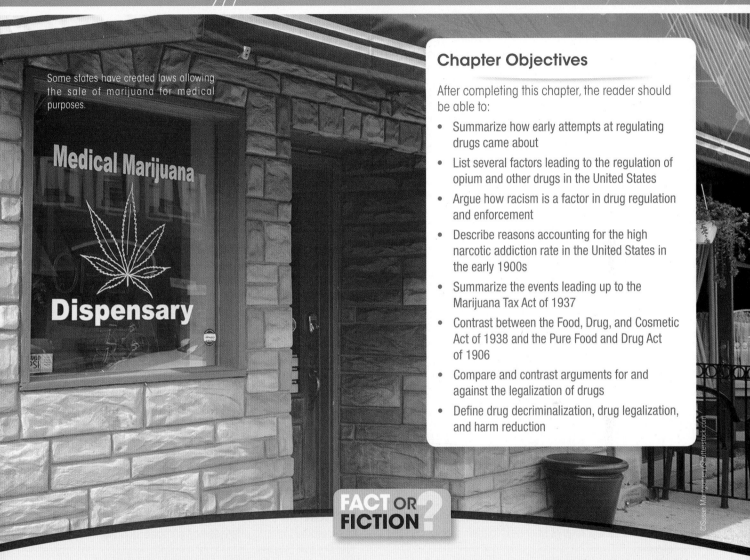

3

Drugs and the Law

Some states have created laws allowing the sale of marijuana for medical purposes.

Chapter Objectives

After completing this chapter, the reader should be able to:

- Summarize how early attempts at regulating drugs came about
- List several factors leading to the regulation of opium and other drugs in the United States
- Argue how racism is a factor in drug regulation and enforcement
- Describe reasons accounting for the high narcotic addiction rate in the United States in the early 1900s
- Summarize the events leading up to the Marijuana Tax Act of 1937
- Contrast between the Food, Drug, and Cosmetic Act of 1938 and the Pure Food and Drug Act of 1906
- Compare and contrast arguments for and against the legalization of drugs
- Define drug decriminalization, drug legalization, and harm reduction

©Susan Montgomery/Shutterstock.com

FACT OR FICTION?

1. When Harvard University was started, students were prohibited from drinking alcohol.
2. At one time, any drug, including cocaine or heroin, could be bought in the United States without a doctor's prescription.
3. The Marijuana Tax Act of 1937 stated that individuals could use marijuana if they paid a federal tax.
4. The federal government has mandated that each state establish clinics to distribute free syringes to drug addicts as a means to prevent the spread of AIDS.
5. The US government spends more money on preventing drug use than on treating people who are drug dependent.

6. In the last 5 years, the number of people incarcerated for drug offenses has decreased.
7. Students are more likely to commit drug law violations on school days than on nonschool days.
8. More people in the United States are arrested for offenses related to marijuana than to cocaine.
9. Marijuana use is lower in countries where marijuana is decriminalized, compared with the United States.
10. The penalties for powder cocaine are more severe than those for crack cocaine.

Turn the page to check your answers

Attempts to regulate and prohibit substances have been around for at least two millennia. One of the first attempts of prohibition, according to Bible script, was when Adam and Eve were told they could eat anything in the garden of Eden except the apple from the tree of knowledge. This early example of prohibition shows us the difficult nature of prohibition even when the directive comes from a higher being!

From the beginning of the New World, attempts have been made to regulate the use of mind-altering substances. The first substance subject to regulation was alcohol. Although moderate alcohol consumption was believed to be beneficial to the mind and body, excessive drinking was discouraged. In Massachusetts in 1645, taverns were fined for selling more than half a pint of wine to a person at one time.[1] Drunkenness resulted in fines for first-time offenders, whereas hard labor and whippings were punishments for chronic offenders.

This chapter will highlight the history of drug regulation and the impact these policies and laws have on society.

Early Drug Regulations

To generate much-needed income, Congress passed an excise tax on whiskey in 1791. Farmers in southwestern Pennsylvania violently objected to the excise tax because they considered whiskey an economic necessity. To squelch this insurrection, President George Washington sent in the militia from several states. This historical event, known as the Whiskey Rebellion, was important not only because the tax produced income for the federal government, but also because the government demonstrated that it had the power to enforce federal laws within a state.[2]

Another drug that fell under government control was opium. The United States signed its first treaty to regulate the international opium trade in 1833. In 1842, the federal government imposed a tax on crude opium shipped to the United States. Taxing imported opium had very little impact on its use.

Fears regarding opium use increased with the importation of Chinese workers to work on the railroad.[3] Large numbers of Chinese workers were migrating to cities and accepting jobs at low wages, which contributed to Chinese hostility. With the influx of the Chinese came the practice of opium dens. In these dens, men and women smoked opium next to the Chinese. It was reported that young men and women were being morally corrupted by visiting opium houses, or dens, although many brothels, where one easily found drugs, already existed.[4] In 1875, San Francisco passed an ordinance prohibiting opium smoking in opium dens. The legislation could have been motivated by racism because there was much anti-Chinese sentiment at the time.[5] Before it was a state, Hawaii passed legislation to curb opium addiction among Chinese immigrants.[6] In 1890, the federal government allowed only US citizens to manufacture opium or import it. Opium poppies were legally grown in the United States until 1942.

This is a common theme in the United States. When immigration occurs at rapid rates, the current

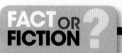

1. **FICTION** The fact is—Many of the original students at Harvard stored kegs of beer next to their supply of wine.

2. **FACT** In the late 1800s and early 1900s, there were no federal laws prohibiting the purchase of cocaine or heroin.

3. **FACT** If people paid a tax to the U.S. Treasury Department, they could use marijuana. The government refused to accept the tax payment.

4. **FICTION** The fact is—The federal government provides no funding for the distribution of free syringes to prevent the spread of AIDS.

5. **FICTION** The fact is—The US government spends five times as much money on drug treatment than it does on drug prevention.

6. **FICTION** The fact is—The number of people incarcerated for drug offenses has climbed steadily over the last 5 years.

7. **FACT** Due to several possible reasons, including access to other students, drug law violations are more likely to occur when school is in session rather than when it is not.

8. **FACT** In recent years, marijuana has been implicated more frequently in arrests than cocaine. The opposite was true in the 1990s.

9. **FACT** Decriminalization of marijuana has not increased its usage in countries that have adopted this policy.

10. **FICTION** The fact is—Current penalties for crack cocaine offenses are 100 times greater than those for powder cocaine offenses, although recent legislation has reduced the differences.

residents become fearful. To control fear, laws are created as a way to control or reduce the impact of immigration. Many early drug laws were attempts at creating laws control minority populations.

Significant Laws

Drug-related laws have had a great impact on society. Yet, the question remains: Do laws against drugs thwart drug-related problems or do they contribute to drug problems?

Pure Food and Drug Act of 1906

During the 1800s, **proprietary drugs** were sold for every possible problem ranging from colds to asthma to alcoholism to sexually transmitted diseases. These drugs were unregulated and contained heroin and cocaine, and were promoted as cures for morphine and alcohol addiction. Moreover, they were reportedly nonaddicting.[7]

Before 1906, patent medicines were largely unregulated. The era between 1890 and 1906 was described as the "golden age of patent medicines." The United States was a free marketplace. Unlike authorities in European countries, the US government had little control over physicians or pharmacists.

Concerns over patent medicines grew in the early 1900s. To regulate improperly labeled and contaminated foods, beverages, and drugs, President Theodore Roosevelt recommended legislation to prohibit the interstate commerce of adulterated and misbranded foods and drugs. Despite opposition from the patent medicine industry, the Pure Food and Drug Act of 1906 passed.

The US Food and Drug Administration (FDA) was created to assess drug hazards and prohibit the sale of dangerous drugs.[8] The law required drug manufacturers to report adverse reactions to their products.

Shortly after Roosevelt's proposal, the putrid conditions of the meatpacking industry were

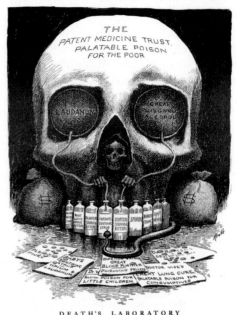

Magazine articles, such as this one in Collier's (June 3, 1905), were influential in the passage of the Pure Food and Drug Act of 1906.

recounted in the book *The Jungle* by Upton Sinclair. Sinclair's account provided further evidence for the need to regulate business.

Another concern was that morphine and other narcotics were being overused in patent medicines. Families were encouraged to avoid patent medicines containing opiates and other drugs. Magazines such as *Collier's* and *Ladies Home Journal* had articles warning of the dangers of patent medicines, especially those containing morphine and cocaine.[9]

The 1906 law allowed the government to enter the drug marketplace. The intent of the law was to regulate what was stated on the drug label. Drug producers were required to indicate whether opiates, cocaine, alcohol, or other psychoactive substances were in their products.[10] The law did not eliminate drugs such as cocaine, alcohol, heroin, and morphine from being included in products, but the amount or proportion of drugs in the medicine had to be listed on the label.[11] The law did not address how drugs

proprietary drugs Drugs that can be purchased without a prescription; over-the-counter drugs

were advertised. Nevertheless, the amount of morphine and cocaine in medicinal preparations was reduced.

Harrison Act of 1914

At the beginning of the 20th century, opiate dependency was believed to have reached its highest rate ever in the United States. With a population of 76 million, the United States had an estimated 250,000 narcotics addicts.[12] Contributing to this high rate of dependency were development of the hypodermic needle, the availability of narcotics via mail-order catalogs and over-the-counter medicines, and narcotic use by soldiers during the Civil War.[13] In 1912, the United States organized an international conference in The Hague, Netherlands to control the opium trade. Several countries agreed to restrict international trade and domestic sale of narcotics.

The need to limit opiate use in the United States resulted in the passage of the Harrison Act. Before that, 29 states had passed laws to control opiate use, and 46 states had enacted laws regulating cocaine. The Harrison Act, written by Dr. Hamilton Wright, allowed a doctor to prescribe narcotics "in the course of his professional practice and for legitimate medical purposes." Doctors were required to register each year and pay a modest fee.[14] Doctors and pharmacists had to keep records of the prescriptions they wrote. Although cocaine is a stimulant, it was classified as a narcotic, and its nonmedical use became illegal. Thus, cocaine became a demonized drug, and its illegality became inevitable.[15]

The law's purported purpose was to govern the marketing and sale of narcotics. It regulated nonmedical narcotic use and made possession of narcotics without a prescription illegal. One medical use was to prevent the withdrawal symptoms that addicts would otherwise have. Eventually, prescribing or taking narcotics to maintain addiction became illegal because it was not seen as a legitimate medical purpose. Addiction was not seen as a disease, but rather as a moral weakness. As a result, many doctors were arrested because they were seen as prescribing drugs to an addict. The adverse publicity ruined the careers of many doctors, even those who were not convicted.

The effects of the Harrison Act were counterproductive. Because people did not have legal access to narcotics, many became delirious from sudden withdrawal. Hospitals treated large numbers of people with drug problems. To obtain drugs, an increasing number of people resorted to criminal activity.[16] A medical problem became a legal problem. Those who were dependent on narcotics had no legitimate or safe place to obtain them. Moreover, medical personnel could not risk helping addicts, under the threat of prosecution.

A 1918 report to Congress noted that opium and other narcotics were still used extensively; that "dope peddlers" had formed a national organization, enabling drugs to be smuggled across US borders; and that the wrongful use of narcotics had increased.[17] To thwart these problems, stiffer law enforcement was recommended. In 1924, heroin was totally prohibited, even for medical purposes. Ironically, after heroin was banned, its black-market use increased greatly.[18]

Marijuana Tax Act of 1937

When the federal government passed the Marijuana Tax Act in 1937, 46 of the 48 states and the District of Columbia already had laws against marijuana. Some believe that passage of the federal law had racist overtones; just as the Harrison Act was motivated by anti-Chinese sentiment, the Marijuana Tax Act might have been linked to anti-Mexican feelings.[19] Many, specifically in the Southwest and West, were fearful of the use distribution of marijuana by the "Mexicans." This law forbade recreational use but not medicinal or industrial uses. An example of industrial use is that the government allowed marijuana seeds to be used in bird food.

Anyone using marijuana was required to pay a tax, and failure to comply meant a large fine or prison term for tax evasion. In essence, using marijuana was not illegal if one paid the tax to use it. Doctors were required to keep detailed records revealing the name of the patient who was provided the prescription for marijuana, nature of the ailment, dates, and the amount prescribed (along with other detailed information). Failure to keep these records had significant consequences for both the doctor and patient who were subject to imprisonment and heavy fines. As a result, many doctors stayed away from prescribing marijuana. To make matters more complicated, the federal government refused to accept the tax on marijuana; thus, by default its use is illegal. Additionally, big liquor producers pushed for the illegalization of marijuana following the end of alcohol prohibition.[20]

The person responsible for state and federal anti-marijuana laws was Henry J. Anslinger, commissioner of the Federal Bureau of Narcotics. Established in 1932, it later became the Drug Enforcement Administration (DEA).[21] Anslinger viewed drug addicts as immoral, vicious people who deserved swift, harsh punishment. State laws against marijuana were comparable to laws applied to heroin, morphine, and cocaine. Until 1971, the federal government labeled marijuana a narcotic.

Media reports sensationalized the hazards of marijuana use, particularly violent behavior, including rape. *Scientific American* described marijuana users as sexually excitable and often vicious. The movie *Reefer Madness* depicted decent, clean-cut young men and women falling into a life of depravity and crime once

ALAMOSA, COLORADO, SEPTEMBER 4, 1936
UNITED STATES TREASURY DEPARTMENT

Bureau of Narcotics

Gentlemen: Two weeks ago a sex-mad degenerate, named Lee Fernandez, brutally attacked a young Alamosa girl. He was convicted of assault with intent to rape and sentenced to 10 to 14 years in the state penitentiary. Police officers here know definitely that Fernandez was under the influence of marihuana.

But this case is one in hundreds of murders, rapes, petty crimes, insanity that has occurred in southern Colorado in recent years.

The laws of this state make the first offense of using, growing, or selling marihuana a mere misdemeanor. The second offense constitutes a felony.

Indian hemp grows wild within the limits of this city. It is clandestinely planted in practically every county in this section. Its use amounts to a near traffic in drugs.

The people and officials here want to know why something can't be done about marihuana. The sheriff, district attorney, and city police are making every effort to destroy this menace. Our paper is carrying on an educational campaign to describe the weed and tell of its horrible effects.

Your bulletins on traffic in opium and other dangerous drugs state that the production and use of Indian hemp are not prohibited by Federal law. Why?

Is there any assistance your Bureau can give us in handling this drug? Can you suggest campaigns? Can you enlarge your Department to deal with marihuana? Can you do anything to help us? I wish I could show you what a small marihuana cigaret can do to one of our degenerate Spanish-speaking residents. That's why our problem is so great; the greatest percentage of our population is composed of Spanish-speaking persons, most of who are low mentally, because of social and racial conditions.

While marihuana has figured in the greater number of crimes in the past few years, officials fear it, not for what it has done, but for what it is capable of doing. They want to check it before an outbreak does occur. Did you read of the Drain murder case in Pueblo recently? Marihuana is believed to have been used by one of the bloody murderers.

Through representatives of civic leaders and law officers of the San Luis Valley, I have been asked to write to you for help. Any help you can give us will be most heartily appreciated.

Very sincerely yours,
Floyd K. Baskette
City Editor, The Alamosa Daily Courier

Questions to Ponder

1. How does this editorial speak the racial undertones of the times?

2. What facts does this article bring forward? What about opinions?

3. How does this article use fear to encourage action?

Source: Schaffer Library of Drug Policy, "The Marijuana Tax Act of 1937: Transcripts of Congressional Hearings." Source: http://www.druglibrary.org/schaffer/hemp/taxact/t10a.htm.

---

they started using marijuana. A popular poster in the 1930s titled "The Assassination of Youth" illustrated the devastating effects of marijuana.[22]

In testimony before Congress, Anslinger described how one young man, Victor Licata, became deranged after smoking one marijuana cigarette and hacked his family with an axe. Anslinger detailed how marijuana leads to addiction, violent crime, psychosis, and mental deterioration.[23] Not surprisingly, the Marijuana Tax Act passed through Congress with little debate.

During the congressional hearings about marijuana, no medical testimony describing its adverse effects was presented. However, the *Journal of the American Medical Association* (May 1, 1937) presented an editorial that was extremely critical of the proposed laws. The editorial stated that even though few physicians prescribed the drug, they should be able to prescribe it as they wished without incurring additional burdens of a tax, recordkeeping, and reporting. Moreover, the cost of this legislation would contribute to the rising cost of sickness. This same editorial expressed doubt that the law would have any effect on nonmedicinal use because antinarcotic legislation had little impact on narcotic and coca use.

The arguments against marijuana consisted largely of newspaper accounts. Dr. William Woodward,

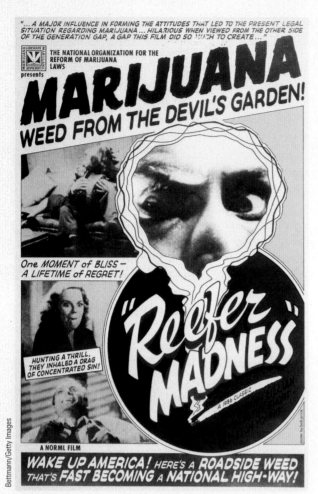

"...A MAJOR INFLUENCE IN FORMING THE ATTITUDES THAT LED TO THE PRESENT LEGAL SITUATION REGARDING MARIJUANA... HILARIOUS WHEN VIEWED FROM THE OTHER SIDE OF THE GENERATION GAP, A GAP THIS FILM DID SO MUCH TO CREATE..."

THE NATIONAL ORGANIZATION FOR THE REFORM OF MARIJUANA LAWS

presents

MARIJUANA
WEED FROM THE DEVIL'S GARDEN!

One MOMENT of BLISS — A LIFETIME of REGRET!

HUNTING A THRILL, THEY INHALED A DRAG OF CONCENTRATED SIN!

"Reefer" MADNESS

A 1936 CLASSIC

A NORML FILM

WAKE UP AMERICA! HERE'S A ROADSIDE WEED THAT'S FAST BECOMING A NATIONAL HIGH-WAY!

The 1930s movie *Reefer Madness* distorted the effects caused by marijuana.

a physician-lawyer representing the American Medical Association (AMA), highlighted this point. He testified before Congress that the many horrific stories circulating about the effects of marijuana had no verifiable proof. Furthermore, Woodward said the law would be a nuisance for the medical profession. The AMA's arguments were disregarded.

The Marijuana Tax Act did not specifically prohibit marijuana. Physicians, dentists, and others could prescribe it by paying $1 per year for a license fee. Druggists were required to pay a license fee of $15 annually, marijuana growers paid $25 annually, and marijuana importers and manufacturers were assessed a $50 annual fee. Nonmedical use, possession, and sale of untaxed marijuana were illegal.

In 1969, the Timothy Leary, a professor and activist, was arrested in Texas for marijuana possession. Marijuana was illegal in the state of Texas. He argued that if he purchased the Marijuana Tax Stamp, he would be self-incriminating himself by admitting to the possession of marijuana. This case went to the Supreme Court who agreed and the Marijuana Tax Act was repealed in 1970.[24]

Food, Drug, and Cosmetic Act of 1938

Before World War II, all drugs except narcotics could be bought over the counter. Efforts to regulate non-narcotic drugs were ineffective until a new antibiotic called **elixir sulfanilamide** reached the market. This product, made by dissolving a liquid form of a sulfa drug in the chemical solvent **diethyl glycol**, was extremely toxic. More than 100 people died from kidney poisoning. Under guidelines of the Pure Food and Drug Act of 1906, a drug manufacturer could not be prosecuted for these fatalities. When the need for some type of regulation became apparent, the 1938 federal Food, Drug, and Cosmetic Act was passed.[25]

The 1938 law differed from the 1906 law in that

- pharmaceutical companies were required to file applications with the federal government demonstrating that all *new* drugs were safe and properly labeled; and
- drug manufacturers had to submit a "new drug application" to the FDA, giving the FDA more authority and responsibility.

Besides listing all ingredients and their respective quantities on the label, instructions concerning proper use of the drug and warnings of the drug's dangers had to be included and written so that the average consumer could understand them.

Limitations of the 1938 Food, Drug, and Cosmetic Act included the following:

- It did not cover drugs that were previously marketed.
- Drugs had to be proven *safe,* but not proven *effective.*
- The federal government had little authority to enact penalties if the information on the labels was not written clearly.
- Drug manufacturers were given the responsibility for determining whether a drug would be sold as a prescription or an over-the-counter drug.
- Drug manufacturers conducted their own tests to determine a drug's effectiveness.

Passage of the 1938 law resulted in the creation of a class of drugs that could be bought only with a prescription. Whether a drug was accorded prescription or nonprescription status was determined by the manufacturer. Thus a drug labeled as a prescription drug by one company could be marketed as an over-the-counter drug by another.

This quizzical situation existed until 1951, when the Humphrey–Durham Amendment was passed. However, neither the 1938 Food, Drug, and Cosmetic Act nor the Humphrey–Durham Amendment allowed for the federal government to oversee the

Bettmann/Getty Images

clinical testing of drugs. The effectiveness of drugs was still determined by the drug manufacturers. In addition, it has only been since 2002 that the FDA required pediatric testing.[26] Previously, drug testing was only done with adults.

Kefauver–Harris Amendments

Efforts to get the federal government more involved in supervising drug testing were stymied until a sedative, used primarily in Europe, came to the United States. This drug, **thalidomide**, was first introduced in Germany in 1958 as an antionvulsive agent and later was used for treating hypertension, migraines, and morning sickness caused by pregnancy. Unfortunately, it altered the development of an embryo's arms and legs, resulting in deformed babies in Europe.[27] This resulted in the implementation of stronger regulations regarding drug testing. The Kefauver–Harris Amendments were passed in 1962, boosting the government's ability to regulate new and existing drugs.

It should be noted here that even though the effects of thalidomide on the fetus are acknowledged, research into its benefits in other areas has continued. The drug could be helpful in treating a myriad of conditions ranging from eye disease (macular degeneration) to rheumatoid arthritis, AIDS, ulcers of the mouth, diabetes, and cancers of the breast, brain, and prostate.[28] In 1998, the FDA approved thalidomide for treating Hansen's disease (formerly known as leprosy). One potential problem, however, is that once a drug is approved for any purpose, physicians can prescribe it for any other purpose. Thus a concern is that the incidence of thalidomide-exposed babies will increase.

The Kefauver–Harris Amendments gave the FDA the authority to withdraw drugs from the marketplace. Also, drug advertisements directed at physicians were required to include the drug's side effects and its contraindicated uses. Although manufacturers still were responsible for drug testing, their testing procedures required prior approval from the FDA.

Extensive drug testing delays the introduction of beneficial drugs. Despite this, most people favor stringent drug testing laws. At the same time, many politicians are putting pressure on the FDA to approve drugs more quickly.

Comprehensive Drug Abuse Prevention and Control Act of 1970

The Comprehensive Drug Abuse Prevention and Control Act, known as the Controlled Substances Act, had the effect of repealing, replacing, or updating all previous federal laws dealing with narcotics and dangerous drugs. Individual states still could impose their own regulations. The law, however, clearly stated that federal enforcement and prosecution take precedence if any illegal activity is involved. The original intent of this law, when presented before Congress, focused on rehabilitation, research, and education. The act expanded community health centers and Public Health Service hospitals for drug abusers. At its final passage, though, the bill emphasized enforcement because of the law-and-order sentiment that prevailed in Congress.

Several important components of this law are worth noting. A commission on marijuana and drug abuse was established to make recommendations subsequent to a 2-year study. Federal mandatory sentences for first-offense possession of an illegal drug were abolished, the possibility of parole was reimplemented, and public records of the conviction were erased. In essence the record was restored to prearrest status, and the violator was legally allowed to deny ever having been arrested on such a charge. Depending on the state, a violator still could receive a 1-year prison sentence or a $5,000 fine, or both, if convicted on a first-offense charge of possession of a controlled substance. Or the offender could receive a 1-year probation instead. The emphasis of the law was to punish the drug dealer, particularly organized dealers, rather than the drug user. A 2004 court decision questioned the application of the Controlled Substances Act to the possession of marijuana for medical purposes.[29] Despite the law's effort to reduce drug use, the United States has the highest rate of illegal drug use compared to 17 countries studied by the World Health Organization.[30]

The Controlled Substances Act of 1970 divided drugs into five categories called schedules (see Table 3.1). Penalties for distributing, manufacturing, and possessing psychoactive drugs depend on which of the five schedules includes the drug.[31] The Justice Department enforces the law, and the US Department of Health and Human Services (DHHS) evaluates drugs to decide the appropriate schedule. The criteria for determining a drug's schedule are as follows:

- The drug's potential for abuse
- Scientific knowledge of the drug
- The drug's capacity to produce psychic or physiological dependence

elixir sulfanilamide An antibiotic that killed more than 100 people in the 1930s

diethyl glycol A chemical solvent

thalidomide A sedative that was found in the 1960s, which caused birth defects including missing or malformed limbs

TABLE 3.1 Drug Schedules

	I	II	III	IV	V
Potential for abuse	High	High	Some, but not as much as drugs on Schedules I and II	Low, less than Schedule III drugs	Low, less than Schedule IV drugs
Medical use	None (marijuana is being used for medical purposes, but it is not authorized by the DEA as having medical application)	Yes	Yes	Yes	Yes
Maximum penalties for illegal manufacturing and distribution	*First offense (narcotics):* 15 years in prison, $25,000 fine, 3 years' probation *Subsequent offenses:* 30 years in prison, $50,000 fine, 6 years' probation *First offense (non-narcotics):* 5 years in prison, $15,000 fine, 2 years' probation *Second offense:* 10 years in prison, $30,000 fine, 4 years' probation	Same as Schedule I	*First offense:* 5 years in prison, $15,000 fine, 2 years' probation *Second offense:* 10 years in prison, $30,000 fine, 4 years' probation	*First offense:* 3 years in prison, $10,000 fine, 1 year probation *Second offense:* $20,000 fine, 6 years in prison, 2 years' probation	*First offense:* 1 year in prison, $50,000 fine, *and* no probation period
Maximum penalties for illegal possession	*First offense:* 1 year in prison and $5,000 fine *Second offense:* 2 years in prison and $10,000 fine; probation may be granted for first offense	Same as Schedule I	Same as Schedule I	Same as Schedule I	Same as Schedule I
Production controlled	Yes		Yes	No	No
Examples	Heroin, LSD, mescaline, marijuana, methaqualone, peyote	Cocaine, methamphetamine, opium, morphine, methadone, codeine	Phencyclidine (PCP), stimulants (those not containing amphetamines), some narcotic preparations, some barbiturates	Diazepam (Valium), phenobarbital, barbital, meprobamate (Equanil, Miltown), some nonamphetamine stimulants not already included	Preparations with small amounts of narcotics, diluted opium and codeine compounds

- The drug's pharmacological effects
- The drug's risk to public health
- The drug's history, duration, scope, and current patterns of abuse
- Whether the drug is an immediate precursor of a substance already controlled under this title

Anti-Drug Abuse Act

The Anti-Drug Abuse Act was signed into law by President Ronald Reagan in 1988. Unlike the Controlled Substances Act, this legislation was directed at the drug user, not just the drug manufacturers or distributors. The point of this law was to reduce drug demand. While previous legislation was directed to curtailing

Category I drugs Drugs determined to be safe, effective, and properly labeled

Category II drugs Drugs generally recognized as unsafe and ineffective or as mislabeled; must be removed from medications within 6 months after the FDA issues its final regulations

Category III drugs Drugs for which data are insufficient to determine general recognition of safety and effectiveness

drug paraphernalia Items that are aids to using drugs

Schedule IV: substances have a low potential for abuse relative to schedule III.

Schedule V: substances have a low potential for abuse relative to schedule IV.

the *supply* of drugs, this law emphasizes stringent punishment of the user. Punishment could be waived if the user completes a drug rehabilitation program or makes an earnest effort to get into a rehabilitation program.

The law greatly increased the federal prison population and led to a new Cabinet position, Director of National Drug Control Policy, commonly known as the "drug czar." The law stipulated that the penalties for possessing crack cocaine were precisely 100 times greater than for powder cocaine. However, in 2010, Congress and President Obama reduced the penalties for crack cocaine arrestees.[32]

The Anti-Drug Abuse Act stipulates that anyone who commits murder or orders someone's murder in conjunction with a drug-related felony can receive the death penalty. Other elements of this law include registration of the following:

- Chemicals used in the manufacture of drugs
- Sales of firearms to felons
- Airplanes

Under this law, drug users are punished more stringently than rapists or robbers.[33] Also, the government can take anything in one's possession at the time of arrest. The effect has been that "in more than 80% of asset forfeiture cases, the owner is never charged with a crime, yet government officials can and usually do keep the seized property."[34] The penalties for drug possession are the following:

- Loss of all federal benefits, such as student loans and grants, for 1 year for a first offense and 2 years after a second offense
- Forfeiture of the car, boat, or airplane in which the drug is found (this may have implications if you lend your car, boat, or plane to someone caught with drugs)
- A civil fine of up to $10,000
- Removal of the individual and his or her family from public housing if that person engages in drug-related activity in or near public housing

---

ON CAMPUS

If a college student who is receiving federal aid is convicted of a drug felony or misdemeanor, federal aid will be withheld for a period for up to 2 years.[1] See Table 3.2. A few studies have shown that this ban does not deter young people from committing drug offenses.

Students affected by this ban are more likely to come from urban lower financial wealth areas. The impact of this ban delays students' likelihood of going to college and increases lower workplace participation, high pregnancy rates, and subsequent convictions rates among these young adults during their ineligibility period.[2] Eligibility for federal aid can strongly impact a college investment decision as the cost of college continues to rise.

Attending college is seen as way to improve one's lifestyle by providing opportunities to improve intergenerational income motility. It is considered one factor that can positively influence a family's wealth potential. This is especially important for low-income, urban youth.

Questions to Ponder

- How does the ban placed on federal aid impact a person's decision to attend college?
- What would you suggest to reduce drug offenses among college bound students?
- How does the current policy place low-income youth at greater risk?

Sources:

1. Office of National Drug Control Policy. US Department of Education. FAFSA Facts (Free Application for Federal Student Aid). Source: https://www.whitehouse.gov/sites/default/files/ondcp/recovery/fafsa.pdf.
2. M.F. Lovenheim, and E.G. Owens, "Does federal financial aid affect college enrollment? Evidence from drug offenders and the Higher Education Act of 1998," *Journal of Urban Economics,* 81 (2014): 1–13.

TABLE 3.2 Drug Offense and Eligibility for Federal Student Financial Aid

Offense	Possession of Illegal Drugs	Sale of Illegal Drugs
First	1 year of ineligibility from date of conviction	2 years of ineligibility from date of conviction
Second	2 years of ineligibility from date of conviction	Indefinite period of ineligibility*
Third	Indefinite period of ineligibility*	Indefinite period of ineligibility *

*Under the law, an indefinite period of ineligibility continues unless your conviction is overturned or otherwise rendered invalid or you meet one of the two early reinstatement requirements specified above.

Source: Office of National Drug Control Policy. US Department of Education. FAFSA Facts (Free Application for Federal Student Aid). Available at: https://www.whitehouse.gov/sites/default/files/ondcp/recovery/fafsa.pdf.

College Students and Drug Convictions

The Anti-Drug Abuse Act has implications for college students. At the present time college students who complete the federal financial aid form, also known as FAFSA, are asked if they have ever had a drug conviction. Students who were convicted of simple possession face a 1-year ban on financial aid. A second conviction of possession results in a 2-year ban on aid, and a third conviction means that one loses eligibility for financial aid indefinitely. A drug-selling conviction means loss of eligibility for 2 years if that is one's first offense. An estimated 200,000 students have lost access to aid since this law went into effect. Some politicians are debating whether this law should continue because they feel it is discriminatory. Children of wealthy parents who are convicted of a drug charge do not need financial assistance to attend college.[35]

Legal Issues

Laws aimed at drug users may been seen as discriminatory laws against people who have a brain disease. Similarly, do these laws actually decrease the need and demand for drugs?

Should people using small amounts of illegal drugs for personal enjoyment receive harsh criminal penalties? What are the advantages and disadvantages of decriminalizing or legalizing drugs? What impact has drug enforcement had on drug use? Should the vast amount of money spent on stopping drugs be used differently?

In trying to answer these questions, political forces take very different stances.[36] Cultural conservatives advocate more emphasis on enforcing drug laws but removing legal loopholes, technicalities, and restrictions. Free-market libertarians think that government is too intrusive, that people have the right to hurt themselves, and that individuals are ultimately responsible for their own behavior. Radical constructionists believe that drug abuse is symptomatic of greater problems in society and that we need to address the underlying social problems if drug abuse is to be curtailed.

Drug Paraphernalia

One way to reduce drug use, logically, would be to make **drug paraphernalia** illegal. Cigarette-rolling papers, water pipes, razors, clay pipes, roach clips, spoons, mirrors, and other products in "head shops," novelty stores, and convenience stores have been used for illegal drugs. Prosecuting individuals for possessing drug paraphernalia is viewed as a deterrent for drug use.[37] Three decades ago, the federal government proposed the Model Drug Paraphernalia Act of 1979. Specifically, the bill attempted to halt the following items:

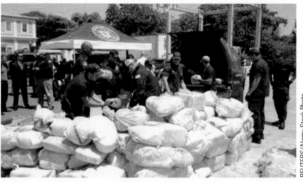

Coastguardsmen alongside Federal Bureau of Investigation, the Drug Enforcement Administration, U.S. Customs and Border Protection and Immigrations and Customs Enforcement law enforcement personnel load 3,591 pounds of marijuana for transportation to a secure facility following an interagency press conference at Sector San Juan, Puerto Rico July 21, 2014. The Coast Guard and federal law enforcement partner agencies announced the interdiction of the motor vessel An Nur, where the motor vessel and the illegal drug shipment, estimated to have a wholesale value of $3.5 million dollars were seized, while the 5-man Guyanese crew was detained for prosecution. (U.S. Coast Guard photo by Ricardo Castrodad, Sector San Juan Public Affairs specialist.)

In February 2003, the federal government conducted Operation Pipe Dream. This federally funded plan, which cost approximately $12 million to fund, concluded with the arrest of 55 people, one of which served a 9-month federal prison sentence, a fine of $20,000, forfeiture of $103,000, and 1 year of probation. Tommy Chong, who is well known for his marijuana-themed movie "*Cheech & Chong*" was arrested and agreed to a plea bargain to prevent his wife and son from being prosecuted.[1]

In 2005, Minnesota Viking Ontario Smith was caught at the airport with the Wizzinator (a penis-shaped device meant to be used to beat a urine test) and dried urine. The President and Vice President of the company, Puck Technology, which produced and sold the Wizzinator, were indicted on charges in 2008 for selling drug paraphernalia. The president was sentenced to 6 months in jail and the vice president was sentenced to 3 years' probation.[2]

Sources:

1. Operation Pipe Dream: 10 Years Later. *The Huffington Post*, February 26, 2014. Available at: http://www.huffingtonpost.com/the-/operation-pipe-dream-10-y_b_2745740.html.

2. J. Sullum, "Bongs Away!," *Reason*, 40, no. 9 (2009).

all equipment, products, and materials of any kind which are used, intended for use, or designed for use, in planting, propagating, cultivating, growing, harvesting, manufacturing, compounding, converting, producing, processing, preparing, testing, analyzing, packaging, repackaging, storing, containing, concealing, injecting, ingesting, inhaling, or otherwise introducing into the human body a controlled substance.[38]

A flaw in this bill was that many household products could be construed as drug paraphernalia. The straws children use to drink milk can be used to snort cocaine, a small change purse could be used to conceal drugs, and some people use cigarette-rolling papers to roll marijuana. Because this bill raised many constitutional questions, it was never adopted. While this law did not come to fruition, there remains the *Federal Drug Paraphernalia Statute, 21 USC 863*, which falls under part of the Controlled Substances Act. Under this act, it is unlawful for people to:[39]

- Sell or offer for sale drug paraphernalia
- Use mail or other interstate commerce to transport drug paraphernalia
- Import or export drug paraphernalia

In the last 10 years, the federal government has cracked down on the sale of drug paraphernalia.

The War on Drugs

The "war on drugs" was coined in the 1970s by President Nixon who believed the way to reduce drug use and abuse in the United States is by reducing the supply. He implemented "Operation Intercept" where he placed over 2,000 border agents at the US/Mexican border. A few years later, Reagan came into office and placed much focus on the "war on drugs" by viewing drugs as a threat to national policy.[40] He created the South Florida Task Force to target cocaine and marijuana smuggling into South Florida from the Caribbean. These efforts did reduce the flow of these drugs into South Florida, but some believe drug traffickers just redirected their routes from South Florida to the Southwest.

In current times, "the presence of law enforcement on the US Mexico border is at historic levels," with increased use of surveillance technology and fencing being used to make it more difficult for smugglers to get into the United States.[41] The United States has put into use drones to monitor drug trafficking activity. However, despite these increased efforts, a report from the Office of the Inspector General found the use of drones were not a cost effective program not able to effectively assess the program's costs and effectiveness.[42]

In 1988, the US Congress proclaimed that the country would be drug free by 1995. This proclamation did not become a reality. Instead, political rhetoric has exacerbated the problem of drugs in the United States. Politicians rely on inflammatory speeches rather than on reasoned responses.[43]

Despite vast amounts of money allotted for drug interdiction, the quantity of drugs interdicted while being smuggled into the United States is minimal. For the fiscal year 2017, President Obama requested $582.7 millions to the Department of Defense, $40.6 billion to the Department of Homeland Security, $29 billion to the Justice Department, and $31.1 billion to the Office of National Drug Control Policy.[44,45,46,47] The monetary expense and human resources employed to combat illicit drug use are enormous. Yet, the war on drugs is being lost. In 1965, according to the DEA, fewer than 4 million Americans had ever used illegal drugs. Today, the number of Americans who have used illegal drugs has exceeded 110 million.

In addition, the number of people who have used cocaine increased 700% in the last 35 years.[48]

Is the war on drugs effective? Some believe this war is really a veiled attempt at social control of urban minority populations. In 2000, according to the Sentencing Project data, African Americans and Latinos represented three-fourths of all drug offenders in state prisons, even though Whites make up a large majority of illegal drug users and dealers.[49] In a book by Michelle Alexander called *The New Jim Crow: Mass Incarceration in the Age of Colorblindness*, she argues the US criminal justice system uses the War on Drugs as a way to promote discrimination and repression among underrepresented populations. She proposes the impact on inner-city African Americans is disproportionate to the actual criminal activity taking place in these areas.[50]

People agree that drug abuse is undesirable. But should drug abuse be treated as a criminal problem or a public health problem? From a public health perspective, the consequences of US drug policies are infection, violence, and criminal injustice.

According to Ethan Nadelmann, a leading proponent of drug reform, government officials should stop wasting taxpayer money on ineffective criminal policies. They should stop arresting drug users and put more effort into reducing overdose deaths and reducing the number of nonviolent drug offenders behind bars.[51]

The Drug Business

Drug seizures are a good measurement to access size of drug markets, drug availability, trafficking patterns, and trends.[52] See Figure 3.1 for information on drug seizures in transit countries. Herbal cannabis production occurs in most countries worldwide and

Main transit countries as reported by recipient countries in major individual drug seizure cases (above 100 g for heroin and cocaine, above 1 kg for cannabis), by drug, 2005–2014

Cocaine (base, salt and crack)			Heroin (base, salt)			Cannabis (herb, resin, oil)		
Transit Countries	Total number of times country mentioned as transit point in individual seizures	Number of recipient countries reporting transit countries	Transit Countries	Total number of times country mentioned as transit point in individual seizures	Number of recipient countries reporting transit countries	Transit Countries	Total number of times country mentioned as transit point in individual seizures	Number of recipient countries reporting transit countries
Argentina	2,101	45	Afghanistan	21	6	Denmark	57	3
Bolivia (Plurinational State of)	530	19	India	44	11	Greece	36	8
Brazil	1,747	56	Kazakhstan	23	1	Morocco	4,308	24
Colombia	1,061	31	Kyrgyzstan	42	3	Netherlands	117	10
Costa Rica	624	34	Netherlands	30	4	Pakistan	76	24
Dominican Republic	1,313	20	Pakistan	3,216	178	Paraguay	117	7
Ecuador	410	22	Spain	29	4	Portugal	28	11
Panama	305	18	Tajikistan	128	4	Saint Vincent and the Grenadines	33	7
Peru	897	25	Turkey	45	7	Spain	846	33
Venezuela (Bolivaria Republic of)	587	27	United Arab Emirates	43	15	Swaziland	32	3

Source: UNODC, major individual drug seizure database. Data presented in the table reflect transit countries as reported by the countries where seizures were made and were not validated by the mentioned transit countries.

Note: *Information provided on the main transit countries reported in major individual drug seizure cases is based on 11,441 cases of cannabis, 11,864 cases of cocaine and 4,041 cases of heroin. This tables lists the ten countries with the highest number of mentions as transit. The figures provided refer to the total number of mentions of the country as the last departure/transit point in major individual seizure cases reported to the UNODC over the 10-year period 2005-2014, and to the number of different reporting countries responsible for those mentions. It should be noted that some major consuming countries did not report on transit and departure countries.*

Figure 3.1 Main Transit Countries:
Which countries would you consider to a problem in the transit of drugs? Why?
Using data from this table, how would you reduce the transit of illicit drugs?

Source: United Nations Office on Drugs and Crime, World Drug Report 2015 (United Nations publication, Sales No. E.15.XI.6).

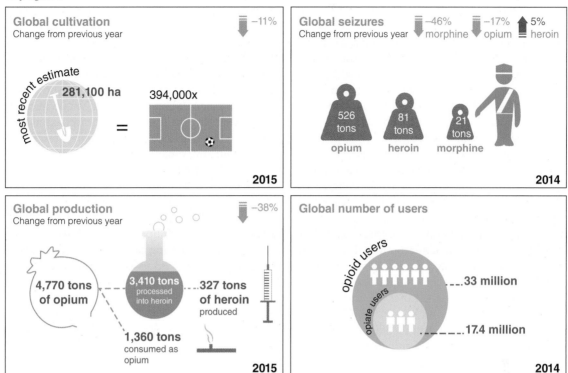

Global cultivation
Change from previous year — −11%

most recent estimate
281,100 ha   **394,000x**   =

2015

Global seizures
Change from previous year — −46% morphine   −17% opium   ▲5% heroin

526 tons opium   81 tons heroin   21 tons morphine

2014

Global production
Change from previous year — −38%

4,770 tons of opium   **3,410 tons** processed into heroin   **327 tons of heroin** produced

1,360 tons consumed as opium

2015

Global number of users

opioid users   opiate users   33 million   17.4 million

2014

Note: Opioids include the non-medical use of prescription opioids and opiates (opiates include opium and heroin).

Figure 3.2 Key Figures in Opium Production

is the most seized drug, considered the largest drug market globally.[53] Other than amphetamine type substances, such as heroin/illicit morphine, quantities of drugs seized in the past decade have remained stable. Figure 3.2 presents trends in opium production. A peak in heroin/illicit morphine seizures was reported in 2011, but has since stabilized. Heroin/illicit morphine and amphetamine-like substances make up the smallest size of drug seizures (on average less than 1kg per seizure). The largest seizures involve cannabis, which average 10 kg confiscated per case. The Americas are where seizures cases are the greatest while Europe has the smallest seizure cases.[54]

South America is the main departure hub for cocaine distribution worldwide, specifically, Bolivia, Columbia, and Peru. Over the past 10 years, the Netherlands, Morocco, and Spain have been the main departure or transit countries for cannabis. In 2010, Afghanistan accounted for more than 90% of the world's illicit opium.[55] Opium and heroin have a long stable shelf-life and can be stored for a long periods of time.

Like ordinary consumers of ketchup or toothpaste, millions of Americans smoke marijuana, snort cocaine, or shoot up heroin without considering the long chain of manufacturers and middlemen who bring to their communities the quality products they demand. The supply lines are tortuous, threading from foreign fields, across seas, and through fissures

in the wall of domestic law enforcement. But the drugs do get through, despite the herculean efforts of the police, courts, and prisons to deter the traffic of mood-altering chemicals. The influx of drugs not only results in thousands of people needing medical care for drug overdoses, but also produces an economic impact on the criminal justice system and the environment.[56]

The demand for drugs in the United States is giving rise to major transnational criminal organizations.[57] Mexican-based criminal organizations are the main supply for illicit drugs in the United States. In 2011, seven main Mexican organizations (Sinaloa Cartel,

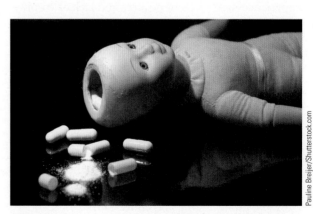

Pauline Breijer/Shutterstock.com

■ Drug carriers use creative methods to carry drugs across the border.

Los Zetas, Gulf Cartel, Juarez Cartel, BLO, LFM, and Tijuana Cartel) are in constant competition with one another to gain control of the US market resulting in extreme violence.[58] Columbia-based criminal organizations involvement in drug trafficking in the United States declined from 2006 to 2011. Heroin and cocaine are the main drugs being trafficked from these areas and usually end up in the East Coast markets. Colombia, the leading producer of cocaine, produces most of its cocaine through 10 major cartels. However, because of a joint operation in which most cartel leaders were extradited and imprisoned, the face of the Columbian cocaine trade has become decentralized: The country's drug trade is now run by numerous small cartels and remnants from the larger cartels.[59]

Within the United States, criminal gangs are responsible for most of the retail distribution of drugs.[60] Gangs in the United States collaborate with Mexican criminal organizations to facilitate drug trafficking networks. It is estimated that the cost of gang suppression, prevention, and correction programs cost the United States more than $5 billion dollars per year. Additionally, between 2005 and 2009 gangs were responsible for almost 4,500 homicides and almost one-fourth of all schools report gang activity.[61,62]

In May 2016, the United Nations Office on Drugs and Crime (UNODC) issued the 2015 World Drug Report, which shows more people are using drugs than ever before, despite the continued increase in money to combat the production and distribution of drugs. The UNODC estimated in 2013 that there were almost 246 million people using an illicit drug, which would amount to about 1 out of every 10 people.[63] This speaks to supply and demand. One must consider what factors contribute to the production and cultivation of drugs in certain countries. What policies are in place to help combat the production of drugs and are they making an impact?

Poverty, economic disadvantage, and unemployment are some of the factors that contribute to illicit crop cultivation and drug production.[64] In areas that experience high levels of poverty and lack of employment, a rise of illicit crop cultivation is seen.[65] A study in Myanmar to determine reasons to illicit opium poppy cultivation suggests the main reason for cultivating the drug was for income. Village headmen reported that the main use of income derived from opium cultivation was to buy food for the village. In addition, most farmers who ceased cultivating opium experienced a significant reduction in income.[65] Other factors that contribute to illicit drug cultivation are lack of security and governance.[66]

How can the government play a role in decreasing illicit drug trade? It seems the answer lies in the ability to control illicit crop cultivation and ensure alternative livelihoods so that a switch can be made from illicit crop cultivation to a legal crop without experiencing a drop in income. Without both of these factors, efforts to reduce illicit crop cultivation will not be successful.

As previously mentioned Afghanistan is a major source of illicit opium cultivation worldwide. In 2000–2001, the Taliban issued a ban on opium cultivation among its controlled territories. While illicit opium cultivation dropped, it negatively impacted the rural economy because a substitute was not provided in its place. Thus unemployment went up significantly and left farmers with no way to pay off accumulated debt. This lead to a large migration out of Afghanistan to Pakistan.[67]

In 2016, Rodrigo Duterte ran and was elected President of the Philippines. Much of his campaign focused on combating the drug problem in the Philippines, which is said to have contributed to his win. It is estimated there are 1.3 million drug users in the Philippines; the most popular drug is methamphetamine, known locally as "Shabu."[68] During his run for election, he promised to suppress crime, drugs, and corruption in government in his first 3 months of presidency. After being elected, he urged citizens to kill drug dealers by saying "Do it yourself if you have guns, you have my support."[69] He has also promised to "fatten the fish in Manila Bay with the bodies of 100,000 criminals."[70] Between July and September 2016, it is estimated that 2,500 people were killed due to the war on drugs. Surprisingly, a survey conducted by Pulse Asia revealed that 91% of Filipinos have a "high degree of trust" in their new leader.[71] It is unclear how this new war on drugs will impact the country and whether it will have an impact on reducing the amount of users in the Philippines.

Conversely, a 2005 opium ban in Nangarhar Province (Southern Afghanistan) provides an example of a government program that works. The ban on opium was accompanied by development in physical and social infrastructure, which resulted in significant economic growth between 2009 and 2011.[72] Farmers initially replaced the opium crop with wheat and onions, but soon replaced those with annual and perennial horticultural crops. As a result of these efforts, many households experienced a growth in annual income.[73]

In response to the worldwide epidemic of drug use, the Global Commission on Drug Policy recommends the end of criminalization for drug use.[74] The rationale is that countries could better regulate the use of drugs while undermining the power of organized crime. To help drug abusers, the commission advocates increasing services and treatment. In addition, it recommends educational activities to prevent the initiation or escalation of drug use.[75]

The economic clout of the drug trade is felt around the world. The increase in the narcotics trade in Eurasia

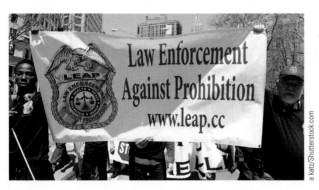

NEW YORK CITY–MAY 2 2015: The 17th annual cannabis parade made its way along Broadway to Union Square Park where activists encouraged legalization of marijuana. LEAP banner

a katz/Shutterstock.com

and elsewhere is fueled by its tremendous profitability. In parts of Asia, drug money is used for lawlessness and bribery. In northern Burma, drug barons finance private armies to protect the fields of opium poppies. Officials in South Korea maintain that Internet use has contributed greatly to international drug trafficking.[76]

A country inundated with money obtained through the sale of illegal drugs is Colombia. Even after billions of dollars were spent on curbing drug production, coca growth by farmers in Colombia rose 27%.[77] The former foreign minister described the enormity of Colombia's drug trade this way:* "The size of this business overwhelms our economy. Just imagine if the United States had a Mafia richer than the federal budget." Drugs from Colombia enter into the United States via Mexico. In the past, these drugs were transported in large fishing trawlers, but because officials have begun frequently intercepting these trawlers, drugs sent to Mexico from Columbia are now usually carried by semisubmersible watercraft.[78]

Halting the flow of drugs is difficult because cocaine sales result in extreme wealth for drug barons, banks' coffers are filled with money from the sale of drugs, and drug money reduces unemployment in Latin American countries. In an ironic twist, when counter-narcotics programs are effective, the cost of cocaine increases.[79] In essence, successful interdiction does not decrease profits.

In addition to domestic production, marijuana is grown in Asia, the Caribbean, and Mexico, although Colombia is the largest exporter. Stopping the drug trade is like sticking a finger in a dike. No sooner is one hole plugged than another hole leaks. As one author writes: "The war on illegal drugs engenders corruption, terrorism, and family breakdown, weakening America while strengthening our enemies."[80]

*L. Kraar, "The drug trade: Think of it as a huge, multinational commodity business with a fast-moving top management, a widespread distribution network, and price-insensitive customers", Fortune, June 20, 1988. http://archive.fortune.com/magazines/fortune/fortune_archive/1988/06/20/70695/index.htm

Preventing drugs from entering the United States or reducing the amount of drugs grown in the country is a matter of demand, not supply. Of the billions of dollars allocated to address drug-related problems, a minority of the money goes to demand reduction and the majority to supply reduction. Until demand decreases, drugs will always be abundantly available. Moreover, the resources of drug dealers for distributing drugs are greater than the resources aimed at interdicting drugs.

Drug Enforcement

Drug enforcement is designed to stem the flow of drugs coming into the United States and to punish users.

Table 3.3 shows the number of drug-related arrests in 2015.[81]

The US government relies on **interdiction** to reduce the flow of drugs. This refers to the "seizure of drugs and smugglers as they travel from the source countries to the United States."[82] Much of the efforts are aimed at reducing the supply coming in from the borders, which is meant to increase the price of illicit drugs with the hopes that the higher price will reduce a person's ability to purchase drugs.[83]

Some believe these efforts have had no impact on the availability and usage of drugs in the United States, as stated in a 1993 Senate subcommittee hearing.[84] More recently, in 2013, it is estimated that only 10% of drugs entering the United States are seized, while the remaining 90% are able to pass through the borders.[85] Additionally, a study in 2013 determined that the price of drugs has dropped while the potency of drugs has increased, which leads one to believe that these national efforts of drug control at the US borders are not working.[86]

Racism and Drug Enforcement

The war on drugs is marred by some racial overtones. In enforcing drug laws in inner-city communities, police officers in Boston and Chicago, among other cities, have obtained questionable search warrants, ignoring the Fourth Amendment protection of people from unreasonable searches and seizures. Also, people of color tend to be stopped and searched more often than others in airports, bus depots, and train stations and on state highways on the basis of "drug courier" profiles. One report noted that Black youths are seven times more likely to be arrested for smoking marijuana or selling drugs than White youths.[87]

There are about 500,000 people in prisons and jails for drug-related offenses. Despite the fact that drug

interdiction the act of preventing movement of a prohibited substance

TABLE 3.3 Annual Number of Arrests for Drug Offenses in the United States By Type of Offense

		Sale/Manufacture					Possession				
Year	Total Drug Arrests	Sale/ Manu. Any Drug	Heroin, Cocaine, and Derivatives	Mari- juana	Synthetic or Manu- factured Drugs	Other Dangerous Nonnarcotic Drugs	Possession Any Drug	Heroin, Cocaine, and De- rivatives	Mari- juana	Synthetic or Manu- factured Drugs	Other Dangerous Nonnarcotic Drugs
2015	1,488,707	239,682	81,879	68,480	26,797	62,526	1,249,025	296,252	574,641	75,924	300,719
2014	1,561,231	263,848	90,551	81,184	29,663	64,010	1,297,383	265,409	619,809	74,939	335,665
2013	1,501,043	265,685	90,063	84,058	28,520	63,044	1,235,358	246,171	609,423	69,048	310,716
2012	1,552,432	276,333	94,698	91,593	29,496	62,097	1,276,099	256,151	658,231	69,859	290,305
2011	1,531,251	278,688	96,469	94,937	27,563	61,250	1,252,563	255,719	663,032	70,438	263,375
2010	1,638,846	296,631	101,608	103,247	29,499	60,637	1,342,215	268,771	750,591	67,193	257,299

Source: "Crime in the United States 2015 - Arrests," FBI Uniform Crime Report (Washington, DC: US Dept. of Justice, September 2016), p. 1, and Arrest Table: Arrests for Drug Abuse Violations.

usage is comparable for Blacks and Whites, Blacks are incarcerated at a rate of 768 out of 100,000 for drug-related offenses while the incarceration rate for Whites is 90 per 100,000.[88] Drug-related incarceration rates for Latinos is 300 per 100,000.[89] In Maryland, 90% of people jailed for drug convictions are Black, even though they make up 30% of the population.[90] The FBI estimates that one-third of Black male babies born in the United States in 2004 will go to prison during their lifetime.[91] It is also possible that racism may lead to drug abuse. One study found that 12-year-old African Americans who experienced racism were twice as likely to use drugs by the time they became teens.[92]

The disparity in drug sentencing becomes particularly apparent when crack cocaine and powder cocaine are discussed. Crack cocaine is more likely to be used by poor people, usually people of color, and powder cocaine is more likely to be used by middle-class people. Data in 2010 show that crack cocaine was used by 0.3% of Whites during the past year while 0.7% of Blacks and 0.2% of Hispanics used crack.[93] Yet, about 85% of people convicted for crack cocaine are Black.[94]

Federal law mandates that a person possessing 5 grams of crack cocaine receive the same sentence as someone with 500 grams of powder cocaine. Many people think this 100-to-1 disparity is unjust because it placed the heaviest penalties on minorities and the poor.[95] In 1995, the US Sentencing Commission recommended lower penalties for crack cocaine, comparable to the penalties for powder cocaine. President Bill Clinton and the Congress rejected the commission's recommendation. However, in 2011, the US Sentencing Commission reduced the penalties for crack cocaine. Instead of a 100-to-1 disparity, crack cocaine sentences are 18 times greater than for powder cocaine.[96]

Minority women who use drugs during pregnancy are subjected to more punishment and stigmatization than nonminority women.[97] One study found that Black women and their newborns were 1.5 times more likely to be tested for illegal drugs than non-Black women.[98] Drug use occurs more or less equally across racial and ethnic groups. A woman from a racial or ethnic minority who uses drugs while pregnant, however, is 10 times more likely to be reported to child protective services than a White woman.[99] Powder cocaine and crack cocaine produce harmful effects to the fetus, too, but crack cocaine has been portrayed in the media as especially deleterious. Nonminority women are more likely to use powder cocaine, and minority women more frequently use crack cocaine. Middle-class women who

People of color tend to be stopped and searched more often in airports, bus depots, and train stations and on state highways on the basis of 'drug courier' profiles.

use cocaine tend to be treated, whereas poor women who use crack tend to be imprisoned. Methamphetamines have replaced crack as the preferred drug for pregnant women and women of child-bearing age.[100]

Mandatory Minimum Drug Sentencing

One proposal for reducing drug-related problems is to mandate minimum drug sentences. Starting in 1984, the US Congress has enacted an array of mandatory minimum penalties specifically focusing on drugs and violent crimes. Politicians from both political parties favor a mandatory minimum sentence for drug offenses because it demonstrates a "get-tough" approach to drug abuse. For example, federal law requires that an individual convicted of possessing one-half kilogram or more of cocaine be sentenced to a prison term of at least 5 years.

Are mandatory minimum drug sentences cost-effective for taxpayers, and do they curtail drug abuse and related consequences? It has been shown that mandatory minimum drug sentences have not acted as deterrents to further crime.[101] One individual who has argued against mandatory minimum drug sentencing is US Supreme Court Justice Anthony Kennedy.[102]

Opponents of mandatory minimum drug sentences argue that they give no latitude to judges to determine appropriate punishments.[103] A defendant's history and circumstances are not taken into account. Moreover, mandatory minimums may violate American standards for justice and equity. The benefit of removing one drug dealer is at best temporary, because there is no shortage of individuals willing to take that person's place, regardless of the possible consequences.

A comprehensive study found that mandatory minimum drug sentences for lower-level dealers were not cost-effective.[104] Less use of cocaine and a reduction of crime are achieved by better enforcement and by providing treatment rather than implementing mandatory minimum drug sentences. One study found that treatment is 15 times more effective for reducing serious crime than mandatory minimum sentencing.[105] Also, the longer low-level, nonviolent drug offenders spend in prison, the greater the likelihood that they will return to prison.[106] With the imposition of mandatory sentences, drug dealers incur more risk and, consequently, increase the cost of cocaine. The authors of the study speculated that mandatory sentences for higher-level dealers might be more cost-effective. Ironically, higher-level dealers are less likely than lower-level dealers to be caught with substantial amounts of cocaine in their possession.

Legislation

What would happen if drugs were legalized? Some argue if drugs were legalized, the United States would save money by eliminating all drug enforcement agencies. Other contend it would hurt Americans by increasing drug availability, thus increasing the number of addicts who would require treatment services. The section below highlights arguments on both sides of the legalization issue.

Con Arguments

Harmful and illegal drug use will never be totally stopped. Still, do drug laws help to prevent drug use, and would **decriminalization** reduce crime? Some argue that legalization would increase drug use,

decriminalization The reduction or elimination of penalties for illegal activities

---

CULTURAL Considerations

Many believe the US policy and actions for reducing drugs have been disproportionately against Black and other minority populations. For example, in Seattle, the majority of those who use and sell drugs are White, however, almost two-thirds of drug-related arrests Black. In Seattle, the majority of arrests are for crack cocaine, which is most often dealt and used by Blacks; however, these only account for an estimated one-third of the city's drug transactions while the majority of drugs on the market are those dealt by and used by Whites. While these arrests and figures may not be racially motivated, they indicate a problem with the typification of "drug dealers," which may arise out of unconscious bias of what a drug dealer looks like.

Questions to Ponder:

■ How can we equalize drug policies so that they are not racially biased?

■ Should we require law enforcement to produce arrest records by racial identity? Should these be required to match the current racial profiles in the city?

Source: K. Becket, K. Nyrop, and L. Pfingst, "Race, Drugs, and Policing: Understanding Disparities in Drug Delivery Arrests," *Criminology,* 44 (2006).

addiction, and drug-related deaths. Herbert Kleber, an adviser to President George H.W. Bush's administration, maintained that the main danger of legalization would be that the lower cost and availability would lead to more use and dependency and that criminal activity would escalate because there would be more users and addicts.[107] Wilson contends that keeping drugs illegal prevents many people from abusing drugs.[108]

According to this line of reasoning, drug legalization would reduce the cost of drugs to somewhere between one-third and one-twentieth of the illegal price. Drug-related crimes might indeed fall, but the number of addicts would rise.[109] Consequently, legalization would result in more dysfunctional addicts who would be unable to support their lifestyles and drug use through legitimate means. And "more users would mean more of the violence associated with the ingestion of drugs."[110]

Portugal decriminalized all psychoactive drugs in 2001 with mixed reviews. On one hand, it seems this new policy reduced drug use among young adults aged 15 to 24.[111] However, in terms of total use, there were increases across the board for all drugs. However, some of the increases were very slight (0.5% compared to 0.9%).[112] Furthermore, the numbers of deaths from drugs decreased to levels much lower than pre-decriminalization time.[113]

Pro Arguments

Some argue that legalization would not eliminate the black market, while others maintain that there would not be enough treatment facilities for the larger number of addicts. It is believed that drug legalization would hurt the Mexican cartels, although it is also believed that they would adapt to other businesses.[114]

Decriminalization is not a panacea. It will not stop the drug crisis, but it could substantially reduce the irrationality and inhumanity of our present punitive war on drugs. The Global Commission on Drug Policy, which includes the presidents of Brazil, Mexico, Colombia, and Switzerland, has called for the legal regulation of drugs to protect drug takers and to save money.[115] Another benefit, according to officials

in the Netherlands, where marijuana use is allowed under certain circumstances, is that the quality of the drug can be assured.[116]

Many activities—for example, hang gliding, parachuting, or driving race cars—can cause harm. Yet, they are not banned. Could not the same argument apply to drug use? The fundamental question is: Should a person be coerced into abstaining from behaviors he or she finds desirable or necessary? If two people buy and sell drugs by mutual consent, is it criminal activity when neither the buyer nor the seller considers himself or herself a victim? The billions of dollars spent on drug enforcement, according to some drug experts, might be put to use more effectively if the money were directed toward education and treatment programs rather than enforcement.[117] Furthermore, some believe legalizing marijuana would increase safety for the user by ensuring quality control and age restrictions.[118]

Does drug use cause criminal activity, or do people who engage in crime also use drugs? The answer is not clear. Some contend that, when drugs are made illegal, their costs increase and there is a corresponding rise in criminal activity.[119] Criminal behavior goes up, not down, when drugs become illegal, whereas their costs would decline if they were legalized.[120]

Twenty years of research showed that street drug users in Miami were involved with criminal activity before using narcotics or cocaine and that drug use per se was not the root cause of criminality.[121] After looking into the link between narcotics and crime, however, the conclusion was that narcotics users are involved extensively with criminal activity, that their crimes against property and others are much greater when they use drugs, and that drug use extends the amount of time they engage in criminal activity.[122]

As the cost of drugs escalates, two possible scenarios can follow:

1. Some people stop or cut down on drug use.
2. Others engage in illegal conduct such as stealing or prostitution to afford drugs.

Table 3.4 identifies the major arguments for and against decriminalizing drugs.

TABLE 3.4 Arguments For and Against Drug Decriminalization

For	Against
Quality of drugs is regulated	Drug use may increase
Less need for jails	More need for treatment
Crime might be reduced	Drug use could be perceived as acceptable
Profit motive is reduced	Drug dealers might target children
Drug users will be treated rather than incarcerated	Drug use is morally wrong
Protection of individual rights	Private drug use affects society
Money is directed to drug education instead of enforcement	Drug users are more likely to be arrested for serious offenses

Prevention

Harm reduction is gaining favor as an approach to preventing drug abuse. Harm reduction, which started during the 1980s in European cities including Amsterdam, Liverpool, and Rotterdam, focuses on reducing the personal and social adverse effects emanating from drug use.[123] It does not address reducing the supply of drugs or punishing the drug user. The goals of harm reduction are to reduce violence associated with the drug trade, lower death rates directly attributable to drugs, and curtail infectious diseases caused by drug use.[124] The concept of harm reduction is also being applied to reducing nicotine dependency. For example, smokeless tobacco or other nicotine-replacement products are viewed as a healthier alternative to smoking cigarettes.[125] This includes the use of e-cigarettes, which has shown promise in its role to reduce harm when used as a tool to reduce tobacco consumption.[126]

Efforts of harm-reduction advocates include providing sterile syringes to people who inject drugs to curtail the spread of HIV infection, as well as educational campaigns and increased treatment. Advocates of harm reduction propose that physicians be allowed to prescribe methadone, heroin, and other drugs to addicts only to prevent addicts from buying drugs on the black market.

One program, the needle exchange program, provides clean needles to injection drug users with the intent of reducing infectious disease among users. Many injection drug users go to "shooting galleries" to inject themselves with drugs and practice unsafe behaviors. In a study on a needle exchange program in California, it was found that users reported a significant decrease in high-risk injection behaviors (i.e., sharing needles) and an increase in the use of sterile needles to inject drugs. These behaviors can significantly reduce the transmission of HIV and Hepatitis C among communities with high rates of injection drug abuse.[127]

In 1982, the Dutch government implemented a policy called **normalization**. Under this policy, using some drugs is not illegal, but it is illegal to traffic in drugs. Small amounts of hashish can be purchased in youth centers and coffee shops, although it remains illegal to buy and use heroin or cocaine. The Dutch believe their policy is pragmatic. The minister of justice contends that the policy removes the sale of hashish from the realm of hard crime and that the illegality of some drugs causes more harm than good.[128]

In recent years, the Dutch coffee shop policies have become more restrictive and there are fewer coffee shops.[129] The new emphasis on restricting marijuana is to stop tourists from buying the drug.[130] Harm-reduction policies may have an impact on attitudes regarding illicit drugs. In a study comparing illicit drug attitudes between the Netherlands (with harm-reduction policies) and Norway (without harm-reduction policies), it was found that people in the Netherlands had higher degrees of attitudes toward drug acceptance compared to Norway.[131] Thus perhaps one unintended consequence of harm reduction policies is an increase in the acceptance of illicit drugs, which may result in an increase of use.

What effect has the Dutch model had on drug use? The Netherlands has less drug use than the United States and other European countries.[132] The use of hard drugs such as cocaine and heroin has declined, and long-term marijuana use has leveled off.[133] In addition to the Netherlands, other European countries have decriminalized marijuana.[134]

More recently, there has been a trend to test drugs at raves, clubs, and dance parties in Europe. The Trans European Drug Information Project is a network of services that are involved in drug checking at recreational settings and report their findings.[135] Information provided at the scene is meant to help the individual understand what substances are in the product purchased to help him/her make better drug-use decisions. Information gathered from these testing sites are used to generate a report that describe current drug trends. Additionally, red alerts are identified (dangerous drugs on the illicit market) and awareness campaigns are presented to the public.

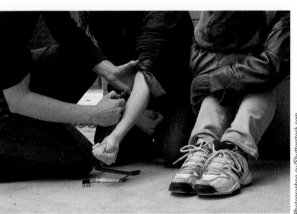

In the 1980s, Switzerland suffered from the highest HIV rate in Western Europe, thanks largely to soaring levels of intravenous heroin use. How the country successfully mitigated this problem—with harm reduction approaches including prescribed heroin, or Heroin Assisted Treatment (HAT)—is instructive.

harm reduction A series of practical interventions that respond to the needs of drug users and the community where they live in an effort to reduce the harm caused by illicit drug use

normalization A term used by the Dutch for the practice of not prosecuting users of soft drugs such as marijuana

For example, in 2012, a toxic chemical was identified in LSD blotter papers. This chemical has been identified in several instances of death. The red alert contained information on the type and look of the blotter paper that is being sold on the streets.[136]

Starting in spring 2004, the Canadian government provided heroin to addicts to reduce heroin-related problems. The Swiss already have a heroin maintenance program. They feel that heroin distribution is one way to reduce the harm associated with heroin.[137] Heroin maintenance programs have produced positive outcomes in Switzerland, the Netherlands, Germany, England, and Denmark.[138] As these strategies illustrate, those individuals who support harm reduction do not support drug use, but they advocate for reducing the dangers associated with drug use.

Summary

The first laws regarding drug regulation had more to do with money than regulation. In the late 1770s Congress passed a tax on whiskey to bring in money that was lost during the Revolutionary War. Since that time, early and contemporary efforts regarding drug laws revolve around concerns for the safety of citizens. Although much of the concern had to do with the safety of products being marketed, a significant portion of drugs laws have been found to have racial roots.

With many drug laws in place, how does the United States go about enforcing these drug laws? The United States has been in a war with drugs since the 1970s. This attempt to eradicate drugs in the United States has proven to be very complicated. With more money being spent on border patrol and attempts to reduce the amount of drugs entering the United States, some have said these strategies have not made a difference in the amount of drug users and abusers.

Many legal issues have evolved concerning drugs. Should drug paraphernalia be banned? Should drug use be decriminalized? Thousands of babies are born to drug-addicted women, and emergency room incidents continue to escalate. The cost of enforcement is enormous, prisons are overcrowded with people arrested on drug-related offenses, and crime and violence are perpetrated by drug dealers and their victims.

One country that decriminalized drugs with some success is the Netherlands. To the Dutch, decriminalization of drugs is pragmatic. They prefer to treat rather than prosecute drug users. Dutch officials contend that drug use not only has stabilized but also has decreased in some cities. The Swiss had the opposite experience.

Thinking Critically

1. Do you view narcotic addiction as a disease or as a crime? If addiction were a medical condition, would you view the addict differently than if addiction were a crime? Should the addict be a patient or an inmate? Why?
2. The case of thalidomide points to the necessity for regulating drugs. Drug regulations, however, can delay beneficial drugs from reaching the marketplace. Should testing procedures be relaxed when certain illnesses, such as AIDS, have a high mortality rate?
3. Students convicted of drug charges are not eligible to receive federal financial assistance. People who commit crimes such as robbery and murder are not denied student aid. Should students who have used drugs be held to a higher standard than others?
4. Many say that some of the current US drug laws were based on racism and used as a way to control immigrants in the country. Do you feel the current laws and enforcement policies reflect racism views? Defend your answer.
5. Legal and physical problems can arise from drug use. Harm may come from the effects of drugs or from their illegal status. If you were asked to reduce the adverse consequences of drugs, would you approach the drug issue as a legal problem or as a public health problem? What is your rationale?

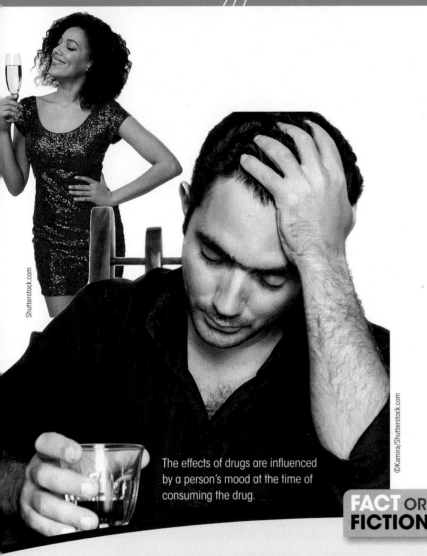

The effects of drugs are influenced by a person's mood at the time of consuming the drug.

Chapter Objectives

After completing this chapter, the reader should be able to:

- Describe how neurons communicate electrically and chemically
- Contrast a dendrite and an axon
- Explain the effects of various neurotransmitters
- Summarize the functions of the reticular activating system, hypothalamus, cerebral cortex, limbic system, basal ganglia, and brain stem
- List and provide examples of the different factors that alter the effects of drugs
- Describe how drugs interact with different systems of the body
- Contrast the sympathetic and parasympathetic branches of the autonomic nervous system
- Describe the additive, antagonistic, and synergistic effects of drugs
- Contrast between pharmacological tolerance, behavioral tolerance, cross-tolerance, and reverse tolerance
- List the mechanisms of how drugs can be administered and discuss the effects of these different routes have on absorption rates

FACT OR FICTION?

1. Marijuana's effects are more profound when it is ingested than when it is smoked.

2. At one time LSD was given to patients in order to study mental illness.

3. People who engage in strenuous exercise actually emit a neurotransmitter that contributes to a "high" feeling.

4. The day of the week on which most heart attacks occur is Monday.

5. The effects of cocaine are the same for men and women.

6. Older men are more affected by a drug's effects than are older women.

7. The number of people aged 50 and older admitted into substance abuse treatment has nearly doubled since the early 1990s.

8. Mixing medications with wine causes more potential health problems than mixing medications with beer.

9. One's mood while taking psychoactive drugs will affect the experience derived from the drug.

10. Women are less likely today than they were 30 years ago to use medicines while pregnant.

Turn the page to check your answers

Different drugs produce different effects within the **psyche** and **soma**, and these effects also differ from one person to another. This chapter addresses the chemical or pharmacological effects associated with drugs. It explores factors that influence how drugs affect people and how people allow drugs to affect them.

Pharmacology

Ancient records show that humans have been using drugs to alter their mood and behavior for a long time.[1] The relationship or interaction between drugs and living organisms is called **pharmacology**. The pharmacology of drugs relates to the way in which they are administered, absorbed, distributed, metabolized, and excreted from the body. Additionally, the self-administration of drugs is dependent on a number of factors including:

- The properties of the drug itself
- The route of administration
- The amount or dosage
- Other drugs in the system
- Previous experience with the drug

Ingesting drugs, for example, produces different effects than inhaling drugs. Chewed tobacco is absorbed differently from smoked tobacco. The effects of injected narcotics are more intense than the effects of narcotics taken in other ways.

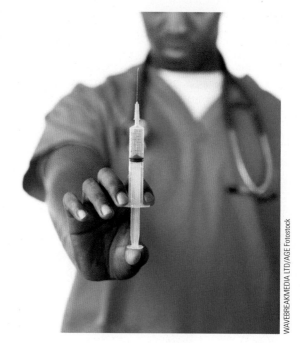

WAVEBREAKMEDIA LTD/AGE Fotostock

Injected drugs reach the brain more quickly than drugs administered by other methods.

Furthermore, drugs that act quickly and produce profound and intense effects are more likely to be abused than are drugs that act slowly. Injected drugs are absorbed quickly, reaching the brain in seconds. However, not all drugs lend themselves to injection. Marijuana cannot be injected because its resin does

FACT OR FICTION?

1. **FACT** New studies now indicate eating cannabis produces a stronger and longer effect compared to smoking it. When ingested, the THC becomes metabolized by the liver, which makes the drug more effective when crossing the blood-brain barrier.

2. **FACT** In the 1950s, it was believed that schizophrenia could be studied by giving LSD to patients.

3. **FACT** During strenuous exercise, the human body produces endorphins, which give the individual a euphoric feeling.

4. **FACT** It is believed that heart attacks occur most frequently on Monday, possibly from a weekend of heavy alcohol use.

5. **FICTION** The fact is—Women are less sensitive to the drug compared to men and had lower levels of cocaine in their blood even when given the same dosage as men. This is even more evident when a

woman takes cocaine during the luteal phase of her menstrual cycle.

6. **FICTION** The fact is—Because they have a higher percentage of fat, which increases the accumulation of drugs, women tend to be more affected by drugs than men.

7. **FACT** Since 1992, the percentage of people aged 50 and older in substance abuse treatment has risen from 6.6% to 12.2%.

8. **FICTION** The fact is—The important factor is how much alcohol is consumed when using medications, not the type of alcohol that is consumed.

9. **FACT** One's state of mind can influence whether a drug's effects are euphoric or dysphoric.

10. **FICTION** The fact is—Pregnant women today are four times more likely to use prescribed medications than they were 30 years ago.

not dissolve in water. Therefore it is less likely to be abused than cocaine or narcotics that can be injected. Similarly, cocaine is more apt to be abused than caffeine because the effects of cocaine are much more powerful. Besides having a different chemical structure from caffeine, cocaine takes effect more quickly because of the way in which it is administered. Injected cocaine produces more powerful effects than snorted cocaine.

Alcohol is metabolized in the liver, and its primary site of absorption is the small intestine. It is removed through exhaling, urinating, and sweating at a rate of three-fourths ounce per hour. If cocaine is snorted, the mucous membranes in the nose absorb the drug quickly, and the effects are felt within minutes. Amphetamines taken orally produce peak effects in 2 to 3 hours and are eliminated in 2 to 3 days, whereas the peak effects from injected amphetamines are felt in less than 5 minutes.

The effects of caffeine are felt in 15 to 45 minutes. It is metabolized by the liver and eliminated primarily by the kidneys. Similarly, nicotine is metabolized by the liver and removed via the kidneys. When marijuana is smoked, about half of its psychoactive substance, tetrahydrocannabinol (THC), is absorbed through the lungs before entering the bloodstream. The organ that initially detoxifies the THC is the liver, and THC is removed primarily through the feces.

Drug Actions

Drugs affect various organs within the body, including the nervous system. The nervous system consists of the **central nervous system (CNS)**, the autonomic nervous system (ANS), and the peripheral nervous system (PNS). The CNS, consisting of the brain and spinal cord, is comprised of nerve cells called **neurons**. Neurons function as messengers in which information is communicated via synapse functions (Figure 4.1). Neurons send messages electrochemically. Transmitting information *between* neurons is accomplished chemically and relaying information *within* the neuron occurs electrically through the exchange of ions. Chemical transmission is much more common than electrical transmission.

The Neuron

A neuron contains two types of nerve fibers: dendrites and axons. **Dendrites** allow nerve impulses to be transmitted to the nerve's cell body (soma), whereas **axons** send impulses away from the cell body. Each neuron has several dendrites but only one axon. Electrical impulses originate in the dendrite and pass through the cell body via the axon. This process is called the **action potential**.

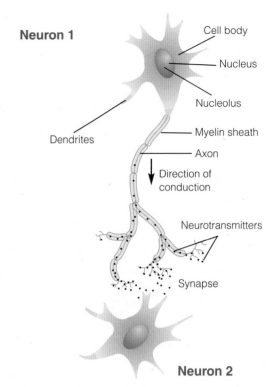

Figure 4.1 Neurons in the Brain

For an electrical message to be sent from the axon of one neuron to the dendrite of another neuron, it must traverse the space, called a **synapse**, between them (Figure 4.2). The message sent through a neuron is electrical, but the process by which an impulse is transmitted from one neuron to another—from the axon of one neuron to the dendrite of another neuron—is chemical. The chemicals used to transmit these messages are called **neurotransmitters**. Neurotransmitters are manufactured within

psyche Refers to the mind

soma From Greek; literally means "body"

pharmacology The professional discipline that studies the relationships and interactions between living organisms and substances within them

central nervous system (CNS) The brain and spinal cord

neurons Messengers in the brain that transmit information via chemical and electrical processes

dendrites Parts of the neuron that allow nerve impulses to be transmitted to the nerve's cell body

axons Parts of the neuron that send nerve impulses away from the nerve's cell body

action potential The procedure by which the nerve impulse is sent down the axon

synapse The space between an axon and a dendrite

neurotransmitters Chemical substances manufactured in vesicles of the brain

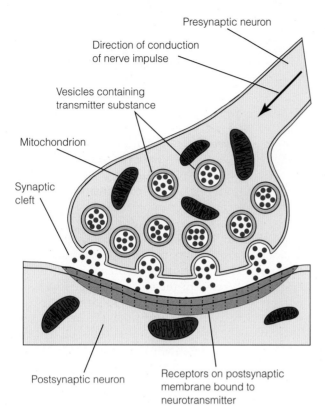

Figure 4.2 Synaptic Transmission

vesicles, which are saclike structures located at the end of axons. In other words, an electrical impulse travels along the axon and when it reaches the tip of the axon it causes neurotransmitters to be released. These chemicals enter the synaptic space between two neurons. Neurotransmitters travel through this space to the dendrites of another neuron and bind to their receptors. This causes the receiving cell to start an electrical impulse.

Drugs are most likely to have their major effect at the synapse. During early phases of drug use, the process of neurotransmission normalizes after the effects of the drugs wear off. However, prolonged or repeated exposure to drugs may lead to permanent neurotransmission abnormalities.[2] Adolescent binge drinking is a risk factor for alcohol abuse as an adult. In a study conducted on rats who were given binge-like alcohol amounts during adolescence found that these rats when matured to adulthood had more extracellular dopamine after being given alcohol. This may help explain the increased risk of abuse for alcohol among adolescents who engage in binge drinking behaviors.[3]

The neuron responsible for causing the neurotransmitter to be released at the synapse is called the presynaptic neuron. The neuron receiving the neurotransmitter is the postsynaptic neuron. Drugs influencing the release, storage, and synthesis of neu-

rotransmitters are classified as presynaptic, and drugs affecting neurotransmitters after they cross the synapse are classified as postsynaptic. Neurotransmitters linked to addiction include dopamine, norepinephrine, gamma-aminobutyric acid (GABA), and serotonin.[4]

Some drugs cause the nerve cell to become more sensitive. As sensitivity increases, activity and excitation of certain neurotransmitters increase. This action is exemplified by caffeine. The opposite effect, in which nerve cells become less sensitive, occurs with sedative-hypnotic drugs. Lessened sensitivity inhibits neurotransmitter release. This process is not as straightforward as it may seem. For example, antidepressants and cocaine produce the same biochemical effect, but their physiological effects differ.

In addition, many nerve cells contain **autoreceptors**, which may be situated on any part of the cell. Autoreceptors act when the nerve cell releases neurotransmitters and alter their synthesis, usually by reducing production of neurotransmitters. This is demonstrated with a drug such as LSD, which activates serotonin autoreceptors. The production of serotonin at the synapse decreases.

To summarize, part of the nerve cell or neuron receives a stimulus, which is converted into an electrical nerve impulse. The nerve impulse is forwarded to the axon, which proceeds to send impulses to terminals, causing chemicals called neurotransmitters to be released. Neurotransmitters traverse the synapse to receptor sites on the next neuron. Some drugs speed up transmission of electrical impulses, and others slow them down. Two drugs that create opposite effects are minor tranquilizers and amphetamines. Minor tranquilizers produce a calming effect. Amphetamines result in increased excitation.

Neurotransmitters

Most drugs affect brain activity by increasing or decreasing the activity of various neurotransmitters. Neurotransmitters enable the brain to receive, process, and respond to information by carrying impulses from one neuron to the next. Precisely how they do this is not well understood. Neurotransmitters affect cognition, our movement, and our emotions.[5] Neurotransmission has been linked to symptoms of major depressive disorder, specifically the neurotransmitters dopamine, norepinephrine, and serotonin.[6] Some research suggests a decreases in the production of serotonin is responsible for depression in some people.[7] Additionally, autopsies performed on people who experienced depression found they had lower levels of norepinephrinergic neurons (responsible for producing norepinephrine) suggesting a link between norepinephrine and depression.[8] However, other studies have found people who are depressed have increased activity in their norepinephrinergic neurons. Lastly, recent research suggests a drop in serotonin triggers a drop in norepinephrine, which may lead to depression.[9] Some scientists are once again using psylocibin and other hallucinogens to determine whether certain types of mental disorders are improved by these drugs.[10] Some of these hallucinogenic drugs have found promise for people suffering from depression and posttraumatic stress disorder.

Some drugs mimic the action of neurotransmitters, and others block their action. The functions of selected neurotransmitters are described on the following pages.

Acetylcholine

Acetylcholine (ACH) is synthesized from a molecule of choline (derived from one's diet and naturally manufactured in the body) and acetyl coenzyme A. It is one of the most common neurotransmitters in the brain.[11] Neurons containing acetylcholine are termed cholinergic and are linked to specific behaviors. Drugs that block the action of ACH receptors are called anticholinergic.

ACH acts as an excitatory transmitter in the skeletal muscles but functions as an inhibitory transmitter in the heart muscle. Drugs that influence ACH can cause various degrees of movement disruption.[12] Some pesticides and nerve gases have been shown to affect ACH functions and can even lead to death.

ACH is also responsible for processing memory and learning.[13] Reduced numbers of ACH receptors in the brain have been associated with Alzheimer's disease, a progressive condition resulting in memory loss. ACH has also been tied to aggression and depression.

A number of hallucinogenic drugs are found in plants and fungi including the *Datura* and the *Amanita muscaria* mushrooms. Species of *Datura* include *Datura solanaceae* and *Datura stramonium* (also known as jimson weed). Species of *Amanita* include *Amanita bisporigera*, *Amanita virosa*, and *Amanita verna*. This is significant because substances in these plants and fungi interfere with the action of ACH and can produce hallucinations. These plants are called **anticholinergic hallucinogens**. Before ACH can be inactivated, the enzyme **cholinesterase** must be present. This enzyme, located in the synapse, is nullified by cholinesterase inhibitors such as nerve gas. The continuous release of ACH resulting from a cholinesterase inhibitor arouses the postsynaptic membrane and can lead to seizures, respiratory depression, and death. Cholinesterase inhibitors are found in the insecticides used on plants, for example. Insecticides contain another highly toxic agent, nicotine, which mimics the action of ACH at the neuromuscular junction.

Serotonin

Serotonin is an inhibitory neurotransmitter situated in the upper brain stem, bowels, and blood platelets.[14] (Figure 4.3). Serotonin plays a role in regulating pain, sensory perception, eating, sleep, and body temperature and is thought to help contribute to feelings of happiness and relaxation.

Many research studies have been conducted to determine if there is a link between serotonin and depression; specifically, low levels of serotonin may contribute to depression. Many of the antidepression medicine available are serotonin reuptake inhibitors (SSRIs), which work by increasing serotonin levels in the brain.[15] It is thought that by increasing levels of serotonin in the brain, symptoms of depression would disappear. However, other studies rebuke theory as such in the case of the study on mice and serotonin. In this study, mice have been genetically altered to prevent the production of serotonin in the brain. What the researchers found is an increase in aggression and compulsive activity in the genetically altered mice, but no signs of depression or depression-like symptoms.[16]

Serotonin syndrome is a potentially life-threatening condition resulting from too much serotonin in the body.[17] It can result from prescribed use of SSRIs and other drugs that influence the amount of serotonin in the body, which include over-the-counter and illicit drugs. Serotonin syndrome or serotonin poisoning can result in death and was responsible for 118 deaths in 2005.[18] Some believe actual death rates are higher than the reported cases.[19] Despite the potential problems with antidepressant drugs such as

vesicles Saclike structure at the end of the axon

autoreceptors Units that alter the synthesis of neurotransmitters after they are released by the nerve cells

acetylcholine (ACH) A neurotransmitter synthesized from a molecule of choline and from acetyl CoA

anticholinergic hallucinogens Substances found in *Datura* and *Amanita muscaria* mushrooms; interfere with the action of acetylcholine to produce hallucinations; species of *Datura* include *Datura solanaceae* and *Datura stramonium* (also known as jimson weed); species of *Amanita* include *Amanita bisporigera*, *Amanita virosa*, and *Amanita verna*

cholinesterase An enzyme necessary for the metabolism of acetylcholine

serotonin An inhibitory neurotransmitter located in the upper brain stem; plays a role in regulating sensory perception, eating, pain, sleep, and body temperature

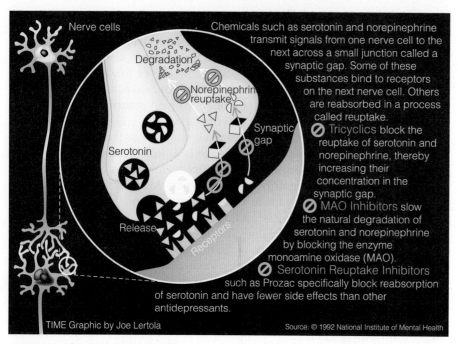

Chemicals such as serotonin and norepinephrine transmit signals from one nerve cell to the next across a small junction called a synaptic gap. Some of these substances bind to receptors on the next nerve cell. Others are reabsorbed in a process called reuptake.

⊘ Tricyclics block the reuptake of serotonin and norepinephrine, thereby increasing their concentration in the synaptic gap.

⊘ MAO Inhibitors slow the natural degradation of serotonin and norepinephrine by blocking the enzyme monoamine oxidase (MAO).

⊘ Serotonin Reuptake Inhibitors such as Prozac specifically block reabsorption of serotonin and have fewer side effects than other antidepressants.

TIME Graphic by Joe Lertola   Source: © 1992 National Institute of Mental Health

Figure 4.3 How the Drugs Work

SSRIs, they are the type of antidepressant most commonly prescribed.[20]

Serotonergic neurons, or tryptaminergic neurons, might prevent overreaction to various stimuli associated with mood, sexual behavior, and motor activity. When functioning improperly, tryptaminergic hormones have been linked to mental illness. Because tryptaminergic neurons affect the release of hormones in the hypothalamus, they monitor the release of hormones from the anterior pituitary gland. These hormones include leuteinizing hormone (LH) and follicle-stimulating hormone (FSH) as well as prolactin, which is responsible for milk production in the nursing mother.

To synthesize serotonin in tryptaminergic neurons, the amino acid tryptophan is needed. High levels of **tryptophan** are found in milk and other protein-rich foods. Drinking warm milk helps a person fall asleep because tryptophan enhances the brain's production of serotonin, which promotes relaxation.

Gamma-aminobutyric Acid

A second type of neurotransmitter that inhibits nerve impulses from being sent from one neuron to another is **gamma-aminobutyric acid (GABA)**. Low levels of GABA have been associated with anxiety, epilepsy, and chronic pain. Drugs such as alcohol stimulate GABA, producing relaxation and feelings of decreased inhibition. Other drugs that increase the action of GABA are barbiturates and minor tranquilizers. The neurological disorder Huntington's chorea and Parkinson's have been linked to low levels of GABA.[21]

Catecholamines

Another group of neurotransmitters is **catecholamines**. Examples of catecholamine neurotransmitters are epinephrine, dopamine, and norepinephrine. Catecholamines function repeatedly because they are reabsorbed by the neuron that discharges them, a process known as **reuptake**. Catecholamines affect emotional states. An increase in catecholamines results in stimulation, whereas a decrease in catecholamines leads to depression. Drugs such as amphetamines and cocaine increase catecholamines initially, but this is followed by a depletion of the neurotransmitters. This explains the mood swings that individuals experience while using these drugs.

Dopamine plays a significant role in emotional, mental, and motor functions. The purpose of this system is to reward natural behaviors (i.e., eating, sex, etc.).[22] Dopamine is what activates the pleasure part in the brain to produce feelings of pleasure to reward behaviors that are needed to continue the human experience, which is why it is associated with eating and sex. When an overproduction of dopamine is present, it produces feelings of euphoria, which is strongly related to drug-seeking behavior.

It is speculated that dopamine can produce hyperactivity and tic and movement disorders such as Tourette's syndrome, affective disorders, and disorders of sexual activity and sexual drive. Dopamine levels are influenced by marijuana, affecting one's perception of pain, movement, and balance. Other drugs that alter dopamine levels include nicotine, heroin, and amphetamines.[23] Excessive dopamine

CASE STUDY: Chocolate vs. Drugs and Dopamine

When a person eats chocolate (and enjoys it), the initial experiences with eating the chocolate releases dopamine levels in the brain. This produces pleasurable and rewarding feelings in the brain, which results in an expectation every time chocolate is eaten. However, after a period of time, the expectation of pleasure derived from chocolate becomes the pleasure feeling, and dopamine is no longer released in the brain when chocolate is eaten.

Contrast this to when an illicit drug is taken, let's say cocaine. Dopamine is released in the brain, up to 10 times the normal level. These high levels of dopamine are very rewarding and encourage users to seek out more cocaine. Now, unlike eating chocolate, cocaine produces higher levels of dopamine each time it is taken, producing more rewarding experiences and encourages the user to take in more cocaine. Furthermore, the brain tries to compensate for the increase in dopamine by desensitizing the

neurons so they are not affected as easily by the surge in dopamine. This is what creates tolerance to the drug. Thus, after using cocaine for a period of time, the increase in dopamine does not produce the same pleasurable feeling compared to the first few times cocaine was used. Thus people are constantly chasing that initial "high" and use more of the drug, more often to gain it.

QUESTIONS TO PONDER:

1. How is dopamine affected by chocolate and cocaine similar and different?

2. What causes regular cocaine users to chase that "initial high"?

3. If a person who was a regular cocaine user were to stop suddenly, do you think they would receive pleasure from other activities that naturally produce dopamine (i.e., sex)? Justify your answer.

Source: D. Hirshman, "Your Brain on Drugs: Dopamine and Addiction." Available at: www.bigthink.com/going-mental/your-brain-on-drugs-dopamine-and-addiction.

---

has been related to schizophrenic symptoms, whereas Parkinson's disease can arise if neurons containing dopamine are destroyed. It has also been found that dopamine has been associated with pathological gambling, compulsive shopping, and hypersexuality.[24] In a study conducted that looked at almost 1,600 people who have experienced pathological gambling, compulsive shopping, and/or hypersexuality, researchers found that almost half of these people were on dopamine receptor agonists.[25] Results from this study indicate dopamine levels may be associated with the behaviors mentioned above. Dopamine receptor agonists are drugs used to mimic the function of the dopamine neurotransmitter and are usually prescribed to people with Parkinson's disease. Parkinson's disease has been associated with lower levels of dopamine in the brain. Another study of 8,000 men showed that those men who drank two or more cups of coffee (a stimulant that increases dopamine levels) daily had a lower risk of developing Parkinson's disease.[26]

In times of acute stress, **epinephrine**, or **adrenaline**, is released into the bloodstream. Epinephrine is integral to the **fight-flight-fright syndrome**. The release of epinephrine speeds up coronary blood flow and heart rate, among other effects. Because epinephrine causes the bronchi to dilate (expand), it is

used to treat asthma. Figure 4.4 diagrams the fight-flight-fright mechanism, which is also called the stress response.

Closely related to epinephrine is norepinephrine, also called noradrenaline. Norepinephrine inhibits target neurons. Depending on the activity level of

tryptophan An amino acid that affects serotonin levels, allowing one to fall asleep more easily

gamma-aminobutyric acid (GABA) A type of neurotransmitter that produces relaxation and sleepiness

catecholamines A group of neurotransmitters that includes epinephrine, dopamine, and norepinephrine

reuptake A process by which a chemical is reabsorbed into the cell from which it was discharged

dopamine A neurotransmitter that affects emotional, mental, and motor functions

epinephrine A natural chemical, also called adrenaline, involved in the fight-flight-fright syndrome

adrenaline A hormone secreted by the adrenal gland in the fight-flight-fright response; another name for epinephrine

fight-flight-fright syndrome Psychological response of the body to stress, which prepares the individual to take action by stimulating the body's defense system

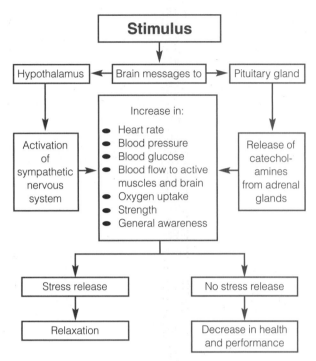

Figure 4.4 Fight-Flight-Fright Mechanism

norepinephrine, a person can be aroused, depressed, or manic. In addition, norepinephrine increases motor activity. Heroin withdrawal symptoms are blocked by decreasing norepinephrine levels. Tobacco and amphetamines stimulate norepinephrine, and antidepressants such as Elavil and Triavil inhibit it. The effect of norepinephrine on mood is not always apparent. Drugs such as mescaline and MDMA (ecstasy) reduce norepinephrine levels. At low doses, however, MDMA acts as a stimulant.

Peptides

Peptides are substances in which sequences of amino acids are linked. Whether peptides are truly transmitters is questionable because they modulate the activity of transmitters. One peptide group consists of **endorphins**, naturally occurring chemicals with opiate-like properties, which are found throughout the body. The term *endorphin* is derived from the words *end*ogenous (naturally occurring) and *morphine. Endorphins in the brain are called **enkaphalins**. The word *enkaphalins* comes from Greek and means "in the head."

Endorphins and enkaphalins, whose actions are similar to those of morphine and heroin, are instrumental in moderating one's perception of pain. High levels of enkaphalins in the brain could be a causative factor in morphine dependency, and the absence of enkaphalins could account for the appearance of withdrawal symptoms. Chronic alcohol use impairs production of these neurotransmitters. Some postulate that alcohol withdrawal may arise from too little enkaphalin and endorphin stimulation.[27] On the other hand, it is speculated that alcohol-dependent people have a preference for sweet foods, which release endorphins.[28]

The brain emits endorphins when the person feels stress or pain. Also, endorphins are believed to be released during strenuous exercise, resulting in the "runner's high." Thus an addiction to running or other forms of strenuous exercise could have a neurochemical basis. Endorphins have been linked to everything from obesity to sexual activity. They ameliorate the emotional response to pain. Opiates release endorphins, and acupuncture and electrical stimulation may cause them to be discharged as well. Table 4.1 provides a synopsis of selected neurotransmitters.

The Central Nervous System

The CNS consists of the brain and spinal cord. Messages are transmitted from the brain to the muscles and organs and back to the brain through the spinal cord. The type of message depends on which part of the brain is sending it. The different parts of the brain and their functions are described next and are illustrated in Figure 4.5.

TABLE 4.1 Effects of Selected Neurotransmitters

Neurotransmitter	Effects
Acetylcholine (ACH)	An excitatory transmitter in the skeletal muscles but an inhibitory transmitter in the heart muscle; affects memory; linked to aggression and depression
Serotonin	An inhibitory neurotransmitter that plays a role in regulating sensory perception, eating, pain, sleep, and body temperature; a factor in hallucinations
Gamma-aminobutyric acid (GABA)	A type of neurotransmitter that produces relaxation and sleepiness
Catecholamines	A group of neurotransmitters that affects emotional states; an increase leads to stimulation and a decrease leads to depression; implicated in mood swings
Peptides	Substances linking amino acids; one type is endorphins, naturally occurring chemicals with opiate-like properties; they moderate perception of pain

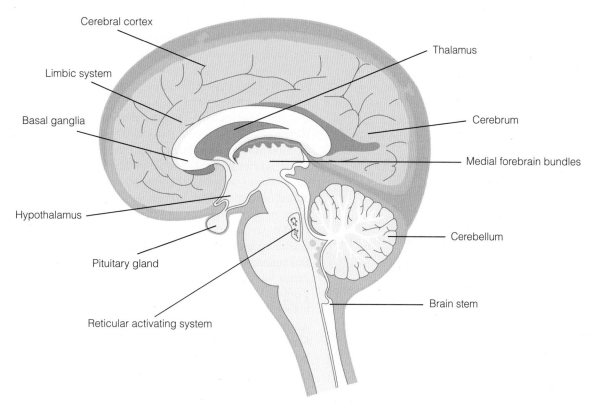

Figure 4.5 Cross Section of the Human Brain

Reticular Activating System

The **reticular activating system (RAS)** is located the brain stem and among other roles plays an important role in sleep and wake cycles. It serves as a portal that all information enters before it enters the brain (except for smell). The RAS system filters out information to allow a person to focus on one piece of information rather than all information being sent to the brain. For an individual to be aroused, the cortex has to be stimulated. The RAS alerts the cerebral cortex of important stimuli and can filter out unimportant stimuli. Stimuli are forwarded to the brain constantly, but the cortex is aroused only if the message is consequential, such as a baby crying. Sleeping through a thunderstorm but waking up to a baby's cry is a function of a properly functioning RAS.

Because the **RAS** has an extensive network of multiple synaptic neurons throughout the brain (like a telephone switchboard), its susceptibility to drugs is high. Many drugs, including barbiturates, LSD, alcohol, and amphetamines, affect the RAS extensively. If the stimuli generate alertness beyond conventional limits, hallucinations occur.

The RAS is involved in helping to focus attention. Hyperactive children are thought to have an underactive RAS, suggesting that they are easily distracted and undermotivated. Stimulants activate the RAS, which filters out extraneous stimuli, enabling the hyperactive child to concentrate on a specific task.

Hypothalamus

Located near the base of the brain, the **hypothalamus** is comparable to a central computer from which many smaller computers receive their directions. The connection between the hypothalamus and the **pituitary gland** makes such communication possible. The pituitary gland regulates hormones

peptides Substances linking amino acids; include endorphins, which are naturally occurring chemicals with opiate-like properties

endorphins Naturally occurring chemicals with opiate-like properties

enkaphalins Endorphins found within the brain

reticular activating system (RAS) Part of the central nervous system; affects sleep, attention, and arousal

hypothalamus Gland situated near the base of the brain; maintains homeostasis; affects stress, aggressiveness, heart rate, hunger, thirst, consciousness, body temperature, blood pressure, and sexual behavior

pituitary gland The "master gland"; responsible for controlling many bodily functions by secretion of hormones that affect many behaviors, and many life-supporting functions originate from the hypothalamus. This helps to keep the body's biological systems in balance, called **homeostasis**. The hypothalamus affects stress, heart rate, hunger, aggressiveness, body temperature, blood pressure, thirst, consciousness, and sexual behavior. It has also been linked to behavioral and chemical dependencies from alcohol to gambling to obesity.

Cerebral Cortex

The part of the brain that distinguishes humans from other mammals is the **cerebral cortex**, which is located in the **cerebrum**. The cortex is essential for most of our thought processes and for understanding information. This encompasses speech, motor movement, sensory perception, hearing, vision, and higher cognitive functions such as fine sensory discriminations, memory, language, abstract thought, and reasoning. The cortex influences personality and how we interpret emotions. The cortex is affected by almost all psychoactive drugs. For example, feelings of euphoria are activated by marijuana.

Limbic System

The **limbic system** combines many diverse structures in the cerebral hemispheres, where circuits relating to varied functions come together. The limbic system serves as the emotional center of the brain. For instance, if a person smells a perfume that his or her mother uses, that person might be reminded of his or her mother. This is largely a result of the ability of the limbic system to store and sort this information and then connect the memory with the emotion. Emotions regulated by the limbic system include sorrow, fear, pleasure, and anger. The limbic system is also the brain's reward circuit and originates within the midbrain called the ventral tegmental area (VTA). When the neurons in the VTA are activated, they release dopamine, which causes a person to feel pleasure.

Cocaine affects neurotransmitters in the limbic system, creating intense feelings of excitement and joy. Childress and colleagues found that the craving for cocaine can be induced by cocaine-related cues that cause activity in the limbic regions of the brain.[29] When cocaine is withdrawn, the outcome is severe withdrawal marked by depression, paranoia, irritability, and craving. However, when certain parts of the limbic system have lesions or are electrically stimulated, emotional disturbances, depersonalization, catatonia (immobility), and hallucinations can occur.

Depressants reduce electrical activity in the limbic system. This produces feelings of tranquility and relaxation rather than depression.

Medial Forebrain Bundle

Along each side of the hypothalamus is a **medial forebrain bundle (MFB)**, which serves as a communication route between the limbic system and the brain stem. By acting on this part of the brain, a part of the limbic system, amphetamines and cocaine produce intense euphoria. This is one reason that people repeatedly use these drugs.

The MFB is significant in sexual response because the sensation of orgasm originates here. Laboratory rats, given the freedom to self-stimulate the MFB by pressing a lever in which electrodes were attached to the MFB, did so until they were completely exhausted. Animals have self-stimulated in preference to sex, food, or water, even though they had to endure electrical shocks to their feet. Humans whose MFB was stimulated while they were being operated on for brain tumors or other brain disorders have exhibited the pleasure response. MFB stimulation also alleviates feelings of depression.

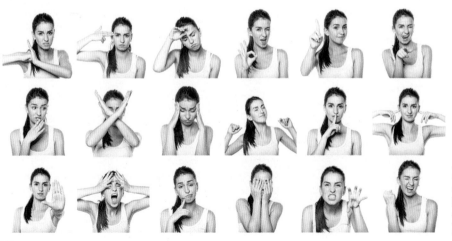

Yurko Gud/Shutterstock.com

The limbic system regulates emotions.

Basal Ganglia

On both sides of the brain and below the cerebral cortex are the **basal ganglia**, which maintain involuntary motor control. The abilities to stand, walk, run, carry, throw, and lift are attributable largely to proper functioning of the basal ganglia. Excessive activity of, or damage to, the basal ganglia, however, can produce rigidity of facial, arm, and leg muscles, as well as spasms and trembling. An example of a condition that destroys the basal ganglia is Parkinson's disease. Drugs prescribed for schizophrenia can precipitate Parkinson's-like behavior. Also, the designer drug China white (fentanyl) has been linked to brain damage similar to that found in patients who have Parkinson's disease, and only small amounts of fentanyl can prove fatal.

Periventricular System

The **periventricular system**, comprised of nerve cells above and to either side of the hypothalamus, is associated with punishment or avoidance behavior. People experience a distinct sense of discomfort or displeasure when the periventricular system is stimulated. When this system is aroused in animals, their behavior slows down or stops. The MFB and the periventricular system are coupled in that stimulation of one inhibits the other.

Brain Stem

The brain stem is located at the point where the brain and spinal cord join. It consists of the **medulla oblongata**, the **pons**, and the **midbrain**. The brain stem is responsible for regulating vital functions such as breathing, heartbeat, dilation of the pupil of the eye, blood pressure, and the vomiting reflex (the body's way of ridding the stomach of toxic substances).

---

homeostasis A condition in which the body's systems are in balance

cerebral cortex Part of the brain involved in intellectual functioning; affects speech, motor movement, sensory perception, hearing, vision, sensory discrimination, memory, language, reasoning, abstract reasoning, and personality

cerebrum Part of the brain that contains the cerebral cortex

limbic system Part of the central nervous system that plays a key role in memory and emotion

medial forebrain bundle (MFB) Serves as a communication route between the limbic system and the brain stem; affects pleasure and reward

basal ganglia Part of the central nervous system

periventricular system Part of the central nervous system implicated with punishment or avoidance behavior

medulla oblongata One of two structures constituting the brain stem; helps control respiration, blood pressure, heart rate, and other vital functions

pons One of two structures constituting the brain stem, connecting the medulla with the brain stem

midbrain Part of the brain stem that connects the larger structures of the brain to the spinal cord

---

In concert with the cerebellum, the brain stem governs muscle tone; with the hypothalamus, it controls the cardiovascular system; and, combined with the RAS, it exerts some influence on arousal.

Drugs affecting the brain stem include alcohol and opiates. These drugs are capable of stopping breathing by depressing the respiratory system. Conversely, stimulants activate the medulla, causing vomiting and nausea.

Table 4.2 summarizes the actions of the parts of the brain discussed here.

TABLE 4.2 Actions of Various Parts of the Brain

Part of Brain	Actions
Reticular activating system (RAS)	Affects sleep, attention, and arousal
Hypothalamus	Maintains homeostasis; affects heart rate, hunger, thirst, consciousness, body temperature, blood pressure, and sexual behavior
Cerebral cortex	Affects speech, motor movement, sensory perception, hearing, vision, sensory discrimination, memory, language, reasoning, abstract thought, and personality
Limbic system	Plays a key role in memory and emotion
Medial forebrain bundle (MFB)	Serves as communication route between limbic system and brain stem; mediates pleasure and reward
Basal ganglia	Affects ability to stand, walk, run, carry, throw, and lift; can produce muscular rigidity of facial, arm, and leg muscles
Periventricular system	Implicated in punishment or avoidance behavior
Brain stem	Regulates vital functions such as breathing, heartbeat, dilation of pupils, and blood pressure, as well as vomiting reflex

The Peripheral Nervous System

Another component of the nervous system, the **peripheral nervous system (PNS)**, encompasses the somatic and autonomic nervous systems. The nerves associated with the PNS lie outside the skull and the spinal cord and serve as transmitting agents that link the brain and spinal cord to the body's extremities.

Somatic Nervous System

The **somatic nervous system** is a collection of nerves that control skeletal muscles and relay sensory information to the CNS and motor information back out. The cranial nerves are involved with our ability to taste, smell, chew, hear, and see, as well as movements of the face and tongue.

Autonomic Nervous System

The **autonomic nervous system (ANS)** regulates blood pressure, gastrointestinal and urinary functioning, body temperature, sweating, and other involuntary bodily functions. It is divided into two branches called the **sympathetic nervous system** and the **parasympathetic nervous system**, which frequently work in opposition to each other. The sympathetic branch relaxes bronchi in the lungs, inhibits intestinal and stomach glands, constricts blood vessels in the skin, increases heart rate, and dilates pupils of the eyes. The parasympathetic branch constricts bronchi, dilates blood vessels of the skin, increases action of the intestinal and stomach glands, decreases the heart rate, and constricts pupils of the eye.

The sympathetic nervous system enables the body to react to situations that require either fighting or fleeing (the fight-flight-fright syndrome) by increasing blood supply to the brain and muscles through the release of adrenaline. During acute stress and excitation, this system is especially active.

The parasympathetic system, in contrast, comes into play during calm situations. It allows the body to achieve a resting state following an emergency. Table 4.3 contrasts the effects of stimulating the sympathetic and parasympathetic systems.

TABLE 4.3 Comparison of Sympathetic and Parasympathetic Systems

Sympathetic Effects	Parasympathetic Effects
Increases heart rate	Decreases heart rate
Constricts blood vessels	Dilates blood vessels
Slows down intestinal action	Increases intestinal action
Dilates pupils	Constricts pupils
Relaxes gall bladder	Constricts gallbladder

Drugs that mimic actions of the sympathetic system are called **sympathomimetics**. Examples are amphetamines, cocaine, and caffeine. Drugs that mimic actions of the parasympathetic system are called **parasympathomimetics**. Examples are nicotine and the hallucinogen *Amanita muscaria*.

Drugs and Major Body Systems

The impact of drugs is not limited to the nervous system. Drugs affect the endocrine, cardiovascular, respiratory, and gastrointestinal systems as well.

Endocrine System

Many structures make up the endocrine system. Because these structures release hormones directly into the bloodstream rather than through ducts, the glands of the endocrine system are called ductless glands. Hormones released by the endocrine system have many effects ranging from stimulating the growth of new tissues to storing nutrients, maintaining homeostasis, and affecting metabolism and sexual behavior. The hypothalamus controls the endocrine system and the pituitary gland, the latter of which has been called the "master gland."

The pituitary gland consists of the anterior pituitary and the posterior pituitary. In females, the anterior pituitary secretes FSH and LH, which cause women's ovaries to produce the sex hormones estrogen and progesterone. Besides regulating the menstrual cycle, estrogen is responsible for development of secondary sex characteristics. In males, FSH and interstitial cell-stimulating hormone (ICSH) produce androgen in the testicles. The primary androgenic hormone, testosterone, is produced in the testes and is necessary for sperm production and development of secondary sex characteristics.

Two hormones released by the posterior pituitary are oxytocin and vasopressin (also known as the antidiuretic hormone or ADH). Oxytocin causes uterine contractions during pregnancy and is administered sometimes to induce contractions during a difficult or slow labor. It has also been associated with bonding and nurturing among both men and women and has been implicated in aggression among outsiders of a group. Vasopressin causes an increase in blood pressure and prevents urine from building up in the kidneys. Recent studies regarding vasopressin have shown a relationship between the hormone and pair-bonding or lifelong attachments in monogamous relationships.[30]

The adrenal glands, another part of the endocrine system, are located at the top of each kidney and secrete adrenaline and cortisol. Adrenaline prepares the body to fight or flee. Cortisol is administered primarily to treat inflammation and to diminish arthritic deterioration of the joints. Unfortunately, cortisol produces a number of undesirable side effects, so synthetic drugs similar to cortisol are being used now.

Cardiovascular System

The heart and blood vessels constitute the cardiovascular system. One arguably could state that the heart is the body's most important organ because people die within minutes when it stops functioning. The heart is responsible for pumping blood throughout the body, delivering nutrients and oxygen through the blood. Drugs that interfere with the heart's ability to contract present a danger. For example, alcohol can cause the heart muscle to degenerate, induce cardiac arrhythmia (irregular heartbeat), and increase blood pressure, which can bring about a heart attack. Heavy, short-term alcohol abuse over several days can cause "holiday heart syndrome," a condition marked by cardiac arrhythmia and symptoms similar to a heart attack.

A drug often implicated in cardiovascular disease is caffeine. Despite popular belief, there is insufficient proof that moderate caffeine use raises the risk of heart disease. A more in-depth look at the research on caffeine and heart disease is included in Chapter 11.

Cocaine has been found to be detrimental to the cardiovascular system. It produces a significant rise in heart rate and blood pressure, thereby increasing the risk for heart attack. Cocaine also is a vasoconstrictor, depriving the heart of needed blood. A particular concern is that cocaine use can produce cardiovascular damage in young people who appear healthy and have no history of heart disease. Further, cardiovascular problems can arise from only small to moderate amounts of cocaine.

Smoked drugs pose a special risk to the cardiovascular system because smoke interferes with the ability of the blood to distribute oxygen. There is much justified concern about the relationship between tobacco and lung cancer. Yet, smokers are far more likely to die from cardiovascular disease than from cancer. A smoker is twice as likely to have a heart attack as a nonsmoker. Nicotine in cigarettes raises the blood pressure, and carbon monoxide makes the heart work harder because the amount of oxygen delivered throughout the body is reduced. A positive note is that people who quit smoking have no greater risk of heart disease than nonsmokers after several years.

Marijuana also produces increased heart rate, called tachycardia. The heart rate is temporarily increased by as much as 50% after marijuana use. Patients with angina pectoris (chest pain related to diminished blood supply to the heart) are more susceptible to angina after smoking marijuana.

Respiratory System

Many drugs interfere with the functioning of the respiratory system. In particular, depressant drugs such as barbiturates, minor tranquilizers, alcohol, and narcotics can have tragic effects because they slow down respiration. Any depressant can cause breathing to stop. Combining depressants with other drugs can have a **synergistic effect**. For example, using alcohol and barbiturates together can be a deadly mix.

Stimulants such as amphetamines and cocaine increase the respiratory rate. Some stimulants can be beneficial. Tea, containing the stimulant theophylline, has been recommended for people with breathing difficulties because it causes the air passages to open.

Smoked tobacco is especially harmful to the respiratory system. Cigarette smoke impedes the cilia from removing mucus and other foreign matter from the lungs. Breathing becomes labored. Close to 70% of the particles in tobacco smoke stay in the lungs. Not only do smokers have more respiratory infections than nonsmokers, but their infections tend to be more severe. Marijuana, too, impairs the ability of the lungs to function properly. Because marijuana is inhaled more deeply and for longer periods than regular tobacco, more particles probably are retained from marijuana. Chronic marijuana smoking results in air passages becoming smaller. In addition, marijuana has as much tar and half as many carcinogens as conventional tobacco.

Gastrointestinal System

The gastrointestinal system, consisting of the esophagus, stomach, and intestines, enables the body to

peripheral nervous system (PNS) Consists of the autonomic and somatic nervous systems

somatic nervous system Part of the nervous system that controls movement of the skeletal muscles

autonomic nervous system (ANS) Part of the peripheral nervous system that is automatic and involuntary

sympathetic nervous system A branch of the autonomic nervous system that releases adrenaline

parasympathetic nervous system Branch of the autonomic nervous system that includes acetylcholine and alters heart rate and intestinal activity

sympathomimetics Drugs that mimic actions of the sympathetic nervous system, which is involved with fight-flight-fright activity

parasympathomimetics Drugs that mimic actions of the parasympathetic system, which allows the body to rest during states of emergency

synergistic effect An enhanced, unpredictable effect caused by combining two or more substances

absorb nutrients and water and remove waste. Gastrointestinal disorders affect millions of people. Upset stomach, ulcers, constipation, and diarrhea are common maladies of modern society. To neutralize stomach acid, antacids containing sodium bicarbonate, calcium carbonate, aluminium hydroxide, or magnesium salts are ingested. Laxatives are used to relieve constipation.

Many drugs contribute to gastrointestinal disorders. Alcohol causes diarrhea, as well as irritation and inflammation of the stomach, small intestine, esophagus, and pancreas. Moreover, it eventually results in malnutrition by interfering with the absorption of nutrients. A combination that is especially harmful to the stomach is alcohol and aspirin, because it can cause excessive internal bleeding. Peyote can produce nausea and vomiting. Although narcotics cause constipation, they can be beneficial, even life-saving, to people suffering from diarrhea—a common cause of death in many underdeveloped countries.

Factors Influencing the Effects of Drugs

The effects of drugs are a function of their pharmacological or chemical makeup. A drug's pharmacology or chemistry, however, does not tell the whole story. Individual and cultural factors play a significant role, too.

Age

Infants and the elderly are more sensitive to the effects of drugs than people between those life stages. Drug actions are prolonged in infants and the elderly because their liver and kidneys are function less effectively making it more difficult to metabolize and excrete drugs.

An increased risk of fractures and falls occur among elderly who are taking SSRIs.[31] Recall, SSRIs are used to treat depression. A little over 10% of the elderly, who require home healthcare or are in a hospital, are depressed.[32] There has been some research that suggests SSRIs many contribute to bone loss in the elderly, but this relationship has not been seen in younger adults.[33]

Two percent of adults aged 55 or older are admitted for treatment from abusing prescription narcotic medications.[34] The American Medical Association calls substance abuse among the elderly a hidden epidemic.[35] It is estimated that 4.4 million older adults will need substance abuse treatment by 2020.[36] Elderly women are more likely than men to be at risk for drug-related problems because they receive more prescriptions. This is partly because women see physicians more often than men do.

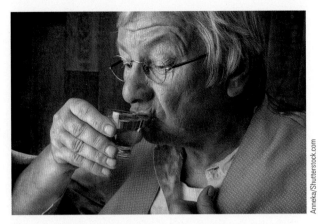

Tolerance for alcohol lessens as people age.

Tolerance for alcohol lessens as people age.[37] Blood alcohol concentrations are higher in the elderly when they drink, because they have less body fluid. The elderly have less lean body mass as a result of aging, which may reduce the distribution of alcohol leading to higher blood alcohol count. Consider someone who has always had two drinks after work, and continues this habit as this person ages. Due to the impact of aging and increased sensitivity to alcohol, these two drinks become enough to make the person drunk.[38] Thus, even though drinking habits have not changed, the effects of alcohol do. One encouraging study, however, reported that older men and women drank less alcohol as they aged.[39] As people age, their percentage of body fat increases. Some drugs accumulate in adipose tissue, increasing the sensitivity to those drugs and the possibility of a toxic reaction. Antidepressant drugs serve as a good example. Although they are effective with 70 to 90% of the elderly who take them, they can precipitate glaucoma, impair the prostate gland, and cause delirium and confusion.

There is also some research showing that elementary-age children respond differently to drugs. The over-the-counter antihistamine diphenhydramine, commonly sold under the trade name Benadryl, has a strong sedating effect on adults. However, researchers in Denver found that this drug did not have a sleep-like effect on children. Moreover, these children scored as well on cognitive tests as children receiving placebos.[40]

Gender

Females and males respond to drugs differently. Differences in how drugs affect men and women are related to fat and water content, not gender per se. Women who weigh the same as men have a higher percentage of body fat and a lower percentage of water, making women more sensitive to the actions of drugs because fat stores drugs and water dilutes the amount of a drug in the bloodstream.

Hormones also make a difference. During the premenstrual phase of the menstrual cycle, women absorb ethyl alcohol more quickly. Females are especially affected by drugs during pregnancy. Many drugs traverse the placental barrier. Because the fetus lacks enzymes and its excretory system is not fully developed, drugs have a greater impact on the fetus than on the pregnant woman. Drugs causing damage to the fetus are called **teratogenic**. Finally, the use of tobacco, coffee, and alcohol during pregnancy increases the risk of miscarriages.

Other drugs react differently in men and women. Ibuprofen, an over-the-counter medication, is more effective in men while opioid painkillers are more effective in reducing pain in women.[41] For treating depression, SSRIs may be more effective for women, while men do better on tricyclics.[42] Lastly, the FDA recently changed its guidelines for prescribing sleeping tablets for women. It seems women have higher levels of the drug in their system after taking it, which would impact driving and other tasks. As a result, the FDA lowered the recommended doses for women.[43]

Dosage

The amount of a drug consumed—the dosage—plays a significant role in the effects of drugs. Before it produces an effect, the drug must be present in a certain amount. The smallest amount of a drug required to produce an effect is called the **threshold dose**. Typically, as the dosage increases, the effects become more pronounced. Because the effects of drugs are not always proportional, they do not affect everyone in the same way. If twice the amount of a drug is administered, it will not necessarily be twice as effective or potent. Some drugs work on an all-or-none basis in that they act either maximally or not at all.

The amount necessary to achieve a specific response is called the **effective dose (ED)**. If a drug is identified as ED 50, it produces an effect in 50% of the population tested. The quantity required to cause death is the **lethal dose (LD)**. The safety of a drug is determined by the difference between its ED and LD.

teratogenic Refers to substances that cause harm to the fetus

threshold dose The smallest amount of a drug required to produce an effect

effective dose (ED) The amount of drug required to produce a specific response

lethal dose (LD) The amount of a drug required to result in death

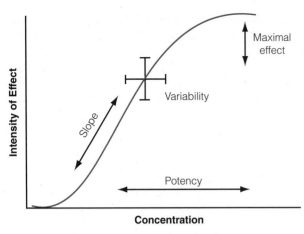

Figure 4.6 Dose-Response Curve

The greater the margin between the ED and LD, the safer the drug. When discussing the effects of drugs at different dosage levels, pharmacologists refer to the **dose-response curve** (Figure 4.6), which plots the specific effects that occur at specific doses. More pronounced effects take place as the dosage level goes up, although age, gender, size, and overall health also matter. Not surprisingly, there is less variability *within* a species than among species.

Purity and Potency

Many health-related problems that drug users experience arise from impurities rather than from the drugs themselves. The quality or **purity** of drugs, which varies greatly among illegal drugs, is a significant factor in the drug's effect. The Drug Enforcement Administration (DEA) found that the purity of heroin purchased in the mid-1970s was about 6%. In the early 1980s, purity was less than 4%, and it was more than 20% in the early 1990s. By 2001, the purity of heroin ranged from 51 to 69%. The purity of cocaine was as low as 53% and as high as 69%.[44]

Potency refers to a drug's ability to produce an effect relative to other drugs. The smaller the quantity required to elicit an effect, the more powerful the drug. Comparing heroin, morphine, and aspirin as pain relievers, heroin is the most potent, followed by morphine, and then aspirin. Thus a smaller amount of heroin than morphine or aspirin is needed to reduce pain to the same degree. Some drugs vary naturally in potency. For example, the percentage of THC, the psychoactive substance in marijuana, ranges from 4 to 9%.

Drug Interactions

The interaction of drugs with other drugs or certain foods can be hazardous. An estimated 25% of admissions to emergency rooms result from interactions between alcohol and medications.[45] Some medicines can cause a person to be sleepy or drowsy and the use of alcohol with these medications may intensify those effects.[46] For example, the herbal preparation, Kava Kava, used for anxiety can cause liver damage and drowsiness when taken with alcohol.

The effects of drugs and food can be additive, antagonistic, or synergistic. Additive effects refer to the sum or cumulative effects of two or more substances mixed together. Combining aspirin and alcohol, for example, increases the risk of intestinal and prolonged bleeding.

Antagonistic drugs negate the effects of other drugs. One commonly prescribed drug that is antagonistic is the antibiotic tetracycline. Mixing it with penicillin, milk, or antacids negates its actions, and penicillin is ineffective when used with milk or antacids. Using barbiturates with diphenhydramine (Benadryl) or dimenhydrinate (Dramamine) negates the effectiveness of both. Minor tranquilizers such as Valium, Miltown, and Librium reduce the effectiveness of oral contraceptives. It has been found that more than 150 prescription and over-the-counter medications interact negatively with alcohol.[47] Therefore, when obtaining a prescription, one should ask a pharmacist or physician about possible drug interactions.

The combination of some drugs has a synergistic effect. The combined effect of taking both drugs is greater than if the drugs' effects are simply added together. One way to illustrate this concept is to consider muscular strength. If a person has enough muscle mass in the bicep to lift 25 pounds of weight and enough muscle mass in the forearm to lift 25 pounds of weight, the person theoretically can lift 50 pounds. Because the muscles in the bicep and forearm work in concert, however, the person may be able to lift 100 pounds instead of 50.

Some drugs have this same type of synergism: Their effects when combined are much greater than the sum of their effects when administered individually. An example of such a synergistic combination of drugs is barbiturates and alcohol. Every year, several thousand people die from combining these two drugs, either accidentally or intentionally. Table 4.4 shows some possible risks of mixing alcohol with other drugs.

dose-response curve Graphic representation of the effects of drugs at various levels

purity Quality of a substance; state of noncontamination of a drug

potency A drug's ability to produce an effect relative to other drugs; the less that is needed to produce a response, the more potent the drug

Taking certain antidepressants with certain foods can result in hemorrhaging and stroke. People who eat foods containing tyramine—such as red wine, beer, chocolate, raisins, and aged cheeses—while taking an antidepressant monoamine oxidase (MAO) inhibitor can experience an increase in blood pressure to perilously high levels. Another dangerous mixture is oral contraceptives and tobacco. Women who smoke and take oral contraceptives have a greater chance of developing a heart attack, stroke, or blood clots. Also, the risk of a heart attack and stroke increases for smokers who are taking medication to relieve hypertension.

TABLE 4.4 Drug Interactions with Alcohol

Symptom/Disorders	Medication (Brand Name)	Medication (Generic Name)	Some Possible Reactions with Alcohol
Allergies/colds/flu	Allegra®, Allegra-D®	Fexofenadin	Drowsiness, dizziness; increased risk for overdose
	Benadryl®	Diphenhydramine	
	Claritin®, Claritin-D®	Loratadine	
	Dimetapp® Cold & Allergy	Brompheniramine	
	Sudafed® Sinus & Allergy	Chlorpheniramine	
	Triaminic® Cold & Allergy	Chlorpheniramine	
	Tylenol® Allergy Sinus	Chlorpheniramine	
	Tylenol® Cold & Flu	Chlorpheniramine	
	Zyrtec®	Cetirizine	
Angina (chest pain), coronary heart disease	Isordil®	Isosorbide	Rapid heartbeat, sudden changes in blood pressure, dizziness, fainting
		Nitroglycerin	
Anxiety and epilepsy	Ativan®	Lorazepam	Drowsiness, dizziness; increased risk for overdose; slowed or difficulty breathing; impaired motor control; unusual behavior; and memory problems
	Librium®	Chlordiazepoxide	
	Paxil®	Paroxetine	
	Valium®	Diazepam	
	Xanax®	Alprazolam	
	Herbal preparations (kava kava)		Liver damage, drowsiness
Arthritis	Celebrex®	Celecoxib	Ulcers, stomach bleeding, liver problems
	Naprosyn®	Naproxen	
Blood clots	Coumadin®	Warfarin	Occasional drinking may lead to internal bleeding; heavier drinking also may cause bleeding or may have the opposite effect, resulting in possible blood clots, strokes, or heart attacks
Cough	Delsym®, Robitussin Cough®	Dextromethorpan	Drowsiness, dizziness; increased risk for overdose
	Robitussin A–C®	Guaifenesin + codeine	
Depression	Anafranil®	Clomipramine	Drowsiness, dizziness; increased risk for overdose; increased feelings of depression or hopelessness in adolescents (suicide)
	Effexor®	Venlafaxine	
	Elavil®	Amitriptyline	
	Lexapro®	Escitalopram	
	Luvox®	Fluvoxamine	
	Prozac®	Fluoxetine	
	Wellbutrin®	Bupropion	
	Zoloft®	Sertraline	
	Herbal preparations (St. John's wort)		
Diabetes	Glucophage®	Metformin	Abnormally low blood sugar levels, flushing reaction (nausea, vomiting, headache, rapid heartbeat, sudden changes in blood pressure)
	Micronase®	Glyburide	
	Orinase®	Tolbutamide	

(continued)

TABLE 4.4 *continued*

Symptom/Disorders	Medication (Brand Name)	Medication (Generic Name)	Some Possible Reactions with Alcohol
Heartburn, indigestion, sour stomach	Tagamet®	Cimetidine	Rapid heartbeat, sudden changes in blood pressure (metoclopramide); increased alcohol effect
	Zantac®	Ranitidine	
High blood pressure	Accupril®	Quinapril	Dizziness, fainting, drowsiness; heart problems such as changes in the heart's regular heartbeat (arrhythmia)
	Hytrin®	Terazosin	
	Lopressor® HCT	Hydrochlorothiazide	
	Lotensin®	Benzapril	
	Minipress®	Prazosin	
	Vaseretic®	Enalapril	
High cholesterol	Crestor®	Rosuvastatin	Liver damage (all medications); increased flushing and itching (niacin), increased stomach bleeding (pravastatin + aspirin)
	Lipitor®	Atorvastatin	
	Pravachol®	Pravastatin	
	Vytorin™	Ezetimibe + simvastatin	
	Zocor®	Simvastatin	
Muscle pain	Flexeril®	Cyclobenzaprine	Drowsiness, dizziness; increased risk of seizures; increased risk for overdose; slowed or difficulty breathing; impaired motor control; unusual behavior; memory problems
	Soma®	Carisoprodol	
Nausea, motion sickness	Dramamine®	Dimenhydrinate	Drowsiness, dizziness; increased risk for overdose
Pain (such as headache, muscle ache, minor arthritis pain), fever, inflammation	Advil®	Ibuprofen	Stomach upset, bleeding and ulcers; liver damage (acetaminophen); rapid heartbeat
	Aleve®	Naproxen	
	Excedrin®	Aspirin, acetaminophen	
	Motrin®	Ibuprofen	
	Tylenol®	Acetaminophen	
Seizures	Dilantin®	Phenytoin	Drowsiness, dizziness; increased risk of seizures
	Klonopin®	Clonazepam	
		Phenobarbital	
Severe pain from injury, postsurgical care, oral surgery, migraines	Darvocet–N®	Propoxyphene	Drowsiness, dizziness; increased risk for overdose; slowed or difficulty breathing; impaired motor control; unusual behavior; memory problems
	Demerol®	Merepidine	
	Percocet®	Oxycodone	
	Vicodin®	Hydrocodone	
Sleep problems	Ambien®	Zolpidem	Drowsiness, sleepiness, dizziness; slowed or difficulty breathing; impaired motor control; unusual behavior; memory problems
	Lunesta™	Eszopiclone	
	Sominex®	Diphenhydramine	
	Unisom®	Doxylamine	Increased drowsiness
	Herbal preparations (chamomile, valerian, lavender)		

Source: *Harmful Interactions: Mixing Alcohol with Medicines* (Rockville, MD: National Institute on Alcohol Abuse and Alcoholism, 2007).

Tolerance

Tolerance has been defined as "a state of progressively decreasing responsiveness to a drug."[48] In developing tolerance, increasing amounts of a drug are required. Tolerance depends on dosage, the type of drug, and frequency of use. Even though a person may require a greater amount of a drug to achieve the desired results, the amount required to cause a fatal overdose does not necessarily increase. The types of tolerance are pharmacological, behavioral, cross-, and reverse tolerance.

Pharmacological Tolerance

Pharmacological tolerance means that the body adjusts to or compensates for the presence of a particular drug. This could arise from the rapid deactivation or excretion of drugs resulting from repeated use. Therefore, to achieve the effect desired, the person has to increase either the amount or the frequency of use.

Depressant drugs provide an example. If the same dosage of a depressant is maintained over a long enough period, that dosage no longer has the desired effect. Similarly, an individual develops tolerance to alcohol, although not everyone has the same tolerance level. Some people are born with naturally higher tolerance levels, suggesting that they can drink more alcohol than others without feeling the effects of alcohol. Likewise, the capacity to reach a state of euphoria from amphetamines declines with regular use, although continued use can produce psychotic-like effects.

Behavioral Tolerance

Behavioral tolerance means that an individual *learns* to adjust to the presence of drugs. After repeated exposure to a drug, experienced drug users are more able to moderate their behavior than people who are less experienced with drugs. Individuals are capable of developing behavioral tolerance more quickly if they are offered an incentive.[49] In a sense, they are conditioned to the effects of the drug. A person who frequently drinks alcohol often can function better under the influence of alcohol than someone who does not drink or one who drinks infrequently.

Cross-Tolerance

Cross-tolerance means that people who develop tolerance to a drug will develop tolerance to chemically similar drugs. If a person becomes tolerant to LSD, for example, he or she will develop tolerance to other hallucinogens, such as mescaline and peyote. Likewise, chronic alcohol users become tolerant not only to alcohol but to other depressants such as barbiturates and minor tranquilizers as well.

Reverse Tolerance

Reverse tolerance means that a drug user will feel the desired effects from lesser amounts of the drug. Hallucinogens and marijuana have been used as examples, though one possible explanation for reverse tolerance in marijuana is that it is stored in fatty tissue and later released as fat breaks down. Also, experienced marijuana users anticipate the drug's effects, and the learning process may play an important role. Reverse tolerance to alcohol seems to occur in the later stages of alcoholism because of progressive liver dysfunction in which the liver enzymes are inadequate to metabolize alcohol.

Set and Setting

Two vital, interlocking components of the drug experience are set and setting. **Set** refers to the drug user's psychological makeup, personality, mood, and

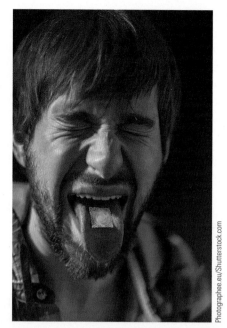

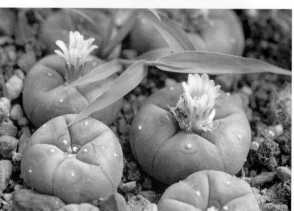

People who develop tolerance to LSD will also have tolerance to mescaline.

expectations when using drugs. **Setting** alludes to the social and physical environment in which drugs are taken. Set, then, deals with the internal environment, and setting relates to the external environment. The

pharmacological tolerance Adjustment or compensation of the body to the presence of a given drug

behavioral tolerance Adjustment or behaviors learned by an individual to compensate for the presence of drugs

cross-tolerance Transference of tolerance to a drug to chemically similar drugs

reverse tolerance A drug user's experiencing of the desired effects from lesser amounts of the same drug

set The psychological state, personality, and expectations of an individual while using drugs

setting The physical and social environment in which drugs are used

effects of drugs on behavior depend greatly on one's attitudes toward drugs, emotional state, and previous experiences with drugs. If a person is depressed or anxious or previously had an unpleasant experience while taking drugs, the effects will be different than if one is in a happy mood or is looking forward to the drug's effects.

Placebos are inert substances capable of producing psychological and physiological reactions. A large percentage of prescriptions given to patients are placebos. They are effective because of expectations for the drug. Placebos may provide relief for 30 to 40% of patients for whom they are prescribed.[50]

The notion of a drug being euphoric or dysphoric depends a great deal on set. For example, people using cocaine who are under stress in their lives may be more susceptible to dysphoria from the drug. Someone in a hospital who is given morphine for analgesic purposes during surgery probably would not describe the effects of morphine in euphoric terms, whereas a person using morphine bought illegally may well describe the effects very differently.

On many college campuses, heavy drinking is associated with football game days. For example, on football game days, fans drink more alcohol and are more affected than nonfans. One study found that males drink more than females but that females experience more adverse consequences. The age group that drank more alcohol was the 21 to 26 age group, as opposed to younger or older age groups.[51]

The portrayal of a drug's effects also is different if drugs are consumed alone or with friends at a party. To a large extent, setting determines set. Taking legal drugs among friends is likely to be viewed as drug *use*. Taking illegal drugs by oneself is likely to be seen as drug *abuse*.

Methods of Administration

How a drug enters the body has a significant bearing on its effects. The route of administration determines how quickly a drug takes effect, the amount of time it is active, its intensity, and how localized its actions are. Drugs enter the body via oral ingestion, injection, topical application to the skin, inhalation, suppositories, and implantation.

Oral Ingestion

Drugs can be consumed in the form of pills, liquids, tablets, or capsules. Though oral ingestion is one of the most convenient, safest, and most common ways to consume drugs, several factors make it difficult to control the dosage level. Once a drug enters the

stomach, its effectiveness is reduced because it mixes with food, acid, and digestive enzymes in the gastrointestinal tract. Any food present slows the rate of absorption of the drug into the bloodstream. Drugs in the form of capsules and tablets must dissolve before they enter the bloodstream.

Some of the disadvantages of taking drugs orally include the following:[52]

- Oral administration is not appropriate in emergencies because drugs are absorbed slowly.
- The slow absorption rate may reduce the amount of the drug to an insufficient level.
- People could fatally choke on a drug if they are not conscious.
- Some ingested drugs cause nausea and vomiting.
- Because conditions in the gastrointestinal tract are changing constantly, drug absorption is variable.

Injection

Parenteral drug use refers to injecting drugs. Injected drugs reach the brain quickly but carry many risks. Drugs such as heroin may not be lethal when they are smoked but may be lethal when they are injected. Injecting drugs with unsterile hypodermic needles poses a risk for infectious diseases including AIDS and hepatitis. Thousands of AIDS infections in women can be attributed to injection drug use. Needle-exchange programs report fewer addicts sharing needles even though the federal government prohibits its drug treatment funds to be used for such programs. Figure 4.7 shows the percentage of males

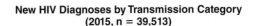

New HIV Diagnoses by Transmission Category
(2015, n = 39,513)

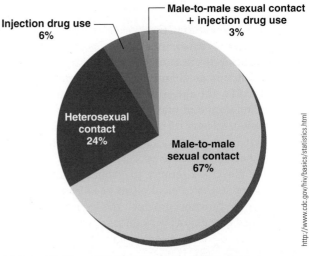

http://www.cdc.gov/hiv/basics/statistics.html

Figure 4.7 New HIV Diagnoses by transmission category-2015

Source: Division of HIV/AIDS Prevention, Viral Hepatitis, STDS and Tuberculosis Prevention/CDC

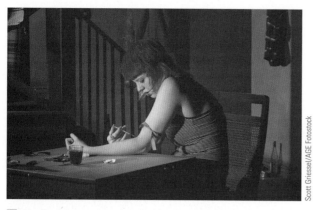

Scott Griessel/AGE Fotostock

■ Health risks are associated with injected drug use.

and females who contracted AIDS through different modes of transmission.

Drugs can be injected intravenously, intramuscularly, or subcutaneously.

Intravenous Injection

In intravenous injection, or mainlining, drugs are administered directly into the bloodstream. Within a minute after injection, the drug is distributed to all parts of the body in high concentration. Consequently, the effects of drugs are experienced quickly and fully when they are taken intravenously.

Further, drugs can be measured precisely when they are administered intravenously. Unlike drugs taken orally, drugs given intravenously do not mix with stomach contents. Thus intravenous drugs do not have to be absorbed first. Although these factors are seen as advantages, repeated intravenous injections increase the risk of clot formation as well as vessel irritation and collapse.

Intramuscular Injection

In intramuscular injection, drugs are injected into muscle tissue. Because muscle tissue serves as a filter, drugs delivered intramuscularly are absorbed more slowly than drugs delivered intravenously. For example, the onset of euphoria after injecting heroin intravenously is 7 to 8 seconds. When it is injected intramuscularly, the onset of euphoria is 5 to

8 minutes.[53] The rate of absorption depends on the muscle receiving the drug. The more blood vessels the muscle has, the more quickly the drug is absorbed. Drugs injected into the deltoid muscle are absorbed more rapidly than the same drugs injected into the buttocks.

Subcutaneous Injection

Injecting drugs just below the layers of the skin is called subcutaneous injection. With this method, also known as skin-popping, drugs are absorbed less evenly. Although subcutaneous injection is safer than intravenous injection, skin irritation and abscesses can occur.

Topical Application

Drugs can be applied to the skin and absorbed into the bloodstream by placing small disks or patches behind the ear or on the arm or chest. Called the **transdermal method**, the use of this method is limited because of the uneven way in which drugs are absorbed. Also, drugs are introduced into the body slowly when applied topically. An advantage to transdermal application is that drugs are absorbed directly into the bloodstream at programmed rates. Transdermal patches have been used to relieve motion sickness, angina pectoris, and nicotine dependency.

Inhalation

Drugs can be absorbed into the bloodstream via the lungs through inhalation. The speed and efficiency of drugs entering the bloodstream are quite high because of the accessibility of the capillary walls of the lung. However, the actual amount of an inhaled drug that reaches the brain is variable. Nevertheless, inhaled drugs reach the brain in 5 to 8 seconds, though the effects usually are brief. Inhaled drugs irritate the lungs.

parenteral drug use Drug administration by injection

transdermal method Administration of drugs by applying them on the surface of the skin

Summary

Drugs alter behavior by the way they affect the central nervous system (CNS). The CNS contains neurons that act as messengers. Consisting of the brain and spinal cord, the CNS has nerve cells, or neurons, that act as messengers. The impulses that pass through the neuron are electrical, and those from the axon

to the dendrite are chemical. To send electrical messages from the axon of one neuron to the dendrite of another neuron, the messages or impulses must cross a space called the synapse.

At the end of each axon are saclike structures or vesicles containing neurotransmitters. Neurotransmitters are chemicals discharged by one neuron that change electrical activity in another neuron. These chemicals have many effects on the mind and body.

Various parts of the brain have their own functions. The reticular activating system (RAS) affects arousal, attention, and sleep. The hypothalamus helps to maintain homeostasis and one's response to stress, and the cerebral cortex enables one to process information and engage in higher-level thinking. The limbic system plays a key role in making a connection between memory and emotion. The medial forebrain bundle (MFB) is the center for pleasure and pain, and the basal ganglia help govern involuntary muscle control. The brain stem is involved in vital functions, including breathing, heartbeat, dilation of the pupils, and blood pressure.

Many factors besides pharmacology account for the way drugs affect people. Age, gender, presence of other drugs, dosage, and setting can help contribute to the ways a drug affects a person.

Another concept relating to the effects of drugs is tolerance. The four types of tolerance are the following:

1. Pharmacological tolerance: A drug has less effect because the body adjusts to the drug based on previous experiences with it.
2. Behavioral tolerance: The person has learned to adapt to the effects of a drug.
3. Cross-tolerance: A person adjusts to drugs that are chemically similar.
4. Reverse tolerance: The person achieves the desired effects of a drug at decreasing levels.

Drugs can enter the body through various means. One of the most common and simplest ways is ingestion. Because ingested drugs mix with the contents in the stomach, their rate of absorption is difficult to control. Drugs injected intravenously are distributed quickly and at high concentrations. Drugs injected intramuscularly are absorbed less quickly, and drugs injected subcutaneously are the least efficiently absorbed.

Thinking Critically

1. An argument for legalizing drugs relates to purity and potency. If drugs were legal, proponents say, there would be more assurance regarding the quality and strength of drugs. What are the arguments against this line of reasoning?
2. A man and a woman both go to a party. They each drink four alcoholic beverages during the party.

At the end of the night, the woman is crying and very drunk. The man, although tipsy, is happy, smiling, and seems more composed. Discuss the reasons why, even though these two people consumed the same drug and same amount, reacted very differently to the drug.

5

Synthetic, Performance-Enhancing, and Other Drugs

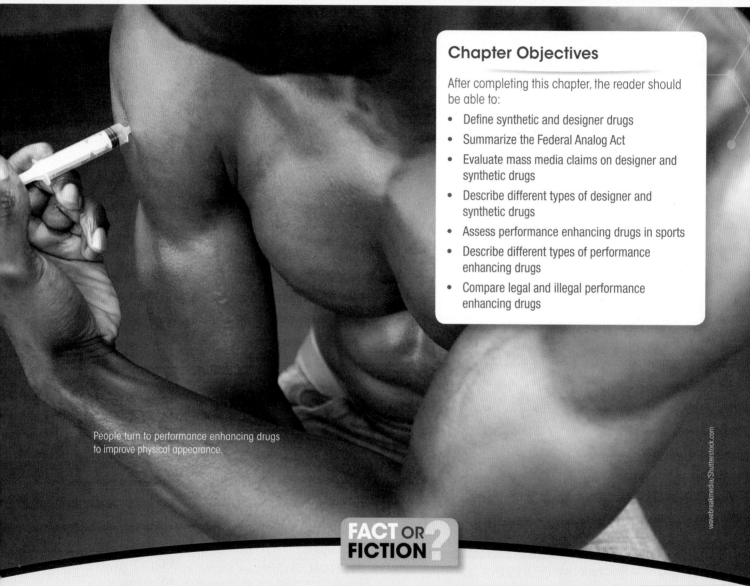

Chapter Objectives

After completing this chapter, the reader should be able to:

- Define synthetic and designer drugs
- Summarize the Federal Analog Act
- Evaluate mass media claims on designer and synthetic drugs
- Describe different types of designer and synthetic drugs
- Assess performance enhancing drugs in sports
- Describe different types of performance enhancing drugs
- Compare legal and illegal performance enhancing drugs

People turn to performance enhancing drugs to improve physical appearance.

wavebreakmedia/Shutterstock.com

FACT OR FICTION?

1. Designer drugs are synthesized from restricted chemicals.

2. The synthetic drug bath salts are related to bath salts (ones you use in the bathtub).

3. Bath salts can turn people into zombies.

4. BZP is 10 to 20 times less potent than amphetamines.

5. In the 1970's MDMA was used as an anxiety reducing drug.

6. Performance enhancing drugs is a relatively new phenomenon.

7. Anabolic steroids have medical benefits.

8. Creatine use has been banned by the NCAA.

9. Caffeine use has no impact on athletic performance.

10. Mexican based criminal organizations are the main suppliers of drugs in the United States.

Turn the page to check your answers

Designer drugs have been in the scene since the 1980s, but have experienced a reemergence in recent years. Media headlines tend to sensationalize these drugs and may overemphasize their use. Manufacturers of designer drugs have historically been able to skirt the law by making minor changes in the chemical sequence, thus staying ahead of the law. Recent changes to the wording of the law made it possible for a substance to remain illegal, even if minor changes were made to its chemical structure.

Performance enhancing drugs have been since the third century as a way to increase physical performance in competitions. Over the past decade, many cases have come up regarding performance enhancing drugs and professional athletes including Olympiads. This chapter will highlight some of the main drugs that belong in this category, their impact on performance, and the effects of these drugs on the body.

The business of drugs continues to be a problem around the world. From producers, to distributers, these supply chains develop as a response to demand. If there was not a demand for drugs, drug businesses would fail. This section will highlight some of the main findings from the World Drug Report 2016 and discuss the impact of policies on the drug business.

Designer Drugs

Someone with knowledge of chemistry may alter the chemical structure of a compound and produce a new drug that not only is psychoactive but also is legal. In recent years, there has been a proliferation of so-called **designer drugs**. The term arose in the 1980s to describe **synthetic drugs** that individuals abused.[1] These drugs often mimic the effects of other drugs. These drugs include bath salts (cathinone), Spice, and BZP (benzylpiperazine). Designer drugs synthesized from common chemicals are usually uncontrolled by the Drug Enforcement Agency. Problems arise regarding the legislation of designer drugs because the chemists who develop them can quickly alter the chemical sequence, making them legal again.

In 1981, an attorney and a paralegal working together did some research and discovered they can create a synthetic drug (heroin) and sell it legally. Their first venture did not turn out a success as they managed to burn down a house and cause leakage of HCl, which resulted in evacuation of much of the area. Arrangements had to be made to properly dispose of the chemical. During the investigation of the fire, personnel came across a binder filed with patents, syntheses, and notes about fentanyl analogs.[2] No arrests were made. A year later, these men tried their luck again, this time creating 4-propyloxy-4-phenyl-N-methylpiperidine (MPPP), which is related to heroin. Due to the slight modification in its structure, it was a legal substance.[3] Unfortunately, they failed to keep the proper temperatures during the process and created a toxic byproduct that caused severe brain damage.[4]

Concern regarding designer drugs began in 1982, when George Carillo, a 42-year-old man, was brought into the Santa Clara Valley Medical Center. He was described as a mannequin because he was unable to move; his body was twisted and drool came out of his mouth. The neurologist at the hospital diagnosed him with Parkinson's, which is highly unusual given the age of the patient; Parkinson's rarely

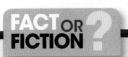

1. **FICTION** The fact is—Designer drugs are created from commonly used chemicals.

2. **FICTION** The fact is—The drug bath salts are not related to the one for use in the bathtub.

3. **FICTION** The fact is—Zombies do not exist.

4. **FACT** Amphetamines are stronger than BZP.

5. **FACT** Psychiatrists prescribed MDMA to clients to reduce anxiety and promote communication. Currently it is approved by the FDA for studies investigating its use for physical pain, psychological trauma in patients dying of cancer, and chronic pain.

6. **FICTION** The fact is—It has been around since the 3rd century. Greek athletes ate mushrooms to enhance their performance.

7. **FACT** They are prescribed to treat hypogonadism, some types of impotence, and to AIDS patients to treat body wasting.

8. **FICTION** The fact is—Creatine is not on the list of banned substances and is one of the most popular supplements on the market.

9. **FICTION** The fact is—In moderate doses (3 cups of coffee), caffeine has shown to improve performance in short term endurance activities.

10. **FACT** In fact, United States gangs are collaborating with Mexican criminal organizations to help them distribute drugs in local areas.

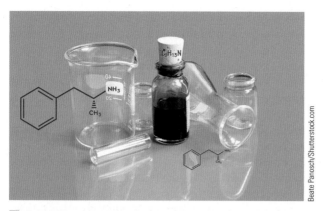

Designer and synthetic drugs were initially difficult to regulate. Once a molecular compound was identified as being illegal, drug producers would change the formula slightly making it legal again. To address this issue, Congress passed the Analog Act.

affects people under the age of 50 and to the extent of the symptoms the patient was displaying, it would have suggested an advanced stage of the disease by at least 10 years. Doctors were puzzled by this case even more when the patient led them to his girlfriend who also had symptoms of the disease. A little later, two brothers, both in their 20s were hospitalized with similar symptoms. These cases had doctors confused until they discovered they had all used a synthetic (and legal) version of heroin type drug.[5]

The problems regarding the legality of this drug arose from the fact that laws regarding legal illegal drugs were related to the exact molecular structure of the drug. For example, if a person changes one thing about a drug's compound, the drug can become legal again.[6] To respond to this problem, in 1986, the US Congress passed legislation curbing the manufacture of these **analogs** in the Federal Analog Act. Under this act, if a chemical is structurally similar to a drug prohibited by the Controlled Substance Act, the chemical is prohibited.[7] These chemicals are classified as Schedule I drugs. The scheduling of these drugs was presented in Chapter 3. Despite these efforts, the business of designer drugs, according to the Drug Enforcement Administration (DEA), exceeds a billion dollars a year.

Mass media sensationalize these designer drugs by reporting them in a manner that is both attention-grabbing and panic-hyping. The use of headlines such as the 2012 Miami story "Zombie Attack" regarding the use of bath salts in an attack invokes panic among readers, which encourages the audience to read articles like this.[8] These articles and news reports often contain information about the accessibility of the drug. One report even showed where to purchase bath salts and provided images on the packaging of bath salts. A potential consequence to this type of reporting is it may actually peak interest in the drug, as

evidenced by a study on Google Trends that showed the search term "bath salts" increased along with the increase in news headlines regarding the 2012 Miami zombie attack article.[9] It is interesting to note that the attack ended up not being related to bath salts or any other type of drug.[10]

In the following section, specific designer drugs will be discussed along with trends and the effects of these drugs.

Synthetic Cathinone (AKA: Bath Salts)

Synthetic cathinones are related to a stimulant in the khat plant.[11] The khat is a shrub in East African and southern Arabia. The people in these regions chew the leaves of this plant for its mild stimulant effects.[12] The synthetic version of these stimulants has been shown to produce effects that are much stronger than the natural version.

Synthetic cathinones are referred to as "new psychoactive substances," which are generally unregulated and are intended to mimic the effects of illicit drugs.[13] These products are sold in small packages and are often labeled "not for human consumption" online or at drug paraphernalia stores. They may also be labeled as "plant food," "jewelry cleaner," or "phonescreen cleaner" and may be advertised under a number of names such as:[14]

- Flakka
- Bloom

BATH SALTS ARE NOT BATH SALTS

"Synthetic cathinone products marketed as "bath salts" should not be confused with products such as Epsom salts that people use during bathing. These bathing products have no mind-altering ingredients."

Source: NIDA, "Synthetic Cathinones ("Bath Salts")", Revised January 2016. Accessed on October 19, 2016 from https://www.drugabuse.gov/publications/drugfacts/synthetic-cathinones-bath-salts.

Designer drugs Term used to describe synthetic drugs that can be abused

Synthetic drugs Drugs that are synthesized by chemicals to mimic illicit drugs

Analog A chemical compound that is similar to an illicit drug

Synthetic cathinones Related to the stimulant in the khat plant related to the stimulant in the khat plant

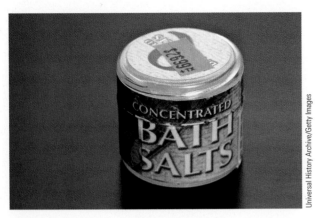

Bath Salts come in appealing containers and usually contain the statement "not for human consumption".

- Cloud Nine
- Lunar Wave
- Vanilla Sky
- White Lightning
- Scarface

The effects of bath salts, which can be smoked, swallowed, snorted, injected, or inhaled, have been compared to those of ecstasy.[15] Bath salts became increasingly popular in Western Europe in 2009 and 2010 before emerging in the United States.[16] The drug has since been made illegal in 28 states, although it can be purchased in convenience stores and head shops. In the first six months of 2011, poison control centers in the United States received 3,470 calls regarding bath salts.[17]

Bath salts react similarly in the brain to stimulants such as cocaine. In a study done on rats, it was determined that the drug 3,4-methylenedioxypyrovalerone (MDPV), commonly found in bath salts, reacts similarly to cocaine in the brain, but has greater potency and efficacy. Furthermore, it produces greater effects than cocaine in locomotor activation (the act of moving from one place to another), tachycardia (fast heartbeat), and hypertension (high blood pressure) in rats.[18] MDPV is the most common synthetic cathinone to be found in people who are admitted to the emergency department after taking bath salts.[19] Symptoms associated with bath salts are:[20]

- Paranoia—extreme and unreasonable distrust of others
- Hallucinations—experiencing sensations and images that seem real but are not
- Increased sociability
- Increased sex drive
- Panic attacks
- Excited delirium—extreme agitation and violence behavior

Media reports regarding bath salts tend to suggest a high prevalence rate with the drug. However, this is not the case. In 2013, a study conducted on university students in Southeast United States found that only about 1% of them reported to using bath salts at least once in their lives.[21] A few years later in 2015, another study was conducted on high school seniors and showed similar results of around 1% of students reporting having used bath salts at least once.[22] This last study showed students who do not live with parents, who earn at least $50 a week (not by a job), and who go out more than four times a week are more at risk for using bath salts. Additionally, people who use bath salts report higher lifetime use of alcohol and marijuana. They are also ten times more likely to use hard drugs such as cocaine, LSD, crack, and heroin.[23]

Synthetic cannabinoids

There are a number of substances that are hyped as legal alternatives to marijuana. They are called **synthetic cannabinoids** because they are related to chemicals found in marijuana plants. They are synthetic chemicals that can be sprayed on dried plants so they can be smoked in a similar fashion to marijuana or sold as liquids to be vaporized and inhaled (much like an e-cigarette).[24] These substances mimic the effects of marijuana without the risk of the user testing positive for marijuana. These drugs come under a variety of names including K2, Spice, Summit, Solar Flare, Yucatan Fire, and Genie.

Easy access and the perceived notion that these are "natural products" that do not cause harm make this drug popular among young people. One study of college students reported that 8% had used the drug.[25] In another study done on substance- and alcohol-dependent inpatients, it was discovered that almost 45% of them were considered synthetic cannabinoid users.[26] In this study, synthetic cannabinoid use was more common among younger people, males, and among those who had fewer years of education.[27]

As mentioned earlier in this section, there persists a notion that synthetic cannabinoids are safe because

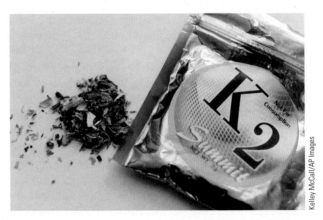

Synthetic marijuana comes in packages that are attractive to young users.

they resemble the natural form of marijuana. Recent studies contradict this notion by providing evidence of not only addiction related to the drug, but the presence of withdrawal symptoms when use of synthetic cannabinoids is discontinued.[28] In a study done on patients receiving treatment services for synthetic cannabinoids, the most common reason for difficulty in stopping drug use was the presence of withdrawal symptoms.[29] This study found the most commonly reported symptoms being anxiety, mood swings, nausea, and loss of appetite with the onset occurring within 1 to 2 hours after the last use. In addition to the presence of withdrawal symptoms, negative outcomes are associated with synthetic cannabinoid use including:[30]

- Severe agitation and anxiety
- Fast, racing heartbeat and higher blood pressure
- Nausea and vomiting
- Muscle spasms, seizures, and tremors
- Intense hallucinations and psychotic episodes
- Suicidal and other harmful thoughts and/or actions

In 2016 through September 30, US poison control centers received 2,075 reports of exposure to synthetic cannabinoids.[31] See Figure 5.1. Adverse effects associated with these drugs include panic attacks, agitation, tachycardia, hypertension, anxiety, numbness, vomiting, hallucinations, tremors, and seizures. These effects can last from 30 minutes to 2 hours.[32]

BZP (Benzylpiperazine)

A lesser known designer drug is **BZP**. It was first synthesized in 1944 as an antiparasitic agent.[33] The effects of BZP are similar to amphetamine effects, but it is 10 to 20 times less potent than amphetamines.[34] Due to the amphetamine-like effects, BZP caught the attention of drug abusers. BZP is often mixed with 1-[3(trifluoro-methyl)phenyl]piperazine (TFMPP), which produces effects similar to MDMA (ecstasy).[35, 36] This drug is promoted at raves as a substitute for MDMA.

The drug first gained popularity in New Zealand, with a reported 44% of college students having used it.[37] From 1999 to 2008, it was a legal drug in New Zealand and was marketed as a legal party pill.[38] Due to the legal nature, users felt it was a safe drug because it was sanctioned by the government. Users also reported the drug was easily accessible and socially acceptable. Furthermore, due to the legal status of the drug, users felt comfortable using higher doses due to the perceived inferior strength of the drug.[39] In 2008, New Zealand changed the legal status of the drug to criminalize its use. The prohibition of BZP in New Zealand resulted in reduced use among young adults. In a survey conducted after the prohibition of the drug, the majority of respondents felt that the drug was harder to obtain and was more expensive compared to prices before prohibition, thus usage of BZP decreased.[40]

There have been no recorded deaths from the sole usage of BZP, but when combined with other drugs (i.e., MDMA and alcohol), the potential for death and hospitalization increase.[41, 42] Ingestion of BZP has been found to produce dissociative states, psychosis, precipitation of mania in schizophrenia, and organ failure.[43]

In the United States, BZP was temporarily labeled as a schedule I drug in 2002 and permanently labeled as a schedule I drug in 2004.[44]

Fentanyl

Fentanyl is the generic name for Sublimaze®, Actiq®, and Duragesic®, a synthetic narcotic developed for its anesthetic properties. It is typically used to help manage pain after surgery and is estimated to be 50 to 100 times more potent than morphine.[45, 46] It is also used to help manage chronic pain for patients who are dependent on and tolerant of opioids.[47] When used in its prescription and legal form, it is administered by injection, transdermal patch, or by lozenges.[48]

The euphoria that fentanyl produces is briefer than the high from heroin. In many instances, fentanyl is combined with other drugs, especially heroin.[49] If one is unaware that fentanyl is mixed into other drugs, there is greater potential for an adverse reaction. The potential for rapid addiction is strong. In California, an estimated 20% of people already dependent on opiates use a powerful derivative of fentanyl nicknamed China white. In 2008, more than 20,179 people went to emergency rooms because of fentanyl.[50] The vast majority of fatal overdoses from fentanyl occurred among males.[51]

People who use fentanyl illegally take it as a powder, spiked on blotter paper, mixed with or substituted for heroin, or as tablets.[52] Fentanyl depresses the respiratory system, decreases the heart rate and blood pressure, and causes constipation. It can be fatal. Death is so swift that needles have been found in people who apparently died while injecting themselves. Whether death is attributable to the drug or to its contaminants is unclear.

Synthetic cannabinoids Related to chemicals found in the marijuana plant

BZP Similar to, but much less potent than, amphetamines

Fentanyl Generic name for the synthetic narcotic used for its anesthetic properties

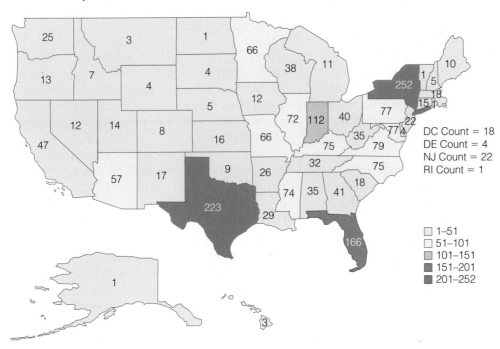

Synthetic Cannabinoid Calls to U.S. Poison Centers (1/1/16–9/30/16)

DC Count = 18
DE Count = 4
NJ Count = 22
RI Count = 1

☐ 1–51
☐ 51–101
▨ 101–151
▩ 151–201
■ 201–252

Please Note:

- These data are only representative of calls received by the poison centers and may not reflect the actual severity of the problem in the United States or any specific geographic location.
- As there is no mandatory reporting, there may be emergency room presentations and hospital admissions of which poison centers are unaware.
- Subject to the above bullets, these numbers are largely reflective of those users/abusers who have experienced adverse effects from the use of these products significant enough to warrant poison center or other health professional intervention; not all individuals who use/abuse such products call poison centers or visit emergency rooms.
- Nevertheless, the data are a good surrogate marker for rising use/abuse patterns and patterns of adverse medical outcomes associated with their use.
- For more information about the American Association of Poison Control Centers (AAPCC) data, please visit: http://www.aapcc.org/data-system/

Figure 5.1 United States Poison Control received thousands of calls each for synthetic cannabinoids.

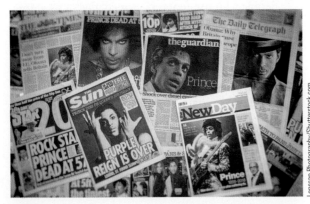

▨ The popstar Prince died in April 2016 from an overdose of Fentanyl.

The popstar Prince died in April 2016 from an overdose of fentanyl. In an investigation into his death, pills containing the drug fentanyl were discovered in his home.[53] These pills were incorrectly labeled as hydrocodone, a narcotic drug used to help manage pain.[54] Fentanyl is a favorite for Mexican cartels and has risen in popularity due to the lucrative nature of the drug and the relative ease in manufacturing it.[55] In fall 2015, Mexico discovered 27 kilograms of fentanyl on a landing strip in Sinaloa, which is equal to almost one ton of heroin.[56] The raid also uncovered almost 20,000 tablets of fentanyl made to look like oxycodone. The men arrested in the raid were members of the drug cartel led by Joaquin Guzman Loera (AKA El Chapo).[57]

When fentanyl is used clinically, side effects include nausea, dizziness, delirium, decreased blood pressure, vomiting, blurred vision, and possible cardiac and respiratory arrest.[58] Its anesthetic effects last 1 to 2 hours, although the effects on respiration last longer. Unfortunately, some patients given a fentanyl patch for moderate pain have used the patch to commit suicide.[59]

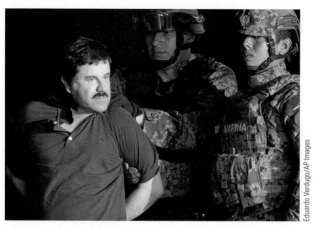

Joaquin Archivaldo Guzman Loera (AKA El Chapo) was ranked as one of the world's most powerful people from 2009 to 2011. After two escapes from jail, he was captured again in 2016.

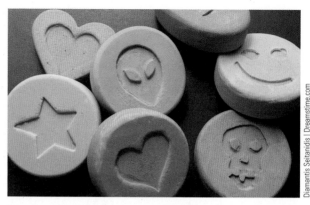

Ecstasy pills come in many creative designs. These simple designs make the user feel the product they are taking is safe.

Meperidine

A dangerous designer drug derived from **meperidine** (Demerol), MPTP is a synthetic derivative of morphine that produces powerful results. Although meperidine has only one-sixth the analgesic potency of morphine, it is highly toxic. It is prescribed to manage severe pain and is available in liquid or pill form.[60] Toxicity is marked by muscle twitching and convulsions. According to government statistics, 782 people were treated in emergency rooms because of meperidine in 2008.[61]

MPTP causes a Parkinson's-like condition that results in paralysis to the brain and nervous system. Symptoms of this condition can be improved, but not cured, through traditional treatment for Parkinson's disease.

Another analog derived from meperidine is **MPPP**. MPPP has the potential to be extremely toxic and leads to the synthesis of MPTP within the body. This was discussed earlier in this section.

MDMA

Also called ecstasy, molly (nickname for molecular), E, XTC, and Adam, **MDMA (***3,4-methylenedioxymethamphetamine***)** is a hallucinogen with amphetamine-like properties.[62] MDMA has been called a "psychedelic amphetamine."[63] First developed in 1914, MDMA is akin to the hallucinogen **MDA**. Intended originally as an appetite suppressant, it received little attention until it resurfaced in the 1960s. LSD and MDMA were available at the same time. LSD, however, did not evoke nausea and vomiting as MDMA did. After being promoted by illicit manufacturers, MDMA became more popular by the mid-1970s. In the 1970s, psychotherapists gave MDMA to their clients to reduce anxiety and facilitate communication. By 1985, production had grown to about 500,000 doses.

Subsequently, MDMA became illegal. Punishment for trafficking could mean a 15-year imprisonment and a substantial fine. Despite its illegality and the substantial penalties associated with it, the demand and cost of MDMA increased throughout the 1990s. In 2014, compared to 2005, its use was down slightly for 8th graders (0.09%) and 10th graders (2.3%) and up slightly for 12th graders (3.6%).[64] See Figure 5.2. There has been some speculation that underreporting of its use is due to misunderstood language on traditional surveys (even though the Monitoring the Future National Survey Results on Drug Use used the word molly on recent surveys and showed little impact on usage reports). In a study conducted in 2016 comparing two surveys—one that included the word molly when questioning MDMA use and one that didn't use the word molly—MDMA prevalence was reported at higher levels on the survey that included the term "molly" in its definition of MDMA. [65]

Today, MDMA is popular in many dance clubs, and is associated with the rave scene. Users claim that it "creates a loving presence and an improved orientation toward intimate relationships. And it deepens meditative calmness."[66] Additionally, many young adults take the drug because of its prosocial and prosexual effects.[67] Some users report an increase in sexual arousal, which may be attributed to increased testosterone and serotonin levels along with greater dopamine activation.[68, 69] Although this drug has been associated with sexual closeness and sexual feelings, there may be a decrease in sexual performance, which has been reported as prolonged along with the absence of orgasm.[70] Regardless, there has been

Meperidine Generic name for the narcotic Demerol

MPPP Analog derived from meperidine

MDMA Hallucinogen with amphetamine-like properties

MDA A member of the amphetamine family

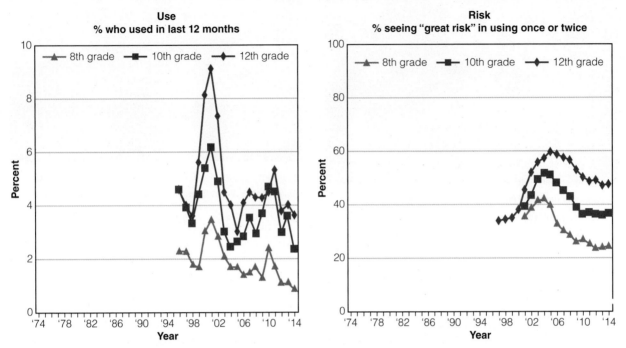

Figure 5.2 Questions to Ponder: What is the relationship between Ecstasy use and perceived risk?

Source: L.D. Johnston, P.M. O'Malley, R.A. Miech, J.G. Bachman, and J.E. Schulenberg, *Monitoring the Future national survey results on drug use: 1975-2014: Overview, key findings on adolescent drug use.* (2015) Ann Arbor: Institute for Social Research, The University of Michigan.

an association made with the use of ecstasy and an increase in risky sexual behavior.[71] One study found MDMA users engage more in risky sexual behaviors compared to alcohol users. Risky sexual behaviors were defined as casual penetrative sex with no condom use among males and females. This study also showed MDMA users engage in sexual activity at a lower age compared with alcohol-only users (16 years of age compared to 17 years of age).[72]

Current research shows that MDMA may affect the brain, although there is much controversy regarding the validity of the research demonstrating brain damage. Most users do not believe that they are harmed by using ecstasy.[73] MDMA has been shown to increase three brain chemicals:[74]

- Dopamine—causes a surge in euphoria and increased energy/activity
- Norepinephrine—increases heart rate and blood pressure
- Serotonin—affects mood, appetite, sleep and other functions (also triggers sexual arousal)

A serious immediate effect is heatstroke because MDMA can trigger convulsions or seizures and widespread blood clotting followed by collapse and coma.[75] Death can result from MDMA use as well. The physical complications that have been reported

include tachycardia, arrhythmias, hypertension, metabolic acidosis, cerebral hemorrhages, convulsions, coma, vomiting, and diarrhea.[76] MDMA use has been associated with overheating, which, although has been seen in nonclub type environments, may be exacerbated in the club environment. [77] Club environments play high-frequency techno music that encourages intense movement via dancing. This may lead to an even higher rise in body temperature along with excessive sweating, which may in turn lead to excessive fluid intake among MDMA users and result in the occurrence of **lethal hyponatremia**. This condition, known as a fatal water overdose, arises from too much water being taken in. The blood cannot accommodate the higher water levels and as a result releases water to the cells that begin to expand resulting in brain edema or brain swelling, which can lead to death.[78] This is especially dangerous when neurons (brain cells) begin to expand because there is not enough room in the brain to accommodate the swelling.[79]

The effects of MDMA can last from 3 to 6 hours with many users taking a second dose once the first one's effects begin to fade.[80] The side effects of MDMA include nausea, sleeplessness, loss of appetite, depression, headache, hangover, jaw clenching, teeth grinding, muscle cramping, blurred vision, and panic.[81] Additionally, some users report symptoms

"In 2002, a 20-year-old, Asian American woman was brought to the emergency room at Harbor-UCLA Medical Center after having taken multiple tablets of ecstasy (3,4-methylenedioxymethamphetamine [MDMA]) and large quantities of water while dancing and drinking excessively during a party the night before. She did not report any symptoms upon returning home after the party. In the morning, however, she was found unresponsive and foaming at the mouth although no seizures were reported. She had rapid and shallow breathing, a weak pulse, and did not respond to painful stimuli. The patient was otherwise healthy, with no medical or surgical history or significant family history. She was not taking any medications and was a college student of good standing.... 12 hours after admission, she was found to have wide-complex tachycardia, which was followed by pulseless electrical activity. Resuscitation efforts were unsuccessful, and the patient expired."

She died from hyponatremia: water overdose

Source: K. Kalanter-Zadeh, M.K. Nguyen, R. Chang, and I. Kurtz, "Fatal hyponatremia in a young woman after ecstasy ingestion", *Nature Clinical Practice Nephrology*, 2 (2006): 283-288.

that can last up to a week following moderate use of the drug that include:[82]

- Irritability
- Impulsiveness and aggression
- Depression
- Sleep problems
- Decreased appetite
- Decreased interest in and pleasure from sex

Regular MDMA use has been associated with psychiatric problems such as anxiety, depression, and psychoses.[83, 84] One study found, through a self-reported questionnaire, a positive correlation between MDMA use and anxiety and psychoticism.[85] Psychoticism is a person who is highly aggressive and exhibits interpersonal hostility. Similarly, another study was done to determine if ecstasy users differed in self-reported rates of depression and anxiety compared to nonecstasy users.

This study separated ecstasy users into two groups: light and heavy users. Researchers found depression rates were lowest in the nonusers group, intermediary in the light users group, and highest in the heavy users group. Similar results were found when analyzing anxiety levels among the three groups.[86] These studies suggest that ecstasy negatively impacts a person's psychological health, although it is not known if people who experience these symptoms had these problems before taking ecstasy or if ecstasy causes these psychological problems. Some studies have found improvements in psychological health after a person has discontinued their ecstasy use. For example, one study found improvements in psychiatric health after 2 years of abstaining from MDMA.[87] In another study on mothers who quit using MDMA, there were significant improvements in depression rates.[88] Users who have quit using MDMA still suffer

ON CAMPUS

Male college athletes report higher rates of performance enhancing drugs compared to non-athlete male college students. Contrary to what one would expect, the use of performance enhancing drugs increased during the off season for male athletes. Similarly, use of social drugs (i.e., tobacco, marijuana, cocaine) were higher during the off season for both male and female athletes. This is true even through athletes are subject to drug testing during the academic year; not just in-season.

Questions to Ponder:

How would you address the use of drugs during the off season for college athletes?

Source: D.A. Yusko, J.F. Buckman, H.R. White, and R.J. Pandina, "Alcohol, tobacco, illicit drugs, and performance enhancers: A comparison of use by college student athletes and nonathletes", *Journal of American College Health*, 57, no.3 (2008): 281-289.

Lethal hyponatraemia Fatal water overdose from taking in too much water

from psychiatric conditions, such as depression, impulsivity, and sleep quality, even after a long period of abstaining from the drug.[89]

Despite concerns regarding its effects, ecstasy does not appear to adversely affect performance on cognitive tests.[90] The US Food and Drug Administration (FDA) has approved studies to determine whether MDMA relieves physical pain and psychological trauma in patients dying of cancer, with chronic pain, and with arthritis. In addition, there is research into whether MDMA is effective for treating posttraumatic stress disorder.[91]

There is evidence that some women who used MDMA during pregnancy had babies with higher rates of congenital abnormalities.[92]

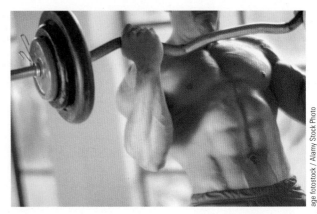

Steroid abuse often begins with an attempt to increase muscle size or to improve appearance.

Performance-Enhancing Drugs

A strong motivation for many people to use drugs is the desire to enhance performance. Society's emphasis on competition could push people into taking drugs to gain an athletic or academic advantage. Likewise, because of the emphasis on sex appeal, some individuals look to drugs to enhance their sexual performance and experience. The effects of drugs, especially anabolic steroids, on performance will be examined here.

Performance-enhancing drugs, also known as **ergogenic aids,** are used to gain a competitive advantage. As early as the 3rd century b.c., Greek athletes ate mushrooms to enhance their performance.[93] In the 1800s, athletes took alcohol, opium, nitroglycerin, and strychnine to improve their performance. American Thomas Hicks won the 1904 Olympic Games marathon after reportedly taking strychnine and brandy, and he was not disqualified.[94] In the 1940s, some athletes and bodybuilders took anabolic steroids to increase their muscle mass and intensify their training regimen.[95]

Drug abuse in sports has become more publicized in the last few years. The media are replete with stories of drug use by athletes during the Olympic Games. Track and field stars such as Marion Jones have blemished careers due to drug use. The Major League Baseball Players Association attracted much adverse attention due to its scandal with performance-enhancing drugs. Because athletes are seen as role models, their fall from grace touches a chord; moreover, drug use by athletes is antithetical to the idea that athletes represent a healthy lifestyle.

The impact of performance-enhancing drugs is evident in baseball. The Major League Baseball Players Association initiated drug testing in 2003. In each season from 1999 to 2001, at least 40 players hit 30 home runs. In 2010, only 18 players hit 30 or more home runs. In 2000, 5,693 home runs were hit (a record number). In 2010, there were 4,613 home runs, nearly a 20% decline.[96] In 2002, former National League Most Valuable Player, Ken Caminiti, believed at least half of all Major League Baseball players were using anabolic steroids.[97] When random mandatory testing was first initiated in 2003, between 5 to 7% of players tested positive for performance-enhancing substances. It is widely believed that this number greatly underestimates those who were using the drug as players were told when they would be tested and certain drugs (human growth hormones) were not detectable in tests.[98]

The type of sport and gender of the athlete have a bearing on the drug of choice. For example, athletes participating in contact sports show preferences for cocaine, crack, and heroin, whereas athletes who engage in noncontact sports prefer amphetamines.[99] The most preferred drug is marijuana regardless of whether the sport is contact or noncontact. In 2009–2010, the number of National Collegiate Athletic Association (NCAA) athletes who tested positive for marijuana was 71, a threefold increase from the previous year.[100] Early in 2015, the NCAA recommended a change in their drug testing policy to exclude recreational drugs from the list of substances being tested for.[101] Proponents for this amendment argue that because these drugs do not impact performance, they should not be tested. Additionally, drug testing among student athletes has not served as a deterrent for drug use, and some wonder the purpose of testing. Lastly, student athletes who test positive for these drugs are more likely to drop out of the sport and out of school.[102] Rather than use testing to deter drug use, the committee recommends education along with interventions and behavioral management programs to address drug use among athletes.[103] The proposal to eliminate street drugs from drug testing was rejected by both the Division II and Division III Management Councils.[104] The focus still remains on

- The Olympic Games have been marred by doping cases. In the summer 2016 Olympics at Rio, Russia was almost banned from competing in the games. In July 2016, the World Anti-Doping Agency conducted an independent investigation on Russia's Ministry of Sport and Federal Security Service which resulted in findings that suggest the Ministry operated as state-wide system to initiate a state-wide doping system and cover the results of positive drug testing samples. By the end of July 2016, the World Anti-Doping Agency decided they will allow Russian athletes if they are able to prove they have not been doping before the Olympic games. It is important to note that athletes from other countries did not have to submit to these guidelines. Moving forward, Russia submitted 389 athletes for consideration and in the beginning of August 2016, 278 of them were eligible to compete in the games.

Questions to Ponder:

- Do you think it was fair for the World Anti-Doping Agency to make Russia prove their athletes were not doping? Should they have made other countries follow the same guidelines? Why or why not?

the creation and implementation of drug education programs to deter drug use among student athletes.

Studies suggest that athletes who use performance-enhancing drugs are more likely to use other illicit substances. In a study conducted on male college athletes, it was discovered that athletes who use a performance-enhancing substance report higher prevalence rates of heavy drinking, cigarette use, marijuana, narcotic, and dietary supplemental use.[105] Is education the answer? As mentioned earlier in this section, the NCAA is investigating the use of substance abuse education to deter drug use among student athletes. Germany introduced the National Doping Prevention Plan to reduce doping by student athletes. The theory behind this program was if student athletes were educated on doping and banned substances, use rates would decline. However, in a study 4 years after the initiation of this program there were no significant changes in doping and banned substance behaviors among athletes who participated in the program. Although knowledge about doping and banned behaviors increased slightly among participants, behaviors did not follow these trends.[106]

Many individuals use sports supplements to enhance their performance or appearance. In Canada, over $1 billion is spent annually on sports supplements.[107] They can be purchased in gas stations as well as grocery and drugstores and over the Internet. Concerns regarding the use of sports supplements include their lack of regulation and absence of research into their long-term effects.

Anabolic Steroids

Prior to their use in athletics, **anabolic steroids** were used by German soldiers during World War II to increase their muscle strength and aggressiveness.[108]

Reports of steroid use by male and female Soviet athletes appeared in 1954. Shortly thereafter, US weightlifters began taking steroids, followed by football players and swimmers.

Anabolic steroids belong to the compound anabolic-androgenic steroids. Anabolic refers to muscle building and androgenic refers to increased male sex characteristics.[109] Anabolic steroids are synthetic substances related to the male sex hormones.[110] They mimic the action of testosterone. Steroids are only legally available through a prescription. They are believed to add bulk and strength if they are taken by motivated people who train intensively and follow a proper diet.[111] Taking testosterone during puberty augments muscle mass and strength, but steroid use later in adolescence stunts growth. Users experience a stimulant-like high and feelings of aggressiveness, which may account for higher intensity while training and competing. Studies on their effects are conducted retrospectively, and factors such as diet, dosage, type of steroid, and level of training make it hard to answer the question conclusively.

Anabolic steroids can be taken orally or intramuscular injections. There are also some topical doses that can be applied and absorbed through the skin. It is estimated that doses used to improve performance are 10 to 20 times higher than doses prescribed by a physician.[112] Some athletes use different techniques

ergogenic aids Substances that provide an athletic advantage, also known as performance-enhancing drugs

anabolic steroids Substances used to increase muscle mass; related to male sex hormones

in their anabolic steroid use to avoid the harmful effects of steroids. These include:[113]

- Cycling—taking doses for a period of time, stopping for a time, and then restarting
- Stacking—combining two or more different types of steroids
- Pyramiding—slowing increasing the dose or frequency of abuse, reaching a peak amount, and then gradually tapering off

These methods have not been shown to reduce the physical risk of steroid use.[114]

Athletes are not the only individuals using steroids. One study reported that college students took steroids to enhance appearance, because their friends took steroids, or to improve physical performance.[115] Among college students, the rate of steroid use has not differed from the early 1990s to the present. Approximately 1% of college students have used steroids for nonmedical purposes.[116] Risk regarding anabolic androgenic steroid use increases from college freshman to college seniors. Results also found that 80% of those who have used an anabolic androgenic steroid once would use it again.[117] Another study found that the average user is a 30-year-old, educated, White male who is not especially athletic.[118] Concern over teenage girls using steroids prompted the US Congress to initiate hearings. However, due to the way survey questions are asked, it is difficult to get a good handle on the extent of steroid use by teenage girls.[119] One survey of high school students reported that only 1.4% used steroids, although 49% believed that they improved athletic performance.[120] Another factor that may influence the use of anabolic steroids is the desire to fit within gender norms. One study found that young boys and men, who conform to gender norms, have higher rates of anabolic steroid use. Furthermore, by age 19, 12% of all males have reported using some type of muscle-building product.[121]

Liver and kidney tumors have been linked to steroids. Within 2 to 8 years of using steroids, 1 to 3% of users develop liver cancer.[122] Other effects in men

KNOWN EFFECTS OF STEROIDS

Both Men and Women	Men	Women
• acne	• increased penis size if used before puberty	• baldness
• increased susceptibility to infections		• decreased breast size
• abrupt mood changes	• more frequent erections	• enlarged clitoris
• hypertension	• atrophied testicles	• increased facial hair
• decreased high-density lipoprotein levels (good cholesterol)	• enlarged breasts	• fluid retention
• effects on liver	• enlarged prostate	• deepened voice
• stunted growth	• infertility	• menstrual irregularities
	• baldness	

are low sperm count, testicular atrophy, high voice, gynecomastia (breast development), infertility, and baldness. These are reversible several months after stopping use of steroids.[123] Even in cases where anabolic-steroid induced hypogonadism is not reversible, most men do not regret their anabolic steroid use.[124] Hypogonadism is an ineffectiveness in the testes resulting in low sperm and/or testosterone. A study looked at men who were diagnosed with hypogonadism, which was believed to be caused from their anabolic steroid use. Of the men, only 16% reported feelings of regret associated with earlier anabolic steroid use that was not related to being diagnosed with hypogonadism. Regret was also not associated with the other side effects of anabolic steroid use such as acne, fluid retention, increased aggression, and mood disorders.[125]

Users display symptoms of depression, panic, anxiety, paranoia, mania, and suicidal behavior. A survey of 7,000 American teenage boys who took steroids indicated a higher level of violent behavior compared to nonusers.[126] This mania has been called **roid rage.** Uncontrollable violence, which occurs for no apparent reason, has also been tied to steroid use. In a study done on weightlifters comparing aggression between those who were anabolic steroid users and nonusers, it was found that anabolic steroid use was associated with increased aggression. However, when conducting personality tests on this sample of weightlifters, those who used anabolic steroids demonstrated traits of antisocial, borderline, and histrionic personality disorders.[127] Additionally, the use of steroids in combination with alcohol has been shown to largely increase the risk of violence and aggression.[128]

At one time anabolic steroids were not considered addictive. However, based on guidelines from the US Sentencing Commission, steroids are now considered addictive.[129] Studies have shown that animals will self-administer steroids when given the chance, and people continue their use despite experiencing negative effects.[130] Users who quit anabolic steroid use report withdrawal symptoms that include mood swings, fatigue, and loss of appetite. Depression has also been associated with the discontinued use of steroids.[131]

Anabolic steroids do have medical benefits when prescribed by physicians. Anabolic steroids were first developed in the late 1930s to treat hypogonadism, a condition in which the testes fail to produce enough testosterone.[132] They are still given to people who have some types of impotence and to AIDS patients to treat the body wasting often associated with that disease.[133]

Human Growth Hormones and Erythropoietin

Human growth hormones (HGH)—which are naturally produced in the body and stimulate protein

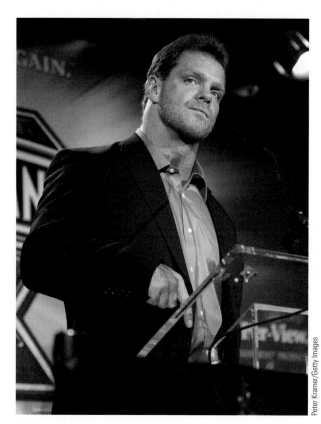

Chris Benoit

synthesis—and **erythropoietin (EPO)** are other drugs used to enhance performance. HGH were first isolated in the 1950s, although it was not until the 1980s that they were used as a doping agent.[134] One study of young male bodybuilders found that 12% used HGH.[135] Starting in 2011, the National Football League (NFL) initiated game-day testing for HGH.[136]

HGH have been given to children who are especially small. Depending on the dosage, children will grow 1.5 to 4 inches,[137] and many of these children feel better about themselves after taking the hormones. In 2008, a bill was introduced into the US Senate to ban HGH for everyone, including children. However, that bill was defeated because of HGH's benefit to some children.[138] It is currently legal to use for children and adults with growth hormone deficiency and for adults with short bowel syndrome and muscle-wasting disease associated with HIV/AIDS.[139]

roid rage Uncontrollable violence associated with use of anabolic steroids

human growth hormones (HGH) Hormones that stimulate protein synthesis; used by athletes to enhance performance

erythropoietin (EPO) Hormone that enhances cardiovascular endurance by increasing red blood cell production

HGH is a polypeptide consisting of 119 amino acids. Every night, the pituitary gland releases HGH into the blood. HGH stimulates the liver to produce the hormone insulin-like growth factor 1(IGF-1), which promotes the growth of bone, cartilage, and muscle. The production of HGH surges during childhood and adolescence but reduces by 50% in adulthood.[140]

Blood doping is defined by the World Anti-Doping Agency as any substance or technique employed to increase one's red blood cell mass, which allows the body to transport more oxygen.[141] In the 1998 Tour de France, the entire Festina team was disqualified on suspicion of human Erythropoietin (rHuEOP) use.[142] EPO is a hormone that increases red blood cell production. An increase in hemoglobin has been shown to increase maximal aerobic power resulting in improved performance.[143] A higher red blood cell count, however, can lead to blood clots, increasing the risk for heart attacks, stroke, and pulmonary embolism. Other side effects are increased bone growth of the jaw, forehead, feet, and hands; increased cholesterol levels; heart disease; impotence; and elevated blood sugar levels.[144] The misuse of EPO may increase the risk for autoimmune diseases.[145]

Creatine

Creatine is a naturally occurring amino acid. An over-the-counter substance that has gained in popularity is the amino acid **creatine monohydrate,** referred to as a nutritional supplement. A number of professional athletes, coaches, and fitness researchers promote its use, although the physiological mechanisms by which it works are not well understood. Creatine is believed to increase water content in muscles, adding to their size and possibly their ability to function. It produces a modest increase in strength.[146] Another study of women between the ages of 58 and 71 who took creatine found that they had significant increases in muscle power and strength without experiencing adverse side effects.[147] A similar study was conducted in 2015 with comparable results. Postexercise creatine supplementation increased lean tissue mass and increased upper and lower body strength compared with resistance training alone in healthy adults between 50 and 71 years of age.[148]

Creatine is one of the most popular nutritional supplements that is taken to improve athletic performance.[149] Some studies show that creatine is effective for improving an athlete's performance. One study of competitive female swimmers found that swimmers propelled themselves more quickly when using creatine, even though their body weight and body composition were unaffected.[150] Other studies of creatine's effects show that one's sprinting ability in hot, humid conditions significantly improved[151] and that anaerobic running capacity is increased for men.[152] On the other hand, creatine supplementation has not been proven to help cardiac patients with physical performance or other health-related

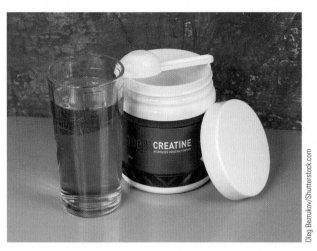

Creatine is considered a nutritional supplement. The FDA does not test it for safety.

measures.[153] One disadvantage is that creatine reduces one's range of movement.[154] Should its use be banned from athletic competition? Among Major League Baseball teams, eight disapproved of creatine use, seven took no position, and one approved it. In the National Basketball Association (NBA), two teams disapproved, eleven took no position, and eight approved. In the NFL, eight teams disapproved, four took no position, and five approved. A higher percentage of football players are believed to use creatine than athletes in other sports.

One benefit of creatine—in a roundabout way—is that it may prevent some people from using anabolic steroids. Another benefit, according to an Australian study, is that creatine may boost brain power in vegetarians.[155] A small study of ten people indicated that creatine may help relieve depression.[156] Moreover, creatine may help the elderly with cognitive functioning.[157] Because creatine is a nutritional supplement and not a drug, the FDA does not scrutinize it for safety. In essence, no regulations are in place regarding its sale and use.[158] Nonetheless, many people perceive creatine as a safe alternative to steroids. Reported side effects of creatine include muscle cramping, dehydration, water retention, and kidney problems. Other side effects are gastrointestinal distress, nausea, and seizures. Three college wrestlers who died in 1997 were believed to be taking creatine, although the relationship between creatine and their deaths could have been coincidental.

Tetrahydrogestrinone

Tetrahydrogestrinone (THG) is a synthetic steroid that athletes are taking to improve athletic performance. THG is made by modifying another anabolic steroid. It is alleged that THG was designed and manufactured by a California company known as Bay Area Laboratory Cooperative (BALCO). BALCO's owner, Victor Conte, claims that THG is not a steroid but a nutritional supplement. Numerous athletes, such as baseball players Jason Giambi and Barry Bonds, football player Bill Romanowski, and track and field athletes including Marion Jones, are suspected of having used THG.[159]

The FDA has not approved THG for use. The FDA has warned individuals not to use THG because the drug has not undergone scientific scrutiny. Despite the lack of testing for THG, the FDA speculates that THG may cause some of the same side effects as steroids.[160] Don Catlin, who heads a drug testing laboratory at the University of California in Los Angeles, fears that other designer drugs that can evade detection may be developed. When THG was first developed, the belief was that it could not be detected by conventional drug testing procedures because it deteriorates quickly. However, with improved drug testing, it can now be detected. Nonetheless, it is difficult for testing to keep up with the changes in the variety of drugs that may be produced.[161]

Despite the stance of the US Anti-Doping Agency (USADA), many athletes taking performance-enhancing drugs do not view themselves as cheaters. Rather, they consider the use of these drugs as a means of getting the edge over their competitors.[162] Though it is not known how extensively THG is used, its consumption is thought to be widespread. Moreover, the public expects to see athletes who are bigger, stronger, and faster. The era of the 250-pound professional lineman is over. Every 2 years when the Olympic Games are held, fans watch to see if world records are broken. Fans get excited when the homerun record is broken. Interestingly, the NBA and the National Hockey League (NHL) have not banned THG.[163]

Androstenedione (Andro)

Another muscle builder that has caught the attention of the public, primarily because it was used by home-run king Mark McGwire, is **androstenedione**.[164] The Major League Baseball Players Association did not forbid players from using androstenedione at that time, even though the NCAA, the NFL, and the International Olympic Committee had banned it. Known as "andro," androstenedione, like creatine, is

creatine monohydrate Natural substance used to increase strength and short-term speed

tetrahydrogestrinone (THG) A designer drug, closely related to the banned anabolic steroids gestrinone and trenbolone

androstenedione Food supplement used for muscle development classified as a nutritional supplement, although it is no longer sold legally.

Androstenedione is a precursor molecule that is just one metabolic step away from testosterone. Its producers claim that androstenedione causes users to generate more testosterone for a few hours after a workout. Androstenedione can be converted into the female sex hormone estrogen as well. In 1999, a randomized controlled trial was conducted to determine if oral androstenedione improved performance in healthy adult athletes. Results from this study showed there were no significant differences between those who took oral andostenedione and those who did not in terms of overall body composition, muscle strength, and muscle fiber analysis.[165]

The effects of androstenedione are similar to those of anabolic steroids. For example, males may experience testicular atrophy, impotence, and breast enlargement. Women who take androstenedione may have increased facial hair, become bald, have deepened voices, and experience abnormal menstrual cycles. Women may also have an increased risk of breast and endometrial cancer.[166] In January 2010, the FDA recalled androstenedione because of its potential side effects.[167]

Stimulants

Cocaine use by collegiate and professional athletes is well documented and is the most frequently detected stimulant found among drug tests of athletes.[168] Cocaine impairs performance requiring hand-eye coordination and concentration. Most athletes use cocaine for social reasons, not to improve performance.

Amphetamines have been used in sports to reduce fatigue and sustain intense exercise. There were reports of amphetamine use in the 1952 and 1956 Olympic Games. By the 1960 Olympics, amphetamine use was rampant. On the first day of competition, a Danish cyclist died and three others collapsed from amphetamine use. This tragedy provided the impetus for drug testing of athletes. In the 1996 Olympics, five athletes tested positive for a banned stimulant.

In 1968, the International Olympic Committee required athletes to submit to drug testing or face disqualification. The US Olympic Committee publishes a list of drugs that result in disqualification. The list includes not only illegal drugs but prescribed and over-the-counter drugs as well.

Concerns over performance-enhancing drugs rose in the United States when professional football players reportedly used amphetamines during competition. The NFL officially banned these drugs in 1971. Although steroids were not seen as a problem at that time, the perception in the NFL has changed and steroids are now banned.

In 1995, the US Supreme Court ruled that high schools have the right to drug test athletes, that the interest of the school outweighs the privacy issues of its students. Also, in preparation for the 2002 Winter Olympics in Salt Lake City, the federal government allocated $3.3 million to support the antidoping program. The drug testing policies of professional sports are outlined in Table 5.1.

In a classic study, 75% of highly trained runners, swimmers, and throwers showed slight improvement after using amphetamines. Even though improvement was slight, amphetamines could account for the margin of difference in highly trained athletes.[169] In a study on rats, those who were given amphetamines were able to run significantly longer compared to those who were not given the stimulant. Rats who were not given the drug experienced a steady increase in core body temperature while those rats given amphetamines experienced a slow-down in temperature.

TABLE 5.1 Professional Sports and Drug Testing

Sport	Policy
National Football League	Players are tested during preseason and tested during season only for *reasonable cause*. Positive test results in outpatient counseling and 30-day probation or 30-day inpatient treatment. After three positive tests a player is banned from the NFL.
National Basketball Association	Testing is limited to cases of *reasonable cause* and random testing of first-year players during preseason. First-time violators who voluntarily seek help receive their salary and free treatment; the second time, they receive treatment but no salary. The third time, they are suspended for life but may petition for reinstatement after 2 years.
Major League Baseball	Players are tested only if they have known involvement with drugs or their contract has a clause. Penalties are handled on a case-by-case basis.
Boxing	World Boxing Council requires testing for world title fights; World Boxing Association does not require drug tests.
Tennis	Men's International Professional Tennis Council conducts drug tests at no more than two tournaments each year; a player testing positive must receive treatment or face a 1-year suspension; three positive tests result in a 1-year suspension.
National Hockey League	NHL has no drug-testing policy.

Results from this study suggest amphetamines may mask or delay fatigue by slowing the rise of body temperature during exercise. This may result in overheating of the muscles.[170] Endurance improved, however, because symptoms of fatigue were masked, not because of improved physiology.

Caffeine is another stimulant that improves endurance, especially short-term endurance. In one study, the length of a bicycle ergometer ride was extended by nearly 20% after the subjects ingested 330 mg of caffeine, equivalent to three cups of coffee. The total energy output of individuals in a laboratory setting who rode for 2 hours was 7% greater after consuming 500 mg of caffeine.[171] Another study showed caffeine use reduced perceptions of exertion and heart rate, although reductions in heart rate go away as intensity is increased. The effects of caffeine on exercise, although present, are very subtle.[172] Currently, the NCAA and International Olympic Committee ban caffeine at specified levels.

The use of caffeine extends beyond professional and college athletes. A number of young people are consuming sports and energy drinks. These drinks are high in caffeine and calories. One effect is weight gain.[173]

Depressants

Depressants such as barbiturates, benzodiazepines (minor tranquilizers), and alcohol are not perceived as ergogenic drugs, though they have been used to improve performance. Benzodiazepines and barbiturates reduce tremors, a quality important to hand steadiness.[174] Weight throwers improved their performance, whereas swimmers were significantly impaired after taking a certain barbiturate. Benzodiazepines impair psychomotor performance, although this becomes less so as tolerance develops. Benzodiazepines hinder driving ability, further demonstrating that these drugs harm performance.[175]

Alcohol significantly reduces psychomotor skills. Some endurance athletes drink beer before competitions because they think it provides carbohydrates for energy. Calories from beer, however, are converted to heat and are not available as energy. Moreover, alcohol results in significant loss of fluid. Alcohol also reduces aerobic capacity, and reaction time, fine and complex motor coordination, balance and steadiness, visual tracking, and information processing are impaired.[176]

Summary

Designer drugs are made from synthetic substances to mimic the effects of illegal drugs. Problems surrounding these drugs came about the difficulty in regulating their legal nature as chemists were able to alter the compounds to skirt away from the law. The Federal Analog Act addressed this issue by the inclusion of any chemical that is similarly structured to a drug classified under the Controlled Substance Act. Use of these drugs continues and they can sometimes be found in local grocery stores.

Performance-enhancing drugs have been around for a long time and used to gain a competitive advantage over others. Perhaps society's emphasis on competition and winning promotes the usage of these drugs as they have been used by some of the nation's top athletes. Risk regarding the use of these drugs are numerous and some would argue they are not worth the risk. Others claim the use of performance-enhancing drugs should left up to the individual.

Thinking Critically

1. Designer and synthetic drugs are often mislabeled to mask the purpose of those drugs (i.e., plant food, jewelry cleaner, etc.). How would you go about regulating a substance that is identified for another purpose? If these products are advertised as "not for human consumption," what responsibility does the company who produces and markets these substances have? Should they be blamed when people use these drugs?

2. As medical improvements and technology advances, it is often difficult for the World Anti-Doping Agency to remain current in policy-making. If an athlete is gaining a competitive edge from a new product that has not been banned, does that constitute as cheating? What if the substance is later banned? Was the athlete cheating?

3. A company called DanceSafe provides onsite testing. People bring their drugs to them and they are tested to determine what the drug contains. They believe college students want to experiment with drugs in a safe manner. They state when the results from the test come back, many students end up throwing away the drug because it contains substances they didn't want to consume. What are your thoughts regarding onsite drug testing? Should it be legal? Do you think it makes taking drugs like ecstasy more safe? Some say it promotes drug usage. What are your thoughts?

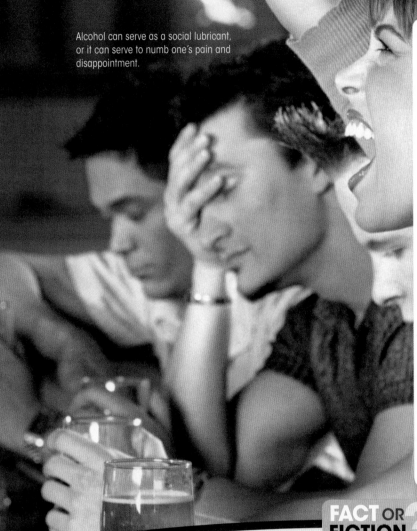

6

Alcohol

Alcohol can serve as a social lubricant, or it can serve to numb one's pain and disappointment.

©Royalty-Free/Getty Images

Chapter Objectives

After completing this chapter, the reader should be able to:

- Identify factors accounting for society minimizing its view of alcohol as a serious drug
- Argue the roles of the Women's Christian Temperance Union, Anti-Saloon League, and National Prohibition Party in alcohol reform
- Describe the events leading up to prohibition, the consequences of it, as well as its repeal
- Compare and contrast patterns of alcohol consumption among ethnic groups
- Compare and contrast patterns of alcohol consumption in the United States to other countries
- Summarize the factors affecting the rate of alcohol absorption
- Explain the effects of alcohol on different systems in the body
- List and describe the effects of alcohol on the fetus
- Evaluate the factors that may contribute to alcoholism
- Argue the influence of culture on drinking patterns
- Describe the effects of alcoholism on adult children of alcoholics

FACT OR FICTION?

1. Nearly 10% of Americans indicated that they have been under the influence of alcohol while at work at least one time during the past year.

2. During Prohibition, alcohol-related deaths increased.

3. Some over-the-counter medicines, such as cough syrups, can contain as much as 10% alcohol.

4. Most college students reduce their binge drinking after graduating from college.

5. Overall, more Blacks drink alcohol than Whites, but Whites are more likely to drink heavily.

6. The younger one is when drinking alcohol for the first time, the more likely one will become a problem drinker.

7. Moderate alcohol drinkers have lower rates of cardiovascular disease than abstainers.

8. By age 11, over 10% of Americans have seen a person drunk, passed out, or using drugs on a social media site.

9. At least one-fourth of people who drive under the influence of alcohol will be arrested.

10. Only two states have a drinking age below age 21 years.

Turn the page to check your answers

No drug in history has had as much impact on the United States or the world as alcohol. Alcohol affects everyone, either by one's own or someone else's use. Attitudes toward alcohol have run the gamut from reverence to dismay. It is believed to be the oldest drug known to humans. Primitive societies used alcohol ritually or socially to deal with anxiety created by an unstable environment. There were, however, instances in which alcohol was seen as a problem. As early as the 1500s, laws were passed in England to regulate "alehouses."[1] Yet, alcohol is not always acknowledged as a drug, because of the following:

1. Alcohol is legal. This could lead one to believe that its effects are not negative or severe. If alcohol were bad for a person, the government would do more to limit its availability.
2. Parents and other role models consume alcohol as part of their lifestyle.
3. Alcohol is shown regularly in the media as a desired beverage.

People drink alcohol for many reasons. They consume it to relax, to reduce their inhibitions, and for pleasure. They use it at family dinners, on festive occasions, at weddings, and to celebrate national holidays. Alcohol is part of the social fabric. It is difficult to think of a drug that serves as many cultural purposes as alcohol—or has caused as much havoc.

In this chapter, we will explore the history of alcohol use in the United States, the role of alcohol in society, the extent of its usage, its effects on the individual, and its impact on the family. Treatment for alcoholism is discussed in Chapter 15.

History of Alcohol Use in the United States

We can trace the history of alcohol beginning with Colonial times, to the temperance movement, to Prohibition, to contemporary use.

Colonial Times

Alcohol use in the United States began when the Puritans disembarked from the Mayflower at Plymouth, Massachusetts. In one speculation, they anchored at Plymouth because their supply of beer and spirits was becoming depleted.[2] Alcohol was an integral component of Colonial life, and attitudes of early settlers toward alcohol were positive. In Colonial times, Americans drank more alcohol than any other time. Alcohol was viewed as being able to cure the sick, contained antiaging properties, and made the world a better place.[3] Not only were beers and wines a part of daily living and used during festive situations, but alcohol was also considered a "good creature from God."

Although drinking in moderation was acceptable, a person could be whipped, fined, and confined to the stocks for drunkenness in Massachusetts and Virginia.[4]

Two factors contributed to the importance of alcohol during Colonial times: sanitation and nutrition. Sanitary practices were lacking. Human and

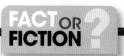

1. **FICTION** The fact is—Fewer than 2% of Americans indicated that they were under the influence of alcohol while at work at least one time during the past 12 months.
2. **FICTION** The fact is—When Prohibition first went into effect, alcohol-related deaths and illness related to alcohol use declined.
3. **FACT** Some medications include as much as 10% alcohol.
4. **FACT** Binge drinking peaks at age 21 and declines after that age.
5. **FICTION** The fact is—More Whites drink alcohol than Blacks, but more Blacks will drink heavily.
6. **FACT** Several studies link alcohol-related problems with the early onset of drinking.
7. **FACT** People who drink no more than one to three drinks per day have less risk of cardiovascular disease than nondrinkers. People who drink more than three drinks per day have a higher risk of cardiovascular disease.
8. **FICTION** The fact is—By age 11, 12% of American children have seen a person drunk, passed out, or using drugs on a social media site.
9. **FICTION** The fact is—Of the estimated 82 million drinking and driving trips in a given year when the driver has a blood alcohol concentration of .08 or higher, about 1.5 million drivers are arrested—less than 2%.
10. **FICTION** The fact is—No state allows alcohol consumption before age 21.

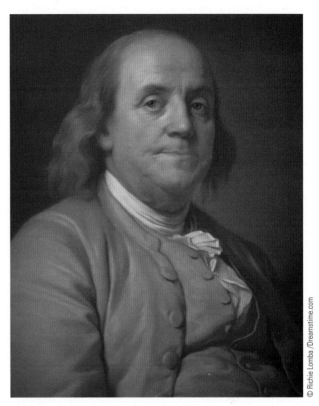

"Beer is living proof that God loves us and wants to see us happy."—Benjamin Franklin

animal waste contaminated drinking wells, and tuberculosis probably was transmitted through cow's milk. Alcohol is a preservative.

Moreover, alcoholic beverages at that time contained important nutrients including vitamins, minerals, and yeast. Early settlers made wine from potatoes, apples, carrots, lettuce, wheat, cranberries, dandelions, squash, and so forth. Beer and wine were

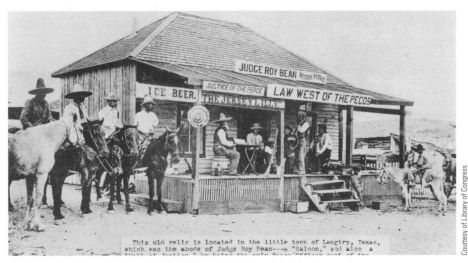

This photograph, circa 1905, depicts a typical saloon interior. The absence of tables allowed more floor space to accommodate customers.

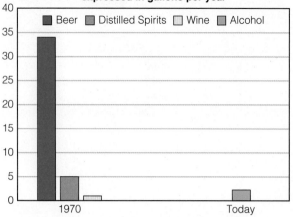

Comparing Alcohol Consumption from 1790 to Today—expressed in gallons per year

Legend: ■ Beer ■ Distilled Spirits □ Wine ■ Alcohol

Figure 6.1 To compare numbers, today, Americans consume about 2.3 gallons of alcohol per year. Compare this to 1790, where the average American drank 34 gallons of beer and cider, 5 gallons of distilled spirits, and 1 gallon of wine per year.

Source: E. Crews, "Rattle-Skull, Stonewall, Bogus, Blackstrap, Bombo, Mimbo, Whistle Belly, Syllabub, Sling, Toddy, and Flip: Drinking in Colonial America", *The Colonial Williamsburg Journal*, (Winter, 2007). Accessed on November 6, 2016 from http://www.history.org/foundation/journal/holiday07/drink.cfm.

necessary drinks instead of recreational beverages. It was not uncommon for children as well as adults to drink alcohol on a daily basis.[5]

Alcohol consumption peaked in the United States in the late 1700s and early 1800s. See Figure 6.1, which illustrates average consumptions rates of American compared to today. Farmers took alcohol into the fields, employers gave it to employees on the job, and aspiring politicians gave alcohol to voters at polling places. Troops of the Continental Army received daily rations of rum or whiskey. Consumption of whiskey was extremely high by the end of the Civil War. Alcohol misuse was one factor that contributed to an increase in suicide throughout the Civil War.[6]

Dr. Benjamin Rush, a signer of the Declaration of Independence, was one of the first people to identify alcoholism as a disease. Before Rush, most people saw excessive drinking as a lack of will.[7] Rush advocated that physicians become abstinent in order to enhance their profession. In his 1784 publication, *An Inquiry into the Effects of Ardent Spirits upon the Human Body and Mind*, Rush described the harmful effects of alcohol.[8] Unfortunately, at the time, his ideas regarding alcohol were not well received, but they did help lead to the temperance movement that followed shortly thereafter.

Temperance Movement

In the early 1800s, a movement to curb the escalating rate of alcohol use and abuse swept through the United States. At this point in time, America was feeling the toll that the Revolutionary War had on society. Many families lost husbands and sons, who were the breadwinners and sole providers. Compounded by high inflation rates and large-scale immigration, the country experienced high levels of poverty and violence.[9] Many people felt hopeless during this time in history and perhaps tried to deal with these feelings by consuming alcohol. Men and women drank alcohol from morning until night, with some historians referring to this age as the "Alcoholic Republic."[10] Public intoxication and binge drinking was at the highest peak, and people recognized the larger problems emanating from uncontrolled alcohol use. Alcohol was seen as a major cause of crime and violence; for example, men who drank too much would steal and beat their wives. These observations led to the temperance movement, the initial purpose of which was to modify alcohol use, not to eliminate it. In essence, alcohol consumption in moderation was acceptable but habitual drunkenness was viewed as sinful.[11]

Dr. Rush did not condemn alcohol, but he was critical of uncontrolled drinking. He argued that alcohol, especially hard alcohol, interfered with the ability

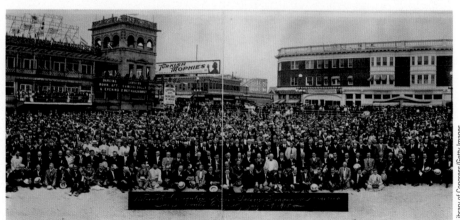

A poster printed for the Ohio Dry Convention in 1917 announced the Anti-Saloon League.

to earn a living and with family life. He believed that alcoholism was both a progressive disease culminating in addiction and a gradual form of suicide.[12]

Beginning in 1808, many independent organizations formed their own temperance groups. Not until 1826, however, did the American Society for the Promotion of Temperance, later called the American Temperance Society, come into being. The purpose of this society was to promote abstinence from alcohol and urged people to sign a pledge of abstinence.[13] Later the Independent Order of Good Templars entered the fray to combat the evils of liquor, recruiting former alcoholics in an effort to promote abstinence. Another group, the Temperance Society, claiming to have 1.5 million members, was a zealous campaigner and put much pressure on politicians. The temperance movement had some success. Through their efforts, alcohol consumption declined (from about 5 gallons per person in the 1830s to under 2 gallons person in the 1840s), and by the mid-1850s individual states had passed legislation restricting the manufacturing and sale of alcohol for nonmedicinal purposes.[14] The temperance movement remained strong until the Civil War, at which time the federal government faced other important issues.

Three influential groups in alcohol reform were the Women's Christian Temperance Union (WCTU), the Anti-Saloon League, and the National Prohibition Party. The WCTU favored social reform, prayer, education, prevention, and legislation for bidding alcohol.[15] The WCTU published journals critical of alcohol, held programs for children, depicting alcohol as a substance to fear and loathe, and was responsible for laws mandating alcohol education.

The Anti-Saloon League grew into a powerful political force, campaigning for candidates who supported controls on alcohol. The National Prohibition Party was a major impetus in getting many states to ban alcohol. From 1880 to 1889, seven states passed prohibition laws and 34 states passed similar legislation between 1907 and 1919, the year national prohibition was signed into law. In the meantime, two states repealed their laws banning alcohol. These events were the imputes to the beginning of the prohibition movement.

Prohibition

Efforts to impose a national ban gathered strength in the early 1900s. Not only did states enact their own legislation, but it was illegal to ship alcoholic beverages to places where the sale and manufacture of liquor was forbidden and to use the postal service to advertise liquor. Sentiment for the federal government to exert control over alcohol was strong.

The United States had been at war since April 1917, and the hysteria that gripped the nation in its crusade in World War I extended the firm belief that liquor sapped the nation's strength and willpower, and even depleted the cereal grains that could be used in bread for feeding the troops and starving Europeans.[16] Additionally, the popularity of saloons was at its highest levels; members of the temperance movement felt

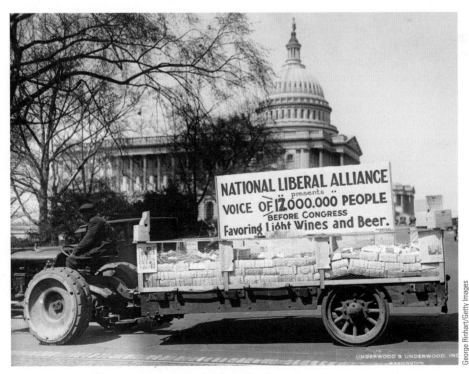

George Rinhart/Getty Images

A poster printed for the Ohio Dry Convention in 1917.

if alcohol were forbidden, husbands would stop spending their family income on alcohol.[17]

The 18th amendment was ratified in 1919 and went into effect on January 16, 1920. The 18th amendment to the US Constitution prohibited the sale, transportation, and manufacturing of alcohol.[18] The Volstead Act (also known as the National Prohibition Act) was created to help carry out the intentions of the 18th amendment. The Volstead Act specifically defined "intoxicating liquors," the language used in the 18th amendment.

Enforcing prohibition proved to be a difficult task and tended to be strictly enforced in rural areas and small towns where many supported prohibition efforts, compared to larger more urban populations.[19] Consumption of alcohol was not illegal and alcohol could be obtained legally for religious purposes and via medical prescriptions.[20] Another problem with the enforcement of prohibition was the year delay between the passage and enactment of the law. Thus many individuals were able to stock up on their supply of alcohol during the year preceding enforcement.[21] While prohibition experienced some successes such as lower rates of alcohol use in the beginning, lower rates of death from alcohol-related deaths, and better work production (less work absenteeism, less worksite alcohol-related accidents, etc.),[22] the problems resulting from prohibition proved to be greater than anticipated.

Consequences of Prohibition

Economics

When the law went into effect, many thought the sales of household goods, clothing, and entertainment costs would increase. Supporters of prohibition expected families would have more expendable income because they were not spending extra money on alcohol. Real estate developers and landlords expected rents to skyrocket as saloons closed, improving neighborhoods.[23] None of these occurred. In fact, a decline was seen among theaters and entertainment industries, while many restaurants failed because they no longer gained a profit from liquor sales.[24] In addition, many people lost their jobs due to the closing of distilleries, saloons, and all alcohol-related trades (i.e., barrel makers, truckers, etc.).[25]

Perhaps one of the largest economic consequences of prohibition was the loss of revenue for local governments and the federal government. Before prohibition, many states relied on liquor taxes to fund their budget. For example, in New York, almost 75% of the state's revenue came from liquor taxes.[26] Once prohibition came into effect, all of that revenue was lost. Loss of liquor revenue also cost the federal government, with some estimates ranging as high as $11 billion. Additionally, the federal government had to put forth extra money to enforce prohibition, with estimates as high as 300 million dollars.[27]

Loopholes

Recall, the 19th amendment did not make it illegal to consume alcohol; it was allowed for religious and medical purposes. Pharmacists were allowed to dispense alcohol for a variety of medical problems (influenza, anxiety, etc.); thus the number of registered pharmacists grew during the era of prohibition. In New York, this amount tripled during the prohibition era.[28] As you can imagine, the number of people suffering from these ailments also increased, as more people went to their local pharmacists for prescription alcohol. More people attended church to gain access to wine. Additionally, there was an increase in self-professed rabbis as they would then have legal access to wine.[29]

With an increase in religion, one would think crime rates would drop due to the improvement of moral character among US citizens, but this was not the case.

Crime

While there were no national crime statistics prior to 1930, some say prohibition contributed to a culture of lawlessness.[30] Prohibition created a large black market for beer in major cities and turned law abiding citizens, who consumed alcohol legally prior 1920, into criminals post-1920. The black market for beer was quite lucrative, contributing to widespread corruption of police and public officials.[31] In Chicago and other large cities, an increase in murders was seen, perhaps due to the disagreements over illegal alcohol production.[32]

The black market for alcohol created conditions conducive for organized crime organizations to thrive. The American mafia grew as they became a large player in bootlegged liquor. The success of these crime organizations relied on good relationships with local

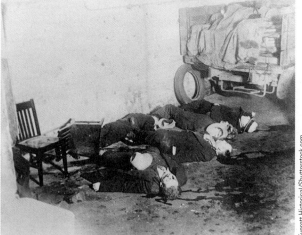

Prohibition led to an increase in organized crime. The Saint Valentine's Day Massacre resulted from a struggle between two gangs for control of crime in Chicago. Seven gangsters of Bugs Moran's gang were killed by Al Capone's in a garage in Chicago on Feb 14, 1929.

Everett Historical/Shutterstock.com

police and public officials, which were developed and maintained through bribes.[33] Al Capone, a crime boss in Chicago, thrived under these conditions. He created a bootlegging international industry consisting of hundreds of breweries and distilleries. He paid off almost every law enforcement agent and public official in the districts, earning over 100 million dollars per year.[34]

It should also be noted that several women's groups opposed prohibition. One group, the Molly Pitcher Club, named after the Revolutionary War heroine, sought to have prohibition overturned because the group found that prohibition led to an increase in violence and lawlessness.[35] In 1929, Pauline Sabin, the first woman to serve on the Republican National Committee, and other influential women formed the Women's Organization for National Prohibition Reform (WONPR). Sabin and WONPR realized that prohibition caused more problems than it cured. The repeal of prohibition was a major platform for the 1932 Presidential election, which contributed to the victory of Franklin D. Roosevelt who promised Americans he would repeal prohibition.[36] The Cullen–Harrison Act was signed by the President in March 1933, allowing the sale of beer (less than 3.2% alcohol) and wine. Later that year, the 21st Amendment was ratified, which repealed prohibition.

Current Alcohol Use

In 2014, a little more than half of all Americans reported to having consumed alcohol.[37] Alcohol use varies greatly, with negative consequences increasing as patterns of alcohol use increase. [38]

Social Drinkers

Most people who drink today are *social drinkers*. Also called "low-risk" drinking, these drinking patterns do not lead to long-term health or social problems, although they may experience immediate risks such as accidents. Social drinkers are able to abstain from alcohol at will.[39]

Problem Drinkers

Problem drinkers engage in risky drinking activity, but can modify their behavior when faced with negative consequences due to their drinking behavior.[40] Problem drinkers sometimes engage in heavy drinking, but are not physically dependent on alcohol and will not experience withdrawal symptoms when abstaining from alcohol.[41] Problem drinkers may engage in **binge drinking** behavior, which is consuming four drinks for women and five drinks for men in a short time period (2 hours).[42] Most people who binge drink are not alcohol dependent. This is

---

FACTS REGARDING BINGE DRINKING

- One in six Americans binge drink about four times a month (coincides with the average number of weekends per month)
- 92% of Americans who drink excessively report to binge drinking in the last 30 days
- Binge drinking is more common among men compared to women
- 90% of underage drinking is in the form of binge drinking
- More than half of the alcohol consumed in the US is in the form of binge drinking

Source: Centers for Disease Control, "Fact Sheet-Binge Drinking." Updated October 16, 2015. Accessed on November 12, 2016 from http://www.cdc.gov/alcohol/fact-sheets/binge-drinking.htm.

---

the most common type of excessive drinking with almost 25% of Americans over the age of 12 engaging in this type of behavior.[43] A person can abuse alcohol and not be an alcoholic. Problem drinkers do not necessarily drink daily or even frequently. See Figure 6.2 for trends related to problem drinkers and binge drinking.

Alcoholics

Unlike the previous drinking behaviors, alcoholics cannot control their drinking behaviors in spite of the negative consequences experienced as a result of alcohol. Considered to be alcohol dependent, alcoholics will experience withdrawal symptoms when abstaining from alcohol. Table 6.1 highlights problem drinking and alcoholism signs. More about alcoholics and alcoholism will be discussed later in this chapter.

Factors Contributing to Alcohol Use

Cost

One factor affecting the extent of alcohol consumption is cost. As costs increase, consumption levels decrease. This can be achieved through raising excise taxes on alcohol. These tax increases are used to reduce harm by reducing excessive alcohol consumption while raising revenue received from these taxes.[44] In a study

---

distilled spirits Beverages such as whiskey, rum, gin, and vodka that are produced by boiling various solutions

binge drinking Consuming five or more drinks for men and four or more drinks for women in a short period of time

TABLE 6.1 Problem and Alcoholism Warning Signs

Signs of Problem Drinking[1]	Signs of Alcoholism[2]
Need alcohol to feel comfortable in social situations	Inability to control drinking after the first drink
Need alcohol to feel good about yourself	Obsessing about alcohol
Need alcohol to feel happy	Repeating unwanted drinking behaviors despite negative consequences
Need alcohol to have a good time	Setting drinking limits and not be able to adhere to them
Need alcohol to escape from problems	Chronic blackouts

Sources: [1]Problem Drinking vs. Alcoholism: Learn the Difference. Alcoholic.org. Accessed on November 12, 2016 from http://www.alcoholic .org/research/problem-drinking-vs-alcoholism-learn-the-difference/.

[2]S.A. Benton, "Social drinkers, problem drinkers, and Alcoholics: Differences and Warning Signs", *Psychology Today* (2009). Accessed on November 12, 2016 from https://www.psychologytoday.com/blog/the-high-functioning-alcoholic/200904/social-drinkers-problem-drinkers -and-alcoholics.

reviewing the effects of alcohol cost and other factors, researchers determined a decrease in overall consumption, decreased alcohol motor vehicle crashes, and a decrease in alcohol-related violence.[45]

Neighborhood

Where one lives can influence alcohol consumption patterns. Living in a more advantaged and educated urban neighborhood has been associated with greater alcohol consumption rates among young adults.[46] Those who live in rural areas are more likely to abstain from alcohol but consume more alcohol per occasion.[47]

Gender

Abstinence, overall, is increasing for men and women. Rates of abstention for both sexes increase as people age but as education and family income go up, abstinence rates go down.[48]

Because more women are seeking treatment, one could surmise that drinking problems among women are increasing. This may be misleading because the stigma of women having drinking problems is diminishing and therefore many women who previously shunned treatment out of fear of being stigmatized are now getting help. However, men have higher rates of alcohol use compared to women. They are more likely to engage in excessive drinking behavior and drink more frequently.[49] Gender roles in America may contribute to this gender disparity regarding alcohol consumption. For example, men may be more likely to drink because it demonstrates masculinity and facilitates aggression.[50] Furthermore, American culture may be more accepting of excessive drinking by men but less accepting of the same behaviors by women. Some also stipulate that women are more likely to successfully quit drinking due to their generally lower levels of drinking (i.e., less alcohol per drinking episode).

In regard to women's drinking patterns, the demographic subgroups that stand out include women who are unemployed, looking for work, or employed part-time outside the home. Drinking problems are

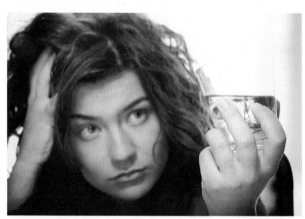

Women who suffer from depression have higher rates of alcohol consumption.

more prevalent among women who are divorced, separated, or not married but living with a partner. Women in their 20s to early 30s as well as women with husbands or partners who drink heavily are at greater risk for becoming problem drinkers. For many women, heavy drinking started after a health problem such as depression or reproductive difficulties.[51]

Ethnicity

Whites typically begin drinking at an earlier age than Blacks and Hispanics. Moreover, Whites progress to alcohol dependence at a faster rate than Blacks and Hispanics.[52] In addition, African American youth are less likely than White or Latino adolescents to drink any alcohol, engage in excessive alcohol use, or develop an alcohol use disorder.[53] Furthermore, African American youth start drinking later and their drinking is less likely to persist throughout adolescence.[54] Alcohol-related mortality is greater for Black and Hispanic men than for White and Asian American men.[55] Black men possibly have more alcohol-related problems than White men because of their higher unemployment rate, discrimination, poor living conditions, and inadequate health care, rather than alcohol use per se.

Among individuals seeking alcohol treatment, Blacks and Hispanics are less likely to seek help than Whites.[56]

Any discussion of drinking patterns among Hispanics is complicated by their cultural diversity. Among the numerous Hispanic groups are Mexicans, Puerto Ricans, and Cubans. In contrast to men and women of Puerto Rican or Cuban origin, Mexican American men and women are more likely to either abstain from alcohol or to drink heavily. Also, Mexican American men and women have more alcohol-related problems than the other two groups. Drinking patterns seem to be affected by **acculturation**. The more acculturated a person becomes, the more he or she follows the drinking patterns of the adopted population.[57]

One study of Caucasian and Asian students found that Asian students were better able to resist social pressure to drink alcohol than Caucasian students.[58] Many Asians have a mutant gene that causes the alcohol-flush reaction when they drink alcohol. Because of this genetic mutation, the liver is less able to metabolize alcohol. Symptoms of the alcohol-flush reaction include facial flushing, heart palpitations, dizziness, and nausea. Consequently, alcohol use and problems are less prevalent among Asian Americans than among all other major racial and ethnic groups in the United States.

Similarly, generalizing about drinking patterns of American Indians is unwise because of tribal diversity. Some tribes have a high incidence of alcohol abuse, and others are primarily abstinent. The research is not consistent. One national study found that Native American adolescents drank more than Hispanics and Blacks but less than Whites.[59] A study of Native American youths in Montana showed that Native American youth began drinking at an earlier age and more heavily than White youths.[60] Because of stress due to perceived discrimination, it was found that 20% of Native American youths begin drinking by age 11 to 12 and that these young people are at greater risk for becoming problem drinkers.[61]

Examining deaths caused by alcohol is one way to assess the extent of alcohol-related problems among American Indians and Alaska Natives. Rates of suicides, accidents, homicides, and especially cirrhosis of the liver—conditions influenced by alcohol—are higher among American Indians and Alaska Natives than the general population. In the last 40 years, the rate of suicide among Native Americans has increased significantly.[62] Native Americans have the highest rates of alcohol-related deaths of all ethnicities in the United States.[63] The high incidence of accidents and homicides is attributed to binge drinking, which is characteristic of some tribes.

It is speculated that American Indians experience a flushing response similar to the flushing reaction in Asians but that it is milder and less unpleasant than the Asian flushing response.[64] This flushing reaction has little effect on drinking frequency or amount.

Sexual Orientation

Those who identify as sexual minorities may experience higher rates of alcohol use. Lesbian women have more than three times greater odds of lifetime alcohol use disorders compared to heterosexual women.[65] On the other hand, one study found that men who identified as being a sexual minority had significantly lower rates of alcohol use disorders compared to heterosexual men.[66] However, another study found an increased risk of alcohol dependence among homosexual men, although there was only a slight increase in risk. [67]

While there are increased risks of alcohol use among sexual minorities, it may have more to do with other characteristics of being in a marginalized subgroup. For example, homosexual persons are more likely to be single and never married, both relationship categories associated with increased risk of alcohol-related problems. Additionally, having children in the household is considered a protective factor against alcohol-related problems, with same-sex couples reporting to having fewer households with children in them.[68] Perhaps the greatest impact on sexual minorities is "minority stress." These are stresses placed on minority populations that are quite different from the stresses placed on nonstigmatized populations. They are chronic, socially based, and include experiences of prejudice, discrimination, and internalized homophobia.[69] These influences and stressors may be the greatest factors in risk of alcohol-related problems.

Other Variables

- College students who are fraternity and sorority members have significantly higher alcohol consumption rates than students who are not affiliated with fraternities and sororities.[70] Among fraternity members, 75% drink heavily compared to nonfraternity peers. Sixty-two percent of sorority members drink heavily compared to 41% of nonsorority peers.[71]
- Binge drinking is more common in households with an annual income above $75,000 than among households with incomes below $75,000.[72]
- Adolescents who are victims of bullying are more likely to drink as a coping mechanism.[73]

acculturation The adaptation and acceptance of cultural and social norms of a new environment

Drinking on Campus

College students drink more alcohol compared to their noncollege-attending peers. To illustrate this point, one study found approximately 32% of college students meet the criteria for alcohol abuse and 6% meet the criteria for alcohol dependence.[74]

The number of arrests on college campuses for alcohol and other drugs has increased dramatically in the last few years. This increase may reflect stricter enforcement policies by college administrators. In a survey of 343 colleges in the United States, 61% responded that they enforced alcohol policies.[75] Many colleges have responded by creating policies that ban alcohol altogether, with approximately 34% of US colleges and universities having a ban on alcohol.[76] However, whether a college campus is considered a "wet" or "dry" campus has little impact on problematic drinking behaviors, although some evidence has shown there is a decrease in alcohol dependence on "dry" campuses.[77]

US colleges are not alone in addressing alcohol use by students. At one Australian university, almost one-half of students drank to harmful or hazardous levels.[78] In Germany, it was reported that 80% of university students drank heavily and that 20% displayed problem drinking.[79]

Drinking Among Older Adults

Even though older Americans have lower levels of alcohol use and abuse, alcoholism is increasing among the elderly. One national survey found that 6.7% of people over age 65 exhibit alcohol abuse or

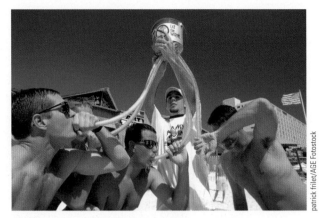
Binge drinking is prevalent on college campuses.

patrick frilet/AGE Fotostock

dependence symptoms.[80] Alcohol abuse among the elderly is not limited to the United States: One report cites alcohol abuse in Britain as becoming epidemic among the elderly.[81] Loneliness and isolation make the elderly more vulnerable to alcoholism. While some older people reduce alcohol use because of different stressors in their lives, for others, those same stressors may result in an increase in alcohol abuse.[82] Also, over one-third of male and female problem drinkers use alcohol to manage pain. Fifteen percent of male nonproblem drinkers and 13% of female nonproblem drinkers use alcohol to manage pain.[83]

Older men are twice as likely as older women to have alcohol-related problems or late-life onset of alcoholism.[84] Older drinkers are more likely to experience hangovers from alcohol use.[85] Despite the increase in alcoholism among the elderly, the

---

ON CAMPUS

Alcohol is a problem on college campus; with more college students engaging in problematic alcohol consumption compared to their non college attending peers. Three-fourths of college students who were sexually assaulted reported being under the influence of alcohol during the assault. One study found 30% of students have claimed to experience a sexual assault while attending college. While the consumption of alcohol does not cause assault, it is associated with higher rates of sexual assault.

Questions to ponder:

In an age where consent is king, and consent must be free and informed, how does one distinguish between intoxicated sex and incapacitated sex?

Alcohol has been shown to lower inhibitions, change what someone does and says, and increase the likelihood of engaging in risky behavior. What do you think is the role of alcohol on a victim and perpetrator of sexual assault?

Source: S. Hepola, "The alcohol blackboard", *Texas Monthly*, 44, no.1 (2016): 112–161.

percentage of abstainers also increases in older age groups.[86] The greater proportion of abstainers among older age groups might be attributed to heavy drinkers' dying before they reach old age. More people aged 55 or older seek treatment for alcohol abuse than do people who are younger than age 55.[87]

Alcoholic Beverages

Alcohol is a central nervous system depressant. Beverage alcohol, or **ethyl alcohol**, should not be confused with **methyl alcohol**, or wood alcohol. Methyl alcohol is extremely toxic and may lead to blindness and death. By using certain yeasts, the carbon, hydrogen, and oxygen of sugar and water are transformed into ethyl alcohol and carbon dioxide. This process, called **fermentation**, yields beverages that are about 14% alcohol.

The percentage of alcohol in a beverage can be increased by **distillation**, a procedure in which a solution containing alcohol is boiled.[88] Alcohol has a lower boiling temperature than other liquids. Therefore, during the heating process, alcohol separates from the solution in the form of steam. The steam is captured in a cooling tube and turns back into a liquid. This distilled liquid contains a higher alcohol content.

To brew beer, sprouted barley is added to cereal grains such as corn, wheat, or rye to change the carbohydrates in the grains into sugar, while yeast changes the sugar into alcohol. The alcohol content of beer is about 5%, and beer advertised as having fewer calories also has alcohol but a smaller percentage.

Fruit juices, particularly those with high sugar content, are used to make wine. The alcohol content of wine ranges from 8 to 14% generally. Wine coolers, a mixture of wine with various carbonated beverages, first introduced in the early 1980s, are about 4% alcohol by volume. Adding alcohol to slightly sweetened wines produces **fortified wines** such as sherry and port. These have higher alcohol content. In the United States, labels on bottles of distilled alcohol, such as rum, gin, and whiskey, indicate the **proof** of the contents. The amount of alcohol is determined by dividing the proof in half. Thus, a bottle that is 80 proof is 40% alcohol. Figure 6.2 shows the equivalent content of alcohol for beer, wine, and hard liquor.

Pharmacology of Alcohol

Alcohol is transformed in the liver into **acetaldehyde** and then to acetate, water, and carbon dioxide. It is eliminated from the body through urine, exhalation,

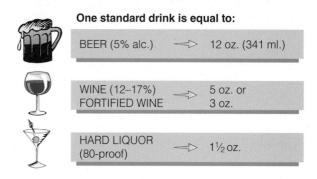

STANDARD DRINK CONVERSION

One standard drink is equal to:

BEER (5% alc.) ⟹ 12 oz. (341 ml.)

WINE (12–17%) FORTIFIED WINE ⟹ 5 oz. or 3 oz.

HARD LIQUOR (80-proof) ⟹ 1½ oz.

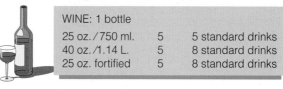

One standard drink represents 13.6 grams of absolute alcohol

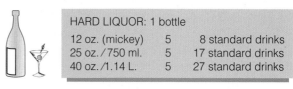

WINE: 1 bottle		
25 oz. / 750 ml.	5	5 standard drinks
40 oz. / 1.14 L.	5	8 standard drinks
25 oz. fortified	5	8 standard drinks

HARD LIQUOR: 1 bottle		
12 oz. (mickey)	5	8 standard drinks
25 oz. / 750 ml.	5	17 standard drinks
40 oz. / 1.14 L.	5	27 standard drinks

For light beer or light wine, standard drinks are calculated in terms of a ratio. For example, 12 oz. of a 2.5% light beer = 0.5 SDs, while 12 oz. of a 4% light beer = 0.8.

Figure 6.2 Standard Drink Conversion

and sweat. Alcohol leaves the body at a rate of approximately three-fourths ounce per hour. An ounce of distilled spirits, a bottle of beer, and a glass of wine all have about the same amount of alcohol.

---

ethyl alcohol The form of alcohol that people consume

methyl alcohol Wood alcohol; not fit for human consumption

fermentation The process of transforming certain yeasts, carbon, hydrogen, and oxygen of sugar and water into ethyl alcohol and carbon dioxide

distillation A heating process that increases alcohol content

fortified wines Beverages produced by adding alcohol to slightly sweetened wines

proof Amount of alcohol in a beverage expressed as twice the percentage of the alcohol content

alcopops Malt, distilled alcohol-containing, or wine-containing beverages that have been flavored with fruit juices or other added ingredients; an example is Mike's Hard Lemonade

acetaldehyde Product of metabolism of alcohol by the liver; also found in tobacco smoke

Three people attend a party. Person A drinks only wine, Person B drinks only beer, and Person C drinks only Vodka. They each have four drinks. At the end of the party which one is more 'drunk'?

The amount of alcohol in a drink can be calculated by multiplying the volume of the drink by the percentage of alcohol it contains. Remember to express percentage of alcohol in its decimal form before doing the multiplication. (5% = .05) *Volume of serving X Concentration of alcohol*

Type of Drink	Volume of serving (in ounces)	Concentration of alcohol expressed as a percent	Concentration of alcohol expressed in decimal form	Total amount of alcohol in ounces
Beer	12	5%	.05	
Wine	5	12%		
Hard Liquor	1.5	40%		

Thus beer and wine are capable of producing the same intoxicating effects as hard liquor.

The primary site of absorption is the small intestine. Several factors affect the rate of absorption. If food is in the stomach, alcohol is absorbed more slowly. Wine and beer are absorbed less quickly than distilled spirits. One exception is champagne, which is absorbed more quickly. This is partly due to the presence of carbon dioxide in champagne. Carbonated drinks are absorbed more quickly. Carbonation increases the pressure on the stomach, which helps force alcohol into the bloodstream via the stomach lining. Thus it does not have to travel to the small intestine to become absorbed into the bloodstream.[89] This effect is seen in not only drinks that are created with carbon dioxide, but also drinks mixed or ingested with a carbonated mixer. The speed at which food travels from the stomach to the small intestine is affected by strong emotions. Emotions such as anger and fear cause food, including alcohol, to be absorbed more quickly.

Males and females absorb alcohol at different rates. Because the average male body is larger and contains more water than the average female, males are less likely to feel the effects from the same amount of alcohol.[90] Another difference is that men have more gastric alcohol dehydrogenase activity, enabling them to metabolize alcohol more quickly than women. Hence, there is a greater buildup of alcohol in women, as alcohol leaves their bodies more slowly.

A woman herself does not always absorb alcohol at the same rate. In the premenstrual phase of her cycle, a woman absorbs alcohol more quickly than at other times. Thus she will feel the effects of alcohol faster. Also, women who take birth control pills absorb alcohol more quickly than women who do not.

The concentration of alcohol in the blood is referred to as **blood alcohol concentration (BAC)** or **blood alcohol level (BAL)**. The effect of alcohol on a person correlates with the percentage of alcohol in the person's bloodstream. Table 6.2 shows the percentage of alcohol in the body, or BAC, based on amount of alcohol consumed and body weight.

If alcohol is consumed at a rate exceeding the rate at which alcohol is metabolized or leaves the body, the BAC rises. As the BAC increases, behavioral and subjective effects become more pronounced. Drinking too much alcohol in a short time can be fatal. A brief summary of alcohol's effects at varying BACs is shown in Table 6.3.

TABLE 6.2 Approximate Blood Alcohol Concentrations

Drinks (per hour)	Body Weight (pounds)							
	100	120	140	160	180	200	220	240
1	.04	.03	.03	.02	.02	.02	.02	.02
2	.08	.06	.05	.05	.04	.04	.03	.03
3	.11	.09	.08	.07	.06	.06	.05	.05
4	.15	.12	.11	.09	.08	.08	.07	.06
5	.19	.16	.13	.12	.11	.09	.09	.08
6	.23	.19	.16	.14	.13	.11	.10	.09
7	.26	.22	.19	.16	.15	.13	.12	.11
8	.30	.25	.21	.19	.17	.15	.14	.13
9	.34	.28	.24	.21	.19	.17	.15	.14
10	.38	.31	.27	.23	.21	.19	.17	.16

Source: Distilled Spirits Council of the United States.

TABLE 6.3 Effects of Alcohol at Varying Blood Alcohol Concentrations

BAC	Effects
0.05%	Less alert; less inhibited; slightly impaired judgment; slight euphoria
0.10%	Slower reaction time; impaired muscle control; reduced visual and auditory acuity; legal intoxication in most states
0.15%	Distorted perception and judgment; impaired mental and physical functions; less responsible behavior
0.20%	Markedly affected psychomotor ability; difficulty staying awake
0.25%	Inability to stand without help; grossly affected ability to comprehend
0.30%	Stuporous state; inability to respond to stimuli; not likely to remember events the next day
0.35%	Completely anesthetized; 1% will die at this BAC
0.40%	State of unconsciousness or coma; half will fatally overdose without medical intervention
0.50%	Deep coma or complete unconsciousness if not already dead

Effects of Alcohol

Alcohol accounts for 10% of all deaths in the United States each year, and the life expectancy of an alcoholic is reduced by 15 years. It affects every organ in the body. Two important factors that determine how alcohol affects the body are frequency of use and quantity consumed. The type of alcohol consumed does not matter. In a study of male and female adolescents, beer, wine, and distilled spirits produced equally damaging physical impairment.[91] In this section, we will examine the acute and chronic effects of alcohol on the brain, liver, gastrointestinal tract, cardiovascular system, and immune system, as well as the relationship between alcohol and cancer. Figure 6.3 illustrates the effects of alcohol on various body systems.

The definition of moderate drinking for men is no more than two alcoholic drinks per day, and for women, it is no more than one alcoholic drink per day. Light drinking would be less than this amount. There is no standard definition of heavy drinking, although a commonly accepted number for binge drinking is consumption of five or more drinks at one sitting for men and four or more drinks at one sitting for women.

Alcohol and the Brain

The brain is highly sensitive to the effects of alcohol. Five to six drinks daily will adversely affect cognitive functioning. The extent of impairment increases with

blood alcohol concentration (BAC)/blood alcohol level (BAL) Percentage of alcohol in the bloodstream

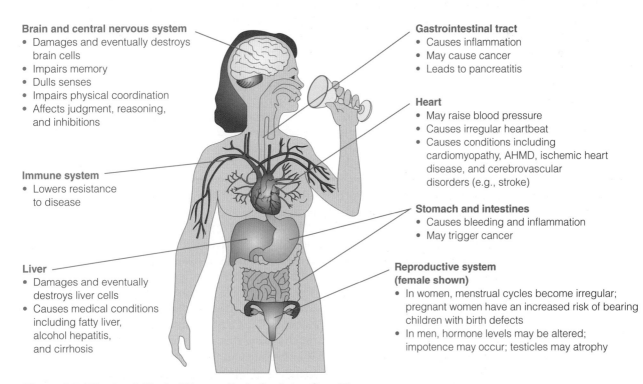

Brain and central nervous system
- Damages and eventually destroys brain cells
- Impairs memory
- Dulls senses
- Impairs physical coordination
- Affects judgment, reasoning, and inhibitions

Immune system
- Lowers resistance to disease

Liver
- Damages and eventually destroys liver cells
- Causes medical conditions including fatty liver, alcohol hepatitis, and cirrhosis

Gastrointestinal tract
- Causes inflammation
- May cause cancer
- Leads to pancreatitis

Heart
- May raise blood pressure
- Causes irregular heartbeat
- Causes conditions including cardiomyopathy, AHMD, ischemic heart disease, and cerebrovascular disorders (e.g., stroke)

Stomach and intestines
- Causes bleeding and inflammation
- May trigger cancer

Reproductive system (female shown)
- In women, menstrual cycles become irregular; pregnant women have an increased risk of bearing children with birth defects
- In men, hormone levels may be altered; impotence may occur; testicles may atrophy

Figure 6.3 Effects of Alcohol Use on Body Systems Over Time

higher levels of consumption. An estimated 15 to 30% of all nursing home patients are admitted because of permanent alcohol-induced brain damage.[92] Alcohol acts on the cerebrum, affecting judgment, reasoning, and inhibitions. It stimulates the release of serotonin, which could account for the disinhibiting effect of alcohol.

Alcohol acting on the cerebral cortex affects motor activity and moods change quickly. Alcohol stimulates the release of dopamine, accounting for feelings of pleasure or euphoria. The senses are impaired when alcohol affects the cerebellum. Many alcoholics experience memory loss and difficulty with problem-solving and decision-making.[93] At some level of consumption of alcohol, the medulla is sedated to the point that respiration could stop.

Alcohol produces brain damage that can be seen using computer tomography imaging. These images look for brain shrinking, which is a way of identifying brain damage. Both alcoholic men and women experience significant brain shrinking because of alcohol consumption, but what is most concerning is alcoholic women who drank for about half the amount of time as men showed similar signs of shrinkage. This suggests the woman's brain is more vulnerable to alcohol compared to a man's brain.[94]

Although drinking small amounts of alcohol daily does not affect memory adversely, occasional large amounts could harm memory. Alcohol use disorders have been associated with a decrease in working memory and episodic memory.[95] Working memory is the brain's way of manipulating short-term information and is associated with decision-making and behavior. Episodic memory is the feeling one gets from remembering a past event. It is more than just a factual set of events, but includes an emotional memory of the event. A study of teenagers in the United Kingdom found that those who used excessive amounts of alcohol suffered from memory problems.[96] Similarly, US middle-school students experienced memory loss after drinking.[97]

Alcohol-induced amnesia usually lasts a short time. Some people appear conscious and even function when they drink, but later, they have no memory of what transpired. This condition, referred to as an alcohol-induced blackout, may be an early indication of alcoholism. Finally, prenatal exposure of the fetus to alcohol possibly affects its attention and memory for the long term even with no more than one drink per day.[98]

One condition resulting from chronic alcohol abuse is Wernicke–Korsakoff syndrome, which occurs in about 20% of chronic alcohol users. This syndrome develops because alcohol impedes the body's ability to utilize thiamine, one of the B vitamins. Brain lesions form on the brain, which are caused by high demands of already depleted vitamin B1 (thiamine) stores.[99] If discovered and treated early, some of the symptoms associated with this syndrome are reversible, but if not treated early on, it may lead to death. The person with this disorder is able to remember events or facts learned early in life but unable to recall recent events or facts. Other characteristics of this disease are disorientation, nerve damage, poor coordination, and rapid horizontal eye movement.

Alcohol and the Liver

Chronic alcohol consumption increases the risk for cancer in many organs, including the liver.[100] Because the liver is the main site of metabolism of alcohol, heavy alcohol use can have devastating effects on that organ. The three main conditions associated with overuse of alcohol are fatty liver, alcohol hepatitis, and cirrhosis. If one already has hepatitis C, then alcohol will exacerbate the condition, resulting in a shorter lifespan. The mean age of death for women with hepatitis C who drink heavily is reduced from 61.0 years to 49.1 years. The comparable reduction for males is from 55.1 to 50.0 years.[101] Cirrhosis is irreversible, even if alcohol use stops. Some signs of fatty liver are evident in 90 to 100% of heavy drinkers, whereas 10 to 35% develop alcohol hepatitis, and 10 to 20% develop cirrhosis.[102] Fatty liver can develop within a few days of heavy drinking. Symptoms of alcohol hepatitis include jaundice (a yellowish skin color), fatigue, low-grade fever, reduced appetite, dark urine, and occasional vomiting and nausea.

Cirrhosis of the liver, a deadly condition in which liver cells are destroyed, occurs in about 10% of long-term heavy drinkers. Deaths from chronic liver disease and cirrhosis have been declining in the United States; in 1970, 17.8 deaths from cirrhosis was reported compared to 12.0 deaths per 100,000 in 2014.[103] Nevertheless, liver cirrhosis remains the 12th leading cause of death in the United States.[104]

Women are more susceptible than men to alcohol-related liver damage despite their lower levels of consumption. Also, women show symptoms of liver disease after shorter time spans of alcohol use. The elderly have seen an increase in alcohol-related liver diseases. Moreover, their prognosis is especially poor.[105] The cirrhosis mortality rate of Hispanics is much greater that Whites and non-Hispanic Blacks.[106] White males and females have lower rates of cirrhosis than non-White males and females.

ALCOHOLIC LIVER DISEASE

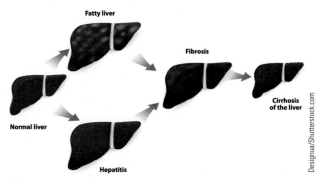

Alcoholic liver disease. Fatty liver, Fibrosis, Hepatitis, Cirrhosis of the liver. illustration. Any kind of alcohol can cause liver damage.

Alcohol and the Gastrointestinal Tract

In moderate amounts, alcohol aids digestion by increasing the secretion of gastric juices in the stomach. Yet, alcohol can irritate the stomach, leading to internal bleeding. When alcohol is consumed on a regular basis, the esophagus and existing peptic ulcers are subject to inflammation.[107] Irritation of the esophagus is marked by chest pain and pain while swallowing. Alcohol abusers have higher rates of esophageal cancer and gastric carcinomas. Because a high proportion of alcohol abusers also smoke, it is difficult to delineate how much damage is attributable to alcohol use and how much is due to smoking. When alcohol is taken with aspirin, the inner lining of the stomach is especially prone to damage. Internal bleeding is especially common when alcohol and aspirin are taken together.

Heavy alcohol use is implicated in an increased risk of tooth decay, gum disease, and loss of teeth.[108] Heavy use has shown to damage the salivary glands and interfere with saliva secretion. Alcoholics may also suffer from inflammation of the tongue and mouth, although it is unclear whether this effect is from the alcohol itself, or from poor nutrition, which is often a symptom of heavy alcohol use.[109]

Heavy alcohol use is implicated in acute pancreatitis, a potentially fatal condition marked by severe abdominal pain, nausea, occasional diarrhea, tachycardia, vomiting, and fever. The pancreas secretes insulin and regulates blood sugar levels. More than three-fourths of chronic pancreatitis cases are related to heavy alcohol consumption. It is believed that alcohol abuse is the major cause of chronic pancreatitis.[110] Development of alcoholic pancreatitis occurs, typically, after 10 to 15 years of heavy drinking.

Alcoholics often incur malnutrition because alcohol interferes with the body's ability to utilize nutrients and also causes diarrhea, which leaches nutrients out of the body. Additionally, people who consume large amounts of alcohol often replace calories from food with alcohol. At least 80% of patients with alcohol-related liver disease have protein energy malnutrition and vitamin defiency.[111] Alcohol alters how the body metabolizes proteins, carbohydrates, lipids (fats), and minerals. Also, alcoholics tend to have poor eating habits and, as a result, often become anemic. Nutritional inadequacies are linked to liver disease, certain forms of cancer, pancreatic disease, and fetal alcohol syndrome in newborns. In young and middle-aged men, chronic alcohol use has been associated with the bone disorder osteoporosis.

Alcohol and the Cardiovascular System

Depending on the level of consumption, alcohol consumption can be both protective and harmful to the heart. Nonetheless, light-to-moderate alcohol use (less than three drinks per day) reduces the risk of heart disease, boosts the good (high-density lipoprotein) cholesterol, and helps prevent type 2 diabetes. Specifically, light-to-moderate users have lower risk of coronary artery disease, ischemic stroke, and heart failure.[112] It has also been shown that women who drink moderately are less likely to become overweight, although the opposite is true for men.[113] Furthermore, in a study among postmenopausal women, it was shown that light-to-moderate drinking may be a protective factor against weight gain and obesity, with wine showing the strongest predictor.[114]

Degeneration of the heart muscle, known as alcoholic heart muscle disease or cardiomyopathy, occurs in about 2% of alcoholics, and less severe forms of this condition are found in most alcoholics. Other conditions include high blood pressure, cardiac arrhythmias, ischemic heart disease (deficient circulation of the blood to the heart), and cerebrovascular disorders such as strokes. Abnormal cardiac rhythms can result from years of heavy drinking, as well as from binge drinking. This "holiday heart syndrome" is more likely to occur around holidays and on Mondays after a weekend of binging. Symptoms of the holiday heart syndrome include irregular palpitations, dizziness, or chest pain and can affect both heavy drinkers and those who seldom drink.[115] Too much caffeine, salt, and lack of sleep are other factors that contribute to this syndrome.[116]

Moderate alcohol consumption (no more than one drink per day for women or two drinks per day for men) has not been shown to cause high blood pressure, although blood pressure rises moderately during drinking. Nonetheless, it has been reported that men with hypertension who drink moderately have a decreased risk of a heart attack.[117] Stroke-like episodes sometimes appear within 24 hours after a drinking binge. People who drink four or more drinks daily have a 62% risk of having a stroke.[118]

Many studies point to a positive relationship between moderate alcohol use and reduced coronary heart disease, particularly for people at risk for heart disease. In fact, regular, moderate alcohol use has been said to reduce the risk of heart disease by 40%. Guidelines published in May 2000 by the US Department of Agriculture indicate that moderate alcohol use can benefit men older than age 45 and women older than age 55 (although the cardiovascular benefits of alcohol were not shown to benefit younger people).[119] The National Institute on Alcohol Abuse and Alcoholism (NIAAA) supports the idea that moderate alcohol use is beneficial cardiovascularly.[120] In a study of 124,000 people, the evidence was clear that moderate alcohol use reduced mortality.[121]

Alcohol and the Immune System

Moderate alcohol consumption has been associated with reduced inflammation and improved response to vaccination.[122] Other studies show moderate alcohol use reduces immunity.[123] Chronic alcoholics are considered immune compromised hosts and are more prone to infections such as pneumonia and peritonitis.[124] Alcohol interferes with the movement of white blood cells, which is important in fighting infections. A type of white blood cells, **T lymphocytes**, which help to resist infections, are notably deficient in alcoholics with severe liver disease.

Alcohol dependence reduces immunity to HIV.[125] One study found that women with HIV tend to drink more alcohol, exacerbating their deterioration.[126] In contrast, a study conducted in 2016 showed drinking patterns among HIV-infected persons to be less compared to the general population. They attribute this to increased awareness of the detrimental effect alcohol has on the antiretroviral drugs used to treat HIV.[127] There is an association between heavy alcohol users and the risk of HIV transmission.[128] Heavy alcohol drinkers are more likely to engage in unsafe sexual behavior, have more sexual partners, and share syringes for other drug use, all of which are risk factors for HIV infection.[129] A study of American and Australian homeless youth found that they were more prone to developing HIV because they were more likely to engage in high-risk behaviors, especially Australian youths.[130] Animal studies demonstrate that HIV infection passes more readily from mother to fetus when drugs such as alcohol are abused.[131]

Alcohol and Cancer

The relationship between alcohol and cancer is complex because the effects vary by quantity and cancer site. The US Department of Health and Human Services released the 14th report on carcinogens, which lists alcoholic beverage consumption as a known carcinogen.[132] Thus the more alcohol a person consumes in a lifetime, the higher the risk of developing alcohol-related cancer. It is estimated that 3.5% of all cancer deaths in the United States are alcohol related.[133] Considerable research links alcohol abuse and certain forms of cancer, especially cancers of the nasopharynx, esophagus, larynx, and liver. A European study of more than 500,000 people found that the risk of colon cancer was 26% higher for those people who had more than two alcoholic drinks per day.[134] A Dutch study indicated that colorectal cancer was related to heavy alcohol use but not to light use.[135] In another study that included 750,000 people, on the other hand, those who drank four to seven glasses of red wine per week were only 52% as likely to be diagnosed with prostate cancer.[136] Similarly, individuals who drank two or more glasses of wine per week had a 40% reduction in developing kidney cancer.[137]

There is a relationship between alcohol consumption and breast cancer. It is estimated that the relative risk for breast cancer increases 7% for every drink per day.[138] Additionally, women who consume two to five drinks per day have 1.5 times the risk of breast cancer.[139] It is estimated that 4% of newly diagnosed cases of breast cancer among women in the United States can be attributed to chronic alcohol use.[140]

Consuming four or more drinks increases the likelihood of oral and pharyngeal cancer five-fold.[141] The same amount of alcohol results in a 30% greater risk for pancreatic cancer.[142] Although alcohol abuse can cause high rates of esophageal cancer even among nonsmokers, alcohol and smoking combined produce a much higher rate, suggesting a synergistic effect.

Beer consumption is related to cancers of the lower gastrointestinal tract. This could be attributable to **congeners**—the nonalcoholic ingredients such as flavoring agents or other residual substances—rather than alcohol itself.

Fetal Alcohol Spectrum Disorders

Fetal alcohol spectrum disorders (FASD) is a general term describing the various effects that occur as a result of women who drink alcohol while pregnant. These effects can be behavioral, physical, and/or mental, see Figure 6.4. In addition, they can produce learning disabilities.[143] The leading known cause of mental retardation is FASD.[144] Unfortunately, diagnosing FASD is difficult because the physical markers for in-utero alcohol use are not apparent. The facial deformities do not always appear.[145]

Alcohol traverses the placenta and interferes with fetal development. The fetus is especially vulnerable during the first trimester of pregnancy. Unfortunately, many women drink alcohol before realizing they are pregnant as most women do not know they are pregnancy until they are four to six weeks into the pregnancy. Three in four women who want to get pregnant as soon as possible report drinking alcohol; thus women are advised to abstain from alcohol while trying to get pregnant.[146] The Centers for Disease Control estimates more than 3 million women are at risk of exposing their baby to alcohol, and there are no safe limits for alcohol use during pregnancy.[147] Yet an estimated 1 in 10 pregnant women consume alcohol while pregnant, with the highest rates among women aged 35 to 44 years old, college graduates, and unmarried women.[148]

In addition to a smaller brain at birth, children with FASD are marked by head and facial anomalies such as a small head, flat cheeks, and thin lips, as well as retarded growth, central nervous system problems, and malformations of many major organs in the body. As these children get older, they exhibit behavioral problems including hyperactivity, short attention span, poor impulse control, and poor coordination. An Australian study found that women who drank more than one drink per day or who engaged in binge drinking had children with learning, attention, and intellectual problems.[149] Children of mothers who used alcohol while pregnant were studied over a period of 25 years. After 25 years, there was a higher likelihood of attention, arithmetic, spatial-visual memory, and IQ deficits as well as increased alcohol problems and psychiatric disorders.[150]

THE NIAAA'S FOUR CRITERIA FOR DEFINING FETAL ALCOHOL SYNDROME:

- Maternal drinking during pregnancy
- A characteristic pattern of facial deformities
- Growth retardation
- Brain damage, which often is manifested by intellectual difficulties or behavioral problems

Source: National Institute on Alcohol Abuse and Alcoholism, *Alcohol Alert* No. 50, December 2000.

Children with FASD also suffer from eye-related problems, although they are not the only people who have eye-related problems from alcohol. Chronic alcoholism is associated with a significantly increased risk of cataracts, color vision deficiencies, and problems with the cornea.[151] Also, there may be a link between prenatal alcohol exposure and iron-deficiency anemia in infancy. The prenatal effects of alcohol may be exacerbated by iron deficiency.[152] FASD is irreversible but preventable.

T lymphocytes Type of white blood cells that help in fighting infections

congeners The nonalcoholic ingredients in some forms of alcohol, such as flavoring agents or other residual substances

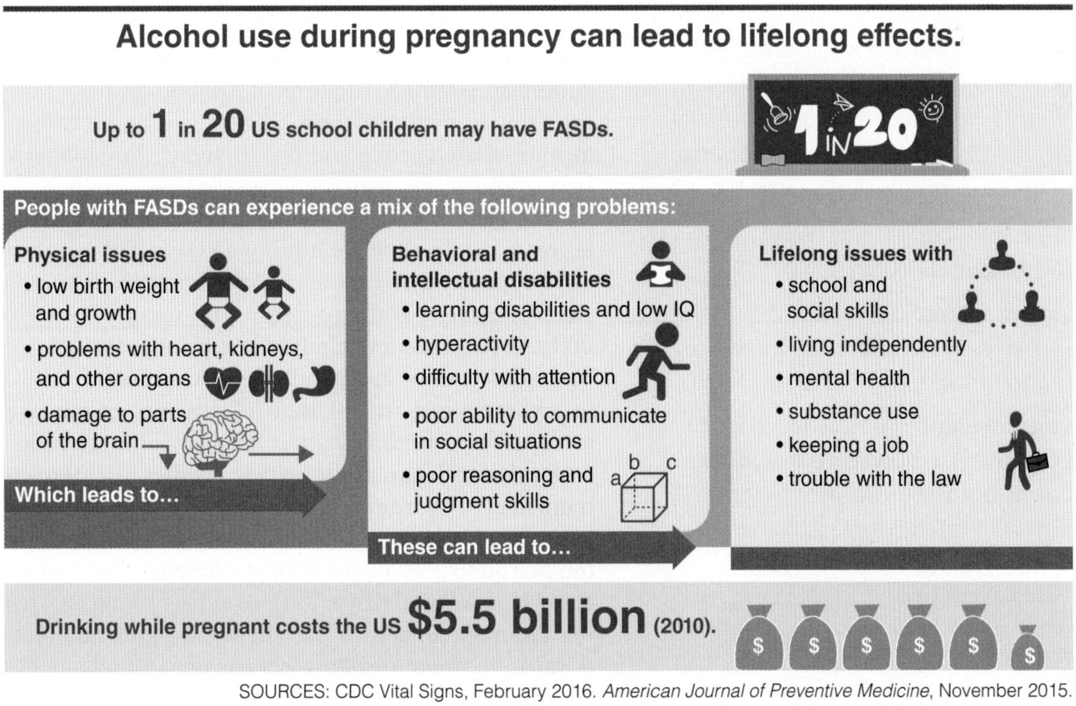
Alcohol use during pregnancy can lead to lifelong effects.
Up to 1 in 20 US school children may have FASDs.
1 IN 20
People with FASDs can experience a mix of the following problems:
Physical issues
• low birth weight and growth
• problems with heart, kidneys, and other organs
• damage to parts of the brain
Which leads to...
Behavioral and intellectual disabilities
• learning disabilities and low IQ
• hyperactivity
• difficulty with attention
• poor ability to communicate in social situations
• poor reasoning and judgment skills
a b c
These can lead to...
Lifelong issues with
• school and social skills
• living independently
• mental health
• substance use
• keeping a job
• trouble with the law
Drinking while pregnant costs the US $5.5 billion (2010).
SOURCES: CDC Vital Signs, February 2016. American Journal of Preventive Medicine, November 2015.

Figure 6.4 Alcohol use during pregnancy has a negative impact on the growing fetus.

Since 1989, the US Surgeon General's office has required that all alcoholic beverages bear a label warning pregnant women of the hazards of drinking. Unlike labels on cigarette packages, these labels are not uniform and are difficult to see. Nevertheless, after the labels were introduced, drinking by pregnant women decreased, although most women who reduced their alcohol consumption were low-risk drinkers.[153] About 5% of pregnant women who drink alcohol also use other drugs. Some drugs like cocaine are especially harmful to the developing fetus, but it is difficult to know the interactive effects of many drugs with alcohol.[154]

A study by the Alan Guttmacher Institute found that half of the doctors it surveyed believe that occasional alcohol use during pregnancy will not increase the risk of adverse outcomes, despite the fact that since the early 1980s the federal government has advised women to refrain from consuming alcohol during pregnancy.[155]

What is the incidence of FASD? On a worldwide basis, it is estimated that 0.97 per 1,000 live births have fetal alcohol syndrome, although it is commonly believed that the rate is much higher.[156] Healthcare

costs for each affected baby is $2,842, but follow-up care would increase that amount significantly.[157] In the United States, FASD rates are considerably higher among Native Americans than among the general population.[158] To quantify exactly how much alcohol the mother has to drink to cause FASD would be difficult. Some women consume two drinks daily and produce children with FASD, whereas other mothers can drink the same amount and not have babies with FASD. Some neurobehavioral problems have appeared with as few as seven drinks per week.[159] A woman who consumes four to six drinks per day has a one-third chance of bearing a child with FASD. One thing is clear, though: The more a pregnant woman drinks, the more likely it is that FASD will develop.

Many women who drink heavily in early pregnancy have higher rates of miscarriages, suggesting that FASD rates may be underreported. A perplexing point is that not all women who drink excessively deliver offspring with FASD. Therefore maternal or genetic factors may account for some women bearing children with characteristics of FASD.

Alcohol-Related Issues

Alcohol has been implicated in violent behavior, suicide, criminal activity, automobile accidents, premature death and disability, and loss of productivity in industry. Next, we will explore underage drinking, caffeinated alcohol, alcoholism, and symptoms associated with alcohol withdrawal.

Underage Drinking

Alcohol is the most widely used drug among American youth.[160] In terms of premature death, disease, injury, property damage, motor vehicle crashes, alcohol-related crime and productivity, the economic cost of underage drinking amounts to $27 billion.[161] By the age of 15, 33% of teens reported to having at least one drink while among 18-year-olds, almost 60% report having at least one drink.[162] Reasons stated among youths regarding underage drinking include seeking new challenges, peer pressure, increased desire for independence, and stress.[163]

More than 4,300 deaths among youth are attributed to underage drinking.[164] This includes 1,580 deaths from motor vehicle crashes, 1,269 from homicides, 245 from alcohol poisoning, and 492 from suicides.[165] High school students who engaged in binge drinking 10 or more times were six times more likely to drink and drive.[166]

Another concern is that there is a significant relationship between drinking before age 13 and suicide attempts, especially among youths with a history of depression.[167] Youth who start drinking before the age

---

CASE STUDY: Drinking and Pregnancy

A pregnant woman walks into a bar...

No, this is not the beginning of some joke, it is now mandated by the State of New York that women may not be refused alcohol at bars or other establishments that serve alcohol. These rights fall under the New York City Commission on Human Rights and 'prohibits unlawful discrimination in employment, public accommodations, and housing on the basis of pregnant or perceived pregnancy".

Questions to ponder:

Should pregnant women be allowed to drink alcohol at public establishments? Should they be limited on the amount of alcohol served?

Some foods are considered unsafe for pregnant women to consume (i.e. raw fish), should food restrictions be placed on pregnant women? How is this different from alcohol restrictions?

Source: NEW YORK COMMISSION ON HUMAN RIGHTS, "NYC Commission on Human Rights Legal Enforcement Guidance on Discrimination on the Basis of Pregnancy: Local Law No. 78 (2013); N.Y.C. Admin. Code § 8-107(22)", Accessed on November 13, 2016 from http://www1.nyc.gov/assets/cchr/downloads/pdf /publications/Pregnancy_InterpretiveGuide_2016.pdf.

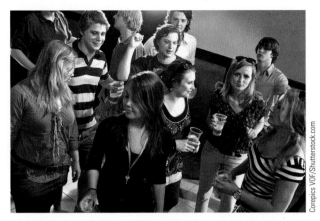
College students drink more alcohol compared to their noncollege peers.

of 15 are four times more likely to meet the criteria for alcohol dependence at some point in their lives.[168]

A vast majority of college students drink alcohol. One study reported that 19.3% injured themselves, 6.6% got into a fight, and 2.0% were coerced into sex at some point in the previous 12 months while under the influence of alcohol.[169] One group that has received little attention is community college students, although their drinking rates are believed to be lower because these students on average are older and tend to have more outside responsibilities.[170] Additionally, greater differences are seen among male college students compared to female college students who tend to drink less.[171] The alcoholic beverage of choice is beer, especially among male adolescents. The health and social costs associated with underage drinking are expected to rise because the number of underage youth will increase during the next decade. A less obvious consequence is economics in that money spent on alcohol is not spent on more constructive pursuits.

In the early 1970s, many states lowered the legal age for purchasing alcohol from 21 to 18. Subsequently, the number of alcohol-related fatalities among people in that age group increased. To address

TABLE 6.4 Problems Associated with Underage Drinking

Underage Drinking can lead to...

✓ School problems (higher rates of absenteeism, poor grades)
✓ Social problems (fighting)
✓ Legal problems (arrest due to underage drinking)
✓ Disruption of normal growth and development
✓ Higher risk for suicide and homicide
✓ Memory problems
✓ Changes in brain development that have long term effects

Source: Centers for Disease Control and Prevention, "Underage drinking". Updated October 2016. Accessed on November 13, 2016 from http://www.cdc.gov/alcohol/fact-sheets/underage-drinking.htm.

this disturbing trend, in 1984, the federal government attempted to standardize the drinking age at 21. States that did not raise the drinking age to 21 risked losing federal highway funds. By 1988, all states were in compliance with the age 21 limit. Addressing drinking by students, especially younger students, is important because it has been demonstrated that the younger one is when drinking is initiated, the more likely one will develop an alcohol dependency.[172]

Caffeinated Alcohol

Alcoholic beverages with caffeine were first introduced in 2005. These drinks, also known as "blackout in a can," ranged in alcohol content from 6.0 to 12.5%.[173] One popular brand, Four Loko, was believed to be responsible for numerous hospitalizations due to alcohol intoxication.[174] Young adults who combine alcohol with energy drinks experience more alcohol-related harm compared to other drinkers.[175] Combining energy drinks with alcohol has been shown to offset fatigue, which may increase the urge to continue drinking.[176] Additionally, some believe combining energy drinks with alcohol reverses the impaired effects of alcohol, but this is not the case. In a study comparing the driving ability of alcohol-impaired individuals and alcohol combined with energy drinks-impaired individuals, it was shown the addition of energy of caffeinated drinks does not improve driving ability or attention/reaction time.[177] It has been shown that caffeinated alcohol adversely affects visual-spatial ability as well as cognitive functioning.[178] Essentially, caffeinated alcohol enables an individual to be awake longer and so he or she is able to drink more. Hence, these drinks result in greater intoxication.[179] In 2010, the US Food and Drug Administration banned adding caffeine to alcohol.[180]

Not everyone supports the ban on caffeine being added to alcohol. There are many examples in which caffeine is mixed with alcohol, such as rum and Coke, Irish coffee, and Red Bull and vodka. According to Jacob Sullum, editor of *Reason* magazine, the proposed ban on Four Loko resulted from only two studies. He maintains that the conclusions drawn from those studies are questionable.[181]

Alcoholism

Alcoholism has many definitions, none of which is universally accepted. Some consider it to be a disease. The disease concept gained popularity with the

blackouts A common symptom of problem drinking; characterized by temporary memory loss

alcoholism Condition in which an individual loses control over intake of alcohol

decline of the temperance movement and the failure of the movement to prohibit alcohol. The notion that alcoholism is a disease identifies the individual as having some kind of personal defect rather than placing the blame on failed social policies. The idea that alcoholism is a progressive disease that follows a series of stages was promoted by E. M. Jellinek. His ideas have been dismissed because most alcoholics do not follow consistent patterns.

The 1994 revision of the *Diagnostic and Statistical Manual of Mental Disorders Fourth Edition* (*DSM-IV*) discarded the term *alcoholism* in favor of **alcohol abuse** and **alcohol dependence**. Alcohol abuse refers to continued drinking despite recurring social, interpersonal, and legal problems. Alcohol dependence is predicated on the presence or absence of tolerance and withdrawal. According to the US Department of Health and Human Services, alcohol dependence is "a disease that is characterized by abnormal alcohol-seeking behavior that leads to impaired control over drinking."[182]

Increasingly, mental health experts are viewing alcohol abuse on a continuum with a range of treatments. Whether alcoholism is considered a disease is important. As a society, we are not likely to hold people at fault for having a disease. Thus, if alcoholism is a disease, drunkenness can be used as a legal defense. Also, if alcoholics run afoul of the law, they receive treatment rather than punishment.

Two common threads that run through the various definitions of alcoholism are the following:

1. Alcoholics are unable to control their drinking.
2. Some physical, social, or psychological consequence will result from their drinking.

In 2013, the American Psychiatric Association updated the DSM manual to version 5. In this new version, there are changes in regards to alcohol use and abuse. In the new edition, alcohol abuse and alcohol dependence now fall under one category: alcohol use disorder (AUD).[183] There are further delineated into classifications of mild, moderate, and severe. Furthermore, anyone meeting two of the eleven criteria during a 12-month period would be classified as having an alcohol use disorder.

See Figure 6.5 for a comparison between the two editions.

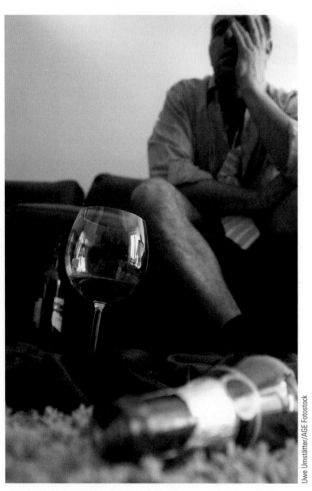

■ Alcoholism affects 1 out of every 10 Americans.

DEFINITIONS OF ALCOHOLISM/ALCOHOLIC

American Medical Association: Significant impairment that is directly associated with persistent and excessive use of alcohol. Impairment may involve physiological, psychological, or social dysfunction.

American Psychiatric Association: Patients whose alcohol intake is great enough to damage their physical health, or their personal or social functioning, or when it has become a prerequisite to normal functioning.

National Council on Alcoholism and Drug Dependency: A disease in which there is impaired control over drinking, preoccupation with alcohol, continued use of alcohol in the face of adverse consequences, and distorted thinking.

American Society of Addiction Medicine: A primary, chronic disease with genetic, psychological, and environmental factors influencing its development and manifestations. The disease is often progressive and fatal. It is characterized by continuous or periodic impaired control over drinking, preoccupation with alcohol, use of alcohol despite adverse consequences, and distortions in thinking, most notably denial.

DSM–IV		DSM–5	
In the past year, have you:		**In the past year, have you:**	
Any 1 = ALCOHOL ABUSE — Found that drinking—or being sick from drinking—often interfered with taking care of your home or family? Or caused job troubles? Or school problems?	1	Had times when you ended up drinking more, or longer, than you intended?	The presence of at least 2 of these symptoms indicates an **Alcohol Use Disorder (AUD).**
More than once gotten into situations while or after drinking that increased your chances of getting hurt (such as driving, swimming, using machinery, walking in a dangerous area, or having unsafe sex)?	2	More than once wanted to cut down or stop drinking, or tried to, but couldn't?	
More than once gotten arrested, been held at a police station, or had other legal problems because of your drinking? ****This is not included in DSM–5****	3	Spent a lot of time drinking? Or being sick or getting over other aftereffects?	The severity of the AUD is defined as:
Continued to drink even though it was causing trouble with your family or friends?	4	Wanted a drink so badly you couldn't think of anything else? ****This is new to DSM–5****	**Mild:** The presence of 2 to 3 symptoms
Any 3 = ALCOHOL DEPENDENCE — Had to drink much more than you once did to get the effect you want? Or found that your usual number of drinks had much less effect than before?	5	Found that drinking—or being sick from drinking—often interfered with taking care of your home or family? Or caused job troubles? Or school problems?	**Moderate:** The presence of 4 to 5 symptoms
Found that when the effects of alcohol were wearing off, you had withdrawal symptoms, such as trouble sleeping, shakiness, restlessness, nausea, sweating, a racing heart, or a seizure? Or sensed things that were not there?	6	Continued to drink even though it was causing trouble with your family or friends?	**Severe:** The presence of 6 or more symptoms
Had times when you ended up drinking more, or longer, than you intended?	7	Given up or cut back on activities that were important or interesting to you, or gave you pleasure, in order to drink?	
More than once wanted to cut down or stop drinking, or tried to, but couldn't?	8	More than once gotten into situations while or after drinking that increased your chances of getting hurt (such as driving, swimming, using machinery, walking in a dangerous area, or having unsafe sex)?	
Spent a lot of time drinking? Or being sick or getting over other aftereffects?	9	Continued to drink even though it was making you feel depressed or anxious or adding to another health problem? Or after having had a memory blackout?	
Given up or cut back on activities that were important or interesting to you, or gave you pleasure, in order to drink?	10	Had to drink much more than you once did to get the effect you want? Or found that your usual number of drinks had much less effect than before?	
Continued to drink even though it was making you feel depressed or anxious or adding to another health problem? Or after having had a memory blackout?	11	Found that when the effects of alcohol were wearing off, you had withdrawal symptoms, such as trouble sleeping, shakiness, restlessness, nausea, sweating, a racing heart, or a seizure? Or sensed things that were not there?	

Figure 6.5 Changes from DSM-IV to 5

Withdrawal

Like other depressants, alcohol can create dependency. Thus an alcohol-dependent person who stops drinking undergoes withdrawal symptoms. The first 5 days of withdrawal are the most severe, although withdrawal symptoms can last for weeks. The craving for alcohol is one obvious symptom of withdrawal. Other characteristics of alcohol withdrawal are the following See Figure 6.6:

1. *Delirium tremens (DTs):* A potentially fatal withdrawal symptom marked by delusions, confusion, and disorientation. The person might feel bugs crawling on the skin. The initial phase of DTs lasts from one day to one week. DTs cannot be cured, and medical supervision is necessary. It is estimated that between 3 and 5% of patients who are hospitalized for alcohol withdrawal experience DTs, with 1 to 4% of these patients dying.[184] During withdrawal, a sedative sometimes is administered to ease the discomfort.

2. *Extreme arousal:* Characterized by anxiety, irritability, absence of hunger, and inability to get to sleep. This state of arousal is actually a rebound effect, as an alcoholic is typically depressed.

3. *Auditory and visual hallucinations:* Visions and imaginary perceptions occur in about one-fourth of alcoholics during withdrawal.

4. *Physiological symptoms:* Include elevated temperature and blood pressure, fast pulse, dilation of pupils, and increased perspiration (may last for

alcohol abuse A state characterized by physical, social, intellectual, emotional, or financial problems resulting from the use of alcohol

alcohol dependence Condition in which one's body requires alcohol or else withdrawal symptoms will occur; also marked by tolerance

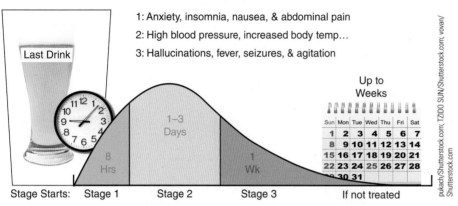

Alcohol Withdrawal Timeline

Last Drink

1: Anxiety, insomnia, nausea, & abdominal pain

2: High blood pressure, increased body temp...

3: Hallucinations, fever, seizures, & agitation

8 Hrs

1–3 Days

1 Wk

Up to Weeks

Stage Starts: Stage 1   Stage 2   Stage 3   If not treated

Figure 6.6 There Are Three General Stages During Alcohol Withdrawal

two or three days), increased sensitivity to sounds and touch, and grand mal seizures.

5. *Cognitive symptoms:* Impaired concentration, memory, and judgment.

Alcohol withdrawal is broken down into stages.[185]

- Stage 1: Anxiety, insomnia, nausea, and abdominal pain. Begins 8 hours after the last drink.
- Stage 2: High blood pressure, increased body temperature, unusual heart rate, and confusion. Begins 24 to 72 hours after the last drink.
- Stage 3: Hallucinations, fever, seizures, and agitation. Beings 72+ hours after the last drink.

Causes of Alcoholism

In the 1800s, a common view of alcoholism was that it was a matter of personal choice. Today, theories explaining the causes of alcoholism range from heredity to sociocultural reasons to differences in biochemistry to personality differences to interpersonal factors. No single theory provides a definitive explanation.[186] A family history of alcoholism is strongly linked to children's alcoholism. According to the *Ninth Special Report to the US Congress on Alcohol and Health* in 1997, "a positive family history for alcoholism is one of the most consistent and powerful predictors of a person's risk for developing the disease." Regardless of the cause for alcoholism, it has been shown that drinking at an early age is associated with later alcoholism. One study found that among alcoholics, 47% had problems with alcohol by age 21.[187] In the following sections, we will examine various theories that seek to explain factors contributing to alcoholism.

Genetics

One way to determine whether alcoholism is genetic is by studying identical twins. Four decades ago, a researcher found that if one identical twin was alcoholic, the chance of the other twin being alcoholic was 71%.[188] It is estimated that the heritability of alcoholism fall between 50 and 80%, suggesting a genetic risk for alcoholism.[189] The odds of fraternal twins both being alcoholic was 32%. More recent twin studies found that the heritability of alcoholism for males was 50%. The heritability for female twins was nil.[190] However, women tend to become addicted to alcohol more quickly than men.[191] In a study looking at young adolescence and young adults, a specific gene (GABRA2) has been linked with an increase in drunkenness, with a greater impact on females compared to males.[192] This may explain the gender difference on the impact of alcoholism and also suggests that drinking alcohol during this developmental stage in life produces a greater risk for having problems with alcoholism later in life.

These studies suggest that genetics could well be a predisposing factor. Twins, however, are socially closer than nontwin siblings and therefore their relationship might lead to imitative behavior. However, Danish twins born to an alcoholic parent but adopted by the age of six weeks to nonalcoholic parents had a higher rate of alcoholism than adopted children born to nonalcoholic parents.[193] Other studies corroborate that children born to alcoholic parents but adopted during infancy and reared by others were at greater risk for alcoholism.[194] Using adoption studies to determine the possible presence of a genetic link to alcoholism has been criticized on the grounds that adoption agencies are biased in how they decide where to place children, and that there is no standard definition of alcoholism.

According to the NIAAA, between 50 and 60% of alcoholism vulnerability has a genetic basis.[195] Recent studies suggest that many genes may play a role in the development of alcoholism,[196] but one of the difficulties is identifying these specific genes. The National Institute on Alcohol Abuse and Alcoholism has funded the Collaborative Studies on Genetics of Alcohol study since 1989 with the hopes of being able to identify specific genes that play a role in alcoholism.[197] To date, many studies have been done to identify specific genes not only to identify genes that influence the risk of alcoholism, but also to help inform treatment decisions regarding the treatment of alcoholism.[198] It is speculated that some neurotransmitters such as serotonin or gamma-aminobutyric acid may be linked to alcoholism.[199] The genetic predisposition to alcoholism may involve a lack of physiological sensitivity to the effects of alcohol, which can lead to heavy drinking.

It is speculated that environmental factors affect the impact of genetics, especially at critical times in one's development.[200] Twins who were maltreated are more likely to become alcoholic. This suggests that genetics and environment both play a role in the development of alcoholism.[201]

Finally, even if genetics is a factor, environmental conditions such as marriage have an ameliorating effect. And, even though the rate of alcoholism among children of alcoholics is higher, most children of alcoholics do not become alcoholics. Practically speaking, children of alcoholics should be mindful of the greater risk but understand that they are not consigned to a life of alcoholism if one or both parents are alcoholics.

Psychosocial Factors

The psychological and social bases for alcoholism include how individuals start using alcohol, the reinforcing qualities of alcohol, and individual traits of people who become alcoholics. Those who believe that alcoholism is a personality disorder view alcoholics as immature and fixated in their development. Most people use alcohol socially and do not progress further. Progression from social drinking to dependence is influenced by one's psychological state and expectations regarding alcohol's effects, the setting in which alcohol is used, and its pharmacological properties. Drinking alone or with others makes a difference in terms of alcohol consumption. For example, individuals are more likely to drink heavily when they are in a group than when they are alone.

A current study found that 20% of alcoholics have a concurrent mood or anxiety disorder. Also, 20% of people with a mood or anxiety disorder had a concurrent substance abuse disorder.[202] The most common disorders associated with alcohol abuse are posttraumatic stress disorder and major depression.[203] Mood disorders and anxiety also play a role in heavy alcohol consumption with one study finding sexual minority groups having higher rates of anxiety and mood disorders, which is related to higher rates of heavy alcohol use.[204] There is research demonstrating that people who lack impulse control have higher rates of alcoholism.[205] For many women, there is a strong relationship between violent behavior and alcohol dependence.[206]

Alcohol problems during adolescence and adulthood have been linked to antisocial behavior in childhood. The relationship between alcohol and depression also occurs among adolescents.[207] However, parents can serve as a protective factor for children with mood disorders by being present in their children's lives and monitoring their children's behavior. One study found that higher rates of alcohol use among children who experienced depression could be offset by increased levels of parental monitoring.[208] Because alcohol produces mild euphoria and reduces anxiety, its use is reinforcing. However, individuals with social anxiety engage in more hazardous drinking when in a party situation.[209]

People's expectations about alcohol have been shown to be predictors of alcohol dependence. Alcohol abusers anticipate the effects of alcohol to be positive. Likewise, if using alcohol is viewed as helpful in coping with negative moods, the potential for abuse is higher. The adolescents at greatest risk for developing alcohol-related problems think alcohol is socially enhancing.

College students who expect positive outcomes from drinking alcohol likewise are heavier drinkers. Abuse is more common among people who believe that alcohol enhances their social and physical enjoyment, potency, aggression, sexual performance and responsiveness, and social competence. However, individuals who expected alcohol to increase their sexual risk-taking behavior did engage in more sexual risk-taking behaviors.[210] Alcohol is linked to sexual behavior. One study of college students found that 32% drank alcohol prior to having unprotected vaginal sex.[211]

One-third of high school students report they are sexually active and one-fourth of these students used alcohol or another drug before their last sexual intercourse.[212] Another study of 18- to 25-year-olds noted that alcohol dependence is associated with a greater

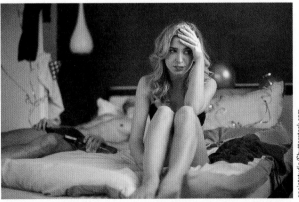

Alcohol consumption has been linked with risky sexual behaviors.

number of sexual partners—ten or more partners.[213] Despite anecdotes about how alcohol makes people appear more attractive, alcohol use does affect one's perception about the appearance of others.[214] Many adolescents expect alcohol to have a disinhibiting effect and, consequently, engage in risk-taking sexual behavior.

Culture

An important variable related to drinking patterns is the attitude of a given culture, subculture, or group that implicitly or explicitly establishes its own rules for behavior. Alcohol abuse is low in any group in which most group members agree on drinking customs, values, and sanctions. Moreover, groups that accept moderate drinking, but not heavy drinking, abuse alcohol less. Among Canadian college students, the degree of alcohol use is dictated by their perceptions of how much other students drink. If they perceive that other students drink a lot, then those students will drink comparably. Likewise, students will limit their drinking if they perceive that other students drink very little.[215] In an international survey of college students in 21 developed and developing countries, the highest rates of drinking were in Belgium, Colombia, Ireland, Poland (men), and England (women).[216]

Religious groups such as Muslims and Mormons advocate abstinence. The greater one's religious commitment, the less likely one is to drink heavily and the more likely one will abstain.[217] When alcohol is used ritualistically (in religious ceremonies or for special occasions) or is consumed for social reasons, heavy drinking is minimal. In contrast, another study found religiosity and religious affiliation do not protect against the development of an alcohol use disorder. These researchers suggest spiritual experiences have a protective factor against developing an alcohol use disorder and may help play a role in treatment of alcohol use disorders.[218] Prayer and mindful meditation, components of spiritual health, provide protective factors against alcohol use disorder and may help those in treatment. Alcoholism rates are higher if alcohol is used for personal reasons such as relaxing or coping with problems.

The European Union (EU) is monitoring binge drinking among teenagers because binge drinking increased from 47 to 57% in Ireland and from 37 to 50% in Norway during the last decade.[219] In a study of adolescent drinking in 30 European countries, it was found that alcohol consumption and violence were less common in Mediterranean countries than other European countries.[220] Also, rates of suicide and heavy drinking among adolescents are higher in northern Europe than in southern Europe.[221] Southern Europeans have higher rates of alcohol con-

The Drinking Age in Selected Countries

Country	Age
Argentina	18
Australia	18
Belgium	16 for beer and wine; 18 for spirits
Brazil	18
Canada	18 or 19, varies by province
China	18
Czech Republic	18
Egypt	18 for beer; 21 for wine and spirits
France	18
Germany	16 for beer and wine; 18 for spirits
Ireland	18
Israel	18
Italy	16
Mexico	18
New Zealand	18
Russia	18
United Kingdom	18
United States	21

Source: International Center for Alcohol Policies

sumption but lower rates of alcoholism. In Russia, meanwhile, where excessive alcohol use is a cultural norm, the rate of suicide is high.[222]

The mere fact that alcohol is available or restricted is not a factor in rates of alcoholism. Forbidding children from drinking small amounts of alcohol does not affect whether they ultimately become alcoholics. Attitudes toward alcohol, reasons for its use, and demonstrating how it can be consumed responsibly are more important in whether children drink abusively. The Cultural Considerations given here shows the age by which one can drink alcohol.

Alcohol and Society

Alcohol can devastate friends, families, neighbors, and others with whom the drinker is involved. The media regularly report family violence, criminal activities, suicides, accidents, and automobile fatalities attributed to alcohol. Violent behavior is dose-related in that the more one drinks, the more likely one is to become violent.[223] Moreover, intoxicated males are more likely than nonintoxicated males to find that using force to obtain sex is acceptable.[224]

Alcohol is the most widely used substance in the United States with an estimated 1 in 12 adults suffering from alcohol abuse or dependence.[225] Additionally, more than 7 million children are living in a household where one parent is abusing alcohol.[226] Moreover, alcoholism is the third leading lifestyle-related cause of death in the United States, and is responsible for an average of 30 years of potential life lost for each death.[227] In a separate study of emergency room patients, it was found that drinking doubles the risk of injury.[228]

Automobile Accidents

The leading cause of death among youth ages 15 to 20 is motor vehicle crashes. Yet, 57% of 16- to 20-year-olds drove a vehicle when they thought that they were over the legal limit.[229] The age group with the highest rate of drunk-driving fatal crashes is 21 to 24. This age group accounts for 35% of all fatal crashes in which the BAC is 0.08 or higher.[230] Among the 3,306 pedestrian fatalities in 2009, 48% of either drivers or pedestrians had a BAC of 0.08 or higher.[231]

In 2015, alcohol-impaired driving fatalities increased by 3.2% compared to 2014.[232] Alcohol-impaired driving accounts for almost 30% of all vehicle fatalities in the United States.[233] In 2015, over 10,000 people died as a result of alcohol-related motor vehicle accidents in the United States (see Table 6.5).[234] Drivers with a BAC of 0.08 or higher are eight times more likely to have a prior "driving while impaired" conviction than drivers with no alcohol.[235]

However, it has been found that revoking a driver's license immediately has more impact than waiting until there is a conviction.[236] One strategy that effectively reduces drinking and driving is the implementation of ignition interlocks.[237] These are devices that use breath analysis to prevent drunk drivers from being able to start their car. Before starting the car,

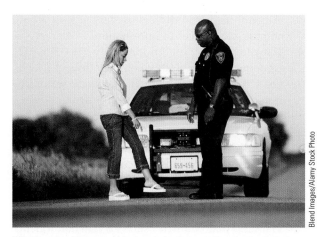

The rate of "driving while intoxicated" convictions in the United States has increased since the late 1990s.

a driver must breath into a device that measures the driver's alcohol level. If the level is higher than the programmed amount, the vehicle will not start. A recent study concluded a reduction of 15% in alcohol-related vehicle deaths in states that use ignition interlocks.[238]

Responsible beverage service laws are requirements or incentives for retail alcohol establishments (i.e., bars, liquor stores) to participate in reducing alcohol-related problems.[239] These establishments participate in training programs aimed at reducing underage alcohol sales and serving already intoxicated customers. Recognizing that having patrons who get into automobile accidents is bad for business, some bar owners have agreed to give out vouchers for taxis to their patrons. To avoid driving after drinking too much, 28% of individuals used a designated driver and 13% called a cab or a ride.[240] However, some studies have found these programs are not effective. A recent study found no association between responsible beverage laws and self-reported binge drinking or alcohol-impaired driving.[241]

The message against drinking and driving has reached to many 16- to 20-year-old drivers. It is estimated that raising the drinking age to 21 has reduced fatalities involving 18- to 20-year-old drivers by 13% and has saved an estimated 19,121 lives since 1975.[242] Gender is an important variable. Males are five times more likely to be involved in fatal car crashes.[243] Alcohol slows down reaction time,[244] and the addition of caffeine to alcoholic beverages does not improve driving performance.[245] Alcohol affects the driver in the following ways:

1. A driver who is under the influence of alcohol processes information more slowly than one who is not.
2. Alcohol-impaired drivers are more likely to look to the center of their visual field and not use their peripheral vision.

TABLE 6.5 Fatalities, by Role, in Crashes Involving at Least One Driver with a BAC of 0.08 or Higher, 2009

Role	Number	Percentage of Total
Driver with BAC = 0.08+	7,281	67%
Passenger Riding w/ Driver with BAC = 0.08+	1,772	16%
Subtotal	**9,053**	**84%**
Occupants of Other Vehicles	1,119	10%
Nonoccupants	667	6%
Total Fatalities	**10,839**	**100%**

3. Alcohol-impaired drivers are less able to attend to multiple sources of information.
4. People who drink moderately (0.05 BAC) underestimate hazards when they drive. In 1998, the US Senate debated whether there should be a national 0.08 BAC standard for drunk driving. Senator Paul Wellstone of Minnesota argued in favor of a 0.08 standard, citing that it would reduce alcohol-related fatalities by 5 to 8%.[246] Senator Jack Reed of Rhode Island concurred, noting that states with a 0.08 standard had 16% fewer fatal automobile deaths.[247] Senator Frank Lautenberg of New Jersey supported the 0.08 standard, claiming that countries such as Canada, Ireland, Great Britain, and Germany have successfully implemented such restrictions.[248] Rick Berman of the American Beverage Institute maintained that the evidence suggesting that a BAC of 0.08 lowers the fatal automobile rate is inconclusive.[249]

Not all US senators believe that a national 0.08 standard is appropriate. In 1998, Senators Trent Lott of Mississippi,[250] Don Nickles of Oklahoma,[251] and Craig Thomas of Wyoming[252] agreed that the issue of drunk driving has to be addressed, but that the federal government should not intervene in the states' right to decide. They asserted that the federal government should not usurp the responsibilities of individual states.

Accidents

One mode of transportation that has become more popular is mopeds. The popularity of mopeds stems in part from the fact that an individual does not need a license to drive one. However, the safety record for mopeds is bad. The BAL of moped drivers has been found to be higher than that of automobile and motorcycle drivers. Moreover, the mortality rate following moped crashes is higher than automobile and motorcycle crashes.[253] Furthermore, in 2014, 30% of all motorcycle accidents resulting in a fatality involved the driver having a BAL of 0.08 percent or higher.[254]

In general, alcohol use is overrepresented among people coming into emergency rooms. One study reported that 38% of women and 48% of men admitted into emergency rooms tested positive for psychoactive drugs, with alcohol the most prevalent.[255] In terms of fire-related fatalities, victims were more likely to have higher BAC levels than survivors of drug-related fires.[256] According to the US Coast Guard, there were 137 fatalities and 302 injuries emanating from alcohol-related boating accidents in 2014.[257] Alcohol use is the contributing factors in fatal boating accidents resulting in 21% of fatalities from boating accidents.[258]

One study found that over 9% of workers were hung over while at work.[259] The International Labor Office estimates that over 30% of all workplace accidents are a result of alcohol consumption.[260] Furthermore, one study found that one-third of all workplaces deaths can be attributed to alcohol use at work.[261] The professions with the highest rate of heavy alcohol users are food service workers (17.4%) followed by construction workers (15.1%).[262]

Suicide

Suicide is among the top 20 leading causes of death in the world.[263] Alcohol and drug abuse are one of the major risk factors associated with suicide.[264] In a meta-analysis of the current literature regarding alcohol use disorder and suicide, it was concluded that alcohol use disorder was associated with suicidal ideation, suicide attempts, and completed suicides.[265]

Among soldiers in the army who commit suicide, which increased throughout the first decade of 2000, 19% involved alcohol.[266] An estimated 32% of veterans who attempted suicide were diagnosed with alcohol abuse or disorder.[267] Adolescents who attempt suicide often suffer from depression and are likely to have initiated alcohol consumption prior to age 13.[268]

Family Violence

Many studies show a relationship between alcohol abuse and intimate partner violence with alcohol use being the strongest predictors for intimate partner violence.[269] Among males and females, violence is likely to be greater on drinking days compared to non-drinking days.[270] Many studies indicate a relationship between alcohol dependence and physical abuse.[271] As the amount and frequency of alcohol use escalate, so does the probability of violence. Conversely, a reduction in intoxication reduces victimization.[272]

Numerous studies show a consistent relationship between alcohol use and dating violence.[273] In one study, one-fourth of youth who went to the emergency room for injuries related to dating violence were under the influence of alcohol.[274] In two-thirds of all homicides, the victim, assailant, or both had been drinking.[275] In an exploratory student among young adults who had perpetrated dating violence, they were asked to describe their feelings on alcohol and if it contributed to dating violence.[276] Many of these perpetrators felt alcohol escalated minor conflict and exacerbated feelings of irritation and anger.[277] Moreover, women who are victims of violence or other traumatic events have higher rates of alcohol dependence.[278]

Alcohol also is related to child abuse, though studies linking the two do not account for variables such as socioeconomic status. In one study, individuals who were abused as children reported higher levels of monthly drinking frequency and problematic drinking behaviors.[279] Additionally, children who were physically abused had higher rates of alcohol

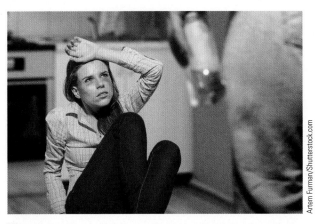
A relationship exists between alcohol use and intimate partner violence.

use disorder compared to nonabused children.[280] A connection has been identified between women who physically abuse children and alcohol abuse or dependency. Yet, cross-cultural studies show that alcohol does not have to lead to aggressive behavior.[281] One could speculate that alcohol is used as an excuse for this behavior. In other words, the relationship between aggression and alcohol use may depend on the culture where alcohol is consumed.

Children of Alcoholics

Children reared by an alcoholic parent carry a burden. Because of the shame and unpredictability of having an alcoholic parent, many children do not bring friends to their homes or have few friends. These children often experience sleep difficulties, depression, loneliness, and stomach problems. Children of alcoholics are more likely to suffer from depression, anxiety, suicidal ideation, substance abuse, and/or interpersonal difficulties.[282] Attention deficit hyperactivity disorder (ADHD) is 2.5 to 3 times more likely to occur in children whose mothers have an alcohol use disorder.[283] It is not unusual for children of alcoholics to lie, suppress feelings, and withdraw from close relationships. Moreover, they may demonstrate anger toward the nondrinking parent for not providing support and protection.[284]

The harmful effects of parental alcohol abuse do not end with childhood. Adult children of alcoholics (ACOAs) find it hard to receive and give love. They devalue themselves, are easily depressed, develop inordinate feelings of responsibility, fear abandonment, handle authority poorly, and feel guilt when asserting themselves.[285] To avoid feelings of failure and self-deprecation, they have a great need to be in control.[286] Children often go to great lengths to hide a parent's drinking problem. Secrecy and denial are key elements of a family with an alcohol problem. However, children of alcoholics will open up if they perceive the listener to be supportive and trustworthy.[287] ACOAs should recognize the following four points:

1. The family affected by alcoholism is not a normal family.
2. Responsibility and blame for an alcoholic family do not rest with them.
3. Growing up in an alcoholic household, although extremely painful, can be a learning experience.
4. ACOAs have to acquire skills to form healthy relationships.

Individuals can find support from the group Adult Children of Alcoholics, which operates similarly to Alcoholics Anonymous. Despite the difficulties, growing up in an alcoholic household does not doom a child to an unhappy, unfulfilling adulthood. Many children are resilient and transcend the frightful situations in which they find themselves.

Although the ACOA movement is beneficial to many people, it does have its detractors. One criticism is that, although ACOA meetings foster support and fellowship, they may also foster feelings of victimhood. This allows some adult children to blame their alcoholic parents for many of the problems they have. Healthy children in healthy families also grow up with conflict and disappointment, and conflict and disappointment during the formative years do not necessarily lead to problems during adulthood. Some studies have found that ACOAs have no more psychological problems than those who are not raised in an alcoholic household.[288] It has been noted that ACOAs do not have higher rates of substance abuse, defensiveness, or codependency.[289] One study found that adolescent sons of alcoholic fathers had strong senses of identity. This may be due to these adolescents maturing at a faster rate than peers.[290]

Summary

No drug is used more extensively or serves as many functions as alcohol. It played an integral role in the early history of the United States, when it was viewed positively because it contained nutrients and because other beverages were often unsanitary. The rum trade was instrumental to the economic prosperity of the United States. Concern over immoderate drinking and alcohol's role in the breakdown of the family eventually led to the temperance movement and to politically active groups such as the Women's Christian Temperance Union (WCTU), the Anti-Saloon League, and the National Prohibition Party.

National prohibition of alcohol, the 18th Amendment, went into effect in 1920. At first it reduced alcohol-related illnesses and deaths. But the law was difficult to enforce, illegal alcohol posed hazards, and there was widespread contempt for the law. In 1933, prohibition was repealed by the 21st Amendment.

Most people who drink alcohol are social drinkers. Drinking behavior varies according to geography, sex, race, and age. Generally, men drink more alcohol than women; some ethnic groups, such as Asian Americans, drink less than other groups, and older people consume less alcohol than younger people. Among college students, about 40% engage in binge drinking on a regular basis.

Alcohol is absorbed primarily in the small intestine. Food in the stomach, carbon dioxide in the beverage, emotional state, and body size affect the rate of absorption. The liver is responsible for metabolizing alcohol. The body metabolizes alcohol at a rate of three-fourths ounce per hour.

Alcohol affects every organ in the body. It affects the brain by altering inhibitions, judgment, coordination, and memory. Alcohol acts on the liver by causing fatty liver, hepatitis, and cirrhosis of the liver. The esophagus and existing peptic ulcers become inflamed from alcohol consumption. Alcohol adversely affects the heart muscle, contributing to poor circulation, raises blood pressure, and increases the risk of stroke. Alcoholics are more prone to infections. Alcohol is associated with cancer of the pharynx, esophagus, larynx, and liver. Women who drink while pregnant can deliver children with fetal alcohol spectrum disorders (FASD), a condition characterized by mental retardation and other physical anomalies.

Alcoholics use alcohol chronically and are unable to control their drinking. They differ from problem drinkers, who consume alcohol infrequently or occasionally but encounter emotional, social, financial, or interpersonal problems when they drink. Alcoholism has been shown to run in families. Studies dealing with twins and alcoholism indicate a possible relationship. Drinking patterns are affected greatly by cultural practices. Cultures that accept drunkenness, allow alcohol to be used for personal reasons, and find intoxication amusing have higher rates of alcoholism.

Everybody in society pays for the problems associated with alcohol. On college campuses, arrests for alcohol offenses increased greatly in the late 1990s. A significant amount of money goes toward treating people with alcohol-related illnesses. Half of all fatalities from automobile accidents are linked to alcohol. Alcohol use is high among those who die from accidents and suicides, and it is connected to family violence. Many children growing up in households in which one or both parents are alcoholics are left with emotional scars.

Most people who drink do so without harm to themselves or others. Yet, too many people have suffered from their own use of alcohol or from the drinking of someone else.

Thinking Critically

1. Drinking behavior is often regulated by social norms. Friends, for example, exert an influence on alcohol use. How would you characterize the norms of your friends regarding alcohol use? Do they accept moderate use? Excessive use? Abstinence? Have your norms changed in response to your friends' norms?

2. Wine coolers are popular with young people. They are sweet and are packaged similarly to soft drinks (in 12-ounce to 2-liter bottles), and advertisements are directed toward young people. What restrictions would you put on advertising and packaging of these alcoholic beverages, if any?

3. Although a person can develop cirrhosis without drinking alcohol, most cases are alcohol-induced. Because many cases of cirrhosis would not occur if people did not drink excessively, should insurance companies and tax dollars pay to treat people whose condition was brought on by their own behavior?

4. Some research shows that moderate consumption of alcohol is healthful. Other guidelines advocate no alcohol intake. Do you think moderate alcohol drinking is healthy or unhealthy, and what is your rationale?

5. Warning labels pointing out the dangers of alcohol on the developing fetus are found on alcohol containers and in places where alcohol is served. Do you think these labels have any value? What are your thoughts regarding alcohol consumption among pregnant women? Would you support alcohol consumption in moderation or complete abstinence? Defend your answer.

6. If alcoholism is accepted as a disease to which a person is genetically predisposed, should an alcoholic be held responsible for developing this disease? If a person has cancer or diabetes, is the person responsible for these conditions? What are the implications of calling alcoholism a disease?

Tobacco

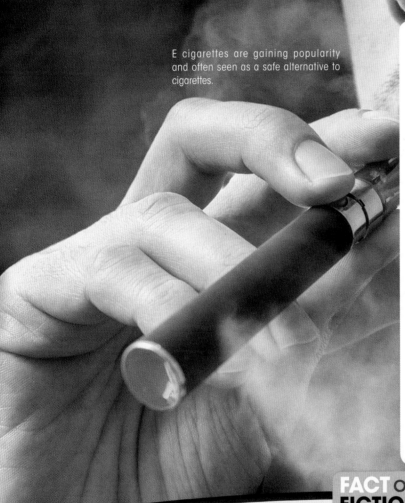

E cigarettes are gaining popularity and often seen as a safe alternative to cigarettes.

vchal/Shutterstock.com

Chapter Objectives

After completing this chapter, the reader should be able to:

- Summarize the importance of tobacco to the US colonies
- Analyze the factors that led to the popularization of cigarettes
- Assess the medical costs linked to tobacco use
- Explain the trends in tobacco use over the past century
- Explain current trends in tobacco among the US population
- Compare and contrast the benefits versus the risks of e-cigarettes from a public health perspective
- Describe the adverse effects caused by secondhand smoke
- Identify the factors associated with tobacco dependence
- Evaluate the connection between tobacco and heart disease, cancer, and respiratory conditions
- Describe the effects of maternal smoking on fetal development
- Appraise the influence of advertising on tobacco use
- List the various smoking cessation techniques and evaluate their rates of success

FACT OR FICTION?

1. In a survey of more than 20,000 Americans, approximately one-half are in favor of totally banning smoking in restaurants.

2. The majority of adults dependent on nicotine started smoking before age 18.

3. The state with the highest percentage of adult smokers is Utah.

4. Less than half as many adults smoke today compared with 40 years ago.

5. The number of people dying from tobacco-related illnesses is about the same as people dying from alcohol-related illnesses.

6. Smokers are more likely to die from heart disease than from lung cancer.

7. Nicotine is absorbed more quickly from cigarettes than from chewing tobacco.

8. More nicotine and carbon monoxide come from the burning end of a cigarette than from what the smoker exhales.

9. The number of retail outlets selling tobacco products to minors has stayed the same for the last 10 years.

10. People who stop smoking by age 35 avoid 90% of the health risks attributed to tobacco.

Turn the page to check your answers

One of the most pervasive and destructive drugs known to humankind is tobacco, and it is legal. It is entrenched in the culture, having played an integral role in the history of the United States, especially in financing the War of Independence. Efforts to regulate tobacco in the United States started in the latter part of the 1800s. Antitobacco legislation was characterized by two themes: (a) fire hazards created by smoking and (b) the morality of smoking.[1] By the beginning of the 1900s, these issues had become less important because of the economic benefits associated with the tobacco industry and states' viewing cigarette taxes as an important source of revenue. In 2013, tobacco sales generated approximately $14.3 billion in tax revenue for federal and state governments.[2] This represents a decrease of about 5% from the 2010, a trend that is expected to continue as prices on tobacco continue to increase, which results in decreased consumption.[3]

In 1995, a US Food and Drug Administration (FDA) proposal to regulate nicotine as a drug was unsuccessful. The current emphasis is on controlling the sale and promotion of cigarettes and smokeless tobacco to minors and publicizing the effects of secondhand smoke. In the adult population, the rate of smoking has declined and is about half of what it was 30 years ago. The public perception of tobacco use has become increasingly negative. What once was simply viewed as a "dirty practice" is seen now as a life-threatening addiction.

Nicotine is the addictive ingredient in tobacco. C. Everett Koop, former US Surgeon General, was the first government official to warn people of the dangers of tobacco. He claimed that nicotine dependence is as powerful as heroin and cocaine dependence. One could argue that nicotine is more addictive because it is more available, but alcohol is as available as nicotine and most drinkers do not become alcoholics, whereas 90% of smokers become dependent.

In 1988, the American Psychiatric Association recognized nicotine dependency as a disorder. Depression is common among smokers, and antidepressants are prescribed for some people who are trying to stop smoking. It is believed that being depressed precedes smoking dependency.[4] In a study of twins, it was found that genetics and environment contributed to smoking dependency.[5]

Nicotine comes from the green tobacco plant, a member of the genus *Nicotiana*. Although this plant has 60 species, only the *Nicotiana rustica* and *Nicotiana*

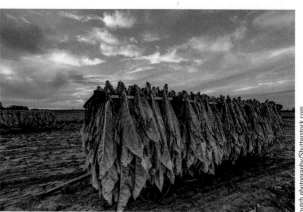

In colonial America, tobacco was seen as a valuable commodity.

FACT OR FICTION?

1. **FACT** Of people surveyed regarding the ban on restaurant smoking, 50.6% support a total ban.

2. **FACT** Eighty percent of nicotine-dependent adults started smoking before age 18.

3. **FICTION** The fact is—Utah has the lowest percentage of adult smokers with 10.4%. Kentucky has the highest percentage at 27.5%.

4. **FACT** In the 1960s, about half of American male adults smoked cigarettes. Today, the rate is less than 25%. Smoking by American women has declined from 34% to 18%.

5. **FICTION** The fact is—More than 400,000 Americans die from tobacco-related illnesses, compared with 100,000 dying from alcohol-related illnesses.

6. **FACT** Heart disease is the leading cause of death associated with cigarettes.

7. **FICTION** The fact is—Chewing tobacco results in quicker absorption of nicotine compared with cigarette smoking.

8. **FACT** Because the burning end of the cigarette is intensely hot, more nicotine and carbon monoxide come from it than from the smoker.

9. **FICTION** The fact is—The number of retail outlets selling tobacco products to minors has been reduced from 20.0% in 2000 to 9.3% in 2010.

10. **FACT** At every age, there are benefits associated with quitting smoking, although there are more benefits if one quits at a younger age.

tabacum species are smoked. The tobacco from these plants is used in cigars, cigarettes, pipes, snuff, and chewing tobacco. This chapter focuses on the history of tobacco, the extent of tobacco use, the medical effects of smoking on oneself and others, and techniques for smoking cessation.

History of Tobacco Use

A stone carving in southern Mexico dating back to between A.D. 600 and A.D. 900 depicts smoke being blown through a pipe. Historians believe that people of that time used tobacco to ward off evil spirits and to communicate with a higher power. During his travels, Columbus received gifts of dried tobacco leaves. Upon returning to Europe, he passed along seeds from the tobacco plant, which the Europeans planted. Tobacco use became popular among Europeans.

At first, only wealthy people used tobacco because it was expensive. In time, tobacco became affordable to most people, and thousands of tobacco shops were operating in London by the early 1600s.

Even though tobacco was well accepted, not everyone was enamored with it. In the 17th century, Pope Urban VIII and Pope Innocent X condemned its use. Sultan Murad IV of Constantinople hanged or beheaded soldiers who smoked, and the czar of Russia slit the nostrils of smokers. Despite these measures, tobacco use continued. When the Thirty Years' War (1618–1648) was in progress, smoking was transported into Eastern Europe.

Tobacco was thought to have medical value.[6] During the plague of 1614, some people thought it warded off the illness. Further, tobacco was used to treat skin diseases; internal and external disorders; injuries; and diseases of the eyes, ears, mouth, and nose. Some people believed smoke could be used to breathe life into another person.

In 1828, when nicotine was isolated and identified as poisonous and addictive, tobacco's reputation as a medicinal agent declined. For the next 30 years, religious leaders, physicians, and educators in the United States and Europe questioned the medical value of tobacco. Moreover, it was attacked for causing mental illness, delirium tremens, impotence, and sexual perversions. Despite the warnings, tobacco continued to be used for pleasure.

Tobacco in the American Colonies

An early settlement in the New World was Jamestown, named after King James I of England. During the early 1600s, the brutal winters and food shortages took their toll on Jamestown residents. As a last resort before abandoning the settlement, Englishman John Rolfe convinced the settlers to plant tobacco. The tobacco crop flourished, and the Jamestown community began to prosper.[7]

Soon thereafter, tobacco farming spread to other communities. Tobacco was established as a valuable commodity and was used as a form of currency. Tobacco farming ultimately contributed to the wealth of many individuals. Ironically, tobacco production, financed by the French government, provided the funds for the colonial settlers to fight the Revolutionary War against England.

Mechanization and Marketing

When the United States was in its infancy, tobacco was used in snuff, cigars, and pipes, not cigarettes. Chewing tobacco was popular, particularly during the expansion westward. While traveling on horses and in carriages, people found it easier to chew tobacco than handle it otherwise. Cigarettes were cheap alternatives to other forms of tobacco.

Until the late 1800s, cigarettes were rolled by hand, and the best workers produced only four cigarettes per minute. This situation changed after the cigarette-rolling machine was patented in 1883. The Duke Company of North Carolina, under the leadership of James ("Buck") Buchanan Duke, bought the rights to the cigarette-rolling machine, which produced 120,000 cigarettes daily. This mass production enabled the Duke Company to cut cigarette prices in half. The cost of a box of ten cigarettes was 5 cents. Other companies soon got into the business of mass-producing cigarettes.

Another influential and innovative person in the tobacco industry was Richard Joshua Reynolds. In 1891, Reynolds put saccharine in tobacco to sweeten it and to give it a longer shelf life. In 1907, he introduced Prince Albert, a new brand of tobacco used for pipes and cigarettes. The promotional literature stated that because the leaves of Prince Albert were sterilized in a licorice casing, it was "the most delightful and harmless tobacco for cigarettes and pipe smokers."

Reynolds introduced other brands, too, including Camel cigarettes. Camels were considered unique because they combined Turkish and domestic tobacco leaves. They were less expensive than other cigarettes, and their popularity skyrocketed. Other companies began to produce cigarettes similar to Camels. The American Tobacco Company came out with Lucky Strike, and Liggett and Myers produced Chesterfield.

The Duke Company extended its marketing campaign to entice women to smoke. Cigarettes were the first of the tobacco products marketed to women. Women who smoked, however, were subject to tarnished reputations. They were seen as promiscuous, and it was rumored that they would grow moustaches and become infertile.

Subsequently, cigarettes were marketed to young males. As an enticement, cigarette companies included colorful cards in their packages, and the cards were traded like baseball cards are traded today. In addition, cigarettes were less costly and milder than cigars, which increased their popularity with this segment of the population.

Opposition and Escalation

One of the first critics of tobacco was physician Benjamin Rush. In 1798, he condemned tobacco for its adverse health effects. Later, the Women's Christian Temperance Union (WCTU) and other groups supported controlling the use and sale of tobacco products. Several states banned the sale of tobacco to children. Wisconsin and Nebraska went further, making possession of cigarettes illegal for children and adults alike. In 1893, Charles Hubbard, the president of the New York Board of Education, was able to get 25,000 New York students to pledge not to smoke until age 21.

Despite efforts to depict cigarette smoking as an undesirable practice, smoking continued to grow in popularity. During World War I, the YMCA, the US Army, and other groups distributed cigarettes to soldiers. After the war, cigarette sales escalated further.

The morality of smoking and concerns about its medical effects took a back seat to the public's desire. Moreover, cigarette taxes contributed to the government's revenue. During World War II, cigarette manufacturers including the makers of Lucky Strike donated cigarettes to soldiers in combat, which was seen as a patriotic gesture.

Costs of Smoking

One factor that has been shown to reduce the demand for cigarettes is an increase in their cost. Many states are currently raising cigarette taxes, with proceeds going to various programs such as smoking prevention, hospital treatment for the uninsured, and school construction. The federal government also amasses substantial tax revenues from tobacco sales. One benefit of raising cigarette taxes is that people are discouraged from smoking. Some argue these tax hikes negatively impact lower-income

Americans whose spending in New York went from 11.6 to 23.6% of their annual income on cigarettes.[8] Additionally, revenue from tobacco prices tend to go down as people find alternative ways to purchase cigarettes See Figure 7.1. This leads to a lucrative black market for cigarettes. Tobacco traffickers are buying cigarettes in low-tax states and are then selling them in high-tax states.[9] Some researchers estimate over 30% of cigarette packs are trafficked or obtained through the black marker.[10] In addition to the casual smuggling of cigarettes, international smuggling of cigarettes has been on the rise as cigarettes are easy to smuggle, generate high profits, and the chances of being caught are low.[11] These black markets have also provided income for illegal terrorists organizations including the Pakistani Taliban, Lashkar-E-Taiba, al-Qaida, Hezbollah, Hamas, FARC, and PKK.[12]

For young people, the Internet became an increasingly popular source for less-expensive cigarettes and created a problem with the process of age verification. To address this problem, in 2010, the federal government signed into law the Prevent All Cigarette Trafficking Act (PACT) designed to require age verification for all tobacco products sold, including online sales.[13] There are still problems regarding age verification regarding online sales of tobacco products. In 2011, officials in New York City filed suit against 32 residents for reselling cigarettes they purchased online.[14] In a more recent study in 2015, researchers conducted an experiment to determine if minors were able to purchase electronic cigarettes online. Results indicate that 76.5% of purchase attempts by minors were successful.[15] Table 7.1 shows the excise taxes on cigarettes and smuggling percentages and changes since 2006.

Extent of Tobacco Use

The use of tobacco has been declining since 1976. In 2014, 14% of 8th graders had smoked within the previous 30 days, which represents a decline of about 81% from 2002.[16]

The rate of smoking increased until 1964, when the Public Health Service issued the publication *Smoking and Health: Report of the Advisory Committee to the Surgeon General*. This report unequivocally identified smoking as a serious health hazard. The percentage of adult Americans who smoke decreased from 42.4% in 1965[17] to 16.8% in 2014.[18] Of those who do smoke, the number of cigarettes smoked per capita has not decreased; people who smoke tend to smoke heavily.[19]

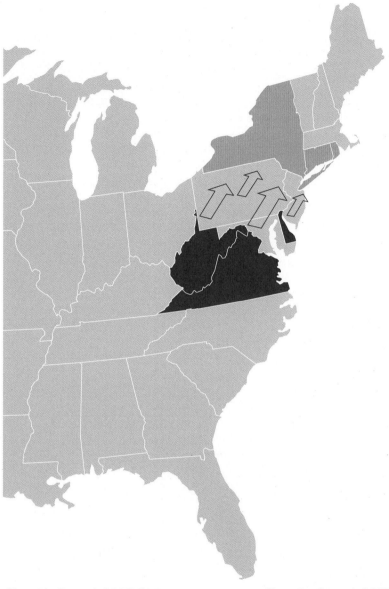

Cigarettes Smuggled INTO States		
State	Excise Tax Rate	Estimated Percentage of Smuggled Cigarettes
New York	$4.35	58.0%
Rhode Island	$3.50	32.0%
Connecticut	$3.40	24.8%

Cigarettes Smuggled OUT of States		
State	Excise Tax Rate	Estimated Percentage of Smuggled Cigarettes
Virginia	$0.30	22.6%
Delaware	$1.60	22.6%
West Virginia	$0.55	19.5%

Source: The Mackinac Center for Public Policy State Cigarette Smuggling as a Percentage of Total State Cigarette Consumption (Legel and Illegal), 2013.

Figure 7.1 Tax Rates on Cigarettes Have an Influence on State Smuggling.

Today, filtered cigarettes are more popular than unfiltered cigarettes. The change to filtered cigarettes began in the 1950s in response to concerns that unfiltered cigarettes would lead to lung cancer.[20] Although levels of **tar** and **nicotine** in

tar A carcinogenic component of tobacco

nicotine Psychoactive component in tobacco responsible for stimulation and tobacco dependence

TABLE 7.1 2013 Cigarette Tax Rates, Smuggling Percentages, and Changes Since 2006

	2013 Tax Rate (per pack)	2013 Consumption Smuggled (positive is inflow, negative is outflow)	2006 Consumption Smuggled (positive is inflow, negative is outflow)	2013 Smuggling Rank (1 is most smuggling, 50 least)	Smuggling Rank Change Since 2006 (e.g., NY changed from #5 to #1, so rank changed +4)	Cigarette Tax Rate Change, 2006-2013
New York	$4.35	+58.0%	+35.8%	1	+4	+190%
Arizona	$2.00	+49.3%	+32.1%	2	+5	+69%
Washington	$3.025	+46.4%	+38.2%	3	+1	+49%
New Mexico	$1.66	+46.1%	+39.9%	4	−2	+82%
Rhode Island	$3.50	+32.0%	+43.2%	5	−4	+42%
California	$0.87	+31.5%	+34.6%	6	+0	No Change
Wisconsin	$2.52	+31.2%	+13.1%	7	+11	+227%
Texas	$1.41	+27.4%	+14.8%	8	+8	+244%
Utah	$1.70	+27.3%	+12.9%	9	+11	+145%
Michigan	$2.00	+25.0%	+31.0%	10	−1	No Change
Connecticut	$3.40	+24.8%	+12.3%	11	+11	+125%
Montana	$1.70	+23.7%	+31.2%	12	−4	No Change
South Dakota	$1.53	+22.3%	+5.3%	13	+15	+189%
Illinois	$1.98	+20.9%	+13.7%	14	+3	+102%
Maryland	$2.00	+20.2%	+10.4%	15	+9	+100%
Minnesota	$1.60	+18.0%	+23.6%	16	−6	+1%
Florida	$1.339	+17.1%	+6.9%	17	+9	+294%
Iowa	$1.36	+16.7%	+2.4%	18	+15	+278%
Kansas	$0.79	+15.0%	+18.4%	19	−7	No Change
Colorado	$0.84	+13.5%	+16.6%	20	−6	No Change
New Jersey	$2.70	+12.9%	+38.4%	21	−18	+13%
Massachusetts	$2.51	+12.0%	+17.5%	22	−9	+66%
Oregon	$1.18	+10.8%	+21.1%	23	−12	No Change
Maine	$2.00	+10.6%	+16.6%	24	−9	No Change
Arkansas	$1.15	+8.5%	+3.9%	25	+6	+95%
Mississippi	$0.68	+8.4%	−1.7%	26	+11	+36%
Ohio	$1.25	+7.1%	+13.1%	27	−8	No Change
Oklahoma	$1.03	+3.0%	+9.6%	28	−3	No Change
Nebraska	$0.64	+2.8%	+12.0%	29	−6	No Change
Louisiana	$0.36	+2.8%	+6.4%	30	−3	No Change
Pennsylvania	$1.60	−0.1%	+12.9%	31	−10	+19%
South Carolina	$0.57	−2.4%	−8.1%	32	+9	+14%
Tennessee	$0.62	−2.9%	−4.5%	33	+5	+210%
Vermont	$2.62	−3.1%	+4.5%	34	−4	+46%
North Dakota	$0.44	−3.7%	+3.0%	35	−3	No Change
Georgia	$0.37	−4.2%	−0.3%	36	−1	No Change
Alabama	$0.425	−7.1%	+0.5%	37	−3	No Change
Kentucky	$0.60	−7.6%	−6.4%	38	+2	+100%
Missouri	$0.17	−13.7%	−11.3%	39	+5	No Change
Indiana	$0.995	−15.5%	−10.8%	40	+3	+79%

(continued)

TABLE 7.1 *continued*

	2013 Tax Rate (per pack)	2013 Consumption Smuggled (positive is inflow, negative is outflow)	2006 Consumption Smuggled (positive is inflow, negative is outflow)	2013 Smuggling Rank (1 is most smuggling, 50 least)	Smuggling Rank Change Since 2006 (e.g., NY changed from #5 to #1, so rank changed +4)	Cigarette Tax Rate Change, 2006-2013
Nevada	$0.80	−18.8%	+4.8%	41	−12	No Change
West Virginia	$0.55	−19.5%	−8.4%	42	+0	No Change
Wyoming	$0.60	−21.0%	−0.6%	43	−7	No Change
Delaware	$1.60	−22.6%	−61.5%	44	+3	+191%
Virginia	$0.30	−22.6%	−23.5%	45	+0	No Change
Idaho	$0.57	−24.2%	−6.0%	46	−7	No Change
New Hampshire	$1.68	−28.6%	−29.7%	47	−1	+110%
Alaska	$2.00	N/A	N/A	N/A	N/A	+25%
Hawaii	$3.20	N/A	N/A	N/A	N/A	+129%
North Carolina	$0.45	N/A	N/A	N/A	N/A	+50%
District of Columbia	$2.50	N/A	N/A	N/A	N/A	+150%

Source: Mackinac Center for Public Policy; Tax Foundation. Available at: http://taxfoundation.org/article/cigarette-taxes-and-cigarette-smuggling-state-2013-0#_ftn1.

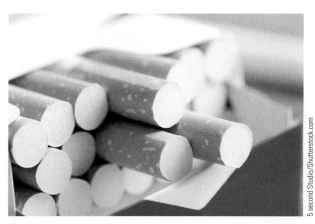

▤ Filtered cigarettes are more common than unfiltered cigarettes.

cigarettes have been sharply reduced, this decrease has contributed to a rise in the number of cigarettes smoked, as smokers seek to take in the same amount of nicotine. People who smoke low-tar and low-nicotine cigarettes inhale more deeply, hold the smoke in their lungs longer, or smoke more of the cigarette.

Demographics of Smoking

More adult males smoke than adult females, although females are gaining on men. Since 1955, smoking rates for White and Black men and women have declined sharply. The drop has been greater for White men than for Black men. See Table 7.2 for smoking prevalence rates by race/ethnicity. The highest percentage of smokers is among those aged between 25 and 44.[21] In addition, groups with the highest smoking rates are those with less than a high school education or GED and among those who live at or below the poverty level.[22]

American Indians/Alaska Natives have much higher prevalence rates compared to other groups in the United States (29.2% compared to 16.8).[23] Some of the factors that may contribute to these higher smoking rates include the use of tobacco for religious ceremonies, the medicinal value placed on tobacco, and the lower cost of tobacco as state and federal taxes are generally not placed on tobacco products sold on tribal lands.[24]

TABLE 7.2 Smoking Rates by Ethnicity in 2014

Race/Ethnicity	Prevalence
American Indian/Alaska Natives (non-Hispanic)	29.2%
Asians (non-Hispanic)	9.5%
Blacks (non-Hispanic)	17.5%
Hispanics	11.2%
Multiple Races (non-Hispanic)	27.9%
Whites (non-Hispanic)	18.2%

Source: Centers for Disease Control and Prevention. Current Cigarette Smoking Among Adults—United States, 2005–2014. Morbidity and Mortality Weekly Report 2015;64(44):1233–1240

A little over 25% of college campuses across the United States are completely smoke-free as many campuses have approved policies that ban the use of tobacco products on campus (including outside areas). These policies have been met with resistance from both smokers and nonsmokers on campus.

One of the possible reasons for this opposition is the smoke-free policy is being debated on an ideological standpoint and not from a public health view. Many feel institutions do not have the moral right to ban the use of a legal product in a legal manner on their campuses.

Questions to Ponder:

While there has been research to link the damaging effects of secondhand smoke, there is limited research on the impact of secondhand smoke while outside. Thus, some would argue that being around a smoker outside does not impose a significant risk to one's health. While there are no safe levels of exposure to tobacco, do you feel enacting a smoke-free environment significantly reduces one's risk of being exposed to secondhand smoke?

Source: B. S. Niemeier, C. B. Chapp, and W. B. Henley, "Improving tobacco-free advocacy on college campuses: A novel strategy to aid in the understanding of student perceptions about policy proposals," *Journal of American College Health*, 62, no.7 (2014): 498–505.

Tobacco companies market their products to women by linking smoking to independence and equality. Also, many women fear that they will gain weight if they stop smoking. It was found that women gained slightly more than 8 pounds following smoking cessation.[25]

Among college students, cigarette smoking has decreased by two-thirds from 1999, with 11% of college students reporting smoking cigarettes.[26] In general, college students smoke less than their noncollege peers and college-bound high school students smoke less than their noncollege-bound peers.[27] The *Monitoring the Future* study party attributes this to lack of academic successes experienced in high school, which may place additional stress on noncollege-bound students.

Women and Smoking

The differences between men and women are diminishing. In 2013, approximately 15.2% of women and 20.5% of men smoked cigarettes.[28] In 1965, 52% of men and 34% of women smoked.[29]

Among women, as with the general population, one's level of education is correlated with smoking behavior. For example, less-educated women (those with an education through 11th grade) are three times more likely to smoke than women with 16 years or more of education.

Annually, cigarettes smoking kills 201,700 women in the United States each year.[30] Smoking is a major cause of coronary heart disease, although that risk declines substantially within 1 to 2 years after cessation. It is estimated that cigarette smoking reduces a woman's lifespan by 14 years. Lung cancer is the leading cause of cancer death among

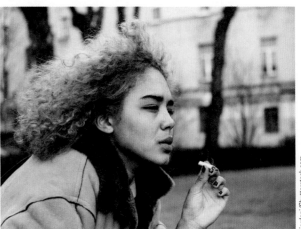

iordani/Shutterstock.com

Tobacco companies target women in their smoking ads by promoting independence among women who smoke.

US women, accounting for 25% of all cancer deaths among women with more women dying from lung cancer than from breast cancer.[31] In addition, smoking is more dangerous for women than men because women cannot repair lung damage as readily as men.[32] Other types of cancer that are more common with women smokers include cancers of the pharynx, bladder, pancreas, kidney, and liver. Women are subject to a number of other medical problems related to smoking. See the box "Women's Health and Smoking" for more information on health problems related to smoking cigarettes.

Smokeless Tobacco

Use of smokeless tobacco—which consists of **snuff** and chewing tobacco—has nearly tripled in the last two decades. In 1986, the US Congress banned television and radio advertisements for smokeless tobacco, but its use continues. However, restrictions on cigarette smoking in the workplace have not resulted in an increase in the use of smokeless tobacco.[33] On the other hand, when the Navy banned cigarette smoking on submarines, there was increased use of smokeless tobacco.[34] In 2012, the Navy took away price discounts on tobacco products sold on bases and now sells tobacco products at market value. The Navy is now considering a ban on all tobacco sales on ships and bases.[35]

The nicotine in smokeless tobacco is absorbed quickly into the bloodstream through the mucous lining of the mouth, making it highly addicting. Thus smokeless tobacco users reportedly have more difficulty stopping than cigarette users do. The nicotine level in one dip of snuff equals that in four cigarettes. Some people argue that smokeless tobacco is a desirable alternative to cigarettes. However, smokeless tobacco has a higher level of NNK, a known carcinogen, than regular tobacco.[36]

Based on the National Survey on Drug Use and Health, about 25.2% of Americans have used tobacco products in the previous month, although only 3.3% used smokeless tobacco in the past month.[37] The age group with the highest percentage of smokeless tobacco use is 18 to 25.[38] States with the highest prevalence of use are Wyoming, West Virginia, Kentucky, and Mississippi.[39] High school athletes are more likely than nonathletes to use smokeless tobacco. Team participation is associated with less use of marijuana, alcohol, and cigarettes but more smokeless tobacco use.[40] One reason is that students perceive smokeless tobacco as less physically damaging than other tobacco products. Most junior high school students and almost half of high school students who use smokeless tobacco believe they are either not at risk or at very little risk.

Although one could argue that smokeless tobacco is less harmful than cigarettes, smokeless tobacco produces many adverse health effects.[41] Besides cosmetic effects including discoloration of the teeth and bad breath, tobacco can cause gum recession, dental cavities, and leukoplakia, a precancerous condition marked by a white patch in the mouth that is reversible once one stops chewing. Chewing tobacco has been linked to cancers of the gum, mouth, larynx, pharynx, and esophagus. The risk of oral cancer is four times greater for smokeless tobacco users than for nonusers. Smokeless tobacco raises the blood pressure for up to 90 minutes after use, constricting blood vessels, and it can cause an irregular heartbeat,

snuff A form of smokeless tobacco

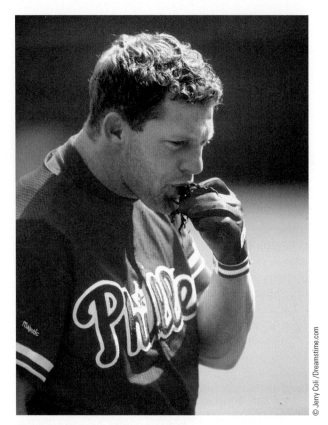

The MLB's new collective bargaining agreement bans chewing tobacco use by new players.

cardiovascular disease, and stroke. One study that looked at the mortality rates of male cigarette smokers who switched to smokeless tobacco found that those who changed to smokeless tobacco had a lower mortality rate but that their mortality rate was higher than former smokers who did not use smokeless tobacco.[42]

Snus

In response to antismoking views, increased taxes on cigarettes and expanding smoke-free ordinances, Reynolds and Altria introduced snus, a new tobacco product. Snus differs from other tobacco products in that it is less carcinogenic, does not require spitting, and is packaged in small pouches that go under one's upper lip. Although 36% of the adult population are aware of snus, only 5.2% have ever used it. Users are predominantly male, employed full time, and younger. Additionally, those who perceive snus to be less harmful than cigarettes are more likely to have used snus.[43]

In test markets where snus was promoted, there was a significant increase in its use. Advertisements for snus are directed primarily at current cigarette smokers. In 2011, Reynolds introduced an advertising campaign for Camel Snus in New York City in response to antismoking laws.[44]

Although snus may appear to be relatively new, it was first manufactured in Sweden more than a century ago. It was not until 30 to 40 years ago that it gained popularity because of improved manufacturing quality.[45] In parts of Northern Europe, snus usage has increased significantly, especially among university students.[46]

Tobacco Use in Other Countries

Smoking has increased greatly in parts of the world, possibly because of lax regulations and aggressive marketing. According to the World Health Organization (WHO), tobacco kills up to half its users and is the leading cause of preventable death in the world. Tobacco accounts for 6 million deaths annually.[47] Another 600,000 deaths are attributed to secondhand smoke.[48] Only one in three countries monitor tobacco use.

Until recently, the Chinese government has done very little to curb smoking. In China, almost 50% of men aged 15 and over smoke daily. Ironically among women in China, only 1.5% smoke daily.[49] About 50% of Vietnamese men smoke. Philip Morris, the producer of Marlboro cigarettes, built a factory in Vietnam to augment its market share in that country.[50] Interestingly, the cost of Western cigarettes in Vietnam ranges between 70 cents and $1, much less compared to prices in the United States. The cost of cigarettes is lower in developing countries than in industrialized countries, and the rates of smoking-related deaths in developing countries are nearly the same as those in developed countries.[51]

Smoking rates in industrialized countries are decreasing, but in underdeveloped countries, the trend is going in the opposite direction. Smoking rates around the world vary from 54% of men and 21% of women in Cuba to 4% in Ethiopia.[52] The WHO is aggressively trying to curb smoking rates throughout the world. Meanwhile, US tobacco companies export more than $2 billion worth of tobacco products. The

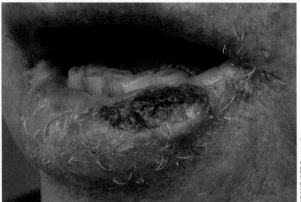

Smokeless tobacco was the cause of this squamous cell carcinoma in the oral cavity

People from underrepresented ethnic/racial groups, lower educational status, and who live at or below poverty level represent the highest population among those who smoke cigarettes.

A recent study was conducted looking at low and middle income countries to determine if there is a relationship among families whose men smoked and human capital expenditures. This study found an inverse relationship among those families that had a smoker and family spending on healthcare and education. Thus families who had a male smoker in them (usually the main financial support for the family) spend less money on healthcare and education costs.

Since 1996, taxes on cigarettes have gone up tremendously (in some states almost 300%). Some would argue these tax increases are negatively impacting groups in society that are already disadvantaged in terms of quality of living, healthcare, and educational opportunities.

Questions to Ponder:

1. Research suggests when cigarette prices goes up, smoking rates decrease. However, among those who choose to continue smoking, there is an additional burden on the family's financial situation. Do you feel increasing taxes on cigarettes places those marginalized populations at an increased risk? Justify your reasoning.

2. With much talk about reducing gender and racial disparities across the United States, what is the role of tobacco in these talks? Tobacco is a public health issue; how does the tax increase on tobacco products improve public health? How does it make it worse?

Source: K. D. Young, M. A. Bautista, and K. Young, "Tobacco use and household expenditures on food, education, and healthcare in low-and middle-income countries," *BMC Public Health*, 15 (2015): 1–11.

US government is pressuring Japan, South Korea, and Taiwan to eliminate restrictions on importation of foreign cigarettes. Unlike cigarette packages in the United States, the packages sent to Asian countries have no warning labels. Traditionally, Asian women have had low rates of cigarette use. Now, though, advertisements for cigarettes are targeting women and adolescents.

Clove Cigarettes and Bidis

An alternative to traditional tobacco cigarettes is clove cigarettes. Manufactured in Indonesia, **clove cigarettes**, also known as kreteks, are made up of 60% tobacco and 40% ground cloves. Typically imported from Indonesia, they are aromatic and give smokers the impression they are safer because one of clove's components, **eugenol**, makes inhalation easier. It anesthetizes the back of the throat and thereby inhibits the coughing reflex that normally accompanies smoking of regular cigarettes. Clove cigarettes also have higher levels of harmful particulates such as eugenol, anethole, and coumarin than conventional cigarettes.[53]

Bidis, clove cigarettes, and kreteks have higher concentrations of nicotine, tar, and carbon monoxide compared to tobacco cigarettes.[54] People who smoke bidis and clove cigarettes have increased risk for acute lung injuries. Additionally, people who smoke clove cigarettes develop fluid in their lungs, bloody phlegm, and wheezing. Less serious effects are respiratory tract infections, shortness of breath, vomiting, and nausea. Both are associated with increased risk for cardiovascular disease, chronic bronchitis, emphysema, cancer, and abnormal lung functioning.[55]

A recent fad, especially among teens, is **bidis**. These small cigarettes from India come in colorful packages and in different flavors. In India, bidis are especially popular because they sell for one-fifth price of what traditional cigarettes sell for.[56] Contrary to popular belief, bidis are not safe alternatives because they contain higher concentrations of nicotine. An estimated 1.2% of high school seniors in the United States smoked bidis in 2014.[57]

clove cigarettes Cigarettes made from tobacco and cloves; contain more tar, nicotine, and carbon monoxide than commercial cigarettes

eugenol Ingredient in clove cigarettes that provides aroma and reduces coughing reflex

bidis Flavored cigarettes from India that have considerably higher concentrations of nicotine than regular cigarettes

Light Cigarettes

In recent years, many smokers have switched to "light" cigarettes, believing that they are a safer alternative to regular cigarettes. Light cigarettes, which are advertised as having less tar and nicotine, were introduced into the US market in the late 1960s and account for the vast majority of the cigarettes sold. In 2011, a federal judge ruled that tobacco companies must admit that they have lied about the dangers of light cigarettes.[58] Although it is stated that light cigarettes deliver less tar and nicotine than regular cigarettes, they do not contain less tar and nicotine. Moreover, when people smoke light cigarettes, they receive about the same amount of nicotine and tar as those individuals who smoke regular cigarettes. Another problem with low-nicotine cigarettes is that smokers compensate for the lower levels of nicotine by changing smoking behaviors to get more of it.[59] In a recent study, researchers looked at the impact of the elimination of descriptors words such as "mild," "low," or "light" on packs of cigarettes to determine if there was an impact on the public's perception on safety for these products. They determined these policies have had little impact on smokers' beliefs regarding a reduction of harm associated with using these products.[60]

One study found that more than a third of smokers switched to light cigarettes to reduce their health risk. Also, many teen smokers believe that light cigarettes are less addictive.[61] Unfortunately, smoking a light cigarette does not reduce one's exposure to the carcinogens in tobacco.[62] Nor is the risk to one's coronary system reduced: Blood pressure and heart rates are no different in light cigarette smokers as compared to regular cigarette smokers.[63]

Not only are light cigarettes marketed as a safer alternative to regular cigarettes, but many people believe that it is easier to quit use of light cigarettes than regular cigarettes. It has been reported, however, that light cigarette smokers actually have a lower rate of smoking cessation than those individuals who smoke regular cigarettes.[64] It is an illusion to think that light cigarettes are safer than regular cigarettes.

Cigars

One trend in the 1990s was the resurgence of cigar smoking. Indicative were magazines devoted to cigar smoking, cigar bars, and restaurants hosting cigar nights. Sales of large cigars have decreased over the past 10 years, but the sales of small cigars, also known as cigarillos, have increased during the same period.[65] The promotion of little cigars is being addressed by attorneys general in 40 states.

TABLE 7.3 Past Month Cigar Use, Percentages from 2010 to 2014

Age	2010	2011	2012	2013	2014
12 or older	5.2%	5.0%	5.2%	4.7%	4.5%
12–17	3.2%	3.4%	2.6%	2.3%	2.1%
18–25	11.3%	10.9%	10.7%	10.0%	9.7%
26 or older	4.4%	4.2%	4.5%	4.1%	3.9%

Source: SAMHSA, Office of Applied Studies, *National Survey on Drug Use and Health*, 2015.

Little cigars, which some people consider to be cigarettes disguised in brown paper, are taxed at a lower rate than cigarettes and have fewer restrictions placed on their promotion.[66] It is believed that flavored little cigars are especially appealing to young people as over 60% of middle and high school students who reported to have used cigars in the past 30 days used flavor cigars.[67] There is some concern among the public health community that cigars and cigarillos will reverse the recent gains in reducing tobacco smoking.[68] Overall, the use of cigars have decreased among high school students. Exclusive cigarette or cigar use decreased by 64% from 1997 to 2013 among high school students.[69] Table 7.3 highlights cigar smoking in the United States by various age groups.

Although many people believe that cigars are a safe alternative to cigarettes, this is not necessarily true.[70] People who switch from smoking cigarettes to smoking cigars continue to inhale with cigars. Many health hazards are associated with cigar smoking. Nicotine levels are higher in cigars than in cigarettes. Cigar smokers have a 34% higher cancer rate than nonsmokers; rates of cancers of the mouth, throat, and esophagus are higher among cigar smokers than cigarette smokers. An increased risk of pancreatic cancer also is associated with cigar smoking.[71]

The lung cancer rate for cigar smokers is higher than that of nonsmokers, but it is lower than that of cigarette smokers. Individuals who smoke several cigars daily have a slightly increased risk for coronary

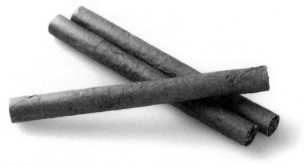

Little cigars have gained popularity in recent years.

heart disease and COPD. The degree of danger is related to how many cigars one smokes and the depth of inhalation.[72]

Hookah

Hookahs are water pipes that are used to smoke tobacco, usually flavored tobacco. The structure consists of charcoal placed at the head of the waterpipe, which is used to cook or bake the tobacco. At the base are single or multiple hoses that are used for the smoker to inhale the tobacco smoke. Hookahs have recently gained popularity over the past few years with many people considering them to be safe alternative to cigarette smoking.[73]

Hookah use was first measured in the *Monitoring the Future* report in 2010, and use was reported at 17.1%. In 2015, use was reported at 19.8%, but it was also found that hookah use is generally light or experimental only.[74] Hookah use has been increasing, partly due to the accessibility of hookahs. In almost 70 out of 100 of the largest cities in the United States, there are exemptions laws that allow hookah smoking in bars and lounges.[75]

Many users feel smoking tobacco through hookahs is less harmful compared to cigarettes. In a study on university students, researchers found over half of those surveyed has used tobacco through hookahs within the past 30 days.[76] Use of hookahs was related to hookah ownership and cigarette smoking, but not alcohol use. Additionally, almost 30% of those who have never used a hookah considered using it in the future.[77]

The dangers associated with tobacco cigarettes are present in hookah use. Hookah tobacco still contains nicotine and the smoke is as toxic as cigarette smoke. Due to the way hookahs are used, smokers absorb more of the toxic substances compared to tobacco cigarettes.[78] For example, during an hour-long hookah session, the average smoker may take up to 200 puffs compared to an average of 20 puffs for one cigarette.[79]

This results in about 90,000 ml of smoke inhaled during a typical hookah session compared with 500 to 600 ml inhaled when smoking a cigarette.[80]

Electronic Cigarettes

Electronic cigarettes are just one type of product listed under Electronic Nicotine Delivery Systems (ENDS). These are devices that allow users to inhale aerosol and other substances.[81] These devices contain a battery and a heating element, which is used to heat liquid that results in the release of aerosol. Many of the liquid cartridges contain flavors and other chemicals.

E-cigarettes is gaining popularity across the United States. According to the *Monitoring the Future* report, 30-day prevalence rates in 2015 were 9.5% for 8th graders, 14% for 10th graders, and 16.2% for 12th graders. These rates are much higher compared to traditional cigarette use.[82] Increase in e-cigarette use can be partly attributed to the lack of perceived risk associated with its use. The *Monitoring the Future* report identified about 16 and 19% of students who perceived a risk with e-cigarette use and compared with around 70% who perceived a risk among tobacco cigarette use.[83] In a study among Canadian e-cigarette users, more than 60% believed they were harmless. Additionally, most of the e-cigarette users in this study reported using the product to quit and reduce their tobacco cigarette use.[84]

E-cigarettes contain nicotine and are not considered a safe product. Nicotine is a highly addictive substance and may harm the developing teenage brain.[85] Currently, e-cigarettes are not regulated by the government. However, beginning in 2018, all ENDS products must comply with newly adopted government regulations, which include adding a warning statement to the product.[86] Many believe e-cigarette vapor is harmless, but this is not the case. Vapors from e-cigarettes contain nicotine, heavy metals, ultrafine particulates, and cancer-causing agents.[87] Table 7.4 highlights the potential benefits and harm of e-cigarettes.

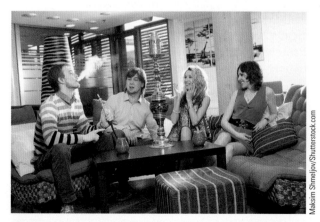

Almost 40% of college studies report having tried hookah smoking

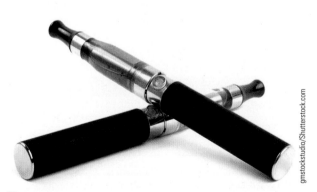

E-cigarettes is the fastest growing tobacco product

TABLE 7.4 Potential Benefits and Harms Associated with E-Cigarette Use

E-cigarette could cause the public health HARM if they...	E-cigarette could lead to public health BENEFIT if...
• Lead to use of nicotine and/or other tobacco products by youth and nontobacco users • Are used by pregnant women • Lead former smokers to relapse to nicotine use or use of other tobacco products • Delay complete smoking cessation among current smokers • Result in nicotine poisoning (e.g., through ingestion, absorption through skin, or inhalation of e-cigarette liquid) • Expose nonusers to secondhand aerosol	• Individual adult smokers switch *completely* from combustible tobacco products to e-cigarettes • They assist in rapid transition to a society with little or no combustible tobacco use

Source: Centers for Disease Control, "E-cigarette Information", Office of Smoking and Health, November 2015. Available at: www.cdc-osh -information-on-e-cigarettes-november-2015.pdf.

Characteristics of Smoking and Smokers

Despite the harm that comes from tobacco products, many people continue to use them, and some people who smoke are unaware of the dangers. Tobacco use tends to have triggers, such as following a meal or while talking on the phone, drinking coffee, or being around other smokers. Unlike most other drugs, cigarettes do not interfere with *most* daily behaviors. A person can read a book, drive a car, and talk to a friend while smoking or chewing tobacco.

Some people use tobacco to be more alert, and others use it to relax. Although using tobacco for stimulation and for sedation seems paradoxical, the state of the smoker and the chemical properties of tobacco play significant roles in their effects. Many smokers describe their first cigarette of the day as extremely pleasurable. Some claim that cigarettes curtail anxiety, sadness, and boredom. Tobacco contains acetaldehyde, a chemical with sedating properties similar to those of alcohol. Thus, depending on one's expectations or desires, tobacco can produce an arousing or a relaxing effect.

Nicotine and Performance

Nicotine improves cognitive performance slightly. The short-term memory and concentration of smokers are enhanced by nicotine for up to a half hour after smoking. Memory, attention, and reasoning ability decline 4 hours after the last cigarette. Because nicotine may improve memory, there is research into its possible benefits for patients with Alzheimer's disease.[88]

Tobacco Use by Young People

Most people begin smoking during childhood or adolescence. Nearly 60% of all new smokers initiate smoking prior age 18.[89] Ninety-nine percent of adult smokers tried smoking by the age of 26.[90] Though it takes an average of 2 to 3 years after one begins smoking to become a regular smoker, the earlier in life one tries a cigarette, the more likely it is that one will become a regular smoker. Yet, it was found that a third of youths who smoked three or four cigarettes a day developed nicotine dependence.[91]

There has been no significant change in overall tobacco use among high school students since 2011.[92] While the use of tobacco cigarettes have gone down, adolescents and young adults have moved to e-cigarettes and other ways to use tobacco products. Table 7.5 highlights tobacco use by middle and high school students.

Factors Associated with Youth Tobacco Use

Social and physical environments

Protobacco media impacts youths' tobacco related beliefs, intentions, and behaviors.[94] Additionally,

TABLE 7.5 Tobacco Use among Middle and High School Students in 2015

	Middle School Students	High School Students
Cigarettes	2.3%	9.3%
Hookahs	2.0%	7.2%
Smokeless Tobacco	1.8%	6.0%
E-cigarettes	5.3%	16%

Source: Centers for Disease Control and Prevention, "Youth and Tobacco Use," Office on Smoking and Health, Updated April 14, 2016. Available at: https://www.cdc.gov/tobacco/data_statistics/fact_sheets/youth_data/tobacco_use/.

media has been shown to influence peer and parental tobacco use by increasing their susceptibility to tobacco use. While tobacco advertising is no longer allowed on television, tobacco companies have found other creative ways to market their materials through depicting smoking scenes on television and in movies. Exposure to smoking in movies has been shown to be a strong predictor of future smoking compared to other types of marketing.[95] In a recent study, researchers found current tobacco use was associated with both exposure to static ads (i.e., tobacco ads in a convenience store) and exposure to tobacco use in television and movies. Static and television ads and movies depicting cigarettes also influence perceptions of peer-tobacco use, which has been shown to be a factor associated with tobacco experimentation.[96]

Youth who grow up in a household where one parent smokes are more likely to smoke as youth. Parents who smoke and are not especially concerned about the effects of smoking are more likely to have children who smoke.[97] Similarly, parents who strongly disapprove of smoking are less likely to have children who smoke.[98] Children of women who smoke during pregnancy have a higher rate of smoking than children whose mothers do not smoke.[99]

Biological and genetic factors

There may be a genetic component that places some more at risk for becoming tobacco users. Some suggest there is a genetic connection between parental smoking and nicotine dependence in adolescents.[100] One study analyzed the TAS2R38 taste receptor, which specifies the ability to taste phenylthiocarbamide (PTC), a bitter compound present in tobacco smoke. This study found PTC tasters were far less common among those who smoke and more common among nonsmokers.[101] Interestingly, this was found for those who identified as European-Americans while the same effect was not found among those who identified as African Americans.[102] In another study looking at environmental exposure (by parents, siblings, and peers) and reward-related candidate gene polymorphisms, researchers discovered exposure to peer smoking was associated with increased liking of smoking. Adolescents who carried the G-variant of a specific gene were more likely to report pleasant sensations associated with smoking.[103]

Mental health

There is a strong relationship between youth smoking and depression, anxiety, and stress.[104] Young people smoke to appear mature, to display independence, to cope with stress, or to bond with peers. Adolescent smoking has a high correlation with psychological distress.[105] Also, there is a strong relationship between depression and smoking.[106] Moreover, it has been demonstrated that there is a connection between nicotine dependence and low self-esteem.[107] A study spanning 25 years showed that adolescents who smoked 20 or more cigarettes daily were several times more likely than those who smoke 20 or fewer cigarettes a day to develop agoraphobia, generalized anxiety disorder, and panic disorder.[108]

Personal perceptions

Youth who have positive expectations from smoking are more likely to smoke. Positive outcomes include using cigarettes to cope with stress or as a weight control mechanism.[109]

Peers seem to be more important than parents in determining whether young people smoke, although children of parents who stop smoking are not as likely to take up smoking and are more likely to quit smoking.[110] The most important factors in whether a teenager smokes are if the teenager's friends smoke, if the perceived benefits outweigh the risks, and if the teenager's household includes smokers.[111] One study found that the influence for smoking starts as early as 6th grade.[112] This is not to suggest that parental smoking is not a factor.

Many young people are under the impression that menthol cigarettes are less harmful than nonmenthol cigarettes. Menthol cigarettes mask the irritation of smoking. Cigarette companies promote menthol cigarettes to young people who disproportionately smoke more menthol cigarettes.[113] It has been shown that young people are insufficiently aware of the adverse effects of smoking.[114]

Other influences

One study found a strong relationship between smoking and early childhood misbehavior. Based on teacher ratings, children who misbehaved most were the most likely to be smokers as adults.[115] Curiosity is given as the most common reason for first trying cigarettes. One predictor of tobacco use among boys is aggressive/disruptive behavior, as early as the 1st grade. A behavioral intervention program to reduce aggressive behaviors had a positive effect on the initiation of smoking.[116]

Other influences that affect youth tobacco use are:[117]

- Low socioeconomic status (including low income or education)
- Lack of skills to resist influences on tobacco use
- Lack of support and/or involvement from parents
- Accessibility, availability, and price of tobacco products
- Low self-image or self-esteem

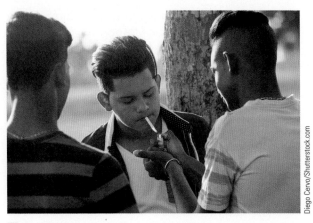

The most important influence on teenagers regarding smoking is peer behavior.

Youth Tobacco Prevention Efforts

When teaching young people about the dangers of tobacco, one challenge is that harmful effects take years to appear, if they show up at all. Therefore teenagers do not contemplate the risks of their behaviors. Although students know of the long-term negative health consequences of tobacco use, this knowledge does not dissuade them from smoking.[118] Emphasizing the short-term or cosmetic effects may have a greater impact. For instance, smoking causes premature wrinkles—a consequence that is of more concern to teens than the more serious long-term effects. Also, teens are more likely to respond to immediate effects such as smelly clothes and bad breath.

Only in the last few years have tobacco prevention programs been evaluated rigorously. Many programs operate on the assumption that if young people have knowledge about the hazards of tobacco, they will not begin to use tobacco or will cease using it. Most programs that are information based have been shown to be ineffective in reducing the onset of smoking. Programs geared toward teaching young people about the social pressures to smoke and how to tactfully refuse cigarettes are more effective as deterrents. This is especially true if tobacco prevention programs are started before smoking is initiated. In the Netherlands, it was shown that a smoking prevention program in the earlier grades had a positive effect as students moved up.[119]

Emphasizing an adolescent's psychological well-being may help because depression and anxiety symptoms play a role in the initiation of smoking.[120] Some smoking prevention programs strive to delay the onset of smoking. School-based smoking prevention programs are more effective when accompanied by antismoking media messages and parental disapproval of smoking.[121] Social influence programs stress the role of peers, culture, and the media. Stressing social influences makes sense because most young people who use tobacco first do so in a social context. Some social influence programs have reduced smoking by adolescents.

Tobacco prevention programs, especially those that operate outside of schools, seem to be more effective with high-risk youths. Community organizations and groups have the potential to reach young people who do not respond to in-school programs. Preventive interventions might be improved by targeting parent, school, and community outcomes with an emphasis on social norms, peer influence, and acceptance of deviant behaviors.[122] Figure 7.2 highlights the rates of nicotine dependence for young smokers.

Nicotine Tolerance and Dependence

When people first attempt to smoke or chew they may experience palpitations, dizziness and nausea, perspiration, and vomiting. However, they build up tolerance quickly, some in a matter of weeks. Most people who use tobacco products continue to do so because nicotine is addictive. The term *addiction*, however, typically is associated with narcotics, not nicotine—which ignores the addictiveness of nicotine. Nonetheless, there is a correlation between nicotine dependence and suicide attempts, especially among those who are persistent smokers and those who have quit but have relapsed.[123]

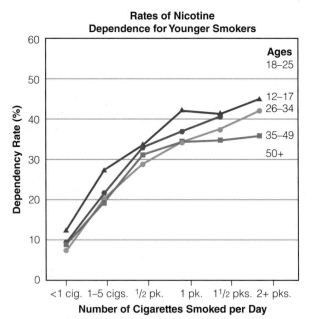

Figure 7.2 Data from the National Household survey on Drug Abuse show that the rate of nicotine dependence is higher among those younger than age 25 than in other age groups and that the dependence in these younger people develops with less exposure to nicotine.

Source: National Household Survey on Drug Abuse.

Tobacco industry documents dating back to the 1960s describe the addictive properties of nicotine.[124] At one time, the US Surgeon General compared nicotine addiction to heroin and cocaine addiction. Nevertheless, the addictive quality of nicotine might be exaggerated in the United States.[125] Half of the people in the United States who have smoked no longer do so. Moreover, most people who quit are able to do so without the benefit of nicotine replacement.

Millions of people smoke 20 to 50 cigarettes daily. Few drugs are used as often. The compulsion for cigarette smoking was illustrated during World War II, when German prisoners of war traded food for cigarettes. Information about the harmful effects of smoking is well known. Most smokers would like to quit, and most are aware that smoking causes cancer.

Despite the desire to quit and the knowledge that cigarettes are detrimental, people continue to smoke. The effects of nicotine are highly reinforcing. Nicotine reaches the brain in a few seconds. To compensate for the reduction of nicotine in the blood, smokers simply light up another cigarette. Not everyone who uses tobacco products becomes addicted, though. The percentage of tobacco users who become addicted is not known. Nevertheless, nicotine addicts exhibit symptoms characteristic of other forms of addiction. They develop tolerance, have a strong desire for continued use, and undergo withdrawal. Rituals connected to smoking, such as lighting a cigarette after eating and when talking on the phone, become ingrained in one's behavior. A sense of comfort comes from rituals, and suddenly stopping these rituals is difficult.

Symptoms of Withdrawal

Although nicotine withdrawal is not fatal and varies from one person to another, the symptoms can be uncomfortable. The severity of withdrawal symptoms is somewhat proportional to nicotine intake: The more one takes in, the greater the withdrawal symptoms. The symptoms are most acute 24 to 48 hours after tobacco use is ended, although the nicotine craving can remain for weeks or even years.

Symptoms of withdrawal include lower heart rate and blood pressure, difficulty maintaining attention, heightened aggressiveness, increased peripheral blood flow, insomnia, tremors, and hunger. Additional symptoms include heart palpitations, headaches, drowsiness, fatigue, and anxiety. The strongest symptom is a craving for nicotine. It has been shown that exercise reduces the craving for nicotine.[126] However, exercise must be continued to have a lasting impact.[127]

Pharmacology of Tobacco

Nicotine is 1 of about 4,000 chemical substances found in tobacco smoke. It has been used as an insecticide (60 mg can cause human death) and is carcinogenic. Nicotine is a stimulant with characteristics similar to those of amphetamines and cocaine. Nicotine injected intravenously is five to ten times more reinforcing than cocaine injected intravenously. Nicotine releases the neurotransmitter **norepinephrine**, which is responsible for producing stimulation. As with other stimulants, depression follows arousal.

Even though nicotine speeds up blood flow to the skeletal muscles, smokers tend to have cold feet and hands because of the constriction of blood vessels. Nicotine also interferes with the ability to urinate and occasionally causes diarrhea.

Nicotine is absorbed almost immediately by the lungs and can reach the brain in as little as 10 seconds. One factor contributing to its addictiveness is the speed with which it works, since drugs that provide immediate relief are more likely to be repeated. Smokers feel the effects of nicotine every time they inhale. One way to reduce nicotine levels may be to smoke fewer cigarettes, but unfortunately, the amount of nicotine taken into the body is not reduced much because smokers will just smoke more of each cigarette.

After nicotine is absorbed in the body, it is distributed quickly throughout. Besides traversing the blood and brain, nicotine passes through the placenta of a pregnant woman to the fetus and has been found in breast milk. The liver metabolizes almost all of the nicotine before it is excreted by the kidneys. Nicotine stays in the body for 8 to 12 hours.

NICOTINE WITHDRAWAL SYMPTOMS

- Lower heart rate
- Tremors
- Aggressiveness
- Hunger
- Heart palpitations
- Headaches
- Anxiety
- Lower blood pressure
- Shorter attention span
- Increased circulation
- Insomnia
- Fatigue
- Drowsiness
- Craving for nicotine

---

norepinephrine A neurotransmitter that may help regulate appetite and reduce fatigue

Physical Effects on the Individual

As early as the 1950s, the tobacco industry was aware that tobacco use was linked to illness. Figure 7.3 depicts the health effects on the human body. It is believed that tobacco manufacturers have the technology to produce cigarettes containing fewer toxic chemicals,[128] but if tobacco companies produce and advertise a safer cigarette, this implies that cigarettes already on the market are unsafe, leaving them open to further litigation.

Today, it is estimated that smoking is responsible for nearly one in five deaths in the United States.[129] Cigarette smoking is one of the leading *preventable* causes of disability and death in the United States. More Americans have died from smoking than from World War II and the Vietnam War combined. Cigarette smoking is the most prominent behavioral cause of lung cancer, other respiratory diseases, and cardiovascular diseases. Cigarette smoking is responsible for more than 480,000 deaths annually.[130] According to the CDC, life expectancy for smokers is on average 10 years less compared to nonsmokers.[131]

Either directly or indirectly, society bears the cost of tobacco-related problems, and smokers pay the price of impaired health. It is estimated that cigarette smoking is responsible for $337 billion in annual health-related economic losses in the United States—$170 billion in direct medical costs and $156 billion in lost productivity.[132,133] As shown in Table 7.6, a greater percentage of smokers compared to nonsmokers miss five or more days of work per month.[134] Moreover, family members of smokers make four more visits per year to healthcare facilities than families of nonsmokers. Nonsmokers pay for the healthcare costs of smokers through higher taxes and insurance premiums.

TABLE 7.6 Percentages of Full-Time Workers Ages 18 to 64 Who Missed 5 or More Days of Work in the Past Month Due to Illness or Injury

Age	Past Month Smokers	Past Month Nonsmokers
18–25	4.5%	3.5%
26–34	3.5%	3.3%
35–44	4.1%	2.6%
45–64	4.7%	3.0%

Source: The *NSDUH Report*, May 17, 2007. Office of Applied Studies, Substance Abuse and Mental Health Services Administration (SAMHSA). Available at: http://www.samhsa.gov /data/2k7/workMissed/workMissed.pdf.

Heart Disease and Strokes

Although cigarette smoking is most often associated with lung cancer, smoking causes more cardiovascular

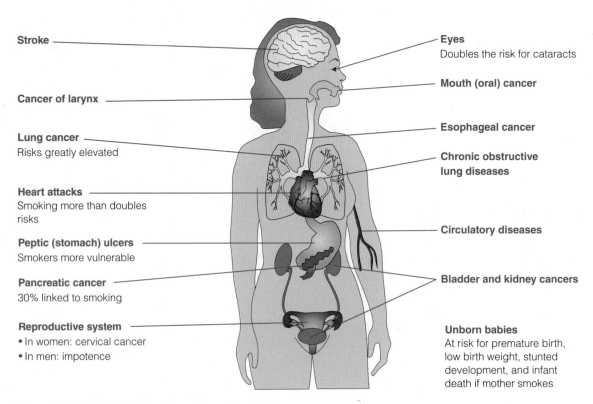

Stroke

Cancer of larynx

Lung cancer
Risks greatly elevated

Heart attacks
Smoking more than doubles risks

Peptic (stomach) ulcers
Smokers more vulnerable

Pancreatic cancer
30% linked to smoking

Reproductive system
• In women: cervical cancer
• In men: impotence

Eyes
Doubles the risk for cataracts

Mouth (oral) cancer

Esophageal cancer

Chronic obstructive lung diseases

Circulatory diseases

Bladder and kidney cancers

Unborn babies
At risk for premature birth, low birth weight, stunted development, and infant death if mother smokes

Figure 7.3 Health Effects of Smoking

Source: B.Q. Hafen and W.W.K. Hoeger, Wellness Guidelines for a Healthy Lifestyle (Englewood, CO: Morton Publishing, 1998), 338.

deaths than cancer deaths. Cigarette smoking is implicated in about one-fifth of all deaths from heart disease each year.[135] Smokers have a 70% higher death rate from coronary artery disease compared to nonsmokers.[136] Each year, 170,000 premature deaths from coronary heart disease are attributed to smoking, and smoking is implicated in 30% of all deaths from coronary heart disease. In the United States, smoking is believed to be the most important modifiable risk factor related to heart disease. Of people younger than age 40 who undergo coronary bypass operations, a majority are smokers. Nonetheless, heart disease due to smoking has declined significantly. When New York City implemented its smoking ban in 2004, the number of people who went to hospitals due to heart attacks declined by 4,000.[137] The risk of a heart attack increases among women older than age 35 who smoke cigarettes and use oral contraceptives. Moreover, the likelihood of experiencing a stroke increases for women who smoke and use oral contraceptives.[138] Also, women smokers who are taking oral contraceptives are more likely to have brain hemorrhages.[139]

Cardiovascular damage is correlated with the frequency and length of time a person smokes. Nicotine raises the heart rate and blood pressure, forcing the heart to work harder. Cigarettes also produce **carbon monoxide**, which impedes the oxygen-carrying capacity of the blood. Because carbon monoxide impairs circulation, cholesterol deposits increase. This can lead to arteriosclerosis, a condition more common in smokers than in nonsmokers. An encouraging point is that the likelihood of a heart attack is significantly reduced following one year of tobacco cessation.[140]

Another condition related to tobacco is Buerger's disease, which can result in amputation of the extremities as a result of poor circulation. Buerger's disease affects mostly young male tobacco users. Tobacco cessation reduces the chances of limb amputation.[141] Smokers also are at greater risk of dying from strokes. Carbon monoxide and nicotine affect the adhesiveness of platelets in the brain, hastening the formation of clots and the possibility of strokes. Finally, nicotine interferes with blood flow to the brain by constricting blood vessels, which can also result in strokes.

Respiratory Diseases

Two common respiratory conditions caused by smoking are chronic coughing (smoker's cough) and shortness of breath. More serious conditions are chronic bronchitis and emphysema, which appear almost exclusively in smokers and are referred to as COPD. Bronchitis develops as a result of smoke irritating the bronchi, or air passages, which go from the windpipe to the lungs. Tar builds up on the cilia (hairlike structures that rid the body of foreign matter), and breathing becomes more labored. Because the cilia become less effective, smokers cough persistently and regurgitate phlegm. Not only does smoking reduce lung functioning during childhood and adolescence, but also the lung functioning of infants is reduced if mothers smoke during pregnancy.[142] An especially puzzling scenario is that of asthmatics who smoke. It was found that high school students with asthma used cigarettes, cigars, marijuana, and inhalants at rates equal to or greater than high school students without asthma.[143] However, a more recent study found no difference in smoking rates among youth who had asthma and those who didn't.[144]

Emphysema is a disabling, incurable disease caused by the lungs' inability to retain normal elasticity and normal amounts of air. The lungs' inability to absorb oxygen as a result of smoking disables the lungs' tiny air sacs, causing shortness of breath. People with emphysema often die from cardiovascular problems. Women are especially vulnerable to respiratory problems. The rates of emphysema and chronic bronchitis are 12 times greater for female smokers than for nonsmokers.[145]

Cancer

Besides carbon monoxide, other gases in tobacco smoke include ammonia, benzopyrene, hydrogen cyanide, nitrosamines, and vinyl chloride. These are just some of the nearly four dozen gases in tobacco smoke that are capable of producing cancer. Most of the cancer-causing substances are found in the tar of tobacco, though nicotine has been implicated in cancer as well. Cigarette packages are required to list levels of tar.

Cancer rates linked to tobacco use are increasing. Cigarette smoking is responsible for at least 30% of all cancers deaths and 80% of lung cancer deaths.[146] More women now die from lung cancer than from breast cancer. Lung cancer is also the most common type of cancer in men. Rates of lung cancer are higher in Black smokers than in White smokers, possibly because Blacks metabolize nicotine more rapidly than Whites, not because they smoke more. In 2016, the American Cancer Society estimates there will be

carbon monoxide Gas in cigarette smoke that interferes with oxygen-carrying capacity of blood

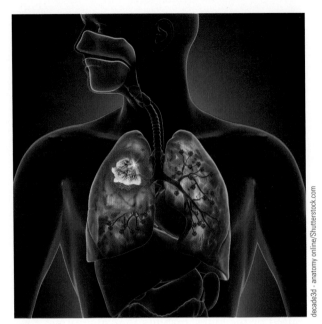

Cigarettes are responsible for 80% of all lung cancer deaths

approximately 225,000 new cases of lung cancer, resulting in about 160,000 deaths among men and women.[147]

Cigarette smoking is the leading risk factor for developing cancers of the larynx, mouth, esophagus, pancreas, and bladder. The chances of developing cancers of the oral cavity, pancreas, esophagus, kidney, larynx, trachea, and bladder are greater among smokers than among nonsmokers. Men who smoked two and a half packs of cigarettes a day for 30 to 39 years had a significantly higher risk of developing non-Hodgkin's lymphoma.[148] Oral and pharyngeal cancers account for almost 8,000 deaths annually in the United States. The warning signs of oral cancer include the following:

- A sore in the mouth that does not heal (most common symptom)
- A white or red patch on the gums, tongue, tonsil, or lining of the mouth that will not go away
- A lump or thickening in the cheek
- A sore throat or a feeling that something is caught in the throat
- Difficulty chewing or swallowing
- Difficulty moving the jaw or tongue
- Numbness of the tongue or other area of the mouth
- Swelling of the jaw that causes dentures to fit poorly or become uncomfortable
- Loosening of the teeth or pain around the teeth or jaw
- Voice changes
- A lump or mass in the neck
- Weight loss

The Impact of Smoking During Pregnancy

The carbon monoxide in tobacco smoke interferes with the fetus. Babies born to women who smoke during pregnancy weigh less and are more likely to be delivered prematurely than babies born to women who do not smoke while pregnant. Pregnant smokers have a higher incidence of spontaneous abortions (miscarriage) than nonsmokers, as well as a higher rate of stillbirths. Exposure to secondhand tobacco smoke increases the risk for lower birthrate, preterm babies, and stillbirths.[149]

One Danish study found that smokers had a considerably higher rate of stillbirths than non-smokers.[150] This study also found women who quit smoking during the first trimester greater reduced their chances of stillbirth risk associated with smoking. Smoking also significantly reduces fertility in women. A Danish study reported that smoking during pregnancy may reduce the likelihood of sons' future fertility by reducing sperm count.[151] It is speculated that DNA in men's sperm may be damaged by smoking, which may decrease fertility or increase miscarriage.[152]

Sudden infant death syndrome (SIDS), in which infants suddenly stop breathing, occurs at a higher rate among babies of women who smoked during pregnancy. According to the Lullaby Trust Organization (formally known as the Foundation for the Study of Infant Deaths), maternal smoking is the most important avoidable risk factor for SIDS.[153] They

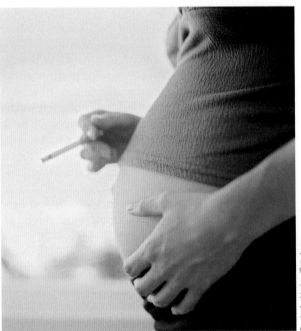

Pregnant woman who smoke increase the risk of having preterm pregnancies and babies with low birth weights.

further estimate 30% of all sudden infant deaths could be avoided if the mother didn't smoke while pregnant. Congenital malformations such as cleft lip and cleft palate are also more likely in children of smokers. There is evidence that children of mothers who smoke during pregnancy have higher rates of psychological problems such as attention problems and hyperactivity, although it is difficult to prove that maternal smoking causes these problems.[154]

The rate of smoking during pregnancy has decreased significantly over the past 20 years. The rate of smoking during pregnancy in 2011 was 10%.[155] An important factor in whether pregnant adolescent girls continued to smoke was having friends who smoke. It was reported that females who initiate smoking prior to age 15 are likely to continue to smoke during pregnancy.[156]

Tobacco and Physical Activity

Although smokers claim they are more alert and aroused after smoking, their ability to engage in physical activity is impaired demonstrably. The mucous membranes of the trachea and the bronchial tubes enlarge as a result of smoking, restricting the ability to get air in and out of the lungs. The alveoli in the lungs receive less oxygen, so respiratory demands, especially during exercise, are harder to meet. Conversely, the role of physical activity in one's lifestyle is important in whether one initiates smoking. A Finnish study found that physically inactive adolescents were more likely to smoke as adults.[157]

Smoking also impairs sexual activity. Carbon monoxide hampers production of the male sex hormone testosterone. Sexual excitement and erection in males diminish because nicotine constricts the blood vessels. The number of sperm in male smokers is reduced significantly, and sperm motility is sluggish. Numerous studies have noted that smoking causes erectile dysfunction in a significant number of men.[158] It has also been reported that smoking impairs normal sexual response in young women.[159]

Passive Smoke

The detrimental effects of tobacco are not limited to smokers. **Passive smoke**, also called involuntary or **environmental tobacco smoke** and secondhand smoke, is a major source of indoor air pollution in the home and workplace. Passive smoke is blamed for 7,300 lung cancer deaths each year.[160] The extent of harm is related to the degree of exposure. Some critics claim that studies linking passive smoking to lung cancer are biased.[161] Nonetheless, the economic impact of environmental tobacco smoke is estimated

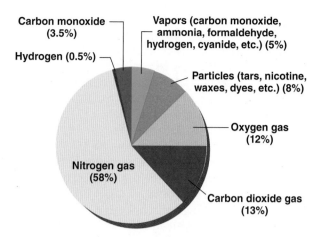

Figure 7.4 Chemical Composition of Mainstream Smoke

at nearly $10 billion in terms of costs for medical care, mortality, and morbidity.[162]

Many nonsmokers report emotional discomfort from being around people who are smoking. Passive smoke is classified as mainstream or sidestream smoke. **Mainstream smoke** is the smoke that smokers exhale after inhaling. Figure 7.4 shows the composition of mainstream smoke. **Sidestream smoke** is the smoke that comes from the burning end of the cigarette, pipe, or cigar. Because sidestream smoke does not pass through a filter and burns at a hotter temperature, it contains more nicotine and carbon monoxide than mainstream smoke. Children of smokers have five times as much cotinine (a byproduct of nicotine) in their urine as children of nonsmokers.[163]

Laws against smoking in public places were precipitated by research pointing out the effects of sidestream smoke. Not only are there more restrictions on indoor smoking, but a number of communities are prohibiting smoking in public parks.[164] The following discussion examines the effects of tobacco smoke on nonsmokers and children of smokers.

Effects on Nonsmokers

Besides irritating the nose and eyes, passive smoke causes many significant health problems. Environmental tobacco smoke has been linked to lung and

passive smoke Tobacco smoke present in the air from someone else's smoking and inhaled by others

environmental tobacco smoke Smoke in the air as a result of someone smoking

mainstream smoke smoke exhaled by a smoker

sidestream smoke Smoke that comes from the burning end of a cigarette, pipe, or cigar

urinary tract problems and to cancers of the liver and pancreas in addition to strokes, coronary heart disease and lung cancer.[165] Passive and active smoke increases the risk of breast cancer.[166] Children who are exposed to cigarette smoke growing up have a higher incidence of atopic dermatitis, a form of eczema.[167] Passive smoke is also linked to type 2 diabetes[168] and multiple sclerosis.[169]

According to a report from the US Surgeon General, for nonsmokers who live with smokers, secondhand smoke increases the risk of heart disease by 25 to 30% and the risk of lung cancer 20 to 30%.[170] As a result of smoking bans, it is estimated that heart attacks have been reduced by 5%.[171] Also, there is some evidence that the risk of dementia increases due to secondhand smoke.[172]

The Environmental Protection Agency officially declared secondhand smoke a carcinogen in 1993.[173] Starting on January 1, 1998, tobacco smoking was prohibited from all bars and taverns in California. Of bartenders studied before and after the ban went into effect, more than half reported no symptoms of respiratory problems, and most showed an overall improvement of respiratory functioning after the ban.[174] Within the general population, the majority of people believe that bars and restaurants should be free of smoke.[175] Like bartenders, it has been demonstrated that casino dealers are adversely affected by passive smoke.[176]

Effects on Children of Smokers

Children of smokers are more likely than children of nonsmokers to get respiratory infections including colds, bronchitis, and pneumonia. One study reported that maternal smoking increased the risk of bronchitis.[177] Yet, many mothers who smoke downplay the harmful effects of their smoking around their children.[178] Children of smokers are adversely affected academically because they are absent from school more often than children whose parents do not smoke.[179]

The incidence of asthma is greater among infants and young children who have been subjected to sidestream smoke. Likewise, there is a relationship between parental smoking and childhood allergies.[180] In fact, the general likelihood of ill health is more significant if both parents smoke. Teenagers have higher rates of asthma and wheezing when exposed to passive smoke.[181] In addition, women who smoke while pregnant have toddlers who are more likely to exhibit more negative behaviors, such as physical aggression and hyperactivity-impulsivity.[182] It has also been shown that preadolescents were more likely to smoke if their mothers smoked during pregnancy.[183] One study found that passive smoke increased the risk

of sickle cell anemia 1.9 times.[184] It has also been reported that passive smoke significantly increased the risk of dental cavities in children.[185]

Rights of Smokers Versus Nonsmokers

Balancing the rights of people who smoke against the rights of people who are opposed to smoking is difficult. Despite the detrimental effects of tobacco on health, should people be penalized for an addiction that is hard to overcome?

Antismoking Legislation

To discourage minors from smoking, federal legislation in 1997 established a minimum age of 18 to purchase tobacco products, and anyone under age 27 must show photo identification. The federal law represents a culmination of much state and local legislation. Numerous legislative efforts to limit smoking were initiated in the 1980s. By the end of 1995, about 1,006 local tobacco control ordinances against smoking had been initiated. The tobacco industry countered by getting state legislators to introduce statewide laws that would take precedence over local laws. Since the decline in cigarette smoking, support to restrict smoking has steadily increased.[186]

Despite the efforts of tobacco companies, the majority of state legislators have supported measures to limit the purchase of tobacco products, especially by minors. Even in Greensboro, North Carolina, home of several large tobacco companies, residents voted to restrict smoking. San Francisco voters approved legislation that forbade smoking not just in public areas but in the private workplace as well. A Massachusetts law stipulated that all new police officers and firefighters were forbidden from smoking—on and off the job. As of September 2012, the FDA will mandate more prominent health warnings on all cigarette packaging and advertisements.[187]

Concerns regarding passive smoking prompted every federal agency to limit or prohibit smoking in public areas and workplaces. In 1994, the US Department of Labor proposed a ban on workplace smoking, affecting about 6 million worksites. The Department of Defense implemented its own ban. In New Zealand, it was found that workers disapproved of smoking in the workplace.[188] In Colombia, restrictions were implemented on cigarette sales and advertising.[189] A Canadian study reported that antismoking legislation banning smoking in restaurants resulted in a 39% decrease in admissions to hospitals due to cardiovascular conditions and a 33% decrease in admissions due to respiratory conditions.[190]

In New York City, tobacco advertisements are banned on all city-owned billboards and on private outdoor advertising media within 1,000 feet of a school. New York City passed a bill prohibiting smoking in public outdoor areas.[191]

Based on support prompted by a statewide initiative, the state of California spent $28 million on an advertising campaign to dissuade individuals from smoking. This initiative passed despite tobacco companies' spending $15 million to defeat it. To finance this antismoking effort, a cigarette tax of 25 cents per pack was implemented. In essence, smokers contributed to the campaign to persuade them to stop smoking. Cigarette sales declined, and lung cancer rates dropped.[192]

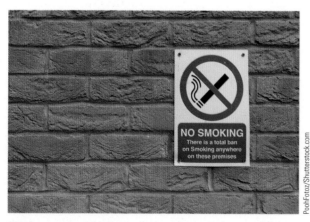

Many companies do not allow smoking on their property; including outdoor areas.

PoohFotoz/Shutterstock.com

In 1990, airline passengers on all commercial flights within the continental United States, including Puerto Rico and the Virgin Islands, were forbidden from smoking. This ban extended to flights to Alaska and Hawaii that were shorter than 6 hours. Foreign airlines flying in the United States have cooperated in the effort to prohibit smoking. Currently, almost all airlines ban smoking on board regardless of the length of travel. Amtrak trains, buses, and stations are entirely nonsmoking.

Exposure to workplace environmental tobacco smoke has been found to double the risk of lung cancer.[193] While there are no federal laws regarding workplace tobacco use, many states have enacted laws to reduce workplace smoking. In 2013, 26 states and the District of Columbia have adopted comprehensive smoke-free workplace laws to reduce exposure to secondhand smoke in the workplace.[194] To reduce workplace smoking, many companies offer financial incentives (in some cases, disincentives) to workers. Some companies require workers who smoke to pay more than nonsmokers toward health insurance costs. Companies and individuals alike benefit from these incentives: The worker is less likely to become ill, health insurance expenses of the companies are lower, and absenteeism is reduced. Another reason that employers may want to prohibit workplace smoking is because of the significant legal risks posed by employees exposed to secondhand smoke. In a number of cases, employers have been sued by employees whose health was compromised by secondhand smoking.[195]

Although no law requires fast-food restaurants to ban smoking, many have implemented their own bans. An estimated 25% of customers and 40% of workers at fast-food restaurants are younger than age 18. Taco Bell restaurants and one-third of the members of the National Council of Chain Restaurants have not allowed smoking since March 1994.

One concern that restaurant owners express is that a smoking ban will result in a significant loss of business; however, a study of the first 13 US cities to ban smoking found no loss in customers.[196] In more recent studies conducted in nine states regarding nonsmoking laws, researchers determined there were no significant adverse economic impacts on restaurants or bars in any of the states included. One state, West Virginia, resulted in a 1% increase in restaurant employment after smoke-free air laws were put into place. When New York City prohibited smoking in restaurants, concern likewise was raised that tourism and restaurant sales would decline. Instead, tourists spent more money.[197] Like New York, the revenues of restaurants in California increased after the ban on indoor smoking went into effect.[198]

The Master Settlement Agreement

If smokers become sick, who is responsible? Should the responsibility lie with tobacco companies or with the smoker? Legislation passed in November 1998 requires the tobacco industry to pay $206 billion among all 50 states. In exchange for this payment, 46 states agreed to end their litigation against the four largest tobacco companies.[199] The purpose of the fine is to compensate states for medical costs resulting from cigarette smoking and to create a $500 million fund to educate young people about the risks of smoking. The Master Settlement Agreement states that tobacco companies are no longer liable for addiction or dependence claims, class action suits, and claims of punitive damages. The people who bear the brunt of this legislation are smokers, because the cost will be passed on to them.

Another aspect of the Master Settlement Agreement is that tobacco companies are totally banned from sponsoring football, basketball, baseball, soccer, and hockey. Some critics contend that the Master Settlement Agreement is a violation of free speech. They assert that constitutional rights are violated.[200] In 2004, then New York Attorney General Eliot Spitzer sued Brown & Williamson Tobacco Corporation for violating the Master Settlement Agreement. Spitzer maintained that Brown & Williamson was promoting KOOL cigarettes through its hip-hop music sponsorship.[201]

Individuals have also sued tobacco companies. In a case in New Jersey, a man was awarded $400,000 for the death of his 58-year-old wife, who died after smoking for 42 years. That award later was overturned, with the court ruling that the woman was 80% at fault for her own death. Critical issues in the case were the absence of health warnings before 1966 and the fact that the woman was not informed properly of the risks. Lawsuits against the tobacco industry have had very little impact on their financial fortunes. Tobacco companies have shifted their promotional activities abroad.[202]

Some maintain that cigarette companies did their own research in the 1950s, which revealed a link between cigarettes and lung cancer, but that this information was not made public. On January 4, 1954, tobacco companies took out full-page advertisements in newspapers throughout the United States with a circulation of 50,000 or more pledging that they would cooperate closely with individuals interested in safeguarding the public's health. Yet tobacco companies continue to court politicians. In many states, money from the Master Settlement Agreement, which was intended for tobacco prevention and cessation, is reallocated by politicians to balance state budgets.[203]

Cessation Techniques

Most smokers say they would like to stop. It usually takes several attempts. The first few months are critical. According to one study, 41% of smokers who want to quit were successful for one day, but less than 5% were able to abstain during the next 3 to 12 months.[204] Seventy percent of smokers say that they want to quit.[205] Withdrawal symptoms can be intense, leading to anxiety and a depressed mood. Most people on average require five to seven attempts to quit before they are successful.[206] One clear benefit of stopping smoking is that children of former smokers are more critical of smoking and are less likely to smoke.[207]

Young adults are more likely than older smokers to successfully quit smoking. This is significant because people who stop smoking by age 30 avoid the long-term effects of smoking.[208] African Americans have lower rates of smoking cessation.[209] Besides race, other factors that reduce the likelihood of smoking cessation are density of tobacco outlets and one's residential proximity to stores selling cigarettes.[210] Additionally, mental health status has been linked to quitting efforts. In one study, those smokers who identified as having a history of mental health conditions were less successful in abstaining from cigarettes compared to those who did not have a history of mental health conditions.[211]

One study found that teenage smokers have a hard time coping with stress without cigarettes and that their friends who smoke often criticize them for trying to stop smoking.[212] Interestingly, less-educated young adult smokers (ages 18 to 24) have higher rates of smoking but attempt to quit smoking at the same rate as more-educated young adult smokers.[213]

Stopping the use of smokeless tobacco is more difficult than quitting cigarettes. A number of smokeless tobacco users switch to cigarettes, although few cigarette users switch to smokeless tobacco.[214]

One reason that people have trouble overcoming tobacco dependency is that many activities trigger smoking. People are cued into smoking when waking up, having a cup of coffee, finishing a meal, talking on the phone, driving a car, or drinking alcohol. Smokers who are active alcoholics are less likely to stop smoking than smokers with no history of alcoholism, suggesting that discontinuing alcoholism may increase the potential for successful smoking cessation.[215]

Many smokers are concerned about gaining weight once they stop. Most weight gain occurs during the first year after quitting. One study involving nicotine gum found that the average gain was about 3½ pounds.[216] A meta-analysis conducted in 2015 confirmed these results and found weight gain and a gain in body mass index (BMI) was associated with quitting, although the effects were greater from those located in North American compared to Asian countries.[217] Quitters who take up exercise experience less weight gain and reduce their potential for cardiovascular damage.[218]

Confidence, not overconfidence, in one's ability to stop smoking is a crucial variable in how long one remains abstinent. Despite the array of smoking cessation programs available, 90% of smokers in the United States who quit do so without benefit of any formal treatment program. Generally, nicotine replacement therapy, such as nicotine gum, nicotine patches, and nicotine inhalers, helps many smokers to stop. On the other hand, drug therapy, aversive techniques, behavior modification, hypnosis, and acupuncture have not been proven conclusively to help.[219] Various cessation techniques are described in the following sections.

Nicotine Gum and Lozenges

If a person is addicted to nicotine, then it would seem logical to fulfill the need for nicotine through a safe source and gradually reduce the need for it. This is the premise of nicotine gum (such as Nicorette) and other nicotine replacement systems. Nicotine gum has been available through prescription since 1984, and beginning in 1996, it could be purchased without a prescription. Nicotine gum reduces withdrawal symptoms associated with cigarettes, but it does not provide the same satisfaction as cigarettes because nicotine gum is absorbed more slowly. Nicotine is absorbed irregularly and unpredictably, limiting its success. In one study in which free nicotine patches or nicotine gum were offered, 53% of smokers indicated they would seriously consider quitting.[220]

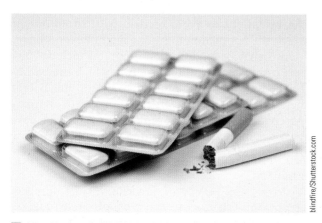

Nicotine gum helps reduce withdrawal symptoms associated with quitting cigarettes

blindfire/Shutterstock.com

One interesting twist is that some people who have never smoked but who have used nicotine gum have become dependent on the gum.[221]

Initially, nicotine gum should be chewed slowly to release the nicotine and then stopped once the taste gets strong.[222] Effectiveness rates vary, but one organization suggests the use of nicotine gum along to quit smoking only has an improvement in success rates by 1%.[223] Lozenges containing nicotine might aid smoking cessation. It has been shown that nicotine lozenges increase the likelihood of smoking cessation by 10% when compared to a placebo.[224] Side effects of nicotine lozenges include insomnia, nausea, hiccups, coughing, heartburn, headache, and gas.[225] When asked if they prefer a nicotine mouth spray to nicotine gum, most smokers preferred the nicotine spray even though the mouth spray was no more effective than the gum.[226]

Nicotine Patches

As of 1996, the nicotine patch, containing 30 mg of nicotine, became available as an over-the-counter drug. Nicotine patches consist of synthetic rubber in which nicotine is slowly dissolved.[227] The patch eases withdrawal symptoms that accompany tobacco cessation. Early studies with the nicotine patch demonstrated that it was effective for helping smokers quit. Various studies found that abstinence rates for those using nicotine patches ranged from 23 to 61% in the first 6 weeks but that success declined afterward.[228]

One study looked at successful quitters among heavy and light smokers. Initially, this study found a significant difference among heavy smokers who used the nicotine patch to aid in quitting. Initially, results were self-reported, but at week 12 of cessation, researchers tested saliva for cotinine levels to verify abstinence. While many smokers self-reported to being abstinent at week 12, saliva tests showed they were currently smoking.[229]

Some users report skin rashes. The biggest drawback, however, is that when people continue to smoke while wearing the patch, they receive dangerously high levels of nicotine. In an out-of-court settlement, the Ciba-Geigy Corporation, which sells the nicotine patch Habitrol, changed its advertisements because consumers believed that the patch is more effective than it actually is. Ciba-Geigy was required to include information that pregnant women, nursing mothers, and people with cardiovascular disease should check with their physicians before using the patch. One current study, however, found that nicotine patches do not increase the risk of coronary artery disease even though many smokers have the misconception that the nicotine patch causes heart attacks.[230]

Nicotine Inhalers

The FDA approved the nicotine inhaler in 1996. Similar to nasal inhalers, the nicotine nasal spray pumps small amounts of nicotine from small tubes into the nose. A common side effect is nasal and sinus irritation. Therefore it is not recommended for people with nasal or sinus conditions, allergies, or asthma. Also, it is not recommended for use exceeding six months.

One study reported that nicotine inhalers were more effective if smokers were given the inhalers by a healthcare provider as opposed to buying the inhalers over the counter.[231] Another study found the combination of using a nicotine patch and a nicotine metered inhaler greatly improved rates of abstinence for six months after initial quit date.[232] One drawback is that the spray can be irritating, although most users adjust to the spray within a couple of days.[233]

Drug Therapy

There are a number of drug therapies that have been developed to treat nicotine addiction. In 1997, the FDA approved the drug Zyban, also known as buproprion and originally prescribed as an antidepressant, for smoking cessation. How Zyban works is unclear, but it does seem to reduce the desire for nicotine. In conjunction with cognitive behavioral therapy, Zyban produced an abstinence rate of 34% after six months for women who also had concerns about their weight.[234] Side effects associated with Zyban are dry mouth, difficulty sleeping, and skin rash. Convulsions and loss of consciousness occur in 1 of every 1,000 people who take the drug. It is contraindicated for people with epilepsy, eating disorders, and women who are pregnant or breastfeeding.

The most recent drug developed for nicotine addiction is varenicline (Chantix). A European study of 551 participants found that nearly 65% were abstinent at the end of the 12-week varenicline treatment.[235] Another study compared varenicline with nicotine replacement therapy for smokers attempting to quit. Results from this study indicate greater success rates among those who were using varenicline treatment compared to nicotine replacement therapy.[236]

Buproprion is also used for major depressive disorders and seasonal affective disorder.[237] Unfortunately, one side effect of buproprion, especially when taken with Prozac, is delirium.[238]

Varenicline has been shown to be three times more effective than a placebo.[239] The drug does not appear to be affected by food and it is well tolerated by users.[240] Despite its effectiveness, the cost of varenicline is a deterrent to some smokers.[241] However, varenicline is more cost effective than other treatment modalities.[242]

Antianxiety drugs have been given to smokers who are trying to quit, and these drugs reduce irritability in these individuals. In a pilot study, Prozac was found to help some individuals maintain their abstinence from cigarettes when it was combined with either group therapy or the nicotine patch.[243] Prozac reduces appetite, and this feature may appeal to people who are concerned about weight gain when they quit smoking. Currently, three vaccines are being developed to prevent nicotine addiction. The vaccinations will be tested to determine whether they are effective for smoking cessation.[244]

Aversive Techniques

One aversive technique is to have smokers engage in **rapid smoking** until they exceed their tolerance levels and become ill. The point is to make smoking an unpleasant experience. This technique is similar to negative reinforcement. An obvious drawback is that it may seriously endanger health, especially of a person with a cardiovascular problem. Another aversive technique is to give the drug taker—in this case, the smoker—an electric shock when he or she is engaging in drug use. This technique has been applied to alcohol treatment, and its benefits are short-term at best.

Behavior Modification

The premise of many programs is to change behaviors linked to smoking. Basically, the smoker learns new or alternative behaviors to use in place of smoking. For example, if a person typically smokes after dinner, he or she could take a walk instead. If someone is accustomed to smoking while talking on the telephone, he or she could keep paper and pencils next to the telephone to doodle in lieu of smoking. People can be taught to avoid or deal with situations in which the temptation to smoke might be a problem. Many behavior modification programs include support groups or a buddy system in which the buddy is called when the urge to smoke strikes. Behavioral therapy programs achieve a cessation rate of approximately 20%. These programs have higher success rates when they are augmented with other types of treatment.[245]

rapid smoking Aversive smoking-cessation technique in which one smokes rapidly to exceed tolerance and becomes ill

Hypnosis

Hypnosis is successful with some people. It seems to work best with people who want it to work; it is most effective with motivated individuals. By the same token, if a person is motivated, the specific program undertaken might not matter. Hypnosis might provide the excuse to motivate people to stop smoking, although hypnosis was not found to be any more effective than other forms of treatment.[246] One study compared the use of relaxation techniques and the use of hypnosis to determine the impact on smoking cessation. No significant difference was observed among the two groups in smoking cessation.[247] One study found that hypnosis as a smoking cessation technique is more effective with men than women.[248]

Acupuncture

The evidence supporting the effectiveness of acupuncture is minimal.[249] The mechanism by which acupuncture stops the desire to smoke is unclear. Nevertheless, advocates of acupuncture claim that it reduces the physical symptoms of withdrawal. They also state that acupuncture reduces the desire for smoking because the process causes endorphins to be released.[250] Acupuncture sessions typically are 30 minutes long, and smokers receive treatment for anywhere from 2 days to 3 months.

Summary

Tobacco played an integral role in the history of the United States because tobacco crops were vital to the survival of the colonial settlement Jamestown, enabling it to prosper. The French government helped finance tobacco farming in the New World, and these funds were used to help the colonies defeat the British during the Revolutionary War.

Initially, tobacco was used in pipes, snuff, and cigars. Cigarette sales increased when the cigarette-rolling machine was developed, because cigarettes became more plentiful and less costly. R. J. Reynolds added saccharine to cigarettes, giving them a sweeter taste and a longer shelf life. At first men used tobacco, then cigarettes were marketed for women, though women were criticized for smoking. Later, young people became the target of cigarette advertisements.

The health cost of tobacco translates to economic loss. Concern over the health effects of tobacco has led to a decline in the percentage of people who smoke. In 1964, when the Office of the US Surgeon General issued its report describing tobacco's hazards, about 50% of adults smoked. Many people subsequently changed to filtered, low-tar, and low-nicotine cigarettes. Light cigarettes deliver the same amount of tar and nicotine as regular cigarettes. They have not been proven to be a safe alternative.

Smoking rates have gone down for men and women alike, though the rate for men has declined more drastically than that for women. Tobacco use correlates with education and occupation. Smoking rates have declined in industrialized countries but have increased in less-developed countries.

Children growing up in homes in which parents smoke are more likely to smoke themselves because parents serve as role models. Peers are an important factor, particularly for adolescents. Teens often follow the behavior of peers with whom they associate. One difficulty in teaching young people about the dangers of tobacco is that the harmful effects take years to appear. Smoking rates have, however, have started to decline among adolescents but may have been replaced by e-cigarette use.

Nicotine is an addictive and carcinogenic component of tobacco. Nicotine is a stimulant that is absorbed almost immediately by the lungs, reduces blood flow, and reaches the brain in seconds. During pregnancy, nicotine is passed to the fetus through the placenta.

Although cigarette smoking is most often associated with lung cancer, smoking causes more cardiovascular deaths than cancer deaths. Smoking increases the risk for strokes, bronchitis, and emphysema. Also, the tar in tobacco increases the risk of cancer. Most deaths from lung cancer are a result of cigarette smoking.

Women who smoke while pregnant deliver babies who weigh less than the typical newborn. Pregnant women also are more likely to have miscarriages and stillbirths, and their babies die more often than others from sudden infant death syndrome (SIDS).

Passive smoke is linked to health problems for nonsmokers. Mates of smokers are more likely to develop heart conditions, and children of smokers are more likely to have respiratory problems.

Smoking cessation is difficult. Because smoking is tied to many other behaviors, breaking the link is difficult. People who quit tend to believe that they were responsible for their success, rather than a program, and they have lower relapse rates.

Thinking Critically

1. In 1989, R. J. Reynolds test-marketed a new cigarette called Uptown, targeted specifically to African American men and women. Although this marketing campaign was dropped, can you find examples of tobacco products promoted more heavily to minorities, young people, or other groups?

2. Televised sporting events such as baseball often show players chewing tobacco. Yet, athletes are seen as role models. Should sport figures be encouraged to publicize the dangers of smokeless tobacco?

3. Nicotine use has been described as a habit and as an addiction. Former US Surgeon General C. Everett Koop claimed tobacco to be as addictive as cocaine and heroin, yet millions of people have quit smoking. Do you believe tobacco use is addictive or is a habit? Why?

4. The cost of health insurance continues to climb. Should smokers be required to pay more for health insurance? How about people who do not exercise or consistently overeat?

5. Nicotine can pass through the placenta and enter the bloodstream of the fetus. What might be done to dissuade women from smoking during pregnancy? Should there be laws created to punish women who smoke during pregnancy? Why or why not?

Chapter Objectives

After completing this chapter, the reader should be able to:

- List and explain the reasons that opium and morphine became prevalent in the United States in the 1800s
- Evaluate the impact of the Harrison Act of 1914 on the type of person who used opiates
- Discuss the factors that have contributed to the increase in abuse of prescription painkillers
- Summarize the impact of reducing narcotic pain prescriptions have impacted narcotic use
- Examine the potential medical dangers related to using nonsterile hypodermic needles
- Defend the purpose of needle-exchange programs and discuss their effect on rates of HIV transmission
- List the factors that influence the intensity of heroin withdrawal
- Evaluate the use of naloxone for overdose cases
- Discuss how narcotic antagonists work
- Explain the medical uses of narcotics
- Compare the advantages versus the disadvantages of methadone maintenance programs

Narcotics provide relief from pain and are among the most addictive drug class.

SanchaiRat/Shutterstock.com

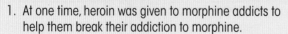

FACT OR **FICTION?**

1. At one time, heroin was given to morphine addicts to help them break their addiction to morphine.

2. More people in the United States die from overdoses of prescription painkillers than from heroin and cocaine overdoses.

3. More students obtain prescription drugs from the Internet than from any other source.

4. Heroin users are likely to become violent while taking the drug.

5. Codeine, which can be found in cough syrup, is a mild narcotic.

6. Heroin is widely abused in the United States.

7. The federal government does not allow federal funds to be used for needle-exchange programs.

8. Women are more likely to die from drug overdoses than men.

9. Although heroin has the reputation of being an extremely addictive drug, it is more difficult to withdraw from alcohol than from heroin.

10. Although methadone is given to patients to treat their heroin addiction, it is possible to become addicted to methadone.

Turn the page to check your answers

The sedating, painkilling, sleep-inducing effects of opium have been noted for several thousand years. Painkilling drugs derived from opium include morphine and heroin. Law enforcement agencies often refer to opium-based drugs as narcotics. The term *narcotic* is derived from the Greek word meaning "stupor."

Throughout history, opium has figured prominently in wars between nations, in the economic vitality of some countries, in medicine, and in the work of lyricists and authors. In the 1800s, opium was plentiful in the United States. More than 70,000 Chinese workers came to the United States in the mid-1800s to build railroads and work in the mines in California. With them came their penchant for smoking opium and for opium dens. Before long, smoking opium was linked to the criminal underworld, and the Chinese were guilty by association.

Morphine use escalated during the 19th century. It was used to relieve pain, diarrhea, and dysentery—conditions that were prevalent during the Civil War.[1] Soldiers routinely injected themselves, and thousands became dependent. Morphine use and dependency were not limited to US soldiers. The drug was used extensively during the Franco-Prussian and Prussian-Austrian wars. Morphine abuse was boosted by development of the hypodermic needle in the mid-1850s. The hypodermic needle hastened the effects of morphine. Also, injected morphine was believed to be nonaddicting.

In the 19th century, no restrictions were placed on what could go into medicines. By 1906, opium and its derivatives were found in more than 50,000 medicines. Drugs containing opiates were used for treating mental illness, headaches, toothaches, coughs, tuberculosis, and pneumonia. Morphine and heroin could

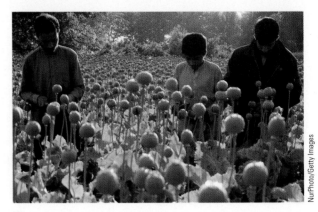

Afghanistan remains the world's largest producer of opium.

be bought in any local store, and prescriptions were not required. People who did not have easy access to stores where drugs were sold could easily get a hypodermic syringe kit and **laudanum**—another form of opium—through a Sears, Roebuck and Company mail-order catalog. Laudanum, which is a mixture of opium and alcohol, was developed in the 1500s by Paracelsus, a Swiss chemist.[2]

The typical patent medicine user was a middle- or upper-class, 30- to 50-year-old, White woman who was genteel and took opiates regularly for medicinal reasons.[3] Patent medicines containing opium and morphine were also used nonmedically, especially by women who frowned on alcohol use during this period of alcohol temperance. Many members of the Women's Christian Temperance Union (WCTU) worked for alcohol reform during the day and took "women's tonics" (containing laudanum) in the evening.[4] Many people continued using these medicines, because they feared the withdrawal symptoms. Ironically, the drug promoted to help people overcome

FACT OR FICTION?

1. **FACT** When heroin was first developed, it was viewed as a cure for morphine addiction even though it is more powerful than morphine.

2. **FACT** Nearly 15,000 Americans have died from prescription painkillers.

3. **FICTION** The fact is—Less than 2% of students receive prescription drugs from the Internet; 70% receive prescription drugs from friends or relatives.

4. **FICTION** The fact is—Heroin puts users in a stupefied state; thus, they are lethargic and nonviolent.

5. **FACT** Although codeine is a regulated drug and a narcotic, it is a cough suppressant.

6. **FICTION** The fact is—Although heroin use has been increasing, only about 0.2% of Americans aged 12 or older are heroin users.

7. **FACT** Beginning in 2015, the federal government now allows federal funding to be used toward NEP (but not the syringes itself).

8. **FICTION** The fact is—More men than women die from drug overdoses.

9. **FACT** Withdrawing from alcohol is more life-threatening than withdrawing from heroin.

10. **FACT** Methadone can be a highly addictive drug.

morphine dependency was heroin. Factors contributing to morphine addiction during the latter part of the 19th century included the following:

- Importation of Chinese workers
- The Civil War
- Development of the hypodermic needle
- Inclusion in patent medicines

By the late 1800s, an estimated 4.59 per 1,000 people were dependent on opiates.[5] This figure is much higher proportionately than today's rate of addiction. The United States was known as the "dope fiend's paradise."

National concern regarding narcotics culminated in passage of the Harrison Act of 1914 (see Chapter 3). Because this law made narcotic use without a prescription illegal, the typical opiate addict shifted from a middle-class woman to a young, lower-class man. In a dramatic change, opiates, which once were viewed as good medicine, now were considered evil. Likewise, perceptions of the opiate addict went from that of an unfortunate victim to one of a deviant criminal who was a threat to society. Following World War I, the British government passed legislation similar to the Harrison Act, restricting the manufacture, sale, possession, and distribution of heroin, morphine, and cocaine.[6]

Extent of Narcotic Use

According to government estimates, in 2014, about 435,000 Americans were heroin users.[7] This amounts to 0.2% of Americans aged 12 and older. Afghanistan is the largest producer of illicit opium, accounting for roughly 70% of global opium production.[8] It is also the largest producer of legal, medical opium.[9] Production went down significantly in 2015, mainly due to poor yields in the county's southern provinces. Myanmar was the second leading producer of opium, accounting for roughly 14% of global opium production.[10] Other prominent producers include Lao People's Democratic Republic, Mexico, Columbia, and Guatemala.[11] In 2014–2015, the Government of Mexico conducted its first opium poppy survey. From this survey, it is estimated around 28,100 ha areas are being used for opium cultivation. However, because this was the first year the survey was conducted, comparisons with previous years are not suitable.[12] Worldwide production levels are shown in Table 8.1.

Use in the United States

During the 1930s, morphine abuse exceeded heroin abuse in the United States. By the following decade, heroin addiction was greater. After World War II, heroin use gradually expanded to ghetto areas in many large cities. Heroin was relatively cheap: A person could get high by buying as little as a dollar's worth. Eventually heroin use spread from poor urban neighborhoods to middle-class suburban areas. Heroin use increased greatly beginning in the late 1960s and early 1970s.

Heroin use has become fashionable in some parts of the country. As a result, heroin-related visits to the

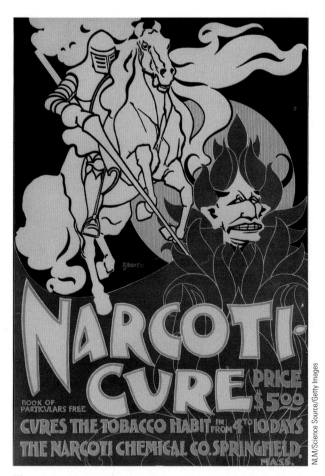

Narcotics were advertised as a cure for addiction to tobacco.

NLM/Science Source/Getty Images

TABLE 8.1 Worldwide Potential Illicit Opium Production, 2005–2009 (Metric Tons)

Country	2005	2006	2007	2008	2009	2015
Afghanistan	445.7	564.4	8000	5500	5300	3300
Burma	380	230	270	340	250	647
Colombia		37	15		17	
Laos	28	8.5	5.5	17	10.6	
Mexico	71	108	149	325	425	

Source: *International Narcotics Control Strategy Report 2016* (Washington, DC: U.S. Department of State, 2016).

laudanum A drug derived from opium

emergency room and deaths in recent years have increased. According to the National Institute for Drug Abuse, there was a sixfold increase in heroin overdose deaths from 2001–2014. Figure 8.1 provides information on deaths from heroin overdoses from 2001 to 2014. Whites comprised the majority of those episodes.[14]

The National Survey on Drug Use and Health reports that 914,000 people aged 12 and older have used heroin in the previous 12 months.[15] Heroin use without a needle has been on the rise.[16] Most heroin users are between the ages of 18 to 25. Table 8.2 shows the percentage of students using heroin in 2015.

Not everyone who uses heroin or other narcotics becomes dependent on them. Some heroin users take the drug occasionally or on weekends. Precise figures on the number of people who fit this description are not available. These users, called **chippers**, take narcotics in a controlled way. Occasional heroin use

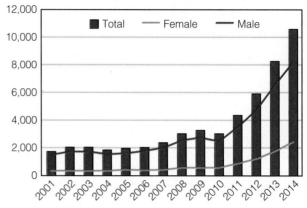

National Overdose Deaths
Number of Deaths from Heroin

Source: National Center for Health Statistics, CDC Wonder.

Figure 8.1 Deaths from Heroin

ON CAMPUS

Alcohol, marijuana, and prescription drug abuse have been the focus of many colleges substance abuse programs. That is slowly beginning to change, especially colleges located in or near cities where heroin use has gone up. In the Rochester region, heroin overdoses has increased fivefold from 2011 to 2014. This is no longer an inner-city problem. Heroin use has increased among college students and colleges are noticing.

At one college, the health center will screen all patients for hard drug use. If a student has hard drugs in their system, they will be referred for treatment. Colleges have initiated recovery communities to help students who are struggling with a hard drug addiction. In 2014, about 100 colleges have created recovery communities.

Questions to Ponder:

When you think of a heroin user, what image comes to mind? How does the image of a college student fit into this? Part of the problem with heroin use on campus is that preconceived notions of a heroin user doesn't fit the typical student on campus. How would you go about educating the college community about heroin use? How would you try to break down stereotypes of what a heroin user looks like?

One college is testing incoming students for hard drug use and then referring those that have hard drugs in their system for treatment. How do you feel about this program? Do you feel colleges should have a drug testing program for new students? Should students who test positive for hard drugs be required to enter a treatment community?

Source: C. Weinberg, "Heroin on Campus", *Inside Higher Ed, April 28, 2014.* Accessed on December 29, 2016 from https://www.insidehighered.com/news/2014/04/28/colleges-confront-increase-use-heroin-students.

TABLE 8.2 Percentage of Students Reporting Heroin Use, 2015

Student Heroin Use	8th Grade (%)	10th Grade (%)	12th Grade (%)
Past month	0.1	0.2	0.3
Lifetime	0.5	0.7	0.8

Source: *Monitoring the Future*, 2015.

contradicts the commonly held notion that a person is either an abstainer or an addict. In an older study comparing compulsive narcotic users to controlled users, controlled users fit the following pattern:

- Seldom used the drug more than once a day
- Could keep opiates around without using them
- Avoided opiates when known addicts were present
- Did not use opiates to alleviate depression
- Seldom, if ever, binged on opiates
- Knew the opiate source or dealer
- Took opiates for recreation or relaxation
- Did not take opiates to escape from life's daily hassles[17]

Generalizing about the extent of heroin addiction is difficult, because patterns of drug abuse deviate sharply. An estimated 65.9% of heroin addicts admitted into treatment are male, and 73% are White.[18] A developing trend is the abuse of narcotics in rural and suburban areas. The increase in abuse is significantly higher in rural areas than in metropolitan areas.[19] Injection is the primary mode for heroin administration in more areas.[20]

During the Vietnam War, US soldiers' use of narcotics generated much concern. Heroin and other drugs were widely available in Southeast Asia. The heroin that service personnel used was 95% pure, inexpensive, and sold openly. Although some soldiers injected heroin, most smoked it after having it mixed with marijuana or tobacco. An estimated 10 to 15% of US troops were addicted to heroin.

To deal with the impending dilemma of massive numbers of addicted service personnel, the military established heroin treatment centers in Vietnam. In conjunction with the military's slogan that addiction "stopped at the South China Sea," every soldier was tested for heroin. This program, called "Operation Golden Flow," required soldiers failing the drug test to attend a treatment program. Ironically, heroin usage was greater in the rehabilitation programs than during active duty.[21] Only about 1 to 2% of the soldiers continued to use narcotics 8 to 12 months after returning to the United States.[22] In the United States, heroin was perceived as a deleterious substance. In Vietnam, soldiers took heroin as a means of escaping from a situation they saw as intolerable.

Heroin simply did not play a role in the life of these soldiers once they returned home. This situation clearly points to the important role of *set* (state of mind) and *setting* to drug-taking behavior.

Worldwide Comparison

It is estimated that there are more than 17 million people worldwide who illegally use opiates.[23] Heroin use has been increasing in Western and Central Europe and North America.[24] Italy has seen a significant increase in heroin prevalence rates, especially among 15-year-old boys, which doubled in 2015.[25] China is believed to have the largest number of narcotic addicts.

Exact figures for the extent of heroin addiction in other countries are difficult to obtain, because many countries deny that they have a drug problem. Also, the covert nature of drug addiction obscures the extent of the problem, and in some countries, penalties for drug use and drug trafficking are not imposed because these crimes are of low priority.[26]

Characteristics of Narcotics

Opiates are narcotics. Law enforcement personnel often use the term **narcotic** to refer to illegal drugs, although many illegal drugs are chemically different from narcotics. Opiates refer to a family of drugs with characteristics similar to opium. A generic term used interchangeably with **opiate** is **opioid**. These drugs may be natural or synthetic.

Opium

The opium poppy, *Papaver somniferum,* which means "the poppy that brings sleep," has been called "the plant of joy." Cultivated throughout Asia and the Middle East, it grows to a height of 3 to 4 feet and has white, red, or purple flowers. After poppies bloom and the petals fall, an egg-sized, round seedpod remains. A white, milky sap exudes from the seedpod after it is cut open. Once the sap dries, a brown, thick,

chippers Nickname for individuals who use narcotics occasionally or on weekends

narcotic An opium-based central nervous system depressant used to relieve pain and diarrhea

opiate A class of drugs derived from opium

opioid A family of drugs with characteristics similar to those of opium

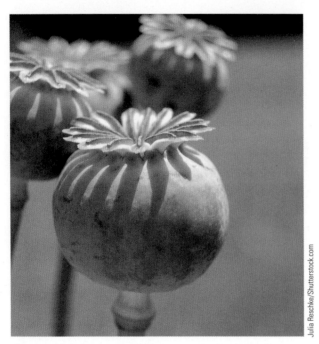
The milky fluid that oozes from the seedpod of the poppy is opium.

and viewed the drug with much reverence. Thus recreational use and addiction were not unusual.

gummy resin forms. This is **opium**. There is only a 10-day window in which opium can be made from the resin of the opium poppy.

Many early civilizations, including Sumeria, Assyria, and Egypt, used opium. The Egyptians gave it to infants, the Greeks and Romans held opium in high regard, and the Greeks sold cakes and candies made from opium. Greek physicians Hippocrates and Galen used opium extensively for medical purposes

Morphine

In 1803, Friedrich Serturner of Germany synthesized morphine from opium and called his discovery *morphium*. The name **morphine** comes from Morpheus, Greek god of dreams. The effects of morphine occur more rapidly than those of opium. Also, morphine is about ten times more potent, although physicians accepted it initially as safer and purer than opium. Another alkaloid that was isolated from opium 30 years later is **codeine**. This word comes from the Greek and means "poppy head." Like morphine, codeine can result in dependency. How morphine is administered and its dosage has a bearing on its effectiveness. If taken orally, it is not very effective. In therapeutic doses, morphine builds up in the spleen, kidneys, lungs, and liver and binds to blood proteins. Its actions last 4 to 5 hours. Almost all morphine passes through the body within 24 hours, but small amounts can be detected in urine for 2 to 4 days. Morphine can traverse the placenta of a pregnant woman and thereby enter the bloodstream of the fetus. Morphine has a profound effect on psychomotor performance, especially on reaction time.[27]

Heroin

Heroin (diacetylmorphine) was first synthesized from morphine in 1874. The word *heroin* is derived from a German word meaning "heroic." Heroin was promoted originally as a cure for morphine

---

CONSIDER This

The typical heroin user in the United States is changing. Many of today's addicts started at the age of 23 and are more likely to live in affluent areas. Many of these addicts were first introduced to opioids though prescription pain pills such as oxycontin. When their prescription ran out, they turned to heroin as a quick and cheaper alternative. During President Clinton's era, the United States consumed 80% of the world's prescription pain pills. Drug overdose was the leading cause of unintentional deaths.

In an effort to curb prescription pain pills, the United States responded by tightening restrictions on prescription pain pills. As a result, while prescription pain pill use went down, heroin use went up, in some areas, it nearly doubled.

Questions to Ponder:

While restricting prescription pain pills reduced the availability of these prescriptions, people have turned to heroin to achieve the same results. How would you go about creating a plan to reduce prescription pain pill abuse and heroin use? Do you think the restrictions on prescription pain pills should be lifted? Explain.

Source: S. Gupta, "Unintended consequences: Why painkiller addicts turn to heroin", *CNN*, Updated June 2, 2016. Accessed on December 29, 2016 from http://www.cnn.com/2014/08/29/health/gupta-unintended-consequences/.

addiction.[28] In a turnabout, morphine later was touted as a cure for heroin addiction.

Heroin was manufactured in 1898 by Bayer, a German pharmaceutical company, which marketed it for ailments ranging from coughs to tuberculosis to bronchitis. Newspaper and magazine advertisements exhorted heroin as a better type of aspirin. When heroin was introduced, it was believed not to be addicting. Now we know, however, that the likelihood of becoming addicted is twice as great for heroin as for morphine.

Heroin can be taken several ways. When smoked, its effects are rapid. Like morphine, it is ineffective when ingested. Individuals who use heroin are more likely to inhale it rather than inject it. Younger abusers tend to use prescription opioids.[29] One is more likely to become addicted when injecting heroin; however, it is a popular misconception that heroin is not addictive when it is smoked or snorted.[30]

Heroin is three to ten times more powerful than morphine. This greater potency results from heroin being much more lipid-soluble than morphine. Also, heroin reaches the brain more quickly and in higher concentrations.

Fentanyl, Methadone, and Other Synthetic Opiates

Synthetic opiates are chemically constructed rather than naturally produced. They elicit effects that are behaviorally similar to those of morphine but bear little chemical resemblance and relieve less severe pain. They differ in duration of action, potency, intensity, and effectiveness. Examples of synthetic opiates are meperidine (Demerol), methadone (Dolophine), oxycodone (Percodan), pentazocaine (Talwin), and propoxyphene hydrochloride (Darvon). These drugs are available only by prescription.

A powerful synthetic opiate that is considerably stronger than heroin, but with similar analgesic effects, is **fentanyl** (Sublimaze). Known colloquially as **China white**, fentanyl carries a much greater risk of a fatal overdose than heroin does due to the opioid receptors location in areas of the brain that control breathing. The potency of fentanyl can cause breathing to stop completely, leading to death.[31] Fentanyl is not amenable to oral use, but it can be injected or snorted. There are a number of clandestine fentanyl labs throughout the United States, although Mexico is the most likely source for it.[32] Fentanyl is often mixed with other drugs, especially heroin. Because it is extremely potent, a small error in diluting or cutting the drug can result in a fatal overdose. Fentanyl has caused some hospitalized patients to experience delirium.[33]

A synthetic opiate widely used as an analgesic in medicine is **meperidine**. Better known as Demerol, meperidine takes effect within 10 minutes after being injected and remains in effect for 2 to 4 hours. It is considerably less potent than morphine. When a pregnant woman is in labor, this drug is preferred over other analgesics because its side effects, especially respiratory depression in newborns, are milder. At one time, meperidine was erroneously believed to be nonaddicting. Other disadvantages to meperidine are that it is not as effective for relieving pain and has adverse interactions with other drugs that could lead to central nervous system problems, including seizures. Meperidine has been found to be the most frequently prescribed inappropriate medication for surgery patients.[34]

Another synthetic narcotic is **propoxyphene hydrochloride** (Darvon). Darvon is related structurally to methadone. It is used primarily to assuage mild pain. At first, Darvon was thought to have few side effects and not to cause dependency. We now know that Darvon can result in dependency, affect intellectual and motor abilities, and even be fatal. In 2009, Xanodyne

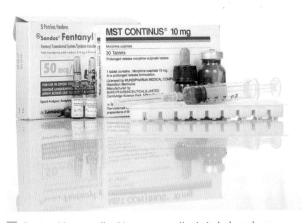

Jes2u.photo/Shutterstock.com

Fentanyl is prescribed to cancer patients to help reduce chronic pain.

opium The plant from which narcotics are derived

morphine An analgesic drug derived from opium; used medically as a painkiller

codeine Mild narcotic that suppresses coughing; a derivative of opium

heroin (diacetylmorphine) A potent drug that is a derivative of opium

fentanyl A synthetic narcotic that is 1,000 times more potent than heroin

China white A synthetic analgesic drug derived from fentanyl that mimics heroin but is considerably more potent

meperidine A synthetic derivative of morphine

propoxyphene hydrochloride A mild narcotic that has the potential to cause dependence

TABLE 8.3 Common Narcotics

Drug	Common Name	Street Name
Heroin	Diacetylmorphine	Snow, Stuff, Harry, H, White Horse, Horse, Hard Stuff, White Stuff, Joy Powder, Scag, Junk
Morphine	Morphine sulfate	Morpho, Miss Emma, Unkie, Hocus, M
Codeine	Codeine, Empirin with codeine, cough syrups with codeine	Schoolboy
Meperidine	Demerol, Mepergan	Doctors
Methadone	Dolophine	Dollies, Methadose
Oxycodone	Percodan, Talwin, Darvon, Pentazone, Propoxyphene	—

Source: Health EDCO, a division of WRS Group, Inc.

conducted a study and determined that even when Darvon was taken at recommended doses, there were significant changes to the electrical activity of the heart.[35] The drug propoxyphene was pulled from the market.[36]

Methadone was first synthesized during World War II by scientists in Nazi Germany as a substitute for morphine. Its effects are comparable to those of morphine, but it is more active when taken orally. The potency of methadone when injected subcutaneously (just below the skin) is equivalent to that of morphine. Methadone can be taken with water or alcohol.

Although methadone is used to lessen severe pain, it is most noted for blocking withdrawal symptoms and euphoric effects from narcotics. Unfortunately, it produces its own euphoria and dependence. Infants born to pregnant women who were prescribed methadone are at risk for developing vision problems.[37] About 5% of infants whose mothers took methadone while pregnant experienced seizures.[38] Table 8.3 lists common narcotics, including their street names.

OxyContin

From 1996 to the present, the number of prescriptions for painkilling drugs has grown dramatically. One drug that has gained much attention is OxyContin, a particularly strong painkiller. OxyContin works by blocking the pain signals from nerves. It allows patients to swallow fewer pills, and it offers patients pain relief that lasts three times longer than other painkillers. It has been shown to be as effective for relieving pain in cancer patients as other painkilling drugs.[39]

OxyContin is not without its risks. In 2012, 16 million people, aged 12 and older, used oxycodone products nonmedically.[40] Thousands of people have become addicted to it. Nonetheless, many women are given OxyContin while pregnant. In one study, almost 30% of pregnant mothers in Tennessee took an opioid while pregnant.[41] The percentage of women taking opioids during pregnancy has doubled over the past 15 years.[42]

The drug's manufacturer, Purdue Pharma, admits that somewhere between dozens and hundreds of people have died from the drug. Purdue Pharma has been trying to address problems with OxyContin through educational sessions with the Drug Enforcement Agency (DEA) and the FDA.

OxyContin has accounted for more than 100,000 emergency room visits.[43] The abuse of OxyContin is especially acute in Appalachia, where addicts are commonly referred to as "pillbillies."[44] West Virginia and Kentucky are in the top ten for number of fatal drugs overdoses from painkillers and opioids.[45] The Kentucky attorney general and other officials have sued Purdue Pharma for millions of dollars to recoup expenses for drug programs and law enforcement.[46] In 2007, Purdue Pharma agreed to pay $634.5 million for understating problems with the drug. In 2010, Purdue Pharma reformulated OxyContin so that it could not be as easily crushed and abused.[47] As a result one study found a 27% decrease in rates of addiction among opioids due to the reformulation.[48]

Physical and Psychological Effects

The feelings derived from narcotics can be induced naturally by the release of endorphins in the brain. Endorphins help regulate a person's response to stress and pain. These are the same chemicals responsible for the so-called runner's high. Opiates mimic endorphins in the brain.

Many dangers associated with narcotics arise from their illegal status. Physical problems related to narcotics frequently result from using these drugs in unclean, unsafe environments. Because of the types of people associated with illegal narcotics, homicide is a threat. Also, because the unregulated use of narcotics is against the law, narcotics often are contaminated. For instance, heroin may be contaminated with other drugs or with substances such as sugar, starch, powdered milk, quinine, and strychnine.

The peril of narcotics is compounded by how they are administered. Sharing needles is a practice fraught with danger. According to the Centers for Disease Control and Prevention (CDC), in 2015, 6% of all new HIV cases that were diagnosed were due to injection drug use.[49] Of course, thousands of HIV cases go undetected and/or unreported.

Medical maladies such as septicemia (blood poisoning), abscesses, hepatitis, HIV/AIDS, and endocarditis (a potentially fatal inflammation of the heart lining) arise from the use of unsterile needles, not from narcotics per se. Death may come within several seconds to users who inadvertently inject air into their veins. Repeated injections into the same vein can lead to its collapse.

Physical Effects

Narcotics cause drowsiness, vomiting, nausea, and difficulty concentrating. The pupils of the eyes constrict to such an extent that this has given rise to the term "pinpoint pupil." Narcotics lower body temperature, dilate blood vessels in the skin, and lower blood pressure. These effects are manifested in a flushed, warm face and neck.

Opiates impede the ability to urinate, and a common and potentially serious side effect from opiates is constipation. Addicts tend to neglect their diet and engage in other poor health habits. In sum, many addicts simply live unhealthy lifestyles.

Users who inject heroin feel intense, immediate reactions. Euphoria is followed by gradually anesthetizing sensations, then sleep and lethargy. Initial users paint a picture of disorientation and discomfort. Some regular users describe feelings of peace and contentment.

When heroin is injected, initial users describe a "rush" similar to a sexual orgasm. The rush tends to last less than a minute, after which feelings of relaxation take over. Despite the sexual euphoria that accompanies injection, heroin addicts have little, if any, sex drive. Both male and female opioid users experience sexual dysfunction; one study showed 33% of male and 25% of female opioid users reporting sexual dysfunction.[50] Moreover, male addicts also have difficulty with achieving an erection.[51] In males, heavy use can retard development of secondary sex characteristics, and in females, menstruation may stop, rendering them infertile. Ironically, during withdrawal, male users sometimes have a spontaneous erection and ejaculation, and women can experience orgasm.

Infants born to women who took narcotics while pregnant exhibit withdrawal symptoms such as irritability, difficulty in feeding, sweating, tremors, stuffy nose, diarrhea, and vomiting. These infants have a shorter gestation and lower birth weight. Numerous studies have shown that pregnant women given narcotic-based medications during the first trimester are more likely to bear children with physical birth defects.[52] One difficulty in knowing whether their children's development is affected is that female addicts often lack parenting skills; thus, it is hard to know whether educational difficulties arose from heroin use or parental inability. Interestingly, the babies of heroin-addicted women adopted or placed in foster homes have *not* been found to be intellectually or developmentally impaired despite low birth weight, small head circumference, and withdrawal symptoms.[53] This suggests that environmental deprivation might play a large role in children's development.

Besides risking infecting their babies, pregnant women who use heroin are more likely to miscarry and deliver prematurely, and the risk of sudden infant death syndrome (SIDS) also increases.[54] Use of opioids during pregnancy may result in neonatal abstinence syndrome.[55] This is a result of the sudden withdrawal of substances (including opioids) during pregnancy.[56] This syndrome impacts the central and autonomic nervous system and gastrointestinal tract and may be quite intense.[57] From 2000 to 2010, there was a five-fold increase in the proportion of babies born with neonatal abstinence syndrome.[58] As a result, babies suffering from neonatal abstinence syndrome require longer hospital stays (on average 16.9 days) and cost hospitals an estimated 1.5 billion dollars.[59] Most of this is paid for by Medicaid as opiate-abusing mothers tend to come from lower-income communities.[60]

Emotional and Social Effects

Narcotics affect emotional and social health. They relieve psychic distress arising from anxiety, hostility, feelings of inadequacy, and aggression. However, the stress of rationalizing and defending one's drug use increases emotional discomfort. Heroin addicts lack the ability to control their impulsivity. They have difficulty regulating their inhibitions and in making decisions.[61] Addicts will take more time to make decisions and frequently make risky decisions.[62] In addition, it is not uncommon for seniors with medical problems to use narcotics to commit suicide.[63]

Users sometimes ignore or become alienated and hostile toward friends and family members who previously were important. The lifestyle of a drug addict makes it difficult to maintain intimacy. It was found

methadone A drug given to heroin addicts to block withdrawal effects and euphoria

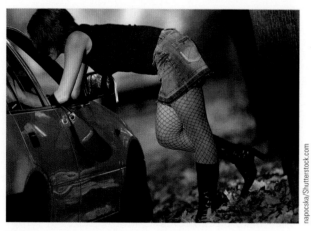

Between 40% and 80% of U.S. prostitutes are addicted to hard drugs such as heroin.

that women who became addicted experienced a profound tragedy as children.[64] One study found women who were addicts had experienced rejection from their female parent, which impacted their self-image.[65] Furthermore, this study also found many women heroin addicts were victims of psychological abuse from peers and friends.[66] In another study looking at the family structure of heroin addicts, it was determined that these families had higher rates of rejection by fathers and mothers and experienced higher rates of stressful events.[67] Heroin-addicted men were more likely to have a history of criminal activity prior to their usage.[68] Whether heroin use preceded antisocial behavior or vice versa is hard to know.

William Burroughs's autobiographical novel *Junky* describes how narcotics make people feel less sociable. Opiates result in lethargy, and users lack motivation. However, instead of claiming that narcotics produce lethargy, lethargic people simply may be more likely to use narcotics. Likewise, whether addicts use heroin to feel euphoria or to avoid dysphoria is unclear.

Heroin use has been associated with criminal behavior, unemployment, and violence. It is not uncommon for heroin users to engage in prostitution, burglary, and theft. An Australian study found a relationship between those with extensive heroin use and criminal involvement.[69]

Needle-Exchange Programs

Although unsafe sexual practices are the most common cause of HIV, it is estimated that one-third of all cases outside of sub-Saharan Africa is due to multiperson use of syringes.[70] Additionally among high- and middle-income countries, injecting drug use is the most common mode of transmission for Hepatitis C.[71] One solution is to get people who

inject drugs to bleach needles or exchange needles for clean ones. Many healthcare personnel favor needle-exchange programs (NEPs) or giving hypodermic needles to addicts at no cost. Prominent groups supporting NEPs are the American Medical Association, the American Bar Association, and the US Conference of Mayors. In the past, the federal government rejected the NEP concept, preferring a criminal justice approach to a public health approach.

Congress banned federal funding for NEPs in 1988 and renewed the ban numerous times until 2016.[72,73] In January 2016, Congress lifted the ban on funding for NEPs. While federal funds cannot be used to purchase syringes, they may be used for other expenses associated with the program.[74] In the United States, NEPs have gained popularity, although their acceptance and funding vary greatly from one municipality to another.[75] One study reported a 5.9% decrease in HIV infection rates in cities with NEPs and a 5.8% increase in cities without NEPs.[76]

An argument against NEPs is that they give the appearance of condoning drug use. Also, because addicts do not want to be identified, many do not benefit from NEPs. Youths who use heroin have a high rate of needle sharing. Therefore services for adolescents who inject drugs might have to be tailored to their needs.[77] Young people who frequent medically supervised injection facilities are more likely to have had medical or legal problems than those who are hesitant to go to such facilities.[78]

The first country to implement an NEP was the Netherlands. Results of NEPs in the Netherlands, Switzerland, and Denmark have been encouraging. Officials in these countries claim that their NEPs have retarded the spread of HIV/AIDS. In Amsterdam, HIV transmission rates were significantly reduced if NEPs were combined with other harm-reduction strategies.[79] Besides reduced HIV infections, Australian officials

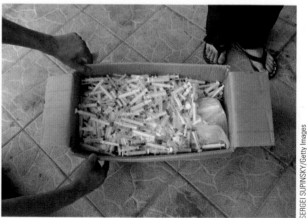

Needle exchange programs are designed to reduce the transmission of AIDS and other diseases.

report reduced hepatitis C infections. Also, Australia saved at least $2.4 billion as a result of NEPs.[80]

NEPs are cost-effective. The lifetime cost for treating HIV infection is $350,000, compared to less than $2 for providing sterile needles.[81] Providing clean needles is estimated to save 30 people each day from contracting HIV infection. Another benefit of NEPs is that they serve as gateways for users to access social and medical services.[82]

Dependency

Physical dependence, psychological dependence, and tolerance develop quickly, although the idea that a person is addicted after trying these drugs one time is a myth. However, after several months of intense

CULTURAL Considerations

In the District of Columbia (DC), injection drug use remains the third leading cause of HIV transmission. This has led to a call for harm reduction programs and policies such as the syringe exchange program (SEP).

One study found the distance to an SEP significantly impacts the behaviors of Latinos' injection behaviors. As the distance increases from a SEP facility, the less likely that person will use the service.

DC has enacted a buffer zone policy that prohibits the distributes of syringes within a 1000 feet of a public or private school. Some believe this impedes the effectiveness of the SEP. One study looked at areas where high intravenous drug use-related activities occurred and found most these activities occurred within the school buffer zones (areas where SEP are not allowed to run).

Questions to Ponder:

Why do you think a school buffer zone exists? Do you believe these buffer zones should continue to exist? Do you believe a SEP in a school buffer zone would encourage intravenous drug use?

Some say these buffer zones in DC disproportionately affect Latinos and other marginalized populations. What are your thoughts?

Source: S. T. Allen, M.S. Ruiz, J. Jones, and M.M. Turner, "Legal space for syringe exchange programs in hot spots of injective drug use-related crime", *Harm Reduction Journal*, 13, no. 16 (2016).

use, some users are capable of taking 40 to 50 times the amount that would kill the person with less tolerance.[83] Another myth is that all addicts are moral degenerates. Numerous studies point out that most addicts maintain some ethical responsibility within their social environment.[84] It has been shown that patients with chronic pain with a past or present substance use disorder were 17 times more likely to become dependent on painkillers than others with chronic pain conditions.[85] Dependency, though, does produce numerous withdrawal symptoms. After withdrawal, the desire for narcotics sometimes persists for years. Withdrawal symptoms appear 8 to 12 hours after the last injection, peaking in 48 to 72 hours. The symptoms have been compared to a bad case of the flu. Although this "flu" is unpleasant, it is not as severe as typically shown in the media.

Withdrawal symptoms, which subside after several days, include the following:

diarrhea	tearing
runny nose	perspiration
constant yawning	restlessness
insomnia	anxiety
muscle aches and pains	irritability
dysphoria	stomach cramps
fatigue	

The hands and legs shake. The person is literally "kicking the habit."

Factors affecting the difficulty of withdrawal include availability of a social support network, the addict's desire to stop, the physical environment during withdrawal, and the convenience and practicality of alternative opiates. Withdrawal from narcotics is not life-threatening, yet many users avoid going through it out of fear. The anticipation of withdrawal could be worse than the physical act of withdrawing. To avoid withdrawal, an addict uses the drug several times daily. Some people think that addicts are really addicted to the *thought* of being addicted, to actually shooting up, and to the lifestyle of an addict. Heroin addicts do not all follow the same path after becoming addicted. In a 33-year study of heroin addicts, it was found that many quit using after becoming addicted while others quit after an extended time. Yet, some addicts continued using heroin for many years.[86]

People can become drug dependent in less than 2 weeks if they take increasing amounts of narcotics. About half of narcotic abusers become dependent. The average amount of time a person is addicted is 6 to 8 years. Dependency may develop because of psychological distress, not because of the pharmacological makeup of narcotics themselves. A study of addicts who abstained from narcotics for 3 years after having been removed from the environment in which they used drugs revealed that they relapsed within a month after returning to their original environment.[88] This implies that addiction is more than a physical phenomenon.

Toxicity

Because opiates depress the central nervous system, they lower respiration, pulse rates, and blood pressure. Narcotics are capable of depressing the respiratory system to the point of death. Even when prescribed, narcotics can be fatal. According to the CDC, half of all opioid overdose deaths involve a prescription opioid.[89]

In many cases of death from narcotic overdose, another drug such as alcohol is present. The synergistic effect of narcotics and other drugs can be fatal. From 1999 to 2014, the deaths from drug overdoses nearly tripled.[90] Death from an overdose of heroin is slow. People who die quickly from an overdose are likely to die from **anaphylactic shock**, a condition caused by an allergic reaction to contaminants such as quinine, which are used to cut or dilute the heroin. Sellers increase their profits by cutting heroin with adulterants such as quinine, cornstarch, and lactose.

Naloxone is an opioid antagonist that has been used for more than 30 years to reverse the effects of an opioid overdose.[91] The recent surge in overdose opioid deaths has resulted in proposals to create a naloxone distribution program. Studies have shown naloxone is effective in reducing the effects of opioid overdoses, even among those who are currently on a methadone program.[92] Other studies have found promising results in reducing opioid overdose deaths by use of naloxone; in a report by the CDC, since 1996 over 50,000 persons were trained to distribute naloxone, resulting in a little over 10,000 overdose reversals.[93] In 2014, the FDA approved Narcan® Nasal Spray, a formulation of a naloxone that comes in a nasal spray for easy administration.[94]

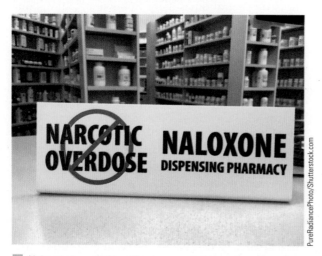

Naloxone is available without a prescription and used to reduce opioid overdose deaths.

Despite evidence to suggest the benefits of naloxone programs to reduce opioid overdose deaths, public opinion regarding these types of programs has been lacking. Widely held negative opinions regarding those who use opioid drugs contribute to the lack of public support regarding naloxone community programs. A lack of sympathy regarding those who use drugs tend to result in a lack of support for these types of programs.[95] Some critics believe the use of these programs will increase opioid overdoses as users will rely on naloxone for life-saving measures if an overdose occurs. Thus far research suggests that opioid use after participating in a naloxone program may be reduced after an overdose event.[96]

Medical Benefits

The word *narcotic* evokes a highly negative response. People are likely to think of narcotics as completely destructive. In medicine, however, narcotics offer a number of benefits. Narcotics have benefited humankind in important ways.

Analgesia

Pain relief is a primary benefit of narcotics. Patients receiving morphine, for example, are still aware of pain, but their perception of pain and their response to it are altered in positive ways. Patients experience the discomfort associated with the pain, but they do not lose consciousness. Opiates block the sensation of pain from being transmitted to the brain and reduce negative feelings connected to the pain. Although narcotics alleviate all types of pain, they are more effective with continuous dull pain than with sharp, intermittent pain. Narcotics are favored over other **analgesics** because they have fewer adverse effects on intellectual and motor ability.

In the United States, morphine is one of the main drugs used for analgesic purposes. A study on rats found morphine can effectively reduce pain for up to 8 hours after a surgical event.[97] Despite concerns about its potential for addiction, morphine effectively alleviates pain. It is used in hospices without negatively affecting survival rates.[98] In England, heroin is commonly used to relieve severe pain, especially the pain associated with cancer. In the United States, use of heroin for medical purposes is illegal. Because there is much concern about the abuse of narcotics, particularly heroin, many people who could benefit from these drugs do not receive them or receive an inadequate dosage.

Gastrointestinal Difficulties

A traveler's worry, "Delhi belly," or "Montezuma's revenge" refers to an intestinal disorder that people commonly experience when traveling abroad. In many less-developed countries, diarrhea is a major cause of death among the young and elderly. Because these countries lack good sanitation, food and water supplies become contaminated, leading to serious infections of the gastrointestinal system.

Narcotics are effective in treating diarrhea. Food passes through the intestinal tract as a result of peristaltic contractions. Narcotics slow down these contractions and the speed at which material is removed from the body. One disadvantage of narcotics is that they may cause constipation. Opioid bowel dysfunction is a common side effect with opioid-induced constipation being the most widely reported effect.[99]

Cough Suppressant

Many people who take medication for coughs have used narcotics without being aware of it. Narcotic agents slow activity of the cough control center, located in the medulla of the brain. The opium derivative codeine has long been used for its **antitussive** properties. Cough medicines with codeine can be obtained on a nonprescription basis, but codeine is now a regulated drug.

Nonopiate drugs such as **dextromethorphan (Delsym)**, which are chemically similar to opiates, often are found in cough preparations today in place of codeine. It is believed that dextromethorphan, also known as DMX, is one of the fastest growing drug problems in the United States. An estimated 10% of teens have abused cough medicine (many containing DMS) to get high.[100] In addition, over 12,000 emergency room visits can be attributed to DMX. Some symptoms of adverse reactions include blurred vision, loss of coordination, stomach pain, and rapid heartbeat.[101] Dextromethorphan also may impair judgment, resulting in injury or fatality.[102] It has been associated with psychosis as well.[103]

Treatment and Support Groups

In 2013, 344,496 heroin users and 163,664 other opiate users checked into treatment.[104] Narcotic addiction is difficult to treat effectively. The **recidivism** (relapse) rate is high, but the longer one is off drugs, the more likely one will remain abstinent. One benefit of treatment is that addicts live longer.[105]

Addicts do not have to be consigned to a lifetime of addiction. Many addicts mature or grow out of drug use. Treatment programs range from psychotherapy to behavior modification to acupuncture to medical intervention. The following sections review several types of treatments. Therapeutic communities are covered in Chapter 15.

Detoxification

Withdrawal from narcotics is not as life-threatening or as severe as many people believe. Most addicts are withdrawn from narcotics gradually, although rapid **detoxification** can be just as effective. Unfortunately, most patients undergoing detoxification fail to complete the program. Freeing one's body of drugs does not remove the person's desire to take drugs.

To help addicts in withdrawal, they receive drugs such as clonidine, buprenorphine, naltrexone, naloxone, and the best known, methadone. Clonidine was used to treat hypertension initially, and it was found also to eliminate some drug withdrawal symptoms. Naloxone reduces the amount of time addicts require to undergo withdrawal, but it triggers withdrawal more suddenly.

Typically, detoxification is completed in 10 to 14 days if it is conducted on an inpatient basis. Federal guidelines allow methadone to be administered for up to 30 days on an outpatient basis, although the time can be extended to 180 days if 30 days is found to be insufficient or if the addict is likely to relapse.

Narcotic Antagonists

Drugs that block narcotics from producing their reinforcing effects are called antagonists. **Antagonists** remove the physical need for opiates, but not the psychic need. They complement psychotherapy or group therapy. Examples are naltrexone, buprenorphine, nalorphine, naloxone, and cyclazocine. Nalorphine and cyclazocine were the first antagonists used, but they have been discarded because of their unpleasant side effects. Naloxone (Narcan) subsequently replaced these drugs because it did not produce dysphoria or physical dependence. The effectiveness of naloxone as an antagonist, however, is limited. It works for a short time only. It is used frequently in emergency situations to handle overdoses from narcotics.

---

anaphylactic shock A condition caused by an allergic reaction to contaminants such as quinine, which are used to cut or dilute heroin

analgesics Drugs that relieve pain

antitussives Drugs that act as cough suppressants

dextromethorphan (Delsym) An over-the-counter nonnarcotic drug found in cough preparations

recidivism Relapse

detoxification Eliminating drugs from the body; usually the initial step in treatment of the effects of alcohol and other drugs

antagonists Drugs that occupy receptor sites and inhibit narcotic activity

Naltrexone (Trexan) is administered orally and is generally effective for a few days. Taking naltrexone negates the effects of heroin injected during the same period. Thus, if a person were to take an opioid while on naltrexone, the effects from the opioid would not be felt. Therefore naltrexone is useful during detoxification. It is not recommended for people who have acute hepatitis or liver failure, because high doses are linked to hepatic toxicity.

Naltrexone is not viewed as a complete form of treatment because addicts crave narcotics after discontinuing medication. Moreover, the dropout rate for individuals receiving naltrexone is substantial because the pill form required either a daily or three time a week regimen.[106] Thus this type of treatment is best for highly motivated individuals. An injectable, long-acting form of naltrexone has been developed.[107] It has been shown to improve rates of abstinence. In a study among opioid dependent prison inmates, those that received the injectable naltrexone in addition with counselling has lower rates of relapse compared to those who only received cousneling.[108] Naltrexone works best when it is used in conjunction with some type of additional reward.

Another drug used to ameliorate withdrawal is **buprenorphine**. The FDA initially approved it to treat pain. It is less addictive than other drugs. It is also a synthetic opioid medication and carries a low risk of overdose.[109] Buprenorphine also reduces the use of cocaine and illicit opiates.[110] Buprenorphine can be taken alone or combined with naloxone. In a recent study looking at the buprenorphine/naloxone combination for addiction treatment, 50% of patients reported they were abstinent 18 months after starting therapy. Additionally, after 3.5 years, fewer than 10% of those on this treatment program met the diagnostic criteria for drug dependence.[111] Pregnant women given buprenorphine were no more likely to bear children with birth defects than were women given methadone.[112]

Methadone and Other Treatments

Since 1960, methadone has been the drug used most frequently to treat heroin addiction. Psychiatrist Marie Nyswander and biochemist Vincent Dole promoted methadone because traditional therapy was ineffective in getting addicts to stop using heroin. Methadone clinics offer individual and group psychotherapy as well as support to addicts. No treatment parallels the effectiveness of methadone. Relative to other forms of treatment, it has been found that methadone maintenance is more cost-effective.[113]

People in methadone maintenance programs do best when it is combined with behavioral treatment.[114] Additionally, people on a methadone maintenance program reduce their use of illegal drugs, especially heroin, and fewer people become HIV positive while receiving methadone. In a study conducted in Australia it was discovered that patients who were in a methadone maintenance program show higher retention rates compared to a buprenorphine program.[115] Prisoners given methadone prior to their release are less likely to engage in HIV sex-risk behaviors compared to those prisoners who received counselling alone.[116] One study indicated that parents in methadone maintenance and a program to address parenting skills are less likely to engage in child abuse.[117] On the other hand, fathers receiving methadone without further help have not been shown to improve parenting skills.[118] Women who take methadone while pregnant have better outcomes including reduced risk-taking behavior and improved infant mortality and morbidity.[119] One negative impact on the infant is reduced fetal growth, as babies born to women on a methadone maintenance program have lower birth rates and low head circumferenes.[120] Women who take methadone while breastfeeding will secrete methadone in breast milk but their infants have not been shown to have greater neurobehavioral problems than infants whose mothers were not on methadone.[121] Nausea and vomiting are the most common complaints of pregnant women on methadone.[122]

Methadone is highly specific to opiate addiction. It does not alter the effects of cocaine, alcohol, benzodiazepines, and other drugs. Methadone maintenance programs have other problems, though. Many addicts resist coming for treatment. Methadone is euphoric for people who are not addicted to heroin. It leads to addiction, though many people consider addiction to methadone preferable to addiction to heroin. Another issue is whether methadone should be a step toward eventual abstinence or whether it is an acceptable lifelong treatment.

The life of a methadone patient is not easy. Methadone has to be administered daily to avert withdrawal symptoms. Methadone patients face discrimination in housing, insurance, and employment. Methadone produces side effects ranging from hallucinations to sexual dysfunction, insomnia, muscle pain, profuse perspiration, frequent urination, nausea, numbness in the extremities, and constipation. Methadone programs have been accused of controlling population growth because the drug has been linked to sexual impotence, and most patients are from disadvantaged backgrounds. Signs and symptoms that the dosage of methadone is too high include drowsiness, euphoria, respiratory depression, pinpoint pupils, and skin flush.

Despite its limitations, methadone maintenance has several advantages. Methadone can be orally administered, it is easy to monitor, it eliminates the need for needles, and it reduces the risk of overdosing. Withdrawal symptoms are prevented for up to 24 hours. Euphoric effects from heroin are blocked for the same amount of time, and patients experience no sedation from methadone.

The longer patients stay in treatment, regardless of the type of substance abuse treatment, the more likely treatment will be successful. Another benefit is that patients are less apt to be hospitalized, saving thousands of dollars.

The FDA monitors methadone maintenance programs closely. Addicts are screened to ensure that they are physiologically dependent on heroin. Adolescent addicts are not eligible to receive methadone except under special circumstances. Addicts can obtain methadone only by enrolling in a maintenance program; no one can receive methadone from private physicians.

Methadone maintenance does not constitute a complete treatment. Rather, it should be viewed as part of a larger treatment. Methadone maintenance does not address the social and psychological factors leading to addiction in the first place. During rehabilitation, patients are advised to participate in constructive activities such as employment, vocational training, volunteer work, or homemaking. A stable source of legal income reduces the likelihood that patients will resort to drug dealing or other criminal activities.

Only a minority of people successfully withdraw from methadone. Individuals who drop out of treatment or who are discharged unfavorably from treatment have a higher rate of death. One factor that has reduced relapse is emphasis on abstaining from heroin. In a 25-year study of patients treated with methadone, 31% of the men who were still alive were using heroin and none of the female survivors were using heroin.[123]

An alternative drug approved by the FDA in 1993 is **levo-alpha-acetylmethadol (LAAM)**. One advantage of LAAM over methadone is that it blocks withdrawal symptoms for up to 3 days. In 2000, 5,715 people were treated with LAAM.[124] Since that time, concerns have been raised about the safety of LAAM. Hence, the federal government has added restrictions to its use.[125]

Heroin addicts treated with methadone prefer LAAM to methadone. LAAM produces fewer significant withdrawal symptoms than methadone, and LAAM could be an effective alternative for patients who do not benefit from methadone. One study found that individuals taking LAAM are more likely to stay in treatment, have lower arrest rates, and are less likely to use drugs than individuals in methadone maintenance programs.[126] With LAAM, addicts are not locked into a routine of daily treatment, though some addicts could be allergic to it.

Narcotics Anonymous

Modeled on the principles of Alcoholics Anonymous, Narcotics Anonymous (NA) is a self-help group that was formed in 1953. It is designed to help people who are addicted to heroin and medically prescribed narcotics. The number of NA group meetings proliferated from 5 in 1964 to more than 67,000 weekly meetings in 2015.[127] Of its members, 59% are male, 74% are Caucasian, 60% are employed full-time, and the average length of clean time is 8.32 years.[128]

Like Alcoholics Anonymous, NA is based on a 12-step model, but the groups are distinctly different. Some people are members of both groups. One difference between the groups is that to members of NA, the problem is not chemical but, rather, the result of one's behavior. Alcoholics Anonymous deals exclusively with alcohol, whereas NA addresses all drugs including alcohol.

naltrexone A narcotic antagonist that blocks the reinforcing effects of narcotics

buprenorphine A synthetic narcotic used to treat narcotic addiction

levo-alpha-acetylmethadol (LAAM) An experimental drug that prevents narcotic withdrawal symptoms for about three days

Summary

Opium and its derivatives are painkilling, sleep-inducing drugs. Narcotic use increased dramatically in the United States in the 1800s because of the Civil War, immigration of Chinese workers, invention of the hypodermic needle, inclusion of opiates in patent medicines, and their easy accessibility. By the end of the 19th century, the typical opiate user was White, middle-class, middle-aged, and female. In 1914, federal legislation made nonmedical use of narcotics illegal which resulted in the typical user to change to young, lower class males. By the 1960s, the cost of heroin escalated, and its purity went down. In the 1970s, narcotic abuse declined. The trend has changed since the 1980s, and the availability and purity of heroin have increased. In 2014, deaths from heroin overdoses rose sixfold compared to 2001. Today, the typical heroin user is a White male, although female use is on the rise.

Not all users become dependent. Some people are chippers—occasional users who can control their use. During the Vietnam War, thousands of service personnel smoked opium, and nearly all ceased using opium after they returned to the United States.

The term narcotic is used by law enforcement personnel to refer to an illegal drug. Opiates and opioids are terms used to describe natural or synthetic drugs similar to opium. Morphine, synthesized from opium in the early 1800s, acts more quickly and powerfully and is more toxic. In the late 1800s, heroin was developed as a cure for morphine addiction and other medical maladies. Synthetic opiates produce behavioral effects similar to those of narcotics. They differ in effectiveness, potency, and intensity. One common potent and dangerous synthetic narcotic is fentanyl.

Opiates mimic endorphins in the brain to which users describe the rush from injecting narcotics in glowing terms. Among the many side effects, however, are vomiting, drowsiness, contraction of the pupils, and constipation. Some users claim to feel less psychic distress, although they still have difficulty relating to others. Physical problems that often accompany association with people in the drug trade arise from drug impurities, unsterile needles, and a generally unhealthy lifestyle. One of the most serious concerns resulting from the injection of drugs is contracting HIV infection, which leads to AIDS.

Although drugs can lead to physical dependency, people have little chance of developing dependency from using a drug just once. Some people become dependent as a means of dealing with distress, rage, and psychic pain.

One reason for addicts not seeking treatment is the fear of withdrawal, characterized by insomnia, diarrhea, irritability, and aches and pains. Withdrawal symptoms have been compared to having a "bad flu" and are generally not as bad as the media portrays them to be.

Despite their drawbacks, narcotics have medical uses. They are effective analgesics, especially for continuous dull pain. Also, they stop diarrhea and suppress coughing.

Treating narcotic addiction has not been especially successful. Recidivism is high. The first step in treatment is detoxification. Ridding the body of narcotics is relatively easy, but the desire to continue drug use remains intense. Narcotic antagonists such as naloxone, naltrexone, buprenorphine, nalorphine, and cyclazocine block the reinforcing effects of narcotics. These drugs work best when coupled with behavioral therapy.

Methadone is the drug most often used to treat narcotic addiction. It blocks the effects of heroin for up to 24 hours. The effectiveness of methadone is questioned, though, because many patients are addicted to drugs other than narcotics and methadone does not block the effects of other drugs. During treatment, addicts are offered social, vocational, and psychological support. Methadone programs are criticized because one addicting drug is replaced by another addicting drug. Moreover, these programs do not reach the root of addiction.

A support group is Narcotics Anonymous (NA). NA is modeled after Alcoholics Anonymous, although NA deals with the process of addiction and not the biological impact of addiction.

Thinking Critically

1. Heroin is one of the most effective painkilling drugs available today, yet in the United States, it is not legal for physicians and hospitals to administer it. Do you think that physicians and hospitals should have the right to administer heroin if conditions warrant? Why or why not?

2. Prescription painkillers help people cope with pain. However, people who take prescribed painkillers can become addicted with just on prescription. Do you think policies should be put into place for people who take prescribed painkillers to receive support while on the prescription? Should there be mandatory counseling or checkins while on a prescription painkiller? Justify your answer.

3. NEPs are controversial. Some people think these programs condone drug use. On the other hand, these programs may reduce the spread of HIV. Who should decide if an NEP needs implemented? Should the decision be made by elected officials, healthcare personnel, clergy, or someone else? Do you support NEP programs? Why or why not?

4. Concern has been raised over using methadone as a substitute for heroin, as both are addictive. Methadone given in a clinical setting, however, is pure, and addicts do not have to engage in illegal activity to afford their drugs. Is using drugs as therapy for other drugs a wise practice? If methadone treatment is given, should users be required to attend therapy sessions?

Sedative-Hypnotic Drugs

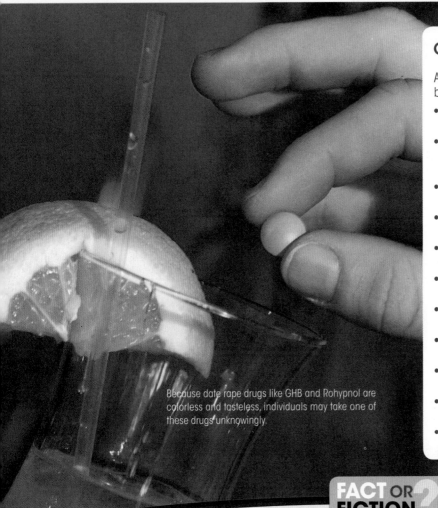

Because date rape drugs like GHB and Rohypnol are colorless and tasteless, individuals may take one of these drugs unknowingly.

Chapter Objectives

After completing this chapter, the reader should be able to:

- Explain the original purposes for which barbiturates were developed
- Contrast between ultrashort-acting, short-acting, intermediate-acting, and long-acting barbiturates
- Discuss the medical applications of barbiturates and their potential side effects
- Define sedative-hypnotic drugs and describe the three main types
- Examine current uses for sedative-hypnotic drugs today
- Summarize the history of methaqualone and dispel the common myths surrounding the drug
- Analyze the medical uses of benzodiazepines and their side effects
- List the various drugs associated with "date rape" and their side effects
- Categorize the classes of inhalants and provide examples for each class
- Describe the extent of inhalant use among adolescents
- List the side effects associated with inhalants

FACT OR FICTION?

1. It is possible to buy prescription drugs through the Internet, although it is illegal to buy them without a prescription.

2. Those who enter treatment for abuse of prescription drugs are better educated than people abusing other types of drugs.

3. Doctors are more likely to prescribe barbiturates for sleep now than they were 20 years ago.

4. The nonmedical use of controlled medications by adolescents is increasing.

5. Withdrawal from barbiturates, while unpleasant, is not life-threatening.

6. People who enter treatment for benzodiazepine abuse are likely to be older than people who enter treatment for abuse of other illegal drugs.

7. When it is used in conjunction with alcohol, the effects of Rohypnol can be fatal.

8. The most common cause of death from inhalants is respiratory depression.

9. More people die from inhaling air fresheners than from inhaling gasoline.

10. Nitrous oxide has been used as an anesthetic by dentists.

Turn the page to check your answers

Sedative-hypnotic drugs derive their name from the relaxing, calming effect they produce in low doses and their sleep-inducing (soporific), hypnotic effect when taken in high doses. Sedative-hypnotic drugs are central nervous system depressants and slow the body's functions. Some users believe they have a stimulating effect because these people become less inhibited after ingesting them.

The three main types of sedative-hypnotic drugs are barbiturates, nonbarbiturate sedatives, and minor tranquilizers. Side effects of these drugs include nausea, lethargy, vomiting, skin rashes, and upset stomach. Other effects are hangover, fever, blurred vision, facial numbness, impaired judgment, poor motor coordination, and a condition resembling dementia. Women are particularly vulnerable to these drugs and are more likely to overdose on medicine for mental health condition.[1] Antidepressants and benzodiazepines send more women to the emergency department compared to men.[2]

As the dosage increases, so does the likelihood of a fatal overdose. Also, people can become physically and psychologically dependent. Once a person stops using the drug, the withdrawal symptoms can be life-threatening.

Barbiturates

These are a class of drugs that are central nervous system depressants. They can produce effects from mild sedation to total anesthesia. Barbiturates have been prescribed as **anxiolytics**, **hypnotics**, and **anticonvulsants**.

In the early 1860s, Germany's Bayer laboratories developed the first barbiturate, although it was not introduced into general medicine until 1903. This depressant, synthesized from chemicals in urine, was initially called **barbital** (all barbiturates in the United States end with the letters *al*). Originally, barbital was effective for inducing sleep. When barbital was

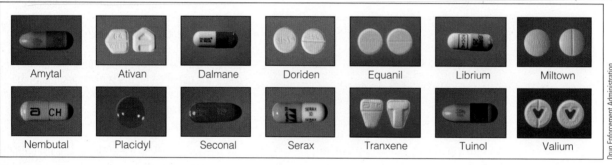

| Amytal | Ativan | Dalmane | Doriden | Equanil | Librium | Miltown |
| Nembutal | Placidyl | Seconal | Serax | Tranxene | Tuinol | Valium |

Depressants come in different shapes and forms.

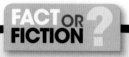

FACT OR FICTION?

1. **FACT** Despite the illegality of buying prescription drugs through the Internet without a prescription, such a practice occurs.

2. **FACT** People who abuse prescription drugs have higher levels of education than people abusing other types of drugs.

3. **FICTION** The fact is—Because sleeping pills interfere with the quality of one's sleep, doctors are less likely to prescribe them today.

4. **FACT** The annual rate of adolescents misusing or abusing controlled medications such as painkillers and stimulants has nearly doubled in the last 15 years.

5. **FICTION** The fact is—Without medical supervision, withdrawal from barbiturates can be life-threatening.

6. **FACT** The average age for admission to treatment for benzodiazepine abuse is 37 compared with 34 for other illegal drugs. People admitted for treatment for benzodiazepines are older than people admitted into treatment for other illegal drugs.

7. **FACT** The effects of the depressant action of Rohypnol increase when used with alcohol.

8. **FICTION** The fact is—The most common cause of death from inhalants is sudden cardiac arrest.

9. **FICTION** The fact is—One study showed that gasoline accounted for more fatalities than air fresheners.

10. **FACT** Nitrous oxide has been given to dental patients as an anesthetic, although its use has declined in recent years.

introduced in 1903, its brand name was **Veronal**. A second barbiturate, **phenobarbital**, was marketed for medical use in 1912. It produced relaxation and relief from anxiety.

Barbiturate use has been declining since 2006, with around 3% of 12th graders, 3% of college students, and 3% of young adults reporting using the drug in 2015.[3] Results from the National Survey on Drug Use and Health (2015) estimates around 0.2% of the population aged 12 and older misuse sedatives.[4]

Types of Barbiturates

Based on their potency and the length of time they act, barbiturates are classified as ultra-short-acting, short-acting (less than 4 hours), intermediate-acting (4 to 6 hours), or long-acting (more than 6 hours). Short-acting barbiturates require less time to take effect than long-acting barbiturates, and their effects do not last as long. Because they act more quickly, short-acting barbiturates are more likely than long-acting barbiturates to be abused. Drugs that take effect rapidly have a higher abuse potential than slow-acting drugs. The length of time that barbiturates act depends on dose, differences among users, and method of administration. A list of selected barbiturates is presented in Table 9.1.

Effects of Barbiturates

Like alcohol, barbiturates produce a depressed, mood-altering action on the central nervous system. They also affect activity of the muscle tissue, the heart, and respiration. In a manner similar to the effects of alcohol, barbiturates can cause confusion, shorter attention span, impaired cognitive functioning, inadequate emotional control, slurred speech, poor judgment, hangovers, and intoxication. Activities such as driving an automobile are ill-advised while a person is using barbiturates because reaction time, hand-eye coordination, and energy levels are affected adversely. Hostility and rage commonly surface after taking barbiturates. As with other drugs, the extent to which barbiturates affect users depends on one's state of mind, the setting in which the drug is used, and the individual's previous experiences with the drug.

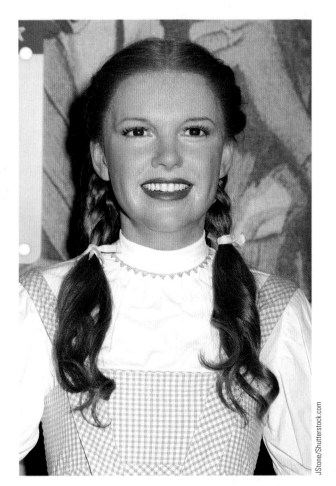

Judy Garland died from a barbiturate overdose.

JStone/Shutterstock.com

Barbiturates sometimes are ingested to ameliorate the effects of amphetamines or to allay the effects of heroin withdrawal. A typical scenario consists of taking amphetamines ("speed") during the day to get charged up ("wired") and barbiturates at night to go to sleep. Actress Judy Garland died from a barbiturate overdose; some say she practiced the habit of using uppers during the day and downers at night.[5] People who take

sedative-hypnotic drugs Class of drugs that produce relaxing to sleep-inducing effects depending on dosage

anxiolytic Also referred to as an antianxiety agent, these are classes of medications that reduce anxiety

hypnotic Also referred to as sleeping pills, these are classes of medications used to induce sleep

Anticonvulsant Also referred to as antiseizure durgs, these are classes of medications used to treat epileptic seizures

barbital A sedative-hypnotic drug used to treat anxiety and nervousness; the original barbiturate

Veronal Brand name for barbital

phenobarbital Second barbiturate developed; produces relaxation and relieves anxiety

TABLE 9.1 Selected Barbiturates

Generic Name	Trade/Brand Name	Type of Barbiturate
pentobarbital sodium	Nembutal	Short-acting
secobarbital	Seconal	Short-acting
talbutal	Lotusate	Short-acting
amobarbital	Amytal	Intermediate-acting
butabarbital	Butisol	Intermediate-acting
phenobarbital	Luminal	Long-acting

barbiturates chronically develop a tolerance to them. Also, people develop a cross-tolerance to chemically similar drugs such as alcohol and minor tranquilizers. If large quantities (800 to 1,000 mg) of barbiturates are taken daily, dependence can result in 4 to 6 weeks.

Potential Hazards

Dangers associated with barbiturates range from fatigue to fatal overdose. Moderate side effects include emotional upset, nausea, vertigo, vomiting, and diarrhea. One study of college students found that those who used sedatives were more likely to experience panic attacks than those who did not use sedatives.[6] Barbiturates can depress breathing, resulting in insufficient oxygen in the blood. Because the heartbeat is depressed, the blood pressure drops. A person can go into shock and fall into a coma or die.

Infants of women who took barbiturates during pregnancy can be born with congenital dependency. As these babies go through withdrawal, they exhibit symptoms similar to those of adults. Barbiturates taken during pregnancy can cause birth defects, brain damage, or death to the fetus because of oxygen deficiency. Studies suggest the risk of fetal abnormalities is approximately 3% if one antiepileptic drug is taken and 17% of two or more antiepileptic drugs are taken.[7] However, women who have epilepsy still need to take a drug to help control the seizures and are advised to work closely with a specialist to help minimize risks.

When taken with other depressants, especially alcohol, barbiturates have a synergistic effect. This may lead to acute toxicity and to death. About 1 in 10 people who overdose on barbiturates or in combination will die.[8] The effects of taking these two drugs together decreases brain activity, which makes it more difficult for the brain to regulate body functions. As a result, the effects of mixing alcohol and barbiturates include:[9]

- Hypothermia
- Respiratory depression
- Lethargy
- Loss of coordination
- Low blood pressure

The brain is not able to handle taking two different depressants drugs and may stop functioning completely. Life-threatening complications can occur, which include hypovolemic shock, respiratory arrest, and coma.[10] Hypovolemic shock occurs when the heart cannot pump enough blood to the body and is considered a medical emergency. Respiratory arrest, the cessation of breathing, is the most common cause of death among people who mix barbiturates and alcohol.[11]

The combination of alcohol and barbiturates can lead to accidental or intentional death. In comparing suicide victims in New York City, those over age 60 were more likely to use barbiturates while younger adults were more likely to use antidepressants.[12] In a similar study, around 2% of overdose suicides in elderly persons were attributed to barbiturates.[13] Another concern is that withdrawal is life-threatening without medical supervision. Withdrawal is marked by profuse sweating, insomnia, muscular twitching, paranoia, vomiting, aches and pains, cramps, quick temper, and, in severe instances, nightmares, hallucinations, and seizures. Possible side effects of barbiturates include the following:

- reduced attention span
- impaired cognitive functioning
- diminished hand-eye coordination
- inadequate emotional control
- nausea
- vomiting
- birth defects
- confusion
- poor judgment
- slurred speech
- vertigo
- diarrhea
- respiratory failure
- violent behavior

Medical Uses

During the 1960s, barbiturates were overprescribed, and thousands of people became dependent on them. Despite the consequences, barbiturates serve several medical functions. They are used primarily as sleeping pills, as well as for certain convulsive disorders and, to a limited extent, for anxiety. The group for whom these drugs are most prescribed is the elderly, although the long-term benefits of these drugs are not well-studied.[14] The percentage of hospitalized older patients who are given sedative-hypnotic drugs to treat insomnia ranges from 31 to 88%.[15] These medicines used to induce sleep for the elderly may not be the best solution as the risk of serious injury, fractures, and dementia are increased.[16] Among children and adolescents, one study in Canada found 66% of physicians prescribed sleep medication for children experiencing sleep disorders.[17] While this medication may be an appropriate treatment method, it is first recommended other behavioral and cognitive therapy be the first line of treatment.[18]

Short-acting barbiturates continue to be used for anesthetic purposes. During surgery, the barbiturate **thiopental (Pentothal)** reduces brain swelling and cerebral pressure and improves blood circulation. In recent years, the number of prescriptions for barbiturates has declined because other drugs are less toxic and less likely to result in dependency.

About one-third of adults report difficulties either falling asleep or staying asleep. The effectiveness of

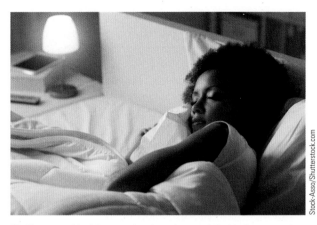

The use of barbiturates for sleep is questionable because they interfere with REM.

barbiturates as sleep agents is questionable, because they interfere with **rapid eye movement (REM)**, which is necessary for a restful sleep.[19] Barbiturates slow brain activity, which prevents people from entering REM sleep.[20] People deprived of REM have difficulty concentrating and can hallucinate. Barbiturate users may experience **rebound insomnia** because one symptom of barbiturate withdrawal is insomnia. People who take sleeping pills often wake up more tired than when they went to sleep. An analogous phenomenon is waking up in the morning after consuming too much alcohol. A person might sleep for hours but wake up exhausted. Therefore barbiturates are counterproductive to sleep over time.

Nonbarbiturate Sedatives

Nonbarbiturate sedatives are depressants that share many of the same characteristics as barbiturates. They increase sedation and sleep while reducing anxiety. Examples of these drugs include chloral hydrate, paraldehyde, bromides, and meprobamate. Except for meprobamate, the history of these drugs dates before the development of barbiturates. Because other drugs are safer than nonbarbiturate sedatives, the latter are rarely used today.

Chloral Hydrate

When used to induce sleep, **chloral hydrate** works rapidly. With a typical dose (1 to 2 g), sleep usually comes in less than an hour, for 8 to 11 hours. Unfortunately, the margin between an effective dose (ED) and a lethal dose (LD) is slight. One study that compared chloral hydrate and music therapy on inducing sleep and sedation in children undergoing EEG testing found that music therapy was a better alternative.[21] In a large study conducted on children aged 6 months to 17 years, the use of chloral hydrate sedation was used to induce sleep to conduct an auditory brainstem response test. The results of this study suggest minimal risk using chloral hydrate when done in the presence of a sedation nurse.[22] Another study was conducted using chloral hydrate sedation on infants undergoing magnetic resonance imaging. This study also determined a relatively low risk of adverse effects using chloral hydrate sedation.[23] However, due to chloral hydrate's risk of hepatoxicity, the American Academy of Pediatrics recommends against its use.[24]

In addition to inducing sleep, chloral hydrate formerly has been given to opiate addicts to enable them to overcome addiction and to alcoholics to help them deal with potentially fatal withdrawal symptoms. Chloral hydrate causes less cardiovascular and respiratory depression than barbiturates at comparable doses. Use of chloral hydrate fell into disfavor because it produces gastric distress, vomiting, and flatulence. Other side effects are unsteadiness, nightmares, and dependency. Chloral hydrate is better known as Mickey Finn or "knockout drops."

Paraldehyde

Paraldehyde has been around for more than 100 years. It is an effective, yet safe, central nervous system depressant. Unlike other depressants, it causes little respiratory depression. In the 1950s, it was given to severely disturbed patients in mental hospitals.

Like chloral hydrate, paraldehyde used to be provided to alcoholics to help manage their withdrawal symptoms. Its biggest drawback was that it produced a terrible smell and taste. Consequently, people who took paraldehyde had extremely bad breath. It is no longer used to treat alcohol withdrawal symptoms.

Paraldehyde is sometimes used to treat seizures in infants and children. This drug is given rectally during seizures that last more than 5 minutes. It has shown to be effective in stopping seizures between 66% and 74% of the time with little risk for respiratory depression.[25]

---

thiopental (Pentothal) A barbiturate that is used as a general anesthetic

rapid eye movement (REM) A stage during sleep that is needed for the sleep to be restful

rebound insomnia A side effect of sleeping pills in which falling asleep becomes more difficult rather than less difficult

chloral hydrate A nonbarbiturate sedative; also called "knockout drops" or Mickey Finns; induces sleep

paraldehyde A nonbarbiturate, sedative-hypnotic drug used with severely disturbed mental patients

Bromides

The discovery of **bromides** dates back to 1826. In the past, bromides were administered to treat schizophrenia and epilepsy. Bromides proved to be unsuccessful. Currently, they are rarely provided as sleep agents, because they build up in the user's body, cause depression, and can be highly toxic. Other side effects include constipation, sedation, violent delirium, mental confusion, headache, dermatitis, psychomotor difficulties, and psychosis.

Meprobamate

Meprobamate was first marketed in 1955 under the brand name **Miltown**. The drug, which is classified as a **minor tranquilizer**, was derived from a muscle relaxant and was one of the first **anxiolytic** drugs used to relieve anxiety. In addition to treating anxiety, meprobamate was prescribed for psychosomatic conditions. One article written in 1957 discussed concerns about the widespread prescribing of meprobamate and other tranquilizers.[26]

The United States clearly was ready for drugs to relieve anxiety because meprobamate was immediately popular. Medical practitioners promptly accepted and prescribed it as a safe alternative to barbiturates. It was given to patients in mental hospitals and was responsible for the release of half of mental patients who were able to lead everyday lives.[27] Sales of Miltown, also known as **Equanil**, exceeded $500,000 in its initial year.

Common side effects include dizziness, agitation, confusion, drowsiness, and fatigue. Some people may experience an allergic reaction the first time they take the drug, which may be life-threatening.[28] Meprobamate is a central nervous system depressant and is metabolized in the liver and excreted though the kidneys. Damage to these organs may occur. Overdose can occur with as little as 12 mg of meprobamate; which has also been used to commit suicide.[29] Blood levels of meprobamate between 1% and 2% are therapeutic, 3 to 10% moderate overdose, and over 20% lethal.[30] Actor and martial arts expert Bruce Lee died from a brain edema (swelling) from an allergic reaction to the painkiller, Equagesic, which contained meprobamate.[31]

It has been reported to cause physical and psychological dependence. At a rate of slightly more than twice the recommended dosage, a person can become physically dependent on meprobamate. Withdrawal from meprobamate is quite severe. Consequently, by 1970, the drug was listed as a controlled substance and the number of refills was regulated. Because of its low margin of safety and the availability of acceptable alternatives, meprobamate is rarely prescribed today.

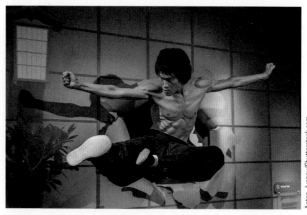

Actor and Martial Arts Expert Bruce Lee died from a drug containing meprobamate.

Methaqualone

In an effort to find a desirable alternative to barbiturates—a drug that can relieve nervous tension and anxiety and promote sleep, yet not produce barbiturate-like hangovers—the pharmaceutical company W. H. Rorer introduced **methaqualone** in 1965. Initially marketed under the brand name **Quaalude**, it also has been called Optimal, Sopor, Parest, Somnafac, and Bi-Phetamine T.

Methaqualone originally was tested in India to treat malaria but was found to be ineffective. Two common street terms for it are "Disco-Biscuits" and "Ludes." During the 1970s, methaqualone gained popularity as a recreational drug and illegal use escalated. Much of the methaqualone bought on the street was manufactured legally but diverted illegally. In the 1970s, they were implicated in numerous high-profile rape cases, including Hollywood director Roman Polanski who was said to have given a 13-year-old girl Quaaludes before having sex with her. He later pleaded guilty to having sex with a minor.[32] More recently, Quaaludes were given media attention when actor/comedian Bill Cosby admitted to giving the drugs to women.[33] They also played a role in the film "The Wolf of Wall Street," which contained several scenes on the recreational/illegal use of Quaaludes.[34]

In 1983, the major manufacturer of methaqualone, Lemmon Pharmaceutical Company, stopped its production. Due to the abuse potential of the drug, Congress banned the production and distribution of the drug in 1984 and placed it in the Schedule I category.[35] It is still produced in some countries and is one of the most widely abused drugs in South Africa.[36]

Misconceptions

Methaqualone had a reputation as an aphrodisiac because of its disinhibiting effect. It was presumed that decreasing inhibition would increase sexual desire.

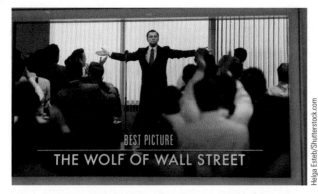

BEST PICTURE
THE WOLF OF WALL STREET

Quaaludes, a popular drug in the 1970s, were prominent in the film "Wolf of Wall Street." After the film aired, Google searches for the word "quaaludes" surged.

Source: E. Bartlett, "Internet searches for 'Quaaludes' drug have gone through the roof since The Wolf of Wall Street", *Metro*, (February 5, 2014). Accessed on March 5, 2017 from http://metro.co.uk/2014/02/05/quaalude-google-searches-spike-the-wolf-of-wall-street-4291908/.

Yet, the drug has no properties that increase the desire to have sex. With a little imagination, nearly any drug can be perceived as an aphrodisiac (just about every drug has been). Methaqualone is no more disinhibiting than alcohol or other central nervous depressants, and it actually interferes with sexual behavior.

When it was approved for medical use, the US Food and Drug Administration (FDA) did not closely monitor methaqualone, because it was thought to be safer than barbiturates and nonaddictive. The FDA was wrong, and the misconception was potentially hazardous. The drug is quite harmful and just as addictive. Withdrawal symptoms, which can be extremely severe, include mania, seizures, vomiting, convulsions, and death. During the 1970s, dozens of people, including the popular musician Jimi Hendrix, overdosed on methaqualone, and thousands were treated in emergency rooms.

Effects

Besides lowering inhibitions, methaqualone induces dreamlike moods at dosage levels of 75 mg. At higher doses, 130 to 300 mg, one might feel anesthetized and fall to sleep—sometimes permanently! Additional effects include the following:

reduced inhibitions	disorientation
diarrhea	drowsiness
menstrual irregularities	headache
depersonalization	pain in extremities
restlessness	anxiety
dry mouth	hangover
paranoia	nosebleeds
anorexia	memory loss

Memory is affected, and this lack of recall may account for some of the accidental overdoses. A person

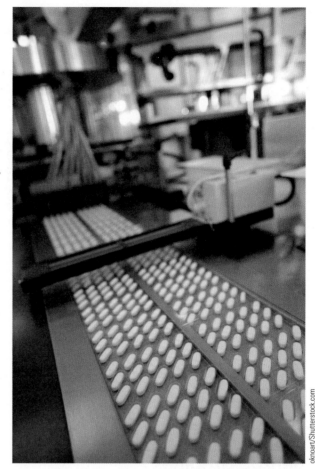

Depressants found on the illicit market are usually legitimately manufactured pharmaceuticals that have been diverted for illegal use.

may not remember taking the drug and, subsequently, ingest more.

In combination with alcohol, methaqualone is especially lethal because these two drugs are synergistic. The number of emergency room visits because of methaqualone overdoses has declined sharply since the late 1970s.

bromides Nonbarbiturate sedatives used to treat epileptic convulsions

meprobamate A minor tranquilizer marketed under the trade names of Miltown and Equanil; also used for treating psychosomatic conditions

Miltown Brand name for meprobamate

minor tranquilizer Drug used primarily to relieve anxiety

anxiolytic Refers to anxiety-reducing drugs

Equanil The first modern drug developed to relieve anxiety

methaqualone A sedative-hypnotic drug that relieves tension and anxiety without barbiturate-like aftereffects

Quaalude Brand name for methaqualone

TABLE 9.2 Medical Uses for Benzodiazepines

Medical Uses	Description
Generalized Anxiety Disorder	Recommendations are for short term treatment not lasting more than a month.
Insomnia	Recommended for short term treatment or an 'as needed' basis
Seizures	First line hospital choice for treating seizures
Alcohol Withdrawal	Most common approach. Helps alcoholics with detoxification and reduces their risk of severe alcohol withdrawal
Panic Attacks	The American Psychiatric Association supports their use for initial treatment of panic disorders. However, the United Kingdom-based National Institute for Health and Care Excellence does not support long use of benzodiazepines for panic disorder

Source: J. Nordqvist, "Benzodiazepines: Uses, side effects, and risks", Reviewed by A. Carter. *Medical News Today,* (August 25, 2016). Accessed on January 16, 2017 from http://www.medicalnewstoday.com/articles/262809.php.

Minor Tranquilizers

Minor tranquilizers were first developed in the 1950s, but the most popular type, called **benzodiazepines**, was not developed until the early 1960s. Also known as anxiolytics, these drugs are used primarily to treat anxiety although they are also effective as anticonvulsant drugs. Today, most users are women, because they are more likely than men to be diagnosed with anxiety disorders. An unfortunate consequence is that anxiety can promote the abuse of mind-altering substances such as minor tranquilizers, alcohol, and other prescribed medications.

Benzodiazepines

Despite their decline in popularity, benzodiazepines are one of the most commonly used drugs in Western societies.[37] Besides reducing anxiety, these minor tranquilizers induce sleep, reduce panic attacks and epilepsy, and control petit mal seizures. See Table 9.2 for medical uses. In the 1950s, they were used in place of barbiturates for treating anxiety and sleep disorders. They are effective as antianxiety and sleep aids on a short-term basis only.

When first developed, these drugs were not thought to cause physical dependency (except in rare instances), withdrawal symptoms, or fatal overdoses. However, benzodiazepines are addictive and produce tolerance and withdrawal symptoms comparable to those for alcohol and barbiturates. Between 15% and 44% of long-term users become dependent on them.[38] One concern is that substance abusers who are given benzodiazepines for a medical problem may become dependent on these drugs.[39]

Taking benzodiazepines at levels higher than recommended causes withdrawal symptoms to appear within a few days after abstinence, and symptoms can occur within 6 months after daily use. These symptoms include anxiety, muscle tension, and insomnia. Ironically, benzodiazepines are taken to reduce anxiety and improve sleep.

Despite their potential harm, benzodiazepines have a wider margin of safety, fewer side effects, and less severe side effects than barbiturates. When taken with barbiturates or alcohol, however, the risk of a fatal overdose increases. Benzodiazepines have been a factor in a number of suicides. A list of commonly prescribed benzodiazepines and their purposes is provided in Table 9.3.

TABLE 9.3 Selected Benzodiazepines

Generic Name	Brand Name	Medical Purpose
alprazolam	Xanax	Panic and anxiety disorders. Most prescribed benzodiazepine in the U.S.
chlordiazepoxide	Librium	Management of alcohol withdrawal syndrome
clorazepate	Tranxene	Hypnotic, sedative used to treat severe anxiety and anxiety disorders
diazepam	Valium	Anxiolytic, sedative, hypnotic, and anticonvulsant with rapid onset. Used to treat panic attacks, insomnia, seizures, restless leg syndrome, and alcohol withdrawal.
flurazepam	Dalmane	Sedative, anxiolytic drug used to treat mild to moderate insomnia
oxazepam	Serax	Used to treat insomnia, anxiety, and control alcohol withdrawal symptoms.
triazolam	Halcion, Apo-Triazo, Hypam, and Trilam	Used as a sedative to treat severe insomnia

Source: J. Nordqvist, "Benzodiazepines: Uses, side effects, and risks", Reviewed by A. Carter. *Medical News Today,* (August 25, 2016). Accessed on January 16, 2017 from http://www.medicalnewstoday.com/articles/262809.php.

Effects of Benzodiazepines[40]

Short-term Effects

Low to Moderate Doses

- Impaired motor control
- Drowsiness, lethargy, fatigue
- Impaired thinking and memory
- Confusion
- Depression
- Altered vision
- Slurred speech
- Vertigo
- Respiratory depression
- Nausea

High Doses

- Slowed reflexes
- Mood swings
- Hostile and erratic behavior
- euphoria

Long-term Effects

- Impaired thinking, memory, and judgment
- Disorientation
- Confusion
- Slurred speech
- Muscle weakness, lack of coordination

Because benzodiazepines have muscle-relaxing properties, they are prescribed for backache, muscle strain, multiple sclerosis, and Parkinson's disease. Benzodiazepines are given to veterans suffering from posttraumatic stress disorder (PTSD) with nearly 30% receiving benzodiazepines.[41] The US Department of Veteran Affairs cautions against the use of benzodiazepines for the treatment of primary symptoms associated with PTSD, as their use has not been shown effective in treating those symptoms.[42] Furthermore, in a recent study regarding women with PTSD, it was discovered that women have a different sensitivity to GABA-A receptor active substances, which results in less effectiveness of benzodiazepines as a sleeping agent.[43]

Although the number of prescriptions for these drugs has declined, their abuse is one of the most serious forms of drug abuse in the elderly population, especially among women. The elderly are at greater risk with for benzodiazepine poisoning due to their impaired metabolism and increased sensitively to benzodiazepines.[44] Furthermore, they are the most frequently ingested drug in self-poisoning among the elderly.[45] In a large cohort study looking at the long term use of benzodiazepines among the elderly, it was discovered that among those who were long-term users of benzodiazepines, they reported lower life satisfaction and more sleep difficulties. Additionally,

those who used benzodiazepines intermittently or chronically reported higher levels of anxiety.[45] Benzodiazepines use in the elderly has been associated with a greater risk of falls and injury among that population.[46] A large cohort-based study found that benzodiazepine use among elderly who had a total hip replacement experienced less positive outcomes compared to those who were not on benzodiazepines.[47] Dialysis patients taking benzodiazepines also experience a higher mortality rate.[48]

Research on the psychological effects of benzodiazepines is inconsistent. Some research has found that they cause rage, hostility, and aggression, but other research points to a decrease in aggression among users. Benzodiazepines interfere with men's ability to attain an erection and achieve orgasm. Women experience less vaginal secretion, although they can be sexually aroused.

The fetus is affected by the mother's use of these drugs. Some children of women who took **Valium (diazepam)** in the first 3 months of pregnancy were more likely to have cleft palates, though subsequent studies contradict this finding. Within hours after delivery, withdrawal symptoms appeared in infants whose mothers used recommended, normal levels of Valium during the first trimester. Some studies have not found the same results and it is recommended that women speak to their doctor regarding benzodiazepine use during pregnancy.[49] Other studies have found women who took benzodiazepines during pregnancy had higher risks of preterm delivery and low birth weight infants.[50]

Similar to fetal alcohol syndrome, some women who took Valium while pregnant had children with **fetal benzodiazepine syndrome**, a condition marked by tremors, a malformed and expressionless face, learning disabilities, poor muscle tone, delayed hand-eye coordination and mental development, hyperactivity, and irritability. The validity of this condition is questioned because many women who take these drugs while pregnant may also be consuming other drugs.

Halcion (triazolam) is another benzodiazepine prescribed for sleep. It is a highly controversial drug because it reportedly produces a number of distressing side

---

benzodiazepines A type of minor tranquilizer; examples are Librium and Valium

Valium (diazepam) A minor tranquilizer

fetal benzodiazepine syndrome A condition of infants caused by the mother's use of benzodiazepine during pregnancy; affected children have malformed face, poor muscle tone, tremors, poor coordination, delayed mental development, and learning disabilities

Halcion A drug used to induce sleep

Ambien, a sleep aid used to replace Halcion, was promoted as less addictive and less likely to leave users feeling groggy after use. Users hailed this drug as the cure for jet lag and it soon became the best-selling sleeping aid in America.

This drug has been implicated in weird behavior that was done in what was later called a sleep trance. Users reported to making phone calls, raiding hotel minibars, shopping online, and answering emails to which later they had no recollection of doing. In a class-action lawsuit by Ambien users, they complained of sleep eating while under the drug's influence. Testimony included examples of clients eating buttered cigarettes and raw eggs while in an Ambien induced sleep.

Later, the drug gained notoriety when Rhode Island Representative Patrick Kennedy crashed into a Capital Hill barrier and blamed Ambien for his car crash. He was later charged with driving under the influence of a prescription drug and served one year probation.

Questions to Ponder:

What is the responsibility of the sleep aid drug makers for impaired behavior? Even if the side effects are listed on the prescription, do you think users or the drug makers are responsible for accidents that may result from the use of their drug?

Source: K. Falkenberg, "While you were sleeping", *Marie Claire*, (September 27, 2012). Accessed on January 16, 2017 from http://www.marieclaire.com/culture/news/a7302/while-you-were-sleeping/.

effects. Writer William Styron described how Halcion exacerbated his depression and how he contemplated suicide while taking the drug.[51] Others report similar experiences. Many people have filed lawsuits against its manufacturer, Upjohn Pharmaceuticals, claiming it caused adverse reactions. There have been reports that people on Halcion and similar drugs have eaten, made telephone calls, and driven while asleep.[52]

Because Halcion interferes with memory, it can lead to accidental overdose. The ability to recall previously learned information is not affected adversely, but learning new information is temporarily more difficult. Other effects include nausea, paradoxical excitement, constipation, and dizziness. Because minor tranquilizers can cause confusion, ataxia (a lack of coordination), and fatigue lasting 1 to 3 hours, operating motor vehicles, using power tools, or running marathons while taking the drug is not advised. Halcion and other sedative-hypnotic drugs increase the risks of accidents because they produce a "hangover" effect after their use.[53] The FDA continues to allow Halcion to be prescribed, although it has been banned in more than a dozen countries.

"Date Rape" Drugs

Rohypnol

A powerful drug related to Valium is **Rohypnol**. Also known as "roofies," "rope," and "roche," Rohypnol (flunitrazepam) has been used in Europe since the 1970s. It acts as a muscle relaxant and at high doses can cause lack of muscle control and a loss of consciousness.[56] It gained a reputation as a "date rape" drug because women have been unknowingly given this colorless, odorless, tasteless drug (usually in alcohol) and then raped. It leaves its victims disinhibited, helpless, and vulnerable. In efforts to help women avoid unwitting ingestion, coasters have been developed to detect drinks spiked with Rohypnol, and three Scottish students have developed a drinking straw that detects date rape drugs like Rohypnol.[55]

Rohypnol is 5 to 10 times more powerful than Valium. On the college campus, Rohypnol sometimes is added to punch during parties. The effects of Rohypnol are greatly enhanced and more dangerous in combination with alcohol. This mixture can cause sedation, muscle relaxation, blackouts, addiction, complete memory loss, and even death. Many Rohypnol users experience amnesia, respiratory depression or arrest, and discoordination, and they have a higher rate of automobile accidents.

The drug takes effect 20 to 30 minutes after ingestion, and the effects last for 2 to 10 hours, depending on the dosage.[57] When one stops using Rohypnol, dependency and withdrawal symptoms include headache, anxiety, muscle pain, confusion, irritability, hallucinations, delirium, convulsions, shock, and even death. Rohypnol is inexpensive and readily available. Two common misconceptions about Rohypnol are that (a) it cannot be detected by urine testing and (b) it is free of adulterants because it comes in sealed packages.

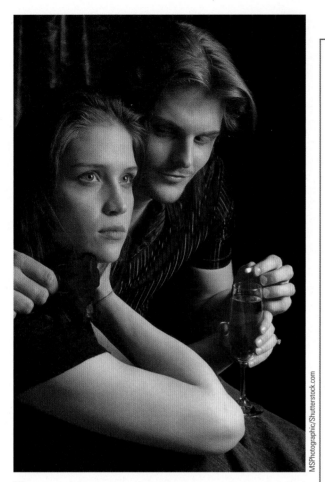

Rohypnol gained the reputation of being a "date rate drug." Drugs are slipped into a victim's drink. Because they are odorless, colorless, and tasteless, detection is difficult.

ON CAMPUS

In a survey done on 6,000 students at three universities, results show nearly 8% of those surveyed said they experienced having their drinks spiked with drugs. Women and men have different perspectives regarding date rape drugs on college campuses. Women believe the motivations behind spiking one's drink to be rape and sexual assault while men believe it is merely just to have fun.

While most agree that sexual assault and rape are crimes of serious nature, some do not believe that slipping a drug in someone's drink as the same type of crime.

Questions to Ponder:

Even if the intent is not rape or sexual assault, do you think slipping a drug in someone's drink is just as serious of a crime as sexual assault? Why or why not?

Source: P. Asinyanbi, "Date rape drugs are a major problem on U.S. college campuses; 80% of victims are women", *Inquisitr*, (May 25, 2016). Accessed on January 16, 2017 from http://www.inquisitr.com/3131341/date-rape-drugs-are-a-major-problem-on-u-s-college-campuses-80-of-victims-are-women/.

Physicians in the United States had been prescribing Rohypnol for insomnia, but in 1996, the federal government passed legislation banning its legal use. Because of its sedative-hypnotic effect, Rohypnol is legally prescribed in 60 countries around the world. As a result, Rohypnol is accessible for illegal use in the United States. Rohypnol, as well as Valium and other prescription drugs, is transported legally across the Mexican border and then illegally diverted.

Currently, Rohypnol is classified as a schedule IV drug.[58] However, penalties related to Rohypnol are the same as those of a schedule I drug.[59] Anyone using Rohypnol or other controlled substances for the purpose of facilitating a crime of violence, including rape, can be sentenced to up to 20 years in prison.

Gamma-Hydroxybutyrate

Another drug referred to as a "date rape" drug is **gamma-hydroxybutyrate**, or **GHB**. Nicknames for GHB include Easy Lay, Grievous Bodily Harm, Gook, and Gamma 10. Like Rohypnol, GHB is odorless, tasteless, and easy to produce. The use of GHB has grown, especially in western states.

GHB has a reputation as an aphrodisiac because it is believed to enhance the sense of touch and sexual prowess. One study reported that 18% of users took GHB to enhance sex while 13% took it to be sociable and another 13% took the drug to alter their consciousness.[60] GHB does cause aphrodisiac effects

Rohypnol A powerful depressant; one of the "date rape" drugs

gamma-hydroxybutyrate (GHB) A type of neurotransmitter that produces relaxation and sleepiness; one of the "date rape" drugs

Andrew Luster, great grandson to cosmetic giant Max Factor was charged with 86 counts related to using a date rape drug on three women and videotaping sex acts. He gave the victims the date rape drug GHB and raped them while they were unconscious at his beachfront home.

Initially sentenced for 124 years, it was later dropped to 50 years with the possibility of parole after 15 years. The judge said 48 years of the sentence was for the sexual assaults and 2 years was for the drug related charges.

Sources:

D. Dimond, "Max Factor heir Andrew Luster: My lawyer made my do it", The Daily Beast, (February 9, 2013). Accessed on January 16, 2017 from http://www.thedailybeast.com/articles/2013/02/09/max-factor-heir-andrew-luster-my-lawyer-made-me-do-it.html.

R. Winton, "Max Factor heir's rape sentence reduced from 124 years to 50" , Los Angeles Times, (April 16, 2013). Accessed on January 16, 2017 from http://articles.latimes.com/2013/apr/16/local/la-me-ln-luster-gets-50-years-20130416.

R. Hernandez, "Andrew Luster gets shorter sentence, change at parole in rape case", Ventura County Star, (April 16, 2013). Accessed on January 16, 2017 from http://www.thedailybeast.com/articles/2013/02/09/max-factor-heir-andrew-luster-my-lawyer-made-me-do-it.html.

in men. In an older study, it was shown that GHB provided disinhibition, heightened sense of touch, enhancement of male erective capacity, and increased orgasm.[61] However, a study years later found that men who consumed GHB experienced difficulty in maintaining stimulated and achieving orgasm.[62] In a 9-year study in the Netherlands, it was reported that nearly one-half of attendees at rave parties who needed first-aid care used GHB in combination with either ecstasy, alcohol, and/or marijuana. Of that number, 22% required medical attention.[63] GHB use (and other club drugs) are not uncommon among gay and bisexual men. Patterns of drug use suggest the use of these drugs to be situational as they are taken at bars, dance clubs, and raves and do not follow a pattern of a substance abuse disorder.[64] However, use of these drugs among bisexual and gay men situationally has been linked with high risk sexual behavior.[65] Some bodybuilders use GHB illicitly as a growth hormone stimulant and/or an anabolic steroid. Both of these are myths as there is no evidence to suggest GHB has any muscle-building effects.[66]

Medically, GHB has been shown to be useful in opiate detoxification. It has been used experimentally to treat narcolepsy. In addition, it has been hypothesized that GHB may be helpful for treating alcohol dependence.[67]

GHB has the potential to be deadly, because it causes the respiratory system to shut down. When GHB is mixed with alcohol, the person may lose memory and consciousness. Other effects are vomiting, nausea, seizures, hallucinations, coma, and respiratory distress. When GHB is combined with alcohol and other central nervous system depressants, the potential for death escalates. Tel Aviv University researchers have developed a sensor to detect the presence of GHB or ketamines in drinks.[68]

Ketamine

Ketamine was developed in 1962 for use in general anesthetics.[69] It was approved for use on humans in 1970 and was considered the battlefield anaesthetic.[70] It is considered a dissociative anesthetic and does not produce a loss of consciousness. Among illicit users of the drug, it has been known to cause hallucinations and produce illusions. It is also commonly used at veterinary clinics.[71] Slang terms for this drug include

CULTURAL Considerations

Chemsex

Chemsex is a term used to describe engaging in sexual activity while under the influence of drugs. The most popular drugs for chemsex include GHB, methamphetamine, and mephedrone. This behavior has increasingly become more popular in London and New York city among men who have sex with men. In a survey in London of more than 1,000 men, almost 20% reported participating in chemsex at some point over the past 5 years.

Risks for chemsex include overdose, becoming physically and psychologically dependent, and engaging in risky sexual behavior.

Source: B. Guarino, "The 'chemsex' scene: An increasingly popular and somethings lethal public-health problem", The Washington Post, May 10, 2016. Accessed on January 17, 2017 from https://www.washingtonpost.com/news/morning-mix/wp/2016/05/10/the-chemsex-scene-an-increasingly-popular-and-occasionally-lethal-public-health-problem/?utm_term=.905b35bb7d65.

Special K, Vitamin K, Super K, Ketaset, Super Acid, and Special LA coke.

Ketamine produces a quick high that lasts about an hour. Users report to feeling "out of their body" and may experience hallucinations.[72] Other side effects include disorientation, drowsiness, increased heart rate, and elevated blood pressure. Due to the anesthetic effects of ketamine, users may injure themselves while on the drug and not realize it, thus compounding the injury.[73] It is currently a Schedule III nonnarcotic substance.

Inhalants

Inhalants are volatile substances that are used to create a mind-altering effect. Inhalant abuse, also called "huffing," was noted during World War I. Compared with many other drugs of abuse, inhalants receive little attention by researchers. Therefore in-depth knowledge about inhalants is limited. The lack of research regarding inhalants could reflect the fact that many inhalant abusers are not in treatment. Studying inhalants is important, because they serve as **gateway drugs**. Also, inhalant abusers are more likely to abuse additional drugs.

Among adolescents aged 12 and 13, inhalants are the most frequently used class of illegal drugs. In 2015, the National Survey on Drug Use and Health included felt-tip pens and computer keyboard cleaners on the list of inhalants. Thus data collected from 2015 are not compared to previous years.[74] Results from this survey suggest approximately 0.2% of the population aged 12 and older were current inhalant users. This drug is most common among adolescents aged 12 to 17.[75] The popularity of inhalants with teens is attributed to their low cost, availability, and size. (Because inhalants come in small packages, they are easily concealed.)

There is a strong relationship between inhalant use and other problem behaviors and sensation-seeking.[76] One study found that young inhalant users were more likely to engage in individual and group fighting.[77] This study also found those with attitudes of lenient parents, friends, and self-attitudes toward substance use were more likely to use inhalants.[78]

Although many inhalants have anesthetic-like properties, they are not considered sedative-hypnotic drugs. Inhalants are classified by how they are used rather than by their effects on the central nervous system. Inhalants are grouped into four classes: volatile solvents, aerosols, gases, and nitrites.[80] Inhalants such as gasoline, paint thinners, plastic cement, Magic Markers, cleaning supplies, glue, and nail-polish remover have no known medical use.

Indications of Inhalant Abuse[81]

- Chemical odors on breath or clothes
- Paint or other stains on face, hands, or clothes
- Hidden empty stray paint or solvent containers
- Chemical soaked rags or clothing
- Drunk or disoriented appearance
- Slurred speech
- Nausea or loss of appetite
- Inattentiveness, lack of coordination, irritability, and depression

Short-term effects include drooling, nausea, sneezing, hypersensitivity, loss of coordination, and coughing. Long-term effects include frequent nosebleeds; liver and kidney damage; sores around the mouth, throat, and nose; weight loss; depression, irritability, and disorientation; paranoia; hostility; and bone marrow abnormalities. Inhalants adversely affect cognitive qualities such as memory and learning.[82] Abuse of solvents is strongly related to antisocial disorders. Moreover, while under the influence of inhalants, users are more likely to engage in more high-risk behaviors.[83] Gasoline sniffing by children is a prominent factor in lead poisoning, which adversely affects physical and mental growth.

Volatile Solvents

These are liquids that vaporize at room temperature. Examples include paint thinners, dry-cleaning fluids, degreasers, gasoline, glues, correction fluid, and felt tip markers.[84] Glue and other solvents are squeezed into paper bags, handkerchiefs, or rags, placed over the nose, and inhaled. The psychoactive agent in glue is **toluene**, which is found in unleaded gasoline and in the glue used for building model airplanes.

Glue sniffing was given scant attention until the 1960s, at which time reports of glue sniffing appeared in newspapers throughout the United States. By warning readers of the dangers of sniffing glue, newspaper articles turned an obscure problem into a major problem. The number of teens inhaling glue increased greatly.

Inhalants are considered gateway drugs. Among inner-city Chicago youths, those who used inhalants by age 16 were much more likely to use heroin than those who used inhalants at a later age.[86] Inhalants often are the first drug abused by children, especially those in poor or rural areas. Some individuals continue to use inhalants as long as 15 years.

> **gateway drugs** Substances that are used before use of more dangerous drugs; alcohol, marijuana, tobacco, and inhalants are considered gateway drugs
>
> **toluene** The psychoactive agent in glue

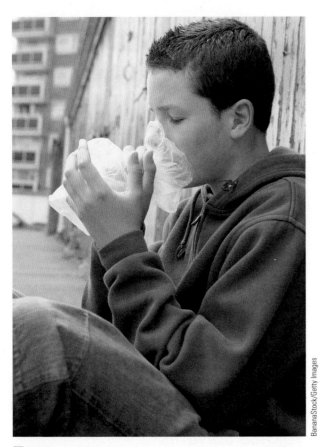

Sniffing an inhalant-soaked rag from a bag is a form of "huffing."

Inhalant users describe the effects as a hazy euphoria, comparable to alcohol intoxication. Some users have violent outbursts, delusions, double vision, disinhibition, ringing in the ears, speech impairment, hallucinations, muscle weakness, disorientation, vomiting, and nausea. These effects are temporary and disappear following exposure to air. A more serious physical threat is immediate cardiorespiratory arrest. Also, solvent sniffing can lead to physical and emotional damage resulting from the lead found in glue and gasoline.

The use of volatile solvents is a district class of abused drugs. One study discovered that 35% of subjects who admitted using volatile solvents met the DSM-IV criteria for substance use disorder, while 28% met the criteria for dependence.[86] Research also suggests volatile solvents can produce addiction pathology similar to cocaine or opiates.[87]

Abuse can lead to major cognitive impairment. Studies have shown chronic users have impaired short-term memory, attention, response inhibition, and problem solving skills. This may be attributed to the loss of white matter in the brain, especially in the frontal and temporal lobes.[88] The use of solvents has been implicated in kidney damage, respiratory system depression, irregularities in the heart (cardiac arrhythmias), and possibly liver damage. Another concern about solvent inhalation is brain damage.

Solvent users can develop anemia and bone marrow damage. Seizures can result from inhaling solvents, and the user may die from heart failure or suffocation. Because inhalants are put into bags and sniffed, the user can pass out and accidentally suffocate.

Aerosols

Aerosols are the most common inhalants in the home. This class of inhalants includes spray paints, deodorant, hair sprays, vegetable oil sprays, and fabric protector sprays.

Gases

This class of inhalants include medical aesthetics and household and commercial gases. **Ether** was marketed commercially in the 18th century as an industrial solvent and an anesthetic. Although the purpose of ether was to eliminate pain during surgery, it was an attractive alternative to alcohol, because it produced intoxication and was less expensive than alcohol. Upper-class Europeans and Americans were the first to use the drug recreationally, but individuals in lower socioeconomic classes soon followed.

Nitrous oxide, a colorless gas with a sweet taste and odor, was discovered by Joseph Priestly and synthesized by Humphrey Davy. A Connecticut dentist, Horace Wells, noted the anesthetic properties of nitrous oxide and incorporated it into his dental practice. When it was given for the first time during surgery, it was considered a dismal failure, because the person to whom the gas was given woke up during the operation and screamed in agony. Despite this early setback, nitrous oxide found its way into medicine. One person who experimented with nitrous oxide was psychologist William James, who contended that it altered his consciousness and that he experienced mystic revelations.

Anesthetic gases render pharmacological effects similar to barbiturates. They provide sedation, pain relief, anxiety relief, and sleep. If people use nitrous oxide in conjunction with alcohol, they receive no greater analgesic effect from this combination. If a patient is given nitrous oxide during surgery, an adequate supply of oxygen is necessary because the decreased oxygen level in the blood can cause irreparable brain damage, a condition called **hypoxia**. Nonmedical use of nitrous oxide (and other inhalants) can lead to hypoxia.

Women given nitrous oxide during childbirth report feeling less anxious during labor.[89] Although nitrous oxide is given to women during labor in Europe, Australia, and Canada, very few hospitals in the United States provide nitrous oxide during labor.

A popular source for nitrous oxide is whippets, small cartridges designed for whipped cream containers. The immediate effects of inhaling nitrous oxide are euphoria, hallucinations, giddiness, and reduced inhibitions. These effects contributed to its nickname, "laughing gas." Also, nitrous oxide impairs cognitive and psychomotor performance. It interferes with memory and concentration. Nitrous oxide may cause death.

Nitrite Inhalants

The final classification of inhalants, the nitrite group, is used for both medical and nonmedical purposes. The three types of nitrites are **amyl nitrite**, **butyl nitrite**, and **isobutyl**. The benefits of nitrites were established more than 150 years ago. In the mid-1800s, amyl nitrite was used as a vasodilator; it relaxed the muscles in the walls of the blood vessels. Subsequently, the drug was used to relieve angina pectoris and to treat congestive heart failure. Also, amyl nitrite is given as an antidote for cyanide poisoning. When inhaled, amyl nitrite alters consciousness and intensifies the sexual experience.

Originally, amyl nitrite came in mesh-enclosed glass ampules called "pearls." As the glass ampules were crushed by the fingers, they emitted a popping sound—hence the nickname "poppers." Nitrites increase intracranial pressure by dilating cerebral blood vessels, producing euphoria.

Like amyl nitrite, butyl nitrite and isobutyl nitrite dilate the blood vessels, but they are not used therapeutically. Butyl nitrite is found in many commercial products such as perfume and antifreeze.

The popularity of inhaling nitrites for sexual purposes—heightened libido, aphrodisiac properties, and prevention of premature ejaculation—escalated in the mid-1970s. At one time, sales of nonprescription nitrites totaled $50 million. One group noted for its use of nitrites is gay males, although use by this group has declined.

Despite the claims of improved sexual performance, no research indicates that nitrites have any direct effect on sexual ability. Since the 1960s amyl nitrites have been popular among men who have sex with men. They use this drug in order to relax the sphincter to achieve enhanced sexual intercourse.[90]

A real danger, however, is that brief exposure to nitrites at moderate dosages suppresses the immune system. Therefore they have been linked to HIV and AIDS.

Side effects of nitrites include pounding headache, nausea, feelings of warmth, drop in blood pressure, throbbing sensations, rapid pulse, and sometimes loss of consciousness. Additional effects are blurred vision, eye irritation, and eye pressure. Crusty lesions may appear where the skin comes into contact with butyl nitrite, suggesting a possible allergic reaction. These lesions can form on the nose, lip, scrotum, and penis. Because nitrites are flammable and explosive, burns are another potential hazard. The tradenames of products containing nitrites, which typically are found in adult bookstores, head shops, and mail-order catalogs, include the following:

Aroma of Men	Heart On
Ban Apple Gas	High Ball
Bang	Jac Aroma
Bolt	Liquid Increase
Bullet	Locker Room
Climax	Mama Poppers
Crypt Tonight	Oz
Cum	RUSH
Discorama	Satan's Scent
Hardware	Toilet Water

ether An inhalant dating back to the late 1700s

nitrous oxide An inhalant also known as laughing gas

hypoxia A lack of oxygen within body tissues; hypoxia can lead to brain damage resulting from an inadequate supply of oxygen to the brain

amyl nitrite An inhalant used to treat angina pectoris and congestive heart failure

butyl nitrite An inhalant no longer used for medical purposes but found in products such as perfume and antifreeze

isobutyl One type of nitrite that is used to treat angina pain; also causes vasodilation, flushing, and warmth

Summary

Just as their name suggests, sedative-hypnotic drugs produce relaxation, and sometimes sleep, depending on the dosage. The three classes of sedative-hypnotic drugs are barbiturates, nonbarbiturate sedatives, and minor tranquilizers. Side effects associated with sedative-hypnotic drugs include nausea, lethargy, vomiting, upset stomach, blurred vision, hangover, fever, and impaired judgment. These drugs can cause physical dependency and severe withdrawal symptoms. The margin of safety between an effective dose and lethal dose is minimal.

Date rate drugs are generally sedative-hypnotic drugs that are given to people before raping them. Two well-known date rape drugs are Rohypnol and GHB. GHB has been implicated in an increasing number of fatalities. These drugs leaves users feeling disinhibited, helpless, and vulnerable and may cause short-term memory problems.

Inhalants with sedative-hypnotic properties are classified as volatile solvents, aerosols, gases, and nitrites. Teenagers, the primary users of inhalants, take them

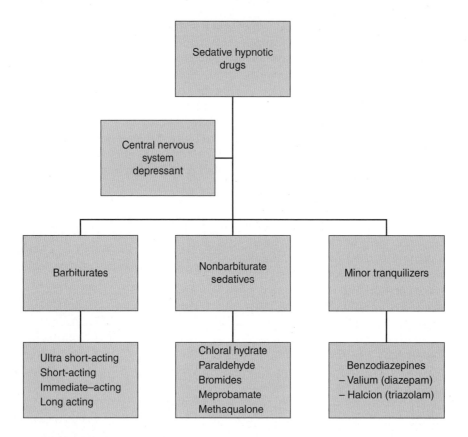

because they are easy to obtain and conceal, work quickly, and are relatively inexpensive. Glue is considered a gateway drug for teenage boys, although an increasing number of girls have begun abusing inhalants. Its effects last about 45 minutes and include intoxication, hallucinations, violent outbursts, seizures, and even cardiorespiratory arrest. Solvents can produce irregular heartbeat, respiratory system depression, anemia, kidney damage, seizures, and death. Some cases of lead poisoning in children have been attributed to solvents.

Two examples of gases inhalants are ether and nitrous oxide. At one time, people used ether as an inexpensive substitute for alcohol. Nitrous oxide eventually found its way into medicine. If it is used during surgery, it is necessary to provide adequate oxygen or patients will suffer from hypoxia. Nitrous oxide also interferes with memory and concentration.

The three types of nitrites are amyl nitrite, butyl nitrite, and isobutyl nitrite. They dilate blood vessels and relax the muscles. Amyl nitrite is available only by prescription. The most common use of nitrites—especially in the 1970s—has been to intensify sexual experiences. Research, however, has not supported this effect. Nitrites can affect the immune system and are linked to HIV. Other effects of nitrites include eye irritation and lesions on the nose, lip, and genitalia.

Thinking Critically

1. Barbiturates are prescribed for people who have difficulty falling asleep. Given that these prescriptions interfere with REM sleep, create an argument for their continued use.

2. A prescribed drug for sleep is Halcion. In one case, a woman taking Halcion killed her mother and blamed the drug and its manufacturer. She was acquitted. Do you think a bad reaction to a prescribed drug is a reasonable defense? Should a person be acquitted for a crime committed while under the influence of a prescribed drug?

3. Adolescents gather information regarding inhalants use from media outlets. Thus, when inhalants are presented in the media, use tends to go up. What are the advantages and disadvantages of newspapers and magazines publishing articles about drugs?

4. Date rape drugs are slipped into a person's drink unknowingly. Do you think bars/bartenders have a responsibility to protect their customers? Should they offer coasters or straws that detect the presence of the drug? If you were developing policy to minimize the risk of a drink being tampered with, what would you include in your policy?

Chapter Objectives

After completing this chapter, the reader should be able to:

- Construct a definition for mental disorder
- Examine special populations at risk for mental disorders
- Elaborate on the connection between mental disorders and substance abuse
- Contrast between psychosis and neurosis
- List the various types of mood disorders
- Identify the risk factors that are faced by ethnic and cultural minorities regarding mental illness
- Compare and contrast the various types of antidepressants
- Elaborate on the conditions for which lithium is most effective
- Judge the effectiveness of antipsychotic drugs
- Explain the dangers associated with abusing and/or mixing psychotherapeutic drugs

Almost 10% of Americans suffer from depression. Antidepressants are generally effective for many people with mild to moderate forms of depression.

TZIDO SUN/Shutterstock.com

FACT OR FICTION?

1. Most people with a mental illness seek professional help for their illness.

2. People with mental disorders are violence and unpredictable.

3. One side effect associated with antidepressants is weight gain.

4. Half of all mental disorders begin to show symptoms during childhood.

5. Personality weaknesses cause mental disorders.

6. In America, ethnic and racial minorities often face cultural and social stressors that may pose greater risk factors for mental illness.

7. A person can never get better from a mental disorder.

8. People with mental disorders are just as productive at work compared to people without mental disorders.

9. Although the number of children in the United States taking antipsychotic drugs has increased, the number of children in other countries taking these drugs has decreased.

Turn the page to check your answers

About one in four adults suffer from mental illness at some point in their lives.[1] Pinpointing precise factors that contribute to the emotional adversities people face is difficult. Mental illness is not caused by one single event but is linked to multiple causes. Possible causes range from childrearing practices, to heredity, to biochemical imbalances, and to our fast-paced and get-ahead-at-any-cost mentality. The DSM-5 (*Diagnostic and Statistical Manual of Mental Disorders, Fifth Edition*) offers the following as a definition:

> A mental disorder is a major disturbance in an individual's thinking, feelings, or behavior that reflects a problem in mental function. Mental disorders cause distress or disability in social, work, or family activities.[2]

Half of all mental conditions begin at age 14, although the normal personality changes associated with adolescence can mimic a mental health condition.[3] Serious mental illnesses include major depression, schizophrenia, bipolar disorder, obsessive compulsive disorder (OCD), panic disorder, post-traumatic stress disorder (PTSD), and borderline personality disorder.[4]

In this chapter, we will examine the concept of mental illness and the drugs used to treat its various forms.

Understanding Mental Illness

In a literal sense, one could say that **mental illness** means an illness of the mind. In this sense, mental illness would be the result of a brain disease or a biochemical imbalance. The famous US physician Benjamin Rush, who lived two centuries ago, speculated that mental illness arises from problems with the blood vessels in the brain. Mental illness, however, involves much more than anatomical structures and hormones. That being said, mental illness implies inappropriate thinking and behavior as well. The word *inappropriate* is subject to individual interpretation. Even if we agree that a person's behavior or thinking may exceed a socially acceptable range, who is to determine what is appropriate? Even the American Psychiatric Association states the difference between what is considered normal and abnormal is often unclear.[5]

Expected responses to stressors are not considered a mental disorder. For example, feeling depressed after a loved one's death is an expected reaction. Additionally, feelings such as anxiety, fearfulness, and anger are normal emotions. However, a mental disorder is characterized as such when it causes prolonged distress in a person's ability to cope with daily life.[6]

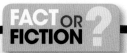

1. **FICTION** The fact is—It is estimated that only about 10% of people with mental illness seek professional help.

2. **FICTION** The fact is—People with a mental disorder are no more likely to be violent compared with people without a mental disorder.

3. **FACT** Weight gain is a common side effect associated with antidepressants.

4. **FACT** Half of all mental disorders begin to show first signs before a person turns 14 years old.

5. **FICTION** Fact is—Many factors contribute to mental disorders including biological factors, life experiences, and family history of mental disorders.

6. **FACT** Negative stressors cause mistrust of mental health services and often prevent minorities from seeking treatment.

7. **FICTION** The fact is—some depression and anxiety disorders only require a person to take medication for a short period of time.

8. **FACT** Studies done found employers who hired people with a mental disorder report good attendance, job motivation, and quality of work.

9. **FICTION** The fact is—The rate of children receiving antipsychotic drugs has more than doubled in some European countries.

Mental disorders are identified through a variety of **symptoms** exhibited by a person. Mental health professionals use guidelines highlighted in the American Psychiatric Associations' guidebook DSM-V to assist in diagnosing mental **disorders**.

Mental Illness and Medicine

Identifying people as mentally ill frequently is left to the judgment of medical personnel, who view illness, regardless of whether it is physical or mental, from a **disease** perspective. This implies that illness results from a **pathogen**—suggesting that mental illness is a disease that has symptoms and a cure. This approach involving symptoms, diagnosis, and cure is the basis for the **medical model**.

The application of the medical model to emotional problems gives rise to some concern. For one thing, behaviors deemed inappropriate or unacceptable might not be the result of any given disease. Many people have difficulties adjusting to the stresses and problems of life. Should they be labeled mentally ill?

One critic of the medical model is psychiatrist Thomas Szasz, who says that the concept of mental illness is a myth.[7] He argues that most people identified as mentally ill do not have any type of disease. If mental illness is a myth, as Szasz contends, should drugs be administered to individuals to regulate their behaviors? The use of drugs in treating mental illness dates back many centuries, although drugs used in the past and present to treat mental illness do not *cure* it. Instead, drugs treat symptoms related to mental illness and moderate people's behavior.

Mental Illness and Special Populations

No group of people is immune to the possibility of mental illness. In America, ethnic and racial minorities often face cultural and social stressors that may

TABLE 10.1 Levels of Mental Illness in Percentages by Demographic Variables 2015

Demographic Variable	Percentage of Any Type of Mental Illness
Male	14.3
Female	21.2
White	19.3
Black or African American	15.4
American Indian or Alaska Native	21.2
Asian	12
Hispanic or Latino	14.5

Source: Substance Abuse and Mental Health Services Administration, "National Survey on Drug Use and Health", 2015.
Accessed on January 22, 2017 from https://www.samhsa.gov/data/population-data-nsduh.

pose greater risk factors for mental illness including racism, discrimination, violence, and poverty. People of low socioeconomic status are more likely than those of higher strata to suffer from a mental illness.[8] Living with racism and discrimination is stressful and negatively affects mental health. These negative stressors cause mistrust of mental health services and often prevent minorities from seeking treatment. Additionally, culture often determines what type of mental health care if any is sought by minorities. See Table 10.1 regarding percentages of mental illness by demographic variables.

One specific group, sexual minorities, or those who identify as lesbian, gay, or bisexual, have a high risk of mental illness compared to those who identify as heterosexual.[10] Those who identify as lesbian, gay, bisexual, transgender, or queer (LGBTQ) are at least two times more likely to have a mental health condition. Additionally, youth who identify as LGBTQ are two to three times more likely to attempt suicide compared to heterosexual youth.[11] Issues faced by these multicultural communities include less access to treatment, less likely to receive treatment, poorer quality of care, and higher levels of stigma. To highlight this point, one survey discovered that 11% of transgender individuals reported being

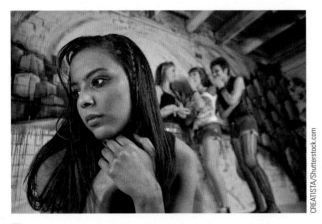

Living with discrimination is a risk factor for mental illness.

CREATISTA/Shutterstock.com

mental illness A disturbance in thinking and/or feelings which impact a person's ability to function

Symptoms An observable or stated behavior

Disorder Applied to a collection of symptoms

Disease Applied when the underlying pathology is known and idenfied

pathogen Any organism that produces disease

medical model The premise that a pathogen is responsible for a person's illness or disease

denied care by mental health clinics due to bias or discrimination.[12]

Adolescents appear to be at risk for experiencing a mental disorder with rates increasing and a larger number of children and adolescents requiring pharmacological, psychotherapeutic treatments, educational interventions, and a variety of other special services.[13] Worldwide, the prevalence rate for youth and adolescents suffering from a mental illness is estimated to be 13.4%.[14] Furthermore, the lifetime prevalence of any mental illness among Americans aged 13 to 18 years old is 46%.[15]

Mental Disorders and Substance Abuse

A relationship exists between mental disorders and substance use and abuse. The term **dual diagnosis** is used to describe someone who experiences both a mental illness and a substance abuse disorder.[16] A person with depression make take illicit drugs to alleviate the symptoms or a person who has a substance abuse disorder may develop a mental disorder due to a change in the person's moods, thoughts, brain chemistry, or behavior.[17]

Roughly one-third of people experiencing a mental illness and half of all people with a severe mental illness also experience substance abuse.[18, 19] Risk factors for the development of these disorders include being male, coming from a lower socioeconomic status, and being a military veteran. Certain drugs of abuse are most common with specific mental health disorders.

Alcoholism is associated with antisocial personality disorder. People with antisocial personality disorder disregard social norms and laws and act in a manner that places themselves before others.[20] Sometimes referred to as sociopathic personality disorder, people with this disorder have a lack of empathy for others, feel comfortable breaking the law, often lie, exploit others, and may harm animals. Estimates reveal that those who drink to excess on a regular basis are 21 times more likely to deal with antisocial personality disorder.[21] A study in India was conducted on males who were seeking treatment for alcoholism. This study found that among those seeking treatment for alcoholism 15% of them presented with antisocial personality disorder.[22] Another study found a positive relationship among college students who practice heavy episodic drinking and antisocial personality disorders.[23]

Other comorbid conditions associated with alcoholism are bulimia, depression, and anxiety. Those diagnosed with bulimia, an eating disorder characterized by binge eating and purging behaviors, have higher rates of alcoholism compared to those who do not have bulimia.[24] That National Institute on

TABLE 10.2 Major Psychiatric Disorders

Psychiatric Disorder	Increased Risk for Substance Abuse
Antisocial personality disorder	15.5%
Manic episode	14.5
Schizophrenia	10.1
Panic disorder	4.3
Major depressive episode	4.1
Obsessive-compulsive disorder	3.4
Phobias	2.4

Alcohol Abuse and Alcoholism estimates that around 10 to 30% of alcoholics have panic disorder and 20% of persons with an anxiety disorder abuse alcohol.[25] It has been suggested that symptoms of depression are likely to develop during the course of alcoholism and will disappear once withdrawal from alcohol is complete (from a few days to a few weeks).[26]

A dual diagnosis needs to be treated from two perspectives. Treatment should include specific inventions for both the substance abuse disorder and the mental illness.[27] Unfortunately, many mental health and substance abuse treatment services do not have sufficient resources to adequately deal with a dual diagnosis. One study sampled a little over 250 programs across the United States and found only 18% of addiction treatment centers and 9% of mental health programs met the criteria for dual-diagnosis capable services.[28] Table 10.2, based on a National Institute of Mental Health study, lists seven major psychiatric disorders and shows how much each one increases an individual's risk for substance abuse.

Types of Disorders
Neurosis
Emotional problems range from anxiety to psychosis. Anxiety and worry are common, normal experiences. When they become disproportionate and interfere with daily life, however, problems arise. When discomfort turns to panic, skepticism turns to fear, and concern turns to unrealistic worry, the person has to deal with these barriers to everyday functioning. Anxiety of this magnitude is often referred to as **neurosis**. In other words, the anxiety has become a

Dual Diagnosis A term to describe when a person has a substance abuse problem and a mental illness simultaneously

neurosis A long-term disorder featuring the symptoms of anxiety and/or exaggerated behavior dedicated to avoiding anxious feelings

With the introduction of the Affordable Care Act (ACA) and expanded access to health care, the hope was to reduce ethnic/racial disparities for mental health and substance abuse treatment. While Whites have benefited from the ACA, racial/ethnic minorities continue to access mental health and substance abuse treatment at significantly lower rates.

A study was conducted to determine the outcome of ACA on racial/ethnic minorities to gather information on disparities for mental health and substance abuse services. Historically, underrepresented groups have lagged behind in access and utilization of mental health and substance abuse services.

This study suggests that although there have been increases in mental health treatment, there has been no improvement in racial/ethnic disparities for mental health and substance abuse treatment. Compared to pre-ACA years, Whites received significantly more mental health services post ACA. Other than those who identified as Hispanic, none of the other racial/ethnic minorities groups received significantly more care after ACA was enacted and there has been no change in racial/ethnic disparities.

Additionally, for all racial/ethnic groups, treatment rates for substance abuse treatment remain very low. Drug and alcohol treatments rates did not increase after the ACA took effect.

Among those who could have benefited from mental health and substance abuse treatment but didn't receive it, the following barriers were stated as causes:

- Cost of care
- No insurance
- Inadequate insurance

Source: T.B. Creedon, and B. Le Cook, "Access to mental health care increased but not for substance use, while disparities remain", *Health Affairs*, 35, no.6 (2016): 1017–1021.

long-term disorder featuring the symptoms of anxiety and/or exaggerated behavior dedicated to avoiding anxious feelings. Sufferers understand that the condition is abnormal. Obsessive-compulsive behaviors, psychosomatic ailments, phobias, and panic attacks are examples. Anxiety typically is treated with anti-anxiety drugs. (A review of antianxiety drugs is included in Chapter 9.)

Psychosis

A **psychosis** is a condition in which the person loses contact with reality. Psychoses are divided into two categories: organic and functional. "Organic" refers to physical causes. Some causes of organic psychoses are excessive use of drugs such as cocaine and alcohol, brain infections, metabolic or endocrine disorders, brain tumors, and neurological diseases.

Functional psychoses are those that have no known or apparent cause. One type is **schizophrenia**. This term, which literally means "split mind," is a misnomer because a schizophrenic does not have two or more personalities. Three symptoms mark schizophrenia: delusions, hallucinations, and a restricted range of emotions.

An estimated 1% of the population are schizophrenic, with women and men being affected about equally. Although heredity is a major factor, schizophrenia may arise from an interaction of environ-ment and heredity. These factors include exposure to viruses, malnutrition before birth, problems during birth, and psychosocial factors.[29] Some scientists believe problems in the development of the brain before birth may lead to faulty connections, which during puberty, could trigger psychotic symptoms.[30] Parents, social factors, nutrition, and environmental chemicals may play a role. Years of alcohol abuse also can lead to schizophrenia-like psychosis.

Mood Disorders

Mood disorders are typified by **depression** at one extreme and **mania** at the other. An estimated 9.5% of adults in the United States have a mood disorder with almost 50% of them being considered severe.[31] See Table 10.3. Women are 50% more likely than

psychosis A severe mental condition marked by loss of contact with reality

schizophrenia A type of functional psychosis; literally, "split mind"

mood disorders Forms of psychosis that affect the person's emotions; can be depression or mania

depression Dejection characterized by withdrawal or lack of response to stimulation

mania A mood disorder characterized by inappropriate elation, an irrepressible mood, and extreme cheerfulness

TABLE 10.3 Common Mood Disorders

Mood Disorder	Primary Symptoms	Prevalence	Possible Cause(s)	Treatment(s)
Major Depression	Persistent extreme sadness and negative emotion; lack of energy; loss of interest in enjoyment of life, sleep disturbances; possible suicide risk.	About 15% of the general population will experience major depression. Estimates of lifetime risk are as high as 25% for some segments of the population (women and college educated persons).	Genetic vulnerability, environmental stress; association with low levels of certain neurotransmitters (serotonin, norepinephrine, and dopamine); hormone imbalances (postpartum depression); negative attributional style.	Drug therapy (antidepressants); cognitive therapy; transmagnetic cranial stimulation; electro-convulsive shock therapy (for extreme cases only); inpatient treatment.
Seasonal Affective Disorder (SAD)	Symptoms same as major depression but occur only in autumn and winter.	About 3% of the general population will suffer from SAD.	Lack of adequate light appears to have an effect on neurotransmitter levels.	Light therapy—extended exposure to bright therapeutic lights on a regular basis.
Dysthymia	Mild but chronic version of major depression.	3% of the general population suffer from dysthymia.	Same as major depression; co-morbidity is common.	Cognitive therapy; antidepressant medication.
Bipolar Illness: Type 1 (mania and depression); Type 2 (low grade mania and depression)	Swings of emotional state from highly energetic and agitated ("manic") to extremely sad and hopeless (depressed).	1% of the general population suffer from some form of bipolar disorder.	Strong, consistent evidence of genetic basis; stress may contribute to onset of symptoms; imbalance of neurotransmitters and brain malformations.	Drug therapy is mandatory (anti-convulsants; antidepressants and antipsychotics are all used); electroconvulsive therapy; supportive psychotherapy and psycho-educational support for patient and family.

Source: Mayo Clinic, "Anti Depressants: Selecting One That's Right for You." Retrieved November 9, 2011 from http://www.mayoclinic.com

men to experience a mood disorder, while Whites are 40% more likely than Blacks and 20% more likely than Hispanics to suffer from mood disorders.[32]

Depression is highly correlated with substance abuse.[33] Similarly, alcohol use and depression are strongly linked. Although alcohol use and depression are associated, it is conceivable that this is because alcohol is used to deal with one's depression.[34] Men

with alcohol dependence had rates of depression three times higher compared to the general population, while alcohol-dependent women were four times as likely to suffer from depression.[35] It is not always clear whether the substance use or the depression came first. Depression can cause substance abuse, but substance abuse also can lead to depression. Women often develop the mood disorder first with addiction following while men develop the addiction first with the mood disorder following.[36]

The prevalence of mental illness among adolescents aged 12 to 17 was 12.5% in 2015.[37] Some 30% of teenagers will suffer from teen depression prior to adulthood. At any one time, between 10% and 15% of teens will have symptoms of teen depression, while 5% will suffer from major depression. While 5.3% of the general population has suffered from a depression lasting for at least one year, the percentage of teenagers who have suffered from a year-long depression is 8.3%. Approximately 20% of teens will experience depression before adulthood with 10 to 15% of teens experiencing some symptoms of depression at any given time.[38] Around 30% of depressed teens also develop a substance abuse problem.[39] About 2% of teens suffer the mild but long-lasting depression

Signs and symptoms of depression

known as **dysthymia,** and 15% of teens suffer from bipolar disorder.[40] Teen depression affects both genders, and all types of backgrounds, but teenage girls seem to suffer from depression more frequently than teenage boys, which may be attributed to the hormonal changes that accompany puberty and issues related to body issues.[41,42] Depression in adolescents has been shown to be associated with family history of depression and experience with a traumatic event.[43] Another group affected by depression is postpartum women. The American Psychological Association reports that up to one in seven women will experience postpartum depression.[44] Risk factors include previous experience with depression or mental illness, having a challenging baby, having a special needs baby, first time motherhood, other emotional stressors, financial or employment problems, and a lack of social support.[45]

Besides adolescents and birthing mothers, the elderly are increasingly susceptible to depression. Risk factors for depression among the elderly are lower concentrations of folate in the blood and nervous system, mental impairment, and dementia.[46] Depression among the elderly is associated with increased thoughts of suicide, especially among those confined to a nursing home.[47]

Researchers have found a relationship between smoking and depression, especially among young female smokers.[48] Depressed people may smoke as a form of self-medication. The relationship between smoking and depression is bidirectional. One study found an association between smoking and depression at all ages. However, this study also found that during the adolescence stage, smoking predicted depression later in life and depression predicted smoking.[49] Confirming these claims, researchers conducted a large literature review and found that in half the studies reviewed, depression was associated with later smoking, and in almost one-third of the studies reviewed, smoking behavior was associated with later depression/anxiety.[50]

Women experience twice the rate of depression as men, regardless of race or ethnic background. An estimated one in eight women will contend with a major depression in their lifetime,[51] but men have higher rates of substance abuse disorders and antisocial personality disorder.[52] Between 20% and 40% of women experience premenstrual syndrome with almost 5% of women experiencing symptoms severe enough to be classified as Premenstrual Dysphoric Disorder (PMDD).[53] Symptoms of PMDD include depression that begins a week prior to menstruation and ends within the first few days of menstruation. Clinical depression affects more than 19 million Americans each year. It is a real illness that can be treated effectively. Unfortunately, fewer than half of the people who have this illness seek treatment.[54]

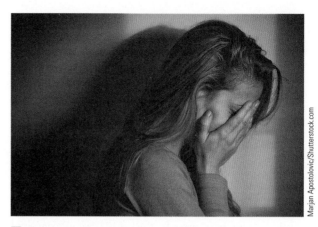

Depression is more common among women.

Some people alternate between mania and depression. This is called **bipolar affective disorder** and it affects almost 2% of the population.[55] Other people have only mania or depression. About 10% of people develop **unipolar depression**, the most common form.[56] Approximately 15% of depressed individuals commit suicide.[57]

Bipolar affective disorder, formerly called manic depression, is marked by alternating periods of mania, depression, and normalcy. It is estimated that one in five patients with depression have bipolar disorder.[58] It is estimated that almost 70% of people with bipolar disorder are misdiagnosed with major depressive disorder.[59] Bipolar disorder affects men and women equally. It usually starts between ages 15 and 25. The exact cause is unknown, but it occurs more often in those who have relatives with bipolar disorder, with some studies showing the heritability of bipolar disorder as twice as high as major depressive disorder.[60]

Some individuals with substance abuse problems are misdiagnosed with bipolar illness.[61] A factor contributing to misdiagnosis is that some people who experience a manic episode have hallucinations or delusions. However, it should be noted that even though drug use may cause such symptoms, bipolar affective disorder cannot be ruled out. Drug abuse may be in some cases a symptom of bipolar disorder. Mania, which can arise suddenly and last for days or months, is characterized by inappropriate elation, an irrepressible mood, and extreme cheerfulness and enthusiasm. A frequent problem among people with

dysthymia Mild, but long-lasting depression

bipolar affective disorder A mental condition characterized by alternating moods of depression and mania; formerly called manic-depression

unipolar depression A mental disorder marked by alternating periods of depression and normalcy

bipolar disorder is noncompliance with medications. One study found that more than 60% do not always take medications as prescribed.[62]

Treatment of Mental Illness Before 1950

Before 1950, remedies for mental illness were crude, unscientific, and even cruel. Mentally ill people were subjected to bloodletting, were given sneezing powder, were flogged and starved, and had hot irons applied to their bodies. In the 1840s, manic patients were treated with cannabis (marijuana) because it brought about euphoria. This treatment was stopped because its benefits were found to be only temporary. In the 1930s, schizophrenic patients were administered insulin to put them into a coma. Insulin treatment might have been effective at first, but subsequent studies indicated a high relapse rate.

Psychoanalysis grew in popularity starting with Sigmund Freud. Today, it is seldom used to treat patients with mental problems.

Eventually, scientists such as Kraepelin, Pinel, and Esquirol devised a classification system of mental illnesses. Drugs such as amphetamines were used with depressed patients and inhaled carbon dioxide and antihistamines were given to patients having other classifications. Some patients received barbiturates and other depressants and slept for a week or more. **Electroconvulsive therapy (ECT)**, first developed in 1938, was used to treat depression and psychosis. Before ECT is administered, the patient is sedated and given a muscle relaxant. ECT involves attaching electrodes to the patient's head and delivering electrical impulses to the brain. Electrical activity in the brain is temporarily interrupted and a seizure within the brain is triggered, generally lasting less than 1 minute.[63] A typical course of treatment is about three times a week until the patient's depressive symptoms improve (6 to 12 weeks).[64] After much apprehension regarding the effects of ECT, it is making a comeback in the treatment of depression.

ECT has raised several concerns, especially in regards to its effects on memory and cognition. In the past, many patients receiving ECT experienced adverse cognitive effects.[65] Significant memory loss was not an uncommon effect. Recent research suggests memory problems were associated more with bilateral ECT in which electrodes are placed on both sides of the head.[66] Conversely, in unilateral ECT, the electrodes are placed on the right side of the brain (opposite from the learning and memory areas), and has been found to be less likely to cause memory problems.[67]

Demographics of Drugs and Mental Disorders

Between 10% and 15% of the general population receive drugs for emotional problems each year. Forty-three percent of all people with mental disorders reside in the United States and Europe.[68] One in three Americans—over 75 million people—will suffer from a mental disorder in any given year. Use of antidepressant drugs has soared nearly 400% since 1988, making the medication the most frequently prescribed therapeutic drug from physician office visits.[69]

Some people are more likely than others to receive medication. Older people are more likely to be prescribed drugs for emotional disorders. Higher levels of medication use also correlate with more education, living by oneself, and higher income. Also, women are twice as likely as men to use prescribed drugs for mental disorders.

Mood Stabilizers

Antidepressants

Depression is a primary factor in thousands of suicides each year. Among US adolescents, suicide is the third leading cause of death.[70] Yet, treating depression is complicated because almost everyone becomes depressed at some time or another—some for understandable reasons. Distinguishing between a temporary period of depression or a situational depression and depression as an emotional disorder requiring medical intervention is difficult. Moreover, determining which depressed individuals will respond to antidepressant medications poses a challenge. Table 10.5 provides a summary of antidepressant medications.

In the past, stimulants were used to treat depression. Depression now is treated with five major classes of drugs—monoamine oxidase inhibitors (MAOIs), tricyclic antidepressants, selective serotonin reuptake inhibitors (SSRIs), serotonin and norepinephrine reuptake inhibitors (SNRIs), and atypical antidepressants that do not fall into one of the above categories.[71]

Although these drugs are effective, some people get discouraged because these drugs sometimes require several weeks to take effect. One study analyzed

psychoanalysis A form of talk therapy based on Freudian principles

electroconvulsive therapy (ECT) Controlled administration of electric shock as a treatment for mental illness

seven therapeutic intervention and found all of them had significant impact in treating depression. The therapeutic interventions analyzed included: interpersonal therapy, behavioral therapy, cognitive-behavioral therapy, problem-solving therapy, socials skills training, psychodynamic therapy, and supportive counseling.[72] One study found that counseling was as effective for treating mild to moderate depression, although a combination of counseling *and* antidepressants appeared to work best.[73]

Monoamine Oxidase Inhibitors

Monoamine oxidase (MAO) is an enzyme found on the outer membranes of subcellular particles known as mitochondria. MAO renders inactive neurotransmitters serotonin, dopamine, and norepinephrine. As antidepressants, MAOIs block the action of monoamine oxidase.

The antidepressant properties of MAOIs were discovered accidentally. First introduced in the 1950s, they were used to treat tuberculosis patients who, on receiving the MAOI **iproniazid**, became energetic. Subsequently, this drug was used with depressed patients even though it proved to be too toxic for treating tuberculosis. The use of iproniazid as an antidepressant was stopped after it was linked to the deaths of 54 people.

The four principal MAOIs currently utilized in the United States are tranylcypromine (Parnate), phenelize (Nardil), isocarboxazid (Marplan), and selegiline (**Emsam**). These medications cannot be combined with SSRIs.

MAOIs are effective only in depressed patients who have high levels of MAO activity. Overall, they have a low efficacy rate.

After patients begin to use MAOIs, 2 weeks or more must pass before the drug relieves the symptoms of depression. MAOIs are not the antidepressant of choice. They are given to patients who remain depressed after being given a minimum of two tricyclic drugs. They work best in patients whose depression becomes more acute as the day progresses (in contrast to many depressed people who feel worse in the morning and improve during the day).

People exhibiting neurotic conditions such as acute anxiety, obsessive-compulsive behavior, and phobias respond positively to MAOIs.[74] Also, individuals who have panic attacks respond better to the MAOI phenelzine than to the tricyclic antidepressant drug imipramine. Rhenelzine also has been used with people who become depressed following romantic rejection—heartbreak. They tend to oversleep, overeat, and have an unstable mood as a result of being rejected.

ON CAMPUS

In a recent literature review conducted by scientist regarding depression and college students, it suggests about one in eight college students suffer from depression. Consistent with other research on depression, more college women suffered from depression compared to college men. Additionally, those students who identified as being a racial/ethnic minority, suffered from depression at higher rates compared to those who identified as White.[1] Another study found that 85% of college students suffering from depression did not receive any type of treatment.[2] Depression can impact student performance and substance use and abuse.

Questions to Ponder

Given that almost 40% 18- to 24-year-olds are enrolled in college, should more resources be provided to private and public higher educational institutions to address the role of depression on campus? How would you go about address depression on college campuses?

Sources:

1. M.A. Whisman, and E.D. Richardson, "Normative data on the Beck Depression Inventory-Second Edition (BDI-II) in College Students", *Journal of Clinical Psychology*, 71, no.9 (2015): 898–907.

2. American College Health Association, "American College Health Association-National College Health Assessment II: Reference Group Summary Spring 2014". (2014).

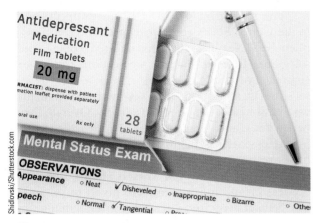

There are many different types of antidepressant drugs that are effective for treating depression.

Another group for which MAOIs seem to work are depressed elderly patients. Elderly patients who cannot tolerate some of the side effects of tricyclics respond favorably to MAOIs.

Side effects of MAOIs include fatigue, dizziness, dry mouth, and drowsiness. Impotence and ejaculatory problems have been reported in men, and some women have difficulty achieving orgasm. A significant and potentially serious side effect of MAOIs is low blood pressure (hypotension). The opposite effect, however, can occur when MAOIs are taken simultaneously with tricyclic drugs, psychostimulants, and L-dopa. This extremely high blood pressure can lead to fever, bleeding in the brain, headaches, and possibly death. Also, dangerous levels of hypertension occur when MAOIs interact with foods containing **tyramine**, an amino acid. The interaction of MAOIs and tyramine produces nausea, a stinging headache, vomiting, palpitations, internal bleeding, skin flush, and death.

One drawback to MAOIs is the strict dietary regimen that patients must follow. People using MAOIs absolutely must avoid foods that contain tyramine.[75] A rise in blood pressure results from the interaction of MAOIs and tyramine, causing the release of catecholamines. This action produces **sympathomimetic effects**, including elevated blood pressure. After a person stops taking MAOIs, the body can take 2 weeks to readjust. Besides high and low blood pressure, other toxic effects include hallucinations, high fever, agitation, and convulsions. Foods rich in tyramine include the following:

aged cheeses	sauerkraut
blue cheese	concentrated yeast extracts
old cheddar	sausage
mozzarella	pickled herring brine
Parmesan	Chinese foods
Swiss	beer and ale
Chianti wine	

MAOIs are dangerous, too, because they interact with certain medications, especially dextromethorphan, found in over-the-counter cough medications, and Demerol. MAOIs are potentially fatal if the individual is taking other antidepressants that affect serotonin, such as Prozac. The recommendation is to wait at least 5 weeks after stopping Prozac before taking MAOIs.

Despite their limitations, MAOIs have some advantages. They do not cause tolerance, psychological dependence, or withdrawal symptoms after their use is discontinued. They are not likely to be abused because they have little effect on people who are not depressed.

Tricyclic Antidepressants

The term *tricyclic* is derived from the chemical structure of **tricyclic antidepressants**, which are shaped like three-ringed compounds. First introduced in the 1950s, these drugs were originally used with psychotic patients, and it was noted that they had an antidepressant effect. They are effective, but have generally been replaced by antidepressants that cause fewer side effects. Other antidepressants are prescribed more often, but tricyclic antidepressants are still a good option for some people. They work by affecting the levels of norepinephrine and serotonin in the brain.[76] In certain cases, they relieve depression when other treatments have failed.[77]

Amitriptyline (Elavil) is used for depression accompanied by agitation. Imipramine (Tofranil) is given for depression involving psychomotor retardation, as well as for agoraphobia, panic attacks, and obsessive-compulsive behavior. Clomipramine (Anafranil) also has been used to treat obsessive-compulsive behaviors.

Tricyclics are superior to MAOIs. The antidepressant action of tricyclics, however, takes 3 to 4 weeks to attain a therapeutic level.[78] These drugs

monoamine oxidase (MAO) An enzyme that deaminates monoamines oxidatively and that functions in the nervous system by breaking down monoamine neurotransmitters

iproniazid A monoamine oxidase inhibitor

Emasam The levorotatory form of the monoamine oxidase inhibitor deprenyl.

tyramine An amino acid that interacts with monoamine oxidase inhibitors to cause very high levels of hypertension

sympathomimetic effects An increase of blood to the brain and muscle, allowing the body to flee or fight

tricyclic antidepressants Drugs that effectively remove the symptoms of acute depression

TABLE 10.4 Tricyclic Antidepressants

Generic Name	Brand Names	Type of Depression
imipramine	Tofranil Janimine Presamine SK-Pramine	Psychomatic retardation
amitriptyline	Elavil Endep	Agoraphobia, panic attacks, obsessive-compulsive behavior
clomipramine	Anafranil Aventyl Pamelor	Obsessive-compulsive behavior
desipramine	Norpramin Pertofrane Adapin Sinequan	Anxiety, panic disorder

© Cengage Learning 2014

accumulate in fatty areas of the body such as the brain and lungs, are excreted primarily in the urine, and are metabolized by the liver. Features of common tricyclic antidepressants are outlined in Table 10.4.

Effectiveness

Symptoms of acute depression are effectively removed in most cases in which the proper dosage of tricyclic antidepressants is taken and adequate time is allowed for the drugs to take effect. Imipramine helped to relieve symptoms of depression including insomnia, listlessness, and loss of appetite in 60 to 70% of patients in one study. In general, antidepressant drugs are 60 to 70% effective for treating major depression.[79] The mood and confidence of patients improve and suicidal thoughts are eliminated.

Tricyclics work best with severe unipolar depression. Patients with bipolar depression who are given tricyclics sometimes go from being depressed to being manic. Consequently, these drugs are not recommended for use in bipolar depression.

Tricyclics seem to be successful in treating a number of disorders besides depression. For patients whose primary symptoms are related to phobias, some tricyclic drugs help facilitate behavioral treatment. Tricyclics are also effective in moderating pain.[80] A recent study looked at the use of tricyclics for ADHD in school-age children and found some them to be effective as an alternative treatment for ADHD when other medications have not proven successful.[81] Moreover, they can be beneficial in treatment of the eating disorder bulimia. Because these drugs do not produce euphoria, they are not used for recreational purposes.

Side Effects

Common side effects of tricyclics are distorted vision, **tachycardia**, dry mouth, constipation, sleepiness, and urinary retention. On standing up, the blood pressure can drop significantly. Confusion and disorientation are other typical effects. Less frequent side effects are rashes (especially in the elderly), jaundice, glaucoma, tremors, and impotence. In children, a small risk exists for cardiotoxicity and sudden death.[82] Another side effect is the development of type 2 diabetes, especially when tricyclics are taken with the newer antidepressants.[83] In a rather large study (n=44,715) looking at the categories of antidepressant medication and later development of type 2 diabetes, almost 7% of patients who were on antidepressant medications later developed type 2 diabetes. This was true for all categories of antidepressants, including tricyclics.[84]

When tricyclic antidepressants are used in combination with alcohol, the risk of a deadly reaction increases. An overdose can result in coma, cardiac difficulties, and respiratory problems. Because another concern is suicide, patients who are contemplating suicide should be assessed before tricyclics are prescribed.

Patients frequently experience side effects during the period before antidepressants take effect. Therefore many discontinue taking the medication before it has a chance to act.

If patients cease taking tricyclics abruptly, they demonstrate withdrawal symptoms such as chills, muscle aches, and malaise. Tolerance to tricyclics does not develop, and psychological dependency is minimal. People who are not depressed are unlikely to take tricyclics because of the undesirable side effects.

Toxicity

Even at low dosage levels, tricyclics can be toxic, and excessive levels of tricyclic antidepressant drugs can be fatal. A therapeutic dosage of imipramine is about 300 mg a day, and a lethal dose is about 2,000 mg. Early warning signs of toxicity include low blood pressure, low body temperature, excitement, seizures, restlessness, reduced breathing, dry skin, flushed face, and coma. The coma can last 1 to 3 days and is followed by confusion and disorientation. Death, which occurs within 24 hours of ingestion, usually results from irregular heart rate (arrhythmia) or from the heart simply no longer working.

tachycardia Faster than normal heart rate

Selective Serotonin Reuptake Inhibitors

A newer family of antidepressants was developed in the 1980s. Known as **selective serotonin reuptake inhibitors (SSRIs)**, these drugs include Prozac, Zoloft, Paxil, Lexapro, and others. These are the most commonly prescribed antidepressants.[85] Serotonin is thought to help regulate mood; where there is a limited amount of serotonin in the brain, depression can occur. Thus SSRIs work by increasing levels of serotonin in the brain by blocking the reuptake of serotonin. This leaves higher levels of serotonin in the brain making it more available.[86] These drugs are widely promoted for treating depression and have other benefits such as reducing aggressive and violent behavior[87] and agoraphobia.[88] Yet, there are several concerns regarding these drugs. The first concern deals with their efficacy. Some studies suggest that pharmaceutical companies exaggerate their effectiveness. However, in a recent study conducted on almost 7,000 depressed adults, researchers found 91% of the patients on an SSRI showed a significant difference in mood.[89] Adverse effects of SSRIs include sexual dysfunction, increase in weight, and altered sleep patterns.[90] Another concern is that these drugs may increase the likelihood of youth suicide, although the evidence indicates that the risk of youth suicide is overstated.[91] In children and adolescents, there appears to be a slight increase in suicide ideations and attempts, but not completed suicides, while in adults the risk of suicide is decreased for those on SSRIs.[92] One study conducted on Danish individuals found the risk of suicide and the use of SSRIs to be highest in the first 3 months after being prescribed the drug and recommends close monitoring on behalf of the physician during those first few months of being on the medication.[93] Pediatric depression is a national problem. Many children who commit suicide suffer

CONSIDER This

Siamese fighting fish, also known as bettas, are extremely territorial fish. Males cannot be housed together for risk of a territorial fight which may result in injury or death. In a recent study, researchers gave Prozac to bettas to determine the effects of the drug on these fish. The drug had a significant impact on the behavior of these fish which included a reduction in aggression and risk taking. These effects lasted even after the drug was removed.

Questions to Ponder

Should aggression in humans be treated using medication? What about in institutionalized settings where violence is high (i.e., prisons, juvenile detention facilities), should drugs be given to residents at these facilities to reduce violence if aggression is the only symptom?

Source: K. Knight, "Prozac makes siamese fighting fish timid", *Journal of Experimental Biology*, 219, no.6 (2016): 771–771.

from depression. It is reported that antidepressants, especially in conjunction with cognitive behavior therapy, actually reduce the risk of pediatric suicide.[94]

Prozac

Every so often a "wonder drug" appears that is supposed to be more effective and less toxic than existing drugs. The antidepressant **Prozac (fluoxetine)** is such a drug.

Contributing to the popularity of Prozac is the fact that it has fewer unpleasant and serious side effects than other antidepressant drugs. The efficacy of Prozac in treating symptoms related to depression, however, does not exceed that of other antidepressants.

In addition to being prescribed for depression, Prozac is used for bulimia and obesity, anxiety, and obsessive-compulsive disorders. Higher doses are required for obsessive-compulsive disorders than for depression.

Prozac reduces symptoms of tension, irritability, and dysphoria in women. It curtails the rate of panic attacks. It does not cause the hypotension, weight gain, or irregular heart rhythms that are common

SIDE EFFECTS OF TRICYCLIC ANTIDEPRESSANTS

• Tachycardia	• Constipation
• Dry mouth	• Urinary retention
• Confusion	• Tremors
• Hypotension	• Rashes
• Disorientation	• Jaundice
• Impotence	• Respiratory problems
• Glaucoma	
• Distorted vision	• Coma
• Sleepiness	• Death

selective serotonin reuptake inhibitors (SSRIs)
A class of antidepressant medications that increase the concentration of the chemical, serotonin, in the brain

Prozac (fluoxetine) An antidepressant drug

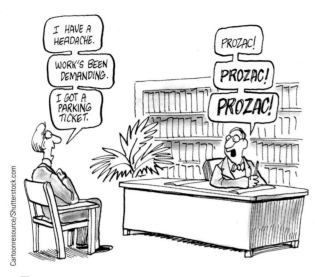

In the 1990s Prozac was the most prescribed antidepressant drug. Popular belief felt it was a cure for anything.

with other treatments. Side effects include headaches, sweating, fatigue, jitteriness, anxiety, stomach upset, nausea, insomnia, dizziness, sexual dysfunction, and reduced appetite. Long-term side effects have not been determined. Some studies suggest Prozac and similar antidepressants may disrupt the hypothalamus region of the brain, an area related to promoting bone growth, resulting in weaken bones and reducing bone density.[95] The use of Prozac has not been limited to humans. It has been given to dogs to help relieve canine depression and compulsive licking. One study in which rats were given Prozac and other antidepressants showed that these drugs actually stimulate the growth of new brain cells.[96]

Prozac has sparked several legal issues. Unhappy consumers have filed lawsuits against the drug's manufacturer, Eli Lilly. One critic, author William Styron, says, "It is Lilly's concerted efforts to minimize such sinister side effects that remain even now indefensible."[62] Because Prozac has been linked to violent behavior, some people have used this information as a criminal defense, claiming they cannot be held responsible for crimes committed while on the drug.

Prozac has been implicated in a number of suicides, but it is unclear if Prozac *causes* violent behavior toward self or others. The issue may hinge on how one views the evidence. Depression can lead to suicide or violence whether or not a person is receiving treatment.

Zoloft

Another popular SSRI is Zoloft (sertraline). Zoloft seems to be as effective as tricyclic antidepressants for treating moderate to severe depression. It is especially effective with elderly patients. Increasing numbers of children, as young as age 5, are given Zoloft and other antidepressants. Zoloft is the most commonly prescribed antidepressant for patients with acute coronary syndrome. Like Prozac, Zoloft is used to treat obsessive-compulsive disorders. However, there is a small risk that Zoloft and other antidepressants may contribute to birth defects.[97] One study found an increase risk (six times as likely) among babies whose mothers took sertraline during pregnancy for persistent pulmonary hypertension compared to mothers who did not take any medication during pregnancy.[98]

Paxil

One of the newest antidepressant drugs is Paxil (paroxetine). It was the most heavily advertised antidepressant between 1999 and 2003.[99] Like the other SSRIs, Paxil increases brain levels of serotonin, the neurotransmitter that affects mood and alertness. In one survey of Paxil users, it was reported that 59% believed that the drug was beneficial, though 21% felt drowsiness or disorientation, 53% experienced decreased sexual interest or performance, and 22% gained weight.[100] The American College of Obstetricians and Gynecologists reports that Paxil taken during pregnancy increases the risk of cardiac malformations and neonatal complications.[101]

The US Food and Drug Administration (FDA) recommended that Paxil not be prescribed for children and adolescents because of the increased risk of suicides. One study indicated that teens and children taking Paxil are 3.2 times more likely to attempt suicide than others taking placebos.[102] GlaxoSmithKline, the company that manufactures Paxil, allegedly failed to disclose data regarding the drug's side effects.[103] Recently researchers reanalyzed SmithKline Beecham's Study 329, which examined the use of Paxil on adolescents with depression. Results from this reanalysis show there were no statistically significant changes between the treatment and placebo group. Additionally, results indicated an increase in suicidal ideation and behavior among those adolescents in the treatment group.[104] GlaxoSmithKline agreed to pay the state of New York $2.5 million to avoid an extended lawsuit.

GlaxoSmithKline distributed a derivative of Paxil known as Paxil CR (Paxil Controlled Release). This new version has several advantages over Paxil. First, it is well tolerated by users and has a low patient dropout rate. In a study conducted in Japan, Paxil CR was shown to be an effective drug for treating depression with almost 70% of the patients being satisfied with the Paxil CR treatment after the 8 weeks of treatment.[105] Besides being used for depression, Paxil CR has been approved for the treatment of social anxiety disorder.[106] In addition, Paxil CR is prescribed for panic disorder and premenstrual syndrome.[107] One other advantage of Paxil CR is that it is sold at 31% of the cost of Paxil.[108]

Lexapro

Currently second in prescriptions written only to Zoloft, Lexapro (escitalopram) is an SSRI antidepressant that was created by Forest Pharmaceuticals and approved by the FDA in August of 2002. Its commercial name is CipraLexapro. It was made from a constituent of Celexa. The medical constituent of Celexa is citalopram HBr.[109] While commonly prescribed to treat depression and anxiety disorders, such as generalized anxiety disorder and major depressive disorder, its off-label investigational uses include the treatment of obsessive-compulsive disorder, panic disorder, social anxiety disorder, PTSD, PMDD, menstrual symptoms such as mood swings and irritability, and compulsive behaviors such as gambling.[110] Like other SSRIs, it works by increasing the amount of available serotonin in the brain. Lexapro, however, has a more selective interaction than many of the other SSRIs. The side effects for Lexapro are essentially the same as the side effects of other SSRIs. However, Lexapro's side effects appear to be less frequent and milder than those caused by other SSRIs and tend to disappear within 2 weeks of starting the drug.[111]

The makers of Lexapro have experienced legal problems regarding marketing of Lexapro as an antidepressant for use with children. In 2004, two separate civil suits alleging illegal marketing of citalopram and escitalopram for use by children and teenagers by Forest were initiated by two whistleblowers.[112] The state of Massachusetts supported the suit in 2009, alleging that a research study showing lack of effectiveness when taken by children was concealed from Forest's own medical advisers and sales personnel, as well as from researchers who conducted a study financed by the company. Forest responded to these allegations by stating that it "is committed to adhering to the highest ethical and legal standards, and off-label promotion and improper payments to medical providers have consistently been against Forest policy."[113]

Atypical

Antidepressants that are not easily categorized are called atypical antidepressants. These include nefazodone, bupropion, mirtazapine, and trazodone. Nefazodone, formerly marketed as Serzone but no longer available in the United States under that name, according to RxList.com, has been reported as causing severe liver failure. It has also been used as an aid for smoking cessation and appetite suppression. Trazodone is a mood elevator. Its side effects may include confusion, concentration difficulties, headaches, and nervousness. Mirtazapine also may cause constipation, dizziness, drowsiness, increased appetite, and weight gain. Less common side effects include seizures, lowered libido, and changes in the menstrual cycle.[114]

Bupropion, also known as Wellbutrin, has been marketed since 1985. Wellbutrin comes in different versions: It can be taken once a day, twice a day, or three times a day. All three formulae are equally effective.[115] Wellbutrin acts by inhibiting the uptake of dopamine and norepinephrine. Besides its use for depression, the drug, under the name Zyban, is used for smoking cessation. It is estimated that 25% of individuals are initially prescribed Zyban to stop smoking. Except in rare instances, people who used Zyban for smoking cessation did not experience adverse side effects.[116]

Wellbutrin has also been approved for seasonal affective disorder. Seasonal affective disorder affects about 5% of all Americans, three-fourths of whom are women.[117] One study found that it helps reduce the risk of depression by 44% if it is taken in the fall prior to symptoms appearing.[118] Unlike other antidepressant drugs, Wellbutrin has not been shown to cause weight gain.

A generic version of Wellbutrin, referred to as Wellbutrin XL, was approved in 2006. In the previous year, it was the highest-selling brand name drug in the United States, totaling $1.3 billion.[119] According to the FDA, this generic version of Wellbutrin is safe, although its manufacturer, Teva Pharmaceutical Industries, came under review for numerous complaints against the drug.[120] The drug is well tolerated by most people, and its side effects are usually mild and temporary. They include loss of appetite, weight loss, dry mouth, skin rash, perspiration, insomnia, ringing in the ears, anxiety, nausea, agitation, and stomach pain.[121] According to the Mayo Clinic, bupropion has fewer sexual side effects than any other antidepressant.[122] The drug should not be used by people with a history of seizures or eating disorders, or by those who are taking MAOI antidepressants.

SNRIs

Serotonin and norepinephrine reuptake inhibitors, or SNRIs, work by blocking the reabsorption (reuptake) of the neurotransmitters serotonin and norepinephrine.[123] There are four types of antidepressants under the SNRI classification: duloxetine, venlafaxine, levomilnacipran, and desvenlafaxine. Side effects are usually mild and go away after a few weeks of treatment. Side effects from SNRIs may include

serotonin and norepinephrine reuptake inhibitors (SNRIs) A class of antidepressant medications that inhibit both the reuptake of serotonin and norepinephrine

nausea, dry mouth, dizziness, headaches, excessive sweating,[124] pain in the eyes, vision blurring, or blindness. They also may cause a variety of other side effects, constipation, insomnia and reduced sexual desire and/or the ability to maintain an erection.[125]

SNRIs include the following:

- **Venlafaxine** (Effexor XR). Venlafaxine may work for some people when other antidepressants have not. It can cause side effects similar to those caused by SSRIs. Venlafaxine can raise blood pressure, and overdose can be dangerous or fatal.
- **Desvenlafaxine** (Pristiq). Desvenlafaxine is similar to venlafaxine and causes similar side effects. Studies have not proven any advantage to desvenlafaxine over venlafaxine, and because venlafaxine is available in a generic form, it is generally a more affordable option.
- **Levomilnacipran** (Fetzima). Levomilnacipran is used to treat depression. It may also help improve sleep and appetite and restore interest in daily living. It may take several months to feel the benefits from this drug. Many people who use this medication do not experience side effects, however, it may raise a person's blood pressure.
- **Duloxetine** (Cymbalta). Duloxetine may help relieve physical pain in addition to depression, but it is not yet clear whether it works better than other antidepressants for pain relief. Duloxetine can cause a number of side effects. Nausea, dry mouth, and constipation are particularly common. Heavy drinkers or those with certain liver or kidney problems are advised against taking duloxetine.[126]

Lithium

A drug used to treat manic symptoms is **lithium**. John Cade, an Australian physician, experimented with lithium to reduce kidney damage in animals and observed that it sedated them. Subsequently, he found that lithium had a similar effect on humans.

Before lithium was introduced, patients with mania had recurring episodes of mood swings. Though Cade's research into lithium's antimanic properties was noted in the 1940s, it received little attention in the United States for 20 years because of the drug's high levels of toxicity. The FDA officially approved lithium in 1970, despite many reservations. When lithium was first administered, many individuals with kidney and cardiovascular problems died. Consequently, physicians were reluctant to prescribe it. Moreover, other drugs such as **chlorpromazine**, with antimanic properties but fewer toxic effects, were available.

Lithium is a positively charged ion that is similar to sodium. It typically is taken orally in salt form and is concentrated in the brain but may accumulate in other body parts such as muscle and bone. It is readily absorbed from the gastrointestinal tract within 8 hours and is excreted in urine. The level of lithium in the body is influenced by the body's sodium level. If a person has a high sodium level, lithium will be readily excreted. If an individual has a low sodium level, high levels of lithium will be retained. One's inability to excrete lithium can lead to toxic levels in the body.

Because lithium has a relatively low margin of safety, administration of the drug is monitored carefully. Its side effects include tremors, excessive thirst, frequent urination, fluid retention, and weight gain. An advantage to lithium is that it has no effect on normal individuals at therapeutic levels.

Effectiveness

Lithium is effective for acute mania and for preventing mania and depression from recurring and has shown to lower suicide in patients who have been diagnosed with bipolar disorder.[127] The maximal benefit is achieved in 1 to 2 weeks, although many patients respond positively in 3 to 4 days. Lithium is especially effective for patients whose manic-depression is genetic. One limitation is that patients have unusually stable moods, even when expressions of emotion are warranted. Lithium typically is prescribed in conjunction with antipsychotic drugs because manic symptoms do not subside for several days.

Lithium prevents symptoms of mania. It is believed that almost two-thirds of patients will relapse into a manic condition within a year of stopping medication.[128] Lithium is effective for people who have unipolar depression and do not respond to tricyclic

Wellbutrin An antidepressant drug that is used to help people stop smoking

Venlafaxine (Effexor XR) An antidepressant drug that acts by inhibiting the reuptake of serotonin and norepinephrine by neurons.

Desvenlafaxine (Pristiq) An antidepressant in a group of drugs called selective serotonin and norepinephrine reuptake inhibitors (SNRIs).

Duloxetine (Cymbalta) A drug used to treat depression and peripheral neuropathy (pain, numbness, tingling, burning, or weakness in the hands or feet) that can occur with diabetes. Duloxetine increases the amount of certain chemicals in the brain that help relieve depression and pain. It is a type of serotonin and norepinephrine reuptake inhibitor.

lithium A psychotherapeutic drug used to treat symptoms associated with mania

chlorpromazine An antipsychotic drug

TABLE 10.5 Antidepressant Medications

Drug Name	Type of Medication	Potential Side Effects
Anafranil Adapin Aventyl Elavil Norpramin Pamelor Pertofrane Sinequan Surmontil Tofranil Vivactil	These medicines are tricyclic antidepressants (TCAs) that work by increasing the available amount of serotonin and/or norepinephrine in the brain.	Dry mouth, blurred vision, increased fatigue and sleepiness, weight gain, muscle twitching (tremors), constipation, bladder problems such as urine retention, dizziness, daytime drowsiness, increased heart rate, sexual problems.
Parnate Nardil Marplan	Monoamine oxidase inhibitors (MAOIs) increase the amount of norepinephrine and serotonin in the brain	Must avoid certain foods and medications to avoid dangerous interactions. Serious side effects may include headache, heart racing, chest pain, neck stiffness, nausea, and vomiting. If you experience any of these symptoms, seek medical care immediately.
Celexa Lexapro Luvox Paxil Prozac Zoloft	Selective serotonin reuptake inhibitors, or (SSRIs), work by increasing the amount of serotonin, a neurotransmitter found in the brain.	Sexual problems including low sex drive or inability to have an orgasm are common but reversible; dizziness, headaches, nausea right after a dose, insomnia, feeling jittery.
Wellbutrin Serzone Trazodone Mirtazapine	Wellbutrin (atypical) may increase the amounts of the neurotransmitters norepinephrine and dopamine in the brain.	Weight loss, decreased appetite, restlessness, insomnia, anxiety, constipation, dry mouth, diarrhea, dizziness Wellbutrin is much less likely to cause the weight gain or sexual problems seen with other antidepressants.
Effexor Remeron Cymbalta	These drugs (SNRIs) increase the levels of the neurotransmitters serotonin and norepinephrine in the brain.	Drowsiness, blurred vision, lightheadedness, strange dreams, constipation, fever/chills, headache, increased or decreased appetite, tremor, dry mouth, nausea. Remeron can be sedating. Cymbalta may increase sweating and blood pressure and also cause fatigue and reduced energy.
Desyrel Ludiomil	These drugs block various neurotransmitter chemicals to some degree.	Desyrel may cause drowsiness, fatigue, tremor, headache, dry mouth, nausea, and vomiting. Ludiomil may cause headache, dizziness, dry mouth, fatigue, daytime sleepiness, and sweating.

© Cengage Learning 2014

antidepressant drugs. Its success varies when it is used to treat premenstrual syndrome, hyperactivity in children, and outbursts of aggression or anger. Lithium minimizes impulsivity. Some research shows that it significantly increases the abstinence period of alcoholics, but other research on lithium use with chronic alcoholics is inconclusive. Some evidence suggests that lithium is useful in managing behavioral problems in individuals with an intellectual disability.[129]

Side Effects

At therapeutic levels, the side effects of lithium include nausea, thirst, excessive perspiration, and hand tremors. After lithium is administered, the body initially loses sodium and potassium; this is followed by sodium and water retention. Lithium users urinate frequently and in large amounts, a condition known as **polyuria**. Also, lithium users consume water frequently and excessively, a condition called **polydipsia**. Polyuria and polydipsia rarely cause significant kidney damage. Additional side effects associated with lithium are vomiting, diarrhea, confusion, weight gain, drowsiness, and muscular weakness.

Side effects that occur less often include **tinnitus** (ringing sounds in the ear), distorted vision, and a metallic taste in the mouth. Increased amounts

polyuria Frequent urination

polydipsia Frequent and excessive consumption of water

tinnitus A condition marked by constant ringing in the ears

SIDE EFFECTS OF LITHIUM

- Nausea
- Excessive perspiration
- Water retention
- Vomiting
- Confusion
- Drowsiness
- Tinnitus
- Kidney dysfunction
- Respiratory depression
- Thirst
- Hand tremors
- Frequent urination
- Diarrhea
- Weight gain
- Muscular weakness
- Distorted vision
- Coma
- Death

of lithium can result in impaired kidney function, respiratory depression, coma, and even death. Taking lithium during pregnancy increases the risk of fetal damage. Also, the drug can be passed to the newborn in breast milk. Lithium does not cause physical dependency or severe withdrawal symptoms, but restlessness and irritability follow cessation of use.

Toxicity

The amount needed for therapeutic purposes (what clinicians call the **therapeutic window)** is small. Three to four times the therapeutic level can cause grave consequences. Yet, carefully monitored patients can take the drug for years. Symptoms of lithium toxicity are intense nausea, tremors, irregular heartbeat, lowered blood pressure, abdominal pain, mental confusion, vomiting, diarrhea, and convulsions. Elderly patients may be at greater risk because they excrete Lithium at a slower rate than younger patients.[130]

Antipsychotic Drugs

Antipsychotic drugs, also known as **major tranquilizers**, are used to treat and manage psychological disorders ranging from psychosis to violent behavior to schizoprenia. Antipsychotic drugs, called **neuroleptics** in Europe, are pharmacologically different from minor tranquilizers and other sedative-hypnotic drugs. Although antipsychotic drugs have been used to relieve anxiety, that is not their primary purpose. Developed in the mid-1950s, antipsychotic drugs are used especially for schizophrenia. They do not *cure* schizophrenia or other forms of mental illness but, rather, treat symptoms associated with mental illness. A mentally ill or schizophrenic person is able to function normally while taking these drugs.

Like many medications, antipsychotic drugs were discovered by accident. French surgeon Henri Laborit noted the calming effect of chlorpromazine, an anesthetic used to ameliorate anxiety and shock during surgery. Chlorpromazine later was given to psychotic patients at a military hospital in Paris. Patients receiving chlorpromazine appeared calm, and their thinking was less disorganized. Moreover, patients did not lose consciousness.

Chlorpromazine was marketed in 1955 in the United States under the trade name **Thorazine**. It is credited with revolutionizing the treatment of people with mental disorders. Despite the proliferation of people diagnosed as mentally ill beginning in the 1950s, the number of hospitalized mental patients in the United States dramatically declined from 600,000 in 1955 to about 150,000 by the mid-1980s, because their illnesses could be better managed by drugs. Newer antipsychotic drugs are not necessarily any more effective, but they may have fewer adverse effects.[131]

Antipsychotic drugs fall into two categories: first-generation antipsychotics and second-generation antipsychotics. First generation antipsychotics include haloperidol (Haldol), trifluoperazine (Stelazine), fluphenazine (Prolixin), and thioridazine (Mellaril). Second-generation antipsychotics include olanzipine (Zyprexa), clozapine (Clozaril), paliperidone (Invega), and quetiapine (Seroquel). To obtain maximum effectiveness, schizophrenic patients have to take antipsychotic drugs for 4 to 6 weeks, although some symptoms of schizophrenia decline within the first week of treatment. Recent studies regarding people with anorexia have shown no improvement in body mass index rates among between those who were prescribed antipsychotics medications and those were not.[132]

Although antipsychotic drugs can be administered by injection, they usually are ingested. Injecting antipsychotic drugs does not offer much of an advantage because they require several days to take effect. Some patients receive injections of antipsychotic drugs so the drug can be released slowly into the bloodstream.

One problem with antipsychotic drugs is that they are absorbed erratically and thus it is difficult to determine an effective dose precisely. These drugs build up in fatty areas in the brain and lungs. Because of their high affinity for lipids, they cross the placenta easily and affect the fetus.

---

therapeutic window The amount of drug needed for therapeutic purposes

major tranquilizers Antipsychotic drugs

neuroleptics The European term for antipsychotic drugs

Thorazine Major tranquilizer used to treat psychosis

Children and Antipsychotic Drugs

An increasing number of children are being prescribed antipsychotic medications. More children in the United States are prescribed antipsychotic drugs more frequently than children in other developed countries. Nonetheless, the use of antipsychotic drugs by children is growing in other countries as well. A recent study found among those children and adolescents who are prescribed antipsychotics, most of them were diagnosed with nonpsychotic mental disorders and boys were prescribed antipsychotic medications at higher rates compared to girls.[133] These drugs are beneficial for treating antipsychotic conditions; however, they also produce adverse effects in children. One study found children who were on antipsychotic medication had lower rates in school performance when compared to a control group of children.[134] Other effects include excessive weight gain, type 2 diabetes, neurological symptoms, digestive problems, and cardiovascular conditions. These effects are more prevalent in females.[135]

Effectiveness

Although schizophrenics receiving antipsychotic drugs almost always show improvement, a small percentage gets worse. While the extent to which patients improve varies widely, symptoms of schizophrenia are greatly reduced in the majority of patients.[136] Patients taking antipsychotic drugs become less belligerent, agitated, and impulsive. Autistic or withdrawn patients sometimes become more responsive and communicative. Delusions, disorganized thinking, and hallucinations disappear, and insight, memory, judgment, appetite, and sleep improve. Improvement is most rapid during the first several weeks of treatment.

Although many people taking antipsychotic drugs relapse, it appears that these drugs reduce violent behavior.[137] For patients having a relapse, psychosocial factors may be the root cause. Stress, interpersonal problems, and overly critical and intrusive relatives increase the risk of relapse. Despite the effectiveness of antipsychotic drugs and the fact that newer antipsychotic drugs have fewer side effects, the rate of noncompliance is very high with only 58% of those prescribed antipsychotics following medication adherence.[138]

Side Effects

Antipsychotic drugs produce many undesirable motor problems, called **extrapyramidal symptoms**. Inappropriate motor movements—**acute dyskinesias**—sometimes appear within a year after treatment begins. Acute dyskinesias take several forms, as follows:

1. **Parkinsonism:** A condition marked by a dull facial expression, weakness in the extremities, tremors, rigidity, and extremely slow and limited movements (**bradykinesia**). These symptoms, resembling Parkinson's disease, appear in about 40% of patients.
2. **Dystonia:** Sudden and involuntary muscle spasms of the head, neck, lips, and tongue. Slurred speech and eyes deviated up are also common.
3. **Akathesia:** Characterized by jerky and uncontrollable constant motion, motor restlessness, and an occasional protruding tongue and facial grimace. This condition is exhibited in about 20% of patients.

Another major side effect, **tardive dyskinesia**, is marked by motor disorders such as involuntary repetitive facial movements, lip smacking, involuntary movement of the trunk and limbs, and twitching. Newer antipsychotic drugs produce fewer side effects. The incidence of tardive dyskinesia varies considerably, although it is more likely to occur with patients who develop their psychosis after age 50 and among females. Symptoms of tardive dyskinesia appear within a year after initiation of antipsychotic drug treatment and sometimes are irreversible.

Numerous, less severe side effects are associated with antipsychotic drugs. Some of these are difficulty urinating, constipation, dry mouth, altered skin pigmentation, changes in heart rate, jaundice, and extreme sensitivity to sunlight and an allergic response in which the patient sunburns easily. Other effects are cessation of menstruation (amenorrhea), weight gain, hypotension, sexual dysfunctions (up to 43% of patients), cardiac arrhythmias, seizures, and

---

extrapyramidal symptoms Neurological symptoms characterized by difficulty walking, shuffling, and inflexible joints

acute dyskinesias Inappropriate motor movements as a side effect of antipsychotic drugs

Parkinsonism A form of acute dyskinesia marked by tremors, weakness in the extremities, and muscle rigidity

bradykinesia Motor movements that are slow and limited

dystonia A type of dyskinesia marked by involuntary and inappropriate postures and muscle tones

akathesia Jerky, uncontrollable constant motion, motor restlessness, occasional protruding tongue, and facial grimace

tardive dyskinesia A side effect of antipsychotic drugs marked by involuntary repetitive facial movements and involuntary movement of the trunk and limbs

metabolic syndrome issues.[139] Additionally, some antipsychotic medications may cause side effects related to physical movement which includes rigidity, persistent muscle spasms, tremors, and restlessness.[140] Many of these side effects are less common with newer antipsychotic drugs. Patients sometimes sleep more at first, but sleep cycles or REM sleep is not altered. Susceptible patients experience an increase in epileptic seizures after taking antipsychotic drugs.

Patients develop tolerance to the side effects of these drugs but do not develop tolerance to therapeutic dosages. Therefore patients do not have to increase the dosage to benefit from the drug. A patient can take antipsychotic drugs for years without having to increase the dosage. The difference between a therapeutic and a toxic level of antipsychotic drugs is considerable. Hence, the risk of a fatal overdose, either accidental or intentional, is low. Antipsychotic drugs do not cause physical dependency, and people do not use them for nonmedical or recreational purposes.

Psychotherapeutic Drug Abuse

Data from the pharmaceutical agencies indicate that at least 50 million Americans report the use of at least one psychotherapeutic drug (tranquilizer, sedative, painkiller, stimulants) at some point in their lifetime. In 2013, approximately 2 million persons aged 12 and older had used psychotherapeutics nonmedically within the past year. This number is lower compared to previous years.[142] Approximately 2 million Americans over the age of 12 report using psychotherapeutic drugs in the past year.

Patients need to understand the dangers associated with abusing and/or mixing prescribed psychotherapeutic drugs with illicit and licit drugs.

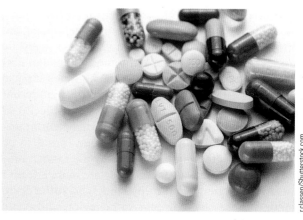

Many times, patients do not fully disclose what drugs they are currently taking to their doctor. Mixing drugs has resulted in accidental overdose.

Unintentional poisoning deaths involving psychotherapeutic drugs, such as sedative-hypnotics and antidepressants, were the leading mechanism of injury deaths in 2014.[143] Emergency rooms across the nation have reported more visits from individuals whose symptoms are caused by abuse of prescription drugs. Accidental overdose and adverse reactions to the drugs account for the majority of these cases. In many instances, it is discovered that the individuals had been abusing multiple drugs of different classes, thus compounding the toxicity and increasing the chance of an adverse reaction.[144]

Because these medications are prescribed by doctors, many assume that they are safe to take under any circumstances. This is not the case. Prescription drugs act directly or indirectly on the same brain systems affected by illicit drugs. Using a medication other than as prescribed can potentially lead to a variety of adverse health effects, including overdose and addiction.[145]

Summary

Mental illness is a vague, ill-defined problem that is increasing in the general population. Its causes can be social, genetic, biochemical, or some combination of these. Mental illness encompasses more than diseases of the brain and central nervous system; it entails behavior or thinking that is considered inappropriate. Social norms often serve as the basis to determine whether a given behavior exceeds what is considered acceptable.

A relationship exists between mental disorders and substance use and abuse. A dual diagnosis refers to a person who has both conditions. People experiencing a comorbid condition need to receive treatment that addresses both the substance abuse disorder and mental illness.

Almost 10% of the US adult population suffer from a mood disorder, with women being affected at higher rates compared to men. Mood disorders include depression, unipolar depression, and bipolar affective disorder.

Between 10% and 15% of the US population receive medication for a mental or emotional problem. Antidepressant drugs are effective for mild to moderate cases of depression, but most people suffering from depression do not seek help for their condition. Five types of drugs used to treat depression are monoamine oxidase inhibitors (MAOIs), tricyclic antidepressants, selective serotonin reuptake inhibitors (SSRIs), serotonin and norepinephrine reuptake inhibitors (SNRIs), and antidepressants that do not categorize easily (atypical).

MAOIs repress the activity of certain neurotransmitters in the brain. They have been found to be largely ineffective and are used only after other antidepressant drugs have failed. They are more effective in elderly patients and in patients who suffer from anxiety, obsessive-compulsive behavior, and panic attacks. One serious side effect is high blood pressure resulting from foods containing tyramine being consumed concurrently with MAOIs.

Tricyclic drugs are more effective in removing symptoms of acute depression and about 60% effective in eliminating symptoms of chronic depression. Tricyclics are also used for treating phobias, chronic pain, and bulimia. Some side effects are irregular heartbeat, confusion, constipation, disorientation, hypotension, and coma. Tolerance and physical dependence do not occur with tricyclic antidepressants, but malaise, muscle aches, and chills appear when treatment is stopped.

Prozac is part of the family of SSRIs that also include Zoloft, Paxil, and Lexapro, and is reportedly more effective and less toxic than other antidepressants. Preliminary research indicates that Prozac is about 60% effective for depression. It is also used for anxiety, eating disorders, and obsessive-compulsive behaviors. Long-term effects have not been established.

Lithium is administered primarily to treat mania. When given initially, it caused a number of deaths in people with kidney and cardiovascular problems. Its effects are altered by the level of sodium in the body. Lithium not only ameliorates the symptoms of mania and depression but also prevents these symptoms from recurring.

It is especially effective with individuals whose mania and depression are genetic. Lithium also is used to treat premenstrual syndrome, hyperactivity, and aggression. It can cause kidney damage, respiratory depression, coma, and death, and taking Lithium during the first trimester of pregnancy increases the risk of a birth defect.

Antipsychotic drugs are particularly helpful in treating symptoms of schizophrenia in adults as well as children. They reduce symptoms in the majority of schizophrenics. As a side effect, some patients exhibit symptoms similar to those of Parkinson's disease. Another side effect, tardive dyskinesia, is marked by involuntary facial movements, which may be irreversible, although one study found that the symptoms were reversed in more than half of patients. Less severe effects include dry mouth, weight gain, constipation, breast development, amenorrhea, sensitivity to light, epilepsy, and sleepiness. Tolerance to and physical dependence on antipsychotic drugs do not develop.

Patients need to understand the dangers associated with abusing and/or mixing prescribed psychotherapeutic drugs with illicit and licit drugs. Using a medication other than as prescribed can potentially lead to a variety of adverse health effects, including overdose and addiction.

Thinking Critically

1. A century ago, mentally ill people were called crazy or lunatics. Today, we are more sophisticated and refer to these people as having mental disorders. Even with the change in terminology, there seems to exist a negative stereotype regarding people with mental disorders. Do you believe the change in terminology altered people's attitudes? When you think of a person who is labeled as having a mental disorder, what comes to mind?

2. Many antidepressants take a period of time to take effect. For example, patients using MAOIs may have to wait at least 2 weeks for the drug to begin to relieve the symptoms of depression. Given that 15% of depressed patients commit suicide, how would you create a treatment plan for people diagnosed with depression?

3. A relationship exists between mental disorders and substance abuse. How would you create a plan at a college to address alcohol use? What mental health services or interventions would you include?

4. Antipsychotic drugs often are effective in reducing symptoms associated with schizophrenia. Not everyone with schizophrenia, however, wants to take the medication. Should people be required to take antipsychotic drugs against their will? Or should they have the choice to decline treatment, even though the drugs may help?

11

Stimulants: Cocaine, Amphetamines, Methamphetamines, and Caffeine

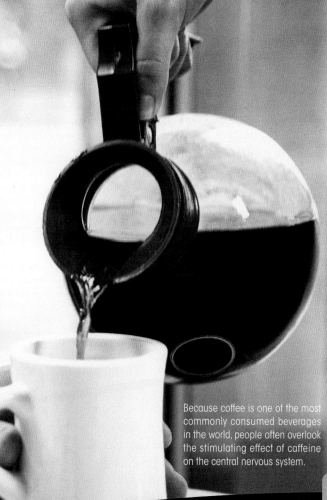

Because coffee is one of the most commonly consumed beverages in the world, people often overlook the stimulating effect of caffeine on the central nervous system.

Creatas

Chapter Objectives

After completing this chapter, the reader should be able to:

- Summarize the extent of illegal stimulant use in the United States
- Distinguish between the different forms of products that contain cocaine including coca leaves, powder cocaine, and crack cocaine
- Contrast the different modes of administering cocaine and how routes of administration impact addiction
- Discuss cocaine use from an historical standpoint and factors that contributed to the rise in popularity during the 1970s and 1980s
- Create an argument why crack cocaine is a more dangerous drug compared to powder cocaine
- Compare the different treatment opportunities for cocaine addiction
- Explain the impact on children who were prenatally exposed to cocaine
- Discuss the medical consequences of amphetamines
- Relate the connection between amphetamines and attention deficit hyperactivity disorder (ADHD)
- Explain the physical and psychological effects of methamphetamines
- Determine whether caffeine is a physically harmful drug

FACT OR FICTION?

1. Cocaine makes sex better.
2. Cocaine does not make you a better athlete.
3. As many people go to emergency rooms for crack cocaine as for powder cocaine.
4. Previously, cocaine was used medicinally as a local anesthetic.
5. The depressant effects of alcohol reduce the stimulating effects of cocaine, making serious side effects less likely to occur.
6. The majority of crack cocaine users are Black while the majority of powder cocaine users are White.
7. Children will eventually outgrow their ADHD diagnosis.
8. Once a person stops using methamphetamines, their brain is able to restore itself to normal.
9. Children with ADHD who are prescribed a stimulant medication are less likely to abuse drugs.
10. Moderate amounts of caffeine can increase cardiovascular endurance.

Turn the page to check your answers ➤

During times of fatigue and lethargy, people sometimes look for substances that will elevate their mood and make them energetic. **Stimulants** provide these effects. They are capable of modifying a person's activity level, mood, and central nervous system. Some stimulants, such as cocaine and methamphetamines, are illegal. Others, such as amphetamines, require a prescription. In addition, legal stimulants such as caffeine and nicotine are among the most widely used drugs in the world. This chapter covers all of the major legal and illegal stimulants except nicotine, which is discussed in Chapter 7.

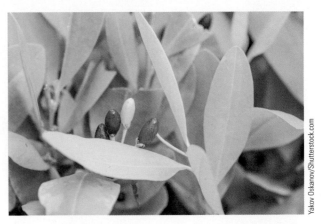

Yakov Oskanov/Shutterstock.com

Cocaine comes from the leaves of the Erythroxylon coca plant.

Cocaine

Cocaine use is at historic lows. In 2016, 2.3% of high school seniors in the United States reported having used cocaine at least one time during the past year. Among 8th-grade students, 0.8% reported having used cocaine, and 1.3% of 10th-grade students indicated having used cocaine at least one time in the previous 12 months.[1] The percentage of high school seniors who have ever used cocaine has declined since the 1980s, when it was the most popular of the illegal stimulants.[2]

Background

Cocaine comes from the leaves of the coca plant, **Erythroxylon coca**. Natives living in the Andes Mountains typically chew the leaves of the coca plant to relieve fatigue, for spiritual reasons, or to enhance well-being. Chewing coca leaves does not seem to cause dependence, possibly because the leaves contain less than 1% cocaine. Also, when coca leaves are chewed or brewed in tea, they do not cause biological harm or social dysfunction.[3] One study suggests that use of coca leaves may enhance physical performance at high altitudes.[4] The researchers of this study believe these enhanced physical performances may be attributed to the flavonoids found in the coca leaf and not the release of cocaine itself since the amount of cocaine present is so small.

The largest producer of cocaine is Colombia. In 2014, US drug agents say they planted 44% more

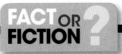

FACT OR FICTION?

1. **FICTION** The fact is—Cocaine increases sexual desire initially and may result in more risky sexual behaviors. Heavy cocaine users may lead to impotence.

2. **FACT** Studies have shown cocaine use before exercising increases the chance of an irregular heartbeat and death.

3. **FICTION** The fact is—Powder cocaine accounts for more than three times as many people going to the emergency room as crack cocaine.

4. **FACT** Although other drugs have replaced cocaine for medical purposes, it has been used as a local anesthetic.

5. **FICTION** The fact is—Alcohol exacerbates the effects of cocaine, increasing the risk of a fatal overdose.

6. **FICTION** The fact is—More than half of all crack and powder cocaine users are White.

7. **FICTION** The fact is—Up to 50% of children who were diagnosed with ADHD will continue to have it in adulthood.

8. **FICTION** The fact is—The brain will start to heal itself; however, studies show that the brain may never fully heal the damage caused by methamphetamines.

9. **FACT** Children, with ADHD, who are effectively treated with stimulant medication have lower rates of substance abuse later in life compared to those with ADHD who are not treated with stimulants.

10. **FACT** Caffeine improves work output marginally.

crops compared to the year 2013 and expect to continue being the world's largest producer and exporter of cocaine.[5] Peru and Boliva are the second and third largest contributors of cocaine. In 2012, the US government supplied money to Columbia for aerial spraying of coca crops. While initially successful, many farmers moved their crop to national parks and indigenous reserves, areas that couldn't be sprayed.[6] It is estimated that two-thirds of the areas coca farms are now located in these off-limit areas.

Properties

Cocaine is a schedule II drug. It is an odorless, crystalline, white powder. It produces intense euphoria, alertness, and energy, as well as inhibits appetite and sleep. As a medical use, cocaine sometimes is put into a mixture called a **Brompton's cocktail**, which is used to manage cancer pain. Also, cocaine is used in surgical procedures on the facial area because that area has many blood vessels and cocaine constricts blood flow and blood vessels. The anesthetizing action takes effect within a minute and lasts up to 2 hours. At one time, cocaine was used to allay withdrawal symptoms from narcotic addiction and to treat depression.

Mode of Intake

Cocaine can be snorted, smoked, or injected. The mode of intake has a bearing on its potential to cause addiction. The more quickly one gets high, the more likely addiction will occur. Injected cocaine reaches the brain the fastest, and euphoria is rapid and intense. Snorted cocaine is absorbed into the bloodstream through the nasal mucous membranes. Most recreational or experimental users snort cocaine

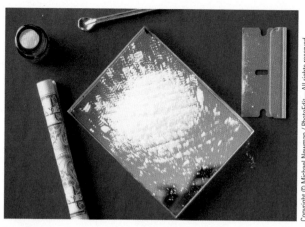

Cocaine paraphernalia includes mirrors, razor blades, and scales used by drug dealers.

initially. It reaches the brain in 10 to 15 minutes, resulting in a "high."

Like injected cocaine, **crack cocaine** reaches the brain in seconds. The immediate reinforcement or reward is critical to addiction. In 2015, crack use among adolescents is 0.1%, which is just slightly higher compared to 2002 when it was at less than 0.1%. Among adults, crack use in 2015 is lower compared to previous years at 0.1%.[7]

Freebasing cocaine started in the mid-1960s. In the **freebase** process, cocaine is treated with an alkaloid to separate it from its hydrochloride salt. Then it is mixed with ether to remove the impurities. Although the euphoria derived from freebasing cocaine is intense and fast, it is brief. The user gets high quickly, at twice the cost for a relatively shorter time. Figure 11.1 depicts different forms of cocaine.

Historical Use

The history of cocaine as a medicinal agent dates back more than 100 years. Cocaine originally was isolated from coca leaves by the German scientist Niemann around 1859. Within several years, Sigmund Freud

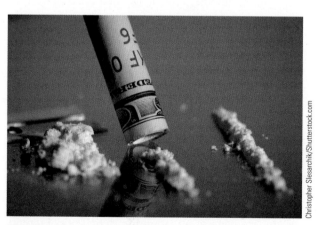

Up to 90% of circulated bills in the United States contain traces of cocaine.

Source: M. Park, "90 percent of U.S. bills carry traces of cocaine", *CNN*, (August 17, 2009). Accessed on March 5, 2017 from http://www.cnn.com/2009/HEALTH/08/14/cocaine.traces.money/.

Stimulants a drug that increases central nervous system activity.

Erythroxylon coca Coca plant from which cocaine is derived

Brompton's cocktail A combination of heroin and cocaine sometimes used to treat terminally ill patients

crack cocaine A variation of cocaine made by heating cocaine after mixing it with baking soda and water

freebase A variation of cocaine in which cocaine is separated from its hydrochloride salt by heating, using a volatile chemical such as ether

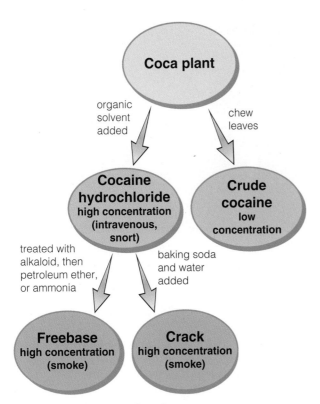

Figure 11.1 Forms of Cocaine

almost every state in the United States had passed laws to control cocaine use. Finally, with passage of the Harrison Narcotic Act of 1914, the federal government officially (although erroneously) designated cocaine as a narcotic.

After the Harrison Act was enacted and nonmedical use of cocaine became illegal, cocaine's use declined. When amphetamines were introduced in 1927, its use declined further. But in the 1970s, its use reemerged. In the succeeding decade, cocaine use increased in Europe and in countries where it had been almost nonexistent. The increase in cocaine use was accompanied by an increase in cocaine-related deaths.

Partly responsible for the rise of cocaine use in the 1970s was the declining popularity of amphetamines and the increased availability of cocaine. During the 1960s, amphetamines had been the drugs of choice. The desire for amphetamines, however, decreased as media campaigns warned people that "speed kills." Cocaine was seen as a safer alternative. Moreover, pharmaceutical manufacturers were limiting supplies of amphetamines.

Also contributing to the interest in cocaine in the 1980s was the fact that movie stars, musicians, and professional athletes reportedly used it. These celebrities established the groundwork for making cocaine glamorous, and it became the "champagne" of drugs. Another factor that furthered the popularity of cocaine was the rejection of the traditional work ethic and middle-class values of the 1950s and 1960s, replaced by a laid-back, relaxed lifestyle; people "mellowed out" and "did their own thing."

A parallel set of values emerged out of the 1970s, with an emphasis on getting ahead, making it to the top, striving to be the best, and being successful. Cocaine delivered feelings of being masterful, competent, and invincible. Thus it satisfied the mood of the time and became the drug of choice for many people.

Current Use

In 2015, an estimated 1.9 million Americans aged 12 and older were current cocaine users, the majority of them between 18 and 25 years of age.[11] Chronic, hardcore drug users—who represent about 20% of drug users—account for two-thirds of the total amount of cocaine used in the United States. Also, males are more likely to use cocaine than women, although women experience greater cravings and are more likely to seek treatment.[12] In one study looking at adult cocaine users, attention deficit hyperactivity disorder (ADHD) was shown to have a higher lifetime occurrence of cocaine use and abuse.[13] Some may attribute this to the higher rates of ADHD in men, increased risk taking, and impulsivity, which

spoke of cocaine in magical terms and recommended it to alleviate opiate addiction, depression, and fatigue, although he eventually stopped using cocaine.[8] Eventually, cocaine use and dependence spread throughout Europe. It became so popular that luminaries including Ulysses S. Grant, Pope Leo XIII, and Sarah Bernhardt touted it. Freud later was held responsible for the "third scourge of humanity" (the first two were alcohol and opiate addiction), whereupon he stopped recommending the drug.

Cocaine was originally included in one of the world's most popular beverages, Coca-Cola. (Coca-Cola derived its name from two of its ingredients: kola nuts and cocaine.) For people opposed to alcohol, Coca-Cola was advertised as a "temperance drink." Coca leaves were also added to a bordeaux wine called Vin Mariani. Even John Stith Pemberton, the original developer of Coca-Cola, invented his own version of cocaine-laced wine called French Coca Wine in 1884.[9] In 1898, druggist Caleb Davis Bradham invented Pepsi-Cola in New Bern, North Carolina, to compete against Coca-Cola. Like Pemberton, Bradham developed the beverage for its medicinal properties.[10]

Despite the widespread use of cocaine by the turn of the 20th century, many people condemned it because it led to dependency. Ironically, the individuals speaking out against cocaine were the same individuals who had promoted it—physicians. By 1914,

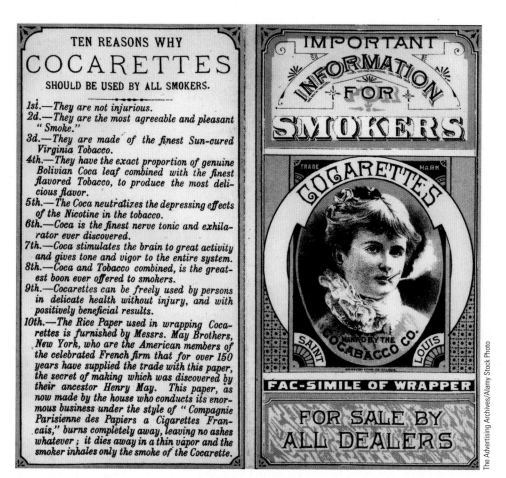

In the late 1800s the Cocabacco Company manufactured cocarettes.

are also risk factors associated with cocaine use.[13] It is important to note that studies have found children who are treated for ADHD using stimulant medications show no signs of an increase in drug abuse later in life. In fact, many studies have found that when individuals are treated with medication for ADHD, they have a lower risk of a substance abuse problem later in life. Conversely, children who are not effectively treated for ADHD have a higher risk for developing a substance abuse problem later in life.[14]

Crack

Crack cocaine emerged in the 1980s, though accounts of its use were noted as far back as the early 1970s. It is the product of mixing cocaine with baking soda and water and then heating the mixture. This simple process produces small chunks or rocks, which can be smoked. Smoking the chunks or rocks produces a crackling sound—hence, the term *crack*. Crack is usually smoked, but it can also be injected. Thus the only difference between cocaine and crack is the removal of hydrochloride, which allows crack to be smoked due to the lower melting point. Because it comes in small units, the cost is low. The euphoria from crack

is brief (about 10 to 20 minutes), and the desire to repeat usage is high. Despite this, most people who use crack once do not continue to use it.

Crack use is a problem among impoverished, inner-city adolescents. Before the less expensive crack form was available, fewer people used cocaine. In one encouraging development, more than 90% of students disapproved of crack cocaine.[15]

In a 2012 survey of those who use crack cocaine, 55% of past month users were White and a little over 12% were Black.[16] However, crack use may be correlated with other problems. In a study conducted in Brazil, those who used crack were more likely to be from low social class areas and have a lifetime use of snorted cocaine.[17] The experience of trauma and sexual assault leads to an increase risk of drug use later in life. In another study, one-third of African American crack users reported having been sexually assaulted at least once in their lifetime.[18] In a study done on women, experiencing physical violence was major risk factor for cocaine, crack, and/or heroin use.[19] In one study, more than 60% of women addicted to crack had been sexually abused, and 70% had symptoms of depression.[20] Similarly, a more recent study looking at long-term opioid and crack use among

CULTURAL Considerations

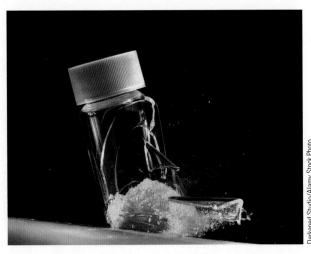

The effects of crack are quick and brief.

Many people feel there is a connection between crack cocaine and violence. In a study completed in 2010, researchers found that crack users reported to be engaged in more violence compared to powder cocaine users.[23] Physical violence in areas such as doing something that could have easily hurt self or others, getting into a fight that came to swapping blows with husband/wife or boyfriend/girlfriend, and hitting someone so hard that you injure that person were higher for crack users. Researchers concluded that individuals who use crack are more likely to engage in all types of violence behaviors compared to users of powder cocaine.[24]

In 1984, laws mandated harsher penalties for individuals arrested for crack cocaine than for powder cocaine. In 2010, the US Sentencing Commission reversed that law. Consequently, that disparity was reduced, and many people who were in prison for charges related to crack cocaine were released. A major factor in the change was that the law was viewed as racially discriminating.

Crack is costly not only to users but to society as well. In a study of crack addicts, many female addicts traded sex for crack, and male addicts traded crack for sex. Also, condoms were used only "sometimes," which has led to high rates of AIDS and associated costs of treatment.

Effects

Cocaine impacts three major neurotransmitters: Dopamine, serotonin, and adrenaline (epinephrine).[25] Dopamine controls the brain's reward and pleasure centers. It also motivates us to take action toward reward seeking behaviors. Cocaine works in the brain by binding to dopamine transporters. This blocks the dopamine reuptake process resulting in an increase of dopamine in the synapse, resulting in the

women found 55% of the women reported having been forced to have sex against their will in their lifetime.[21] In some instances, crack is used to deal with stress.[22] One trend is that fewer people being arrested are testing positive for the presence of crack.

The Action of Cocaine

Normal Synapse

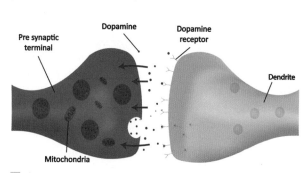

Synapse with Cocaine

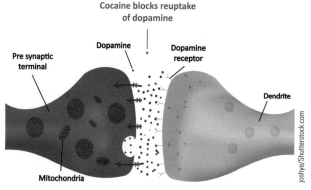

Cocaine blocks the reuptake of dopamine which causes a buildup of dopamine in the synapse.

pleasurable effects from cocaine use.[26] However, the brain only has a limited supply of dopamine; once the dopamine is used up, it takes a while for the brain to produce more. This leaves the user feeling depressed and fatigued.[27] Serotonin influences mood, appetite, and anger. The buildup of serotonin in the brain leaves the cocaine user feeling a sense of confidence. As mentioned earlier, cocaine also impacts adrenaline, which is part of the fight or flight response. An increase of adrenaline in the brain leaves the user feeling energized and increases a person's heart rate and blood flow to skeletal muscles.[28]

A study conducted in 2015 points out another mechanism to the actions of cocaine.[29] Cocaine also impacts the glial cells, which are part of the brain's immune system. Cocaine attaches to the glial cells and triggers an inflammatory response in the brain, further exciting neurons and increasing the amount of dopamine in the brain.[30]

The physical effects of cocaine depend on how the drug enters the body. Some cocaine users place the drug under their tongue, allowing quick absorption. When it is snorted, cocaine is absorbed readily through the mucous membranes of the nose (which have a rich supply of blood vessels) and quickly enters the bloodstream. The peak phase of a cocaine high when taken in this way occurs in 10 to 20 minutes. Intravenous injection produces a high in about 30 seconds and lasts about 10 minutes. Injection, however, is the least common method of taking cocaine.

A variation is the **speedball**, an injected mixture of cocaine and heroin. This mixture carries a higher risk of dependency and overdose, and speedball users have higher rates of psychopathology and HIV infection than other cocaine abusers. Also, when cocaine is used in conjunction with fentanyl, a narcotic more powerful than heroin, there is an increased likelihood of a fatal overdose.[31]

Physical Consequences

When cocaine is snorted, irritations to the nasal membranes, hoarseness, sore throat, and inflamed sinuses are common. Because cocaine is an anesthetic, the nasal passages, throat, and palate become numb from frequent snorting. Snorting leads to sneezing, congestion, burns, sores, and upper respiratory infections including pulmonary congestion, bronchitis, and pneumonia. In extreme cases, people who chronically snort cocaine incur septal necrosis, in which the cartilage separating the two nostrils is destroyed. Snorting cocaine can also lead to a loss of smell and is associated with an elevated risk of mortality. In a recent study comparing the telomere length of elderly women and women addicted to crack cocaine and who had experienced an early life stress, it was shown the women addicted to crack cocaine and who experienced an early life stress had shorter telomeres compared to the elderly non-dependent group.[32] Shortened telomeres are associated with aging-related diseases and organ deterioration. In another study

speedball Injectable combination of heroin and cocaine

conducted over 20 years, it was discovered people who reported a lifetime use of cocaine had elevated mortality risk due to external causes (poisoning, suicide, homicide, and unintentional injury) and elevated mortality due to infectious diseases.[33]

When the effects of cocaine wear off, blood pressure and respiration descend below normal levels, precipitating withdrawal symptoms and an increased desire to take more cocaine. Malnutrition is a problem because cocaine users have less interest in food. People who smoke freebase cocaine often cough up a tarry residue. Freebasing cocaine can cause significant lung damage such as acute bronchoconstriction.[34] Smoked cocaine, especially crack, can produce chest pain, rapid heart rate, irregular heart contractions, circulatory failure, blood pressure that increases to the point of hemorrhaging, or congestive heart failure and death. Injected cocaine carries different risks than snorted cocaine. Besides AIDS, injected cocaine has been linked to inflammation of the heart lining (endocarditis) and liver (hepatitis). The prevalence of HIV is more than two times greater in crack cocaine users than in nonusers.[35]

Cocaine-related crime, abuse rates, and numerous overdose incidents continue to be a burden. Drug users report more criminal behavior compared to nondrug users.[36] One study found those who use cocaine regularly were 6.5 times more likely to commit an acquisitive crime.[37] An acquisitive crime is defined as an offense where the offender gains a material item from the crime (i.e., drugs, money, jewelry).

Psychological Effects

Because the psychological effects of cocaine are subjective, they are open to interpretation. Descriptions of the psychological effects of cocaine are based on interviews with users whose objectivity is questionable. The psychological mosaic of cocaine abusers includes frenzied mood swings, delusions of extraordinary abilities, distortions of perspective, and impaired memory and mental functioning. Because their perspective of the world is dramatically altered, cocaine users claim they are in control, exhilarated, and confident. These delusionary reactions have prompted people to call cocaine "the big lie."

People under the influence of cocaine manifest many social deviations. Some cocaine users become engrossed in repetitive, compulsive behaviors without being aware of what they are doing. Users become detached and neglect personal hygiene, friends, jobs, and schoolwork.

Some cocaine users describe the pleasure they derive from cocaine use as orgasmic. Cocaine often is used as a prelude to romance. Ironically, excessive use actually interferes with sexual pleasure. Like alcohol, it might increase the desire for sex but diminish the ability to perform.

Men and women have different reasons for using cocaine. Women are more likely to use cocaine for depression and stress and have more difficulty overcoming addiction. Women are also more likely to use cocaine to feel sociable, whereas men use it for physical energy.[38]

In the extreme, cocaine psychosis is marked by severe depression, paranoia, rage, thoughts of suicide, and aggressive and violent behavior. Cocaine-induced seizures and psychosis may result from excessive dopamine.[39] Seizures have a direct relationship with cocaine use and for some, can be induced by small quantities of cocaine.[40] Most of these seizures are benign. Psychiatric patients who abuse cocaine and alcohol together have a higher likelihood of homicidal behavior than those who abuse only cocaine or only alcohol. Also, cocaine use can exacerbate the symptoms of posttraumatic stress disorders.

Feelings of paranoia can trigger bizarre behavior that mimics schizophrenia. Some users hallucinate that their arms and legs are getting longer or think they are having an out-of-body experience.

Cocaine diminishes one's need for sleep and the ability to go to sleep. Changes in perception

---

PHYSICAL EFFECTS OF COCAINE

- Elevated blood pressure
- Excessive perspiration
- Nausea, vomiting, abdominal pain
- Headache
- Tightened muscles (including muscles controlling bowel movements)
- Slower digestive process
- Anorexia
- Nutritional deficiencies
- Rapid pulse
- Faster breathing rate
- Increased body temperature
- Urge to urinate, defecate, belch
- Inflammation of trachea and bronchi
- Hoarseness or laryngitis
- Chronic wheezing and heavy coughing
- Coughing up pus, mucus, blood
- Seizures
- Hallucinations

- Talkativeness
- Mood swings
- Hallucinations
- Repetitive behaviors
- Extreme depression
- Neglect of personal hygiene
- Rage and violent behavior
- Delusions
- Distorted perceptions
- Depersonalization
- Suicidal ideation
- Paranoia

occur, distance becomes distorted, and colors intensify. The user may feel bugs crawling on or under the skin, called *cocaine bugs* or formication. People reportedly have tried to rid themselves of these bugs by burning their arms and legs with cigarettes or matches or by scratching themselves constantly.

Dependence

Not all cocaine users, even those who have taken cocaine over several years, experience dependence and withdrawal. Nevertheless, cocaine users build up tolerance to effects of the drug. Unfortunately, users do not develop tolerance to health risks such as seizures, heart attacks, or strokes. Research has not found a "cocaine personality" that accounts for dependency. However, studies have found some associations with users who develop cocaine dependence. Recall from Chapter 10 that many substance abusers experience comorbid conditions. One study looked at cocaine-dependent users who also experienced personality disorders. Among these participants, there was an association with elevated frontal systems-related behavioral symptoms.[41] This area of the brain is associated with executive functioning, which plays a role in attention control, inhibitory control, working memory, reasoning, and problem solving. Participants in the aforementioned study had lower executive functioning compared with cocaine users and nonusers who did not present with comorbid conditions.[42] In another study among cocaine-dependent persons, almost 30% of them had suffered from a traumatic brain injury in their lifetime.[43] This suggests an association with decreased brain functioning and an increased risk for cocaine use. The pleasure derived from cocaine use is self-reinforcing, and some users go on "coke runs," or binges. Perhaps dependency arises not from the desire to feel euphoric but, rather, from the desire not to feel dysphoric.

Cocaine users do not have the classic withdrawal symptoms that narcotic addicts exhibit. Moreover, the withdrawal symptoms associated with cocaine are not life-threatening. Symptoms following cessation of cocaine use include depression, lack of energy, poor appetite, less pleasure from activities, restlessness, and agitation. Scientists are working on the development of a vaccine for preventing addiction to cocaine and other drugs. The concept is to train one's immune system to extinguish the drugs prior to their affect on the nervous system.[44]

Chronic cocaine users demonstrate three phases following abstinence:[45]

1. Intense craving, agitation, anorexia, and deep depression (the "crash"), which can last from 9 hours to 4 days. The desire for cocaine may actually increases over time during withdrawal.[46]
2. Withdrawal, during which the person is incapable of feeling normal pleasure, but depression moderates and sleeping becomes easier, can last up to 10 weeks; although signs and symptoms of moderate cocaine withdrawal tend to stabilize over 7 to 10 days.
3. Extinction, during which improvement is considerable, but periods of depression and occasional craving can last for months and even years.

One study discussed two type of cocaine-dependent persons; type A and type B. A type A-dependent person is one who started using cocaine later in life and does not have a family history of drug abuse. Conversely, a type B-dependent person started using cocaine earlier in life and often has a family history of drug abuse.[47] As one would expect, type B-dependent persons experience stronger withdrawal symptoms and are less successful in treatment programs.

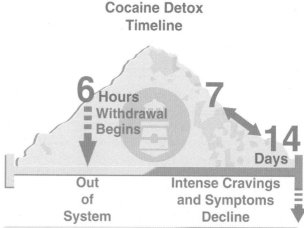

Cocaine Detox Timeline

6 Hours — Withdrawal Begins

Out of System

7

14 Days

Intense Cravings and Symptoms Decline

"Extinction" phase. During this period, which can last for 30 or more weeks, cravings tend to pop up intermittently, often fueled by certain triggers.

Cocaine withdrawal occurs in three phases.

A controversial drug given to cocaine addicts is the African hallucinogen **ibogaine**, which allegedly works by blocking withdrawal symptoms while suppressing the craving for drugs.[48] Ibogaine is structurally similar to serotonin and may help with cocaine addiction in a similar manner as naloxone helps with opioid addiction (see Chapter 8).[49] In addition to research regarding cocaine, ibogaine is being tested to determine whether it is effective for treating narcotic, alcohol, and tobacco dependence. Evidence of its effectiveness is limited to animal studies and unconfirmed reports from individuals. However, in a recent retrospective study conducted in Brazil, where ibogaine is unregulated, drug-dependent patients treated with ibogaine had significantly longer periods of abstinence compared with those who were not treated with the drug.[50] In 2014, the Governor of Vermont addressed the need for ibogaine in the treatment for heroin dependence.[51] Vermont Representative Paul Dame introduced Act H.741, requesting funding for ibogaine clinical trials.[52] Ibogaine is a schedule I drug in the United States, and is legal in other countries. The National Institute on Drug Abuse states there is no long-term proof that it works.

Propranolol, a drug used to treat high blood pressure, has shown promise in helping cocaine addicts. Propranolol eases withdrawal symptoms, making it easier for cocaine addicts to remain in treatment and may also work in reducing cues tied to cocaine dependence.[53] One study looked at the effect of propranolol and cocaine cravings and discovered that propranolol reduced cravings for cocaine more so than the placebo group. Thus patients who received propranolol during treatment exhibited less cravings for cocaine compared to those who did not receive propranolol.[54] Disulfiram, a drug used to treat alcoholism, has also shown potential as a treatment for cocaine addicts. However, some studies have shown no benefits for using disulfiram in the treatment of cocaine-dependent persons. For example, one study found the use of disulfiram along with contingency management for adherence and abstinence (CM) provided no additional benefits compared to using CM alone.[55] Because depression is common among drug-dependent persons, sometimes antidepressants are provided to help treat withdrawal symptoms. While this treatment prototype has been found effective for alcohol-dependent persons, the use of antidepressant medication for cocaine-dependent individuals has been met with mixed results with more studies showing no favorable outcomes for those treated with antidepressant medication.[56]

Death from Cocaine

Because cocaine can cause irregular heartbeat (cardiac arrhythmias), high blood pressure, and chest pains, it can trigger heart attacks. It is capable of destroying the heart muscle by disrupting its blood supply (myocardial infarctions). Coronary artery disease leading to death is relatively common in cocaine users; in fact, cocaine has been shown to increase

---

CONSIDER This

Ibogaine

Ibogaine therapy for the treatment of substance abuse disorders is controversial. In the United States, Ibogaine is a schedule I drug. However, some countries have no regulations on the drug (i.e., Mexico and South Africa) and is used in medical settings to help treat withdrawal symptoms from substance abuse.

Ibogaine has shown some promise for the treatment of substance abuse disorders. Some studies have found that one dose of ibogaine reduces acute withdrawal symptoms without the need for further treatment. In rats and mice, ibogaine treatment results in reduced self-administration of morphine, cocaine, and alcohol.

There is controversy surrounding the drug as some deaths were attributed to ibogaine ingestion. Most of the deaths were attributed to pre-existing conditions, seizures from acute withdrawal, and taking a drug while under the influence of ibogaine.

Methadone, a controlled substance used to treat opioid addiction is not without risk. Some say the risk of death associated with methadone treatment is higher compared to ibogaine treatment.

Questions to Ponder

Ibogaine does carry risk, but is the risk worth the chance of quitting a drug of abuse?

Source: A, R. Kenneth M.D., M. Stajic, Ph.D., and J. R. Gill, M.D., "Fatalities temporally associated with the ingestion of ibogaine. *Journal of Forensic Sciences*", 57, no. 2 (2012).

calcium deposits in the body, resulting in an increase in cocaine-related coronary deaths.[57] Cocaine users have a higher incidence of myocardial infarction (aka: heart attack) with an increase of 24-fold in the first hour after cocaine use.[58] It is estimated that cocaine contributes to about one in every four myocardial infarctions in persons aged between 18 and 45 years old.[59] Some deaths result from "body packing," a method of smuggling cocaine by which it is placed in condoms or plastic bags and swallowed. Often the bags break and the cocaine leaks into the intestines.

Some fatalities from cocaine use result from uncontrolled seizures, strokes, or paralysis of breathing muscles. A lethal dose of cocaine has not been determined precisely. Some people die from relatively low levels.

When death strikes, it tends to come quickly. Some victims do not reach medical facilities in time to receive medical attention. Rates from cocaine deaths have increased and are estimated to be about 2.13 per 100,000 in 2015.[60] Recent data regarding these deaths have suggested the increase is due to a combination of taking heroin and opioids along with cocaine and are not attributed to cocaine alone. Furthermore, the data suggests the increase in the use of fentanyl with opioids are contributing to the death rate from taking cocaine and opioids.[61]

People who inject cocaine are in danger of contracting HIV infection and the eventually fatal AIDS. A person with a weakened immune system is more susceptible to bacterial or viral infections such as pneumonia and meningitis, as well as cancer. In some cities, cocaine and other drugs are injected in places called **shooting galleries**. Because of the illegal status of cocaine and the clandestine nature of shooting galleries, educating addicts about the need to discard needles safely or how to clean needles properly is not easy.

Cocaine and Pregnancy

It is estimated that about 5% of pregnant women use one or more illegal substances.[62] Each year, there are around 750,000 cocaine-exposed pregnancies.[63] Compared with other pregnant women, those who use cocaine drink more, smoke more, have worse nutritional intake, and generally are in poorer overall health. Blood flowing through the placenta delivers oxygen to the fetus. Cocaine constricts blood vessels and thereby blood flow and oxygen. Also, cocaine can cause detachment of the placenta, as well as premature labor, by stimulating uterine contractions, and women who use cocaine during pregnancy have higher rates of spontaneous abortion. Women who use cocaine during pregnancy experience poorer birth outcomes such as preterm birth, low birth weight, and small head circumference.[64]

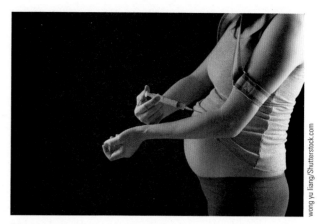

wong yu liang/Shutterstock.com

Should women who test positive for cocaine while pregnant be incarcerated?

In children who were exposed to cocaine prenatally, studies suggest negative effects in attention, executive functioning, language, and behavior.[65] A study conducted on cocaine-exposed children used magnetic resonance imaging (MRI) on children at 7 and 14 years of age. Results from this study found that although overall IQ did not seem to be different in cocaine-exposed children, there were negative effects on perceptual reasoning IQ and visual motor skills. Furthermore, in children exposed to cocaine neonatally, they is decreased grey matter in the occipital and parietal lobes compared to noncocaine-exposed children. This study also found children who were exposed to cocaine neonatally had an increased risk of substance misuse later in life.[66] Another study noted that boys who were prenatally exposed to cocaine had difficulty regulating emotion and exhibited a lack of inhibitory control.[67]

Some babies of women who use cocaine while they are pregnant have neurological problems, perhaps caused by strokes before birth. Cocaine-exposed babies have higher rates of congenital heart defects, lower birth weights, and seizures, and they are more at risk for sudden infant death. Cocaine-exposed babies tend to be born with smaller heads, which often reflect smaller brains. Determining whether these effects result from the mother's cocaine use or from poor prenatal care is difficult. Also, fetal development can be affected by alcohol consumption, cigarette smoking, and other drugs, as well as environmental factors such as poverty, poor nutrition, homelessness, violence, and crime.

Media articles have warned that social and psychological consequences will surface as prenatally

ibogaine A hallucinogen that is used to treat cocaine dependence

shooting galleries Places to buy and inject drugs

exposed children enter school. These children are expected to be irritable, hyperactive, and difficult to console. While these dire forecasts are overexerted, there are some concerns with children who were exposed to cocaine neonatally.[68] Condemning these drug-exposed children with labels indicating a permanent handicap is premature.

One study looked at adolescents at the age of 15 years who were exposed to cocaine in utero during the first trimester of pregnancy. This study analyzed three domains including behavior, cognitive, and growth. For the behavioral domain, the adolescents who were exposed to cocaine reported more delinquent behavior problems including damage and theft. Additionally, these adolescents reported poorer mood outcomes. For the cognitive domain, the cocaine-exposed adolescents performed poorer on the Children's Category Test compared to nonexposed adolescents. Other cognitive tests showed similar outcomes for both groups. For the growth outcomes, prenatal exposure to cocaine was associated with reduced weight, height, and head circumference that persisted to 15 years of age.[69] Not all hope is lost; the cognitive development of infants whose mothers stopped using cocaine after giving birth was higher than for infants whose mothers continued to use drugs.[70] In addition, home environments that are mentally stimulating lessen the prenatal effects of cocaine.[71]

Amphetamines

Amphetamines have played an important role since first marketed in 1927. During World War II, they were given to American soldiers to help them overcome fatigue, heighten their mood, and improve their endurance.[72] They do, however, produce side effects that are disadvantageous in combat. Hitler's bizarre behavior near the end of World War II, in which he was alternately depressed and happy, is speculated to have been caused by amphetamines.

Early Applications

When amphetamines were developed, they were effective in treating asthma. Under the name **Benzedrine**, amphetamine was sold in inhalers. The user would open the inhaler, put the concentrated amphetamine liquid on a cloth, and inhale it. Eventually, the inhalers were used nonmedically, and the US Food and Drug Administration (FDA) banned amphetamines in inhalers in 1959.

Amphetamines have been used for treating depression, for increasing work capacity, and for treating **narcolepsy**. Narcoleptics fall asleep

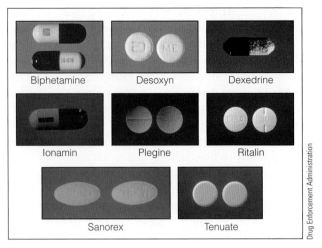

There are a variety of amphetamines on the market today.

spontaneously and sometimes sleep for long periods. It was noted that narcoleptic patients given amphetamines were not hungry. The drug then was used to suppress appetite and ward off fatigue. Beginning in the late 1930s, it was given to hyperactive children. During World War II, American airmen in Great Britain often took Benzedrine pills.[73] Before meeting Soviet Premier Nikita Khruschev in 1961, President Kennedy was believed to have used amphetamines to maintain his energy.[74] In the 1960s, there were 20 million prescriptions written for amphetamines for weight-loss purposes.[75] Amphetamines and amphetamine-like drugs are still used to treat obesity.[76]

Pharmacology

Amphetamines can be administered by ingestion, injection, snorting, or inhalation. When taken orally, they produce peak effects in 2 to 3 hours. The half-life is 10 to 12 hours, and they are not totally eliminated from the body for about 2 days.

The effects are felt more quickly—usually within 5 minutes—when they are injected. Because tolerance to amphetamines develops quickly, many users do not derive pleasure from the drug. Therefore they increase the dosage or go on binges to maintain their high.

Because amphetamines increase activity of the sympathetic nervous system, they are classified as sympathomimetic drugs. Their physiological effects are similar to those in people who are emotionally aroused: increased respiration and perspiration, higher blood pressure and body temperature, increased blood flow to the extremities, and dilation of the pupils.

Amphetamines are absorbed by the blood and distributed rapidly. Their chemical structure is similar to that of the neurotransmitters norepinephrine and dopamine. Amphetamines stimulate receptor sites for these neurotransmitters which releases dopamine and norepinephrine. In addition, they block the reuptake of these neurotransmitters, causes a buildup in the synapse.[77] By stimulating norepinephrine receptors, the drug makes the individual feel more alert. When dopamine receptors are stimulated, the person becomes euphoric and more active.

Amphetamines are removed from the body in two ways:

1. They are excreted through urine after being transformed by liver enzymes.
2. They are deactivated and removed by adding molecules to the amphetamine compound.

Potential psychological effects of amphetamines include paranoia, violence, restlessness, agitation, hallucinations, confusion, and anxiety. Amphetamines may increase the likelihood for producing seizures. One study looked at patients who experienced seizures after taking amphetamines. Of those who experienced a seizure, 40% had a risk factor for epilepsy and for most, sleep deprivation may have contributed to the seizures.[78] Possible physical effects are tremors, tinnitus (ringing in ears), dry mouth, excessive perspiration, increased blood pressure, poor coordination, and convulsions. Amphetamines are especially harmful to the cardiovascular system and can cause cardiac arrest. Intranasal use of amphetamines elevate blood pressure and heart rate more quickly than amphetamines taken orally.[79] Evidence indicates that amphetamine use may increase the risk of stroke, especially when taken in large doses without a prescription.[80] Individuals hospitalized due to amphetamines or methamphetamines are at an increased risk for Parkinson's disease.[81] Not all effects are detrimental. Amphetamines appear to help memory gain in multiple sclerosis patients.[82]

The Amphetamine Trade

Japan and Sweden have had far more severe problems with amphetamine abuse than the United States. To maintain production during World War II, Japanese workers were given amphetamines. As the war ended, massive amounts of the drug remained. To reduce this surplus, pharmaceutical companies sold amphetamines without prescription. This led to amphetamine abuse and medical problems. About 2% of Japan's population was abusing the drug. By the mid-1950s, the Japanese government curtailed production of the drug and provided more treatment, education, and punitive measures. This effort helped to reduce abuse.

Amphetamine abuse was a serious problem in Sweden in the 1940s, necessitating stringent

EFFECTS OF AMPHETAMINES

Psychological	Physical
• Paranoia	• Tremors
• Violent behavior	• Tinnitus
• Restlessness	• Dry mouth
• Agitation	• Excessive sweating
• Confusion	• High blood pressure
• Anxiety	• Poor coordination
• Hallucinations	• Convulsions
	• Cardiac arrest

regulations. Although the abuse of orally ingested amphetamines declined, a segment of hardcore users began injecting amphetamines intravenously. The Swedish government dealt with this dilemma by providing narcotics and stimulants to abusers. Within two years, this program was considered a failure. By 1968, Sweden had banned amphetamines and other stimulants.

Although people in the United States could legally obtain amphetamines in the 1930s, amphetamines were also available illegally. The main users were truck drivers and college students. Truck stops often served as distribution sites. In addition, amphetamines were obtained easily by prescription to treat depression or obesity. Hospital emergency rooms would administer amphetamines to people who had overdosed on sleeping pills. Because of indiscriminate prescribing, the federal government imposed regulations in 1965 to limit their access.

Amphetamines had been so available that every man, woman, and child could be supplied several times daily. They represented about 8% of prescriptions in 1970. By this time, the drug subculture was in place, especially in San Francisco, and drug use flourished for several years before it began to decline.

During the well-known "Summer of Love" in San Francisco in 1967, young people gathered to protest the Vietnam War, decry prejudice and poverty, engage in "free love," and take mind-altering drugs, primarily marijuana and LSD. Within a short time, heroin and amphetamines replaced marijuana and LSD as the drugs of choice. The "flower child" was supplanted by the "speed freak."

Benzedrine An amphetamine used to treat nasal congestion and asthma

narcolepsy Condition in which the person involuntarily falls asleep; commonly called sleeping sickness

Consequences of Amphetamine Use

Like cocaine, amphetamines do not produce classic withdrawal symptoms similar to those with narcotics or barbiturates. Still, most people who are dependent on amphetamines experience withdrawal, continue using them despite problems, cannot stop, develop tolerance, and give up other activities to use amphetamines. Many of the withdrawal symptoms subside within a couple of weeks, but sleep disruption can continue for up to 4 weeks.[83]

After several days of moderate to heavy use, individuals crash. This condition is marked by symptoms opposite to the effects of amphetamines—lethargy, exhaustion, depression, and hunger. Symptoms of amphetamine withdrawal, though not life-threatening, are undeniable. Within hours after an individual stops taking large doses, energy levels decline, mood is altered, and sleep may follow, for up to 24 hours. On waking, the user feels depressed. One study found a strong association between those who inject cocaine and amphetamines and suicide attempts.[84]

Stimulants can improve mental and physical performance. For simple tasks, amphetamines are effective, but for tasks requiring complex thinking, such as problem-solving and decision-making, they are counterproductive. Because high doses affect judgment and decision-making skills negatively, they can cause severe behavioral problems.

One way in which amphetamines have been shown to influence judgment is that users are less likely to use condoms when engaging in sexual behavior. One study found methamphetamine and amphetamine use to be significantly associated with HIV infection among men who have sex with men in high-income countries.[85]

In some instances, users act compulsively and repetitiously. Laboratory animals given high doses have been known to turn in circles continuously or gnaw at the bars of their cages. Gross motor skills improve at the same time as fine motor skills are impaired. Athletes who need speed and strength benefit more from amphetamines than athletes who have to be accurate, although the risks outweigh the benefits. One group of people who are currently using amphetamines is professional baseball players. Although Major League Baseball is concerned about players using steroids, an increasing number of players are taking amphetamines. However, many players are obtaining prescriptions to take the drugs legally. In 2006, 28 players received amphetamines because they were diagnosed with ADHD. In 2007, that number jumped to 103. In 2010, 105 players, about 8% of all players, received medication for ADHD. In 2015, nearly 10% of all baseball players had a amphetamine prescription for ADHD.[86] The adult prevalence of ADHD in the US population is about 4 to 6%.[87] Some believe these exemptions for amphetamines use among baseball players is a way to gain a competitive edge to the game. Others believe the increased rate is due to the fact that children who have ADHD are drawn to competitive sports as an outlet for their hyperactivity.[88]

Amphetamine psychosis, a condition marked by paranoia, aggressiveness, fearfulness, disordered thinking, mania, and hallucinations, is a significant problem related to chronic use. Suspicion and paranoia often lead to hostile and violent behaviors. In reality, the violent behavior might be caused by sleep deprivation, which also can result in suspiciousness and paranoia. Some evidence suggests that use of amphetamines can cause brain damage and exacerbate Tourette's syndrome and tardive dyskinesia.

The dosage of amphetamines required to generate side effects varies among individuals, though beginning users are more likely to have side effects because they have less tolerance. As little as 2 mg can produce negative side effects in some people, whereas other people can take 15 mg before having adverse effects.

"Speed kills," a popular slogan of the 1960s, alluded to the potential consequences of taking amphetamines. Amphetamine abusers can die from their risk-taking behavior while under the drug's influence, from suicide resulting from the severe depression following a "run," or from the associated unhealthy lifestyle in which nutrition and health are neglected. Few people actually die from an overdose, although people can incur irregular heartbeat, heart stoppage, and strokes during heavy usage.

Methamphetamines

After World War II, **methamphetamines**, popularly known as **speed**, began to be widely abused in the United States. Rates for use and abuse have been declining since 1999. In 2016, prevalence rates for methamphetamine use among 8th, 10th, and 12th graders were at an all-time low with rates being 0.4% for both 8th and 10th graders and 0.6% for 12th graders.[89] Like amphetamines, this more potent version has been used to treat narcolepsy, suppress appetite, and relieve the symptoms of Parkinson's disease. Methamphetamines, however, are more likely than amphetamines to be used for nonmedical purposes. Crystals of methamphetamine, known as "ice," are put into the glass bowl of a pipe and heated from below. The vapors then are inhaled. When methamphetamines are taken like this, the person feels the effects in a few seconds.

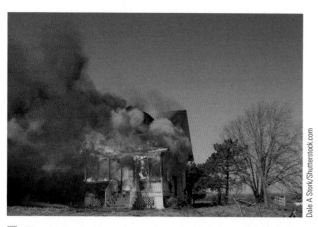

Dale A Stark/Shutterstock.com

Chemicals used to make methamphetamines are highly flammable causing labs to explode.

"Speed freaks" go on binges, shooting up every few hours over a 5- or 6-day period before crashing and then sleeping from 12 hours to 4 days.

Clandestine Methamphetamine Laboratories

The three main types of harm associated with methamphetamine labs are (1) physical injury from explosions, fires, chemical burns, and toxic fumes; (2) environmental hazards; and (3) child endangerment.[90] Methamphetamine labs can explode due to the processing of chemicals at extremely high temperatures. Moreover, safety procedures and adequate ventilation are often overlooked. Not only is the lab a danger to the people making the drug, but police sometimes will trigger explosions when entering a lab. A common way for methamphetamine labs to be discovered is when a fire or explosion occurs.

As indicated, methamphetamine labs pose environmental hazards. For every pound of manufactured methamphetamine, 5 to 6 pounds of hazardous waste are produced.[91] The waste may be disposed of by pouring it down the drain, dumping it along roads, placing it in streams or lakes, or by burning it. Sanitation workers can experience adverse reactions due to their exposure to the hazardous waste. Contamination from hazardous waste can remain in the soil or water supply for many years. One study of methamphetamine labs found that one-fourth of people involved with these labs suffered some type of injury.[92]

Children living in a space that produces illicit methamphetamines is a great cause of concern. Even with decontamination protocols in place, chemicals produced by clandestine methamphetamine labs can stay in drywall, clothing, and children's toys for a long period.[93] Children are at an increased risk due to exposure to these chemicals due to their rapidly developing central nervous and endocrine systems and accelerated rates of bone and organ growth.[94] While clandestine lab incidents are going down, there were almost 9,400 incidents in 2014, down from a little over 12,000 in 2013.[95]

In the United States, methamphetamines have become the number-one drug problem in rural areas per the Drug Enforcement Agency. A strong relationship has been found between counties with the greatest pseudoephedrine sales and clandestine labs.[96] In 2005, the federal government enacted the CMEA (Combat Methamphetamine Epidemic Act), which placed restrictions on the over-the-counter purchase of pseudoephedrine, a drug required to make methamphetamines.[97] Besides production in clandestine laboratories in the United States, however, Mexico has become a major source for the drug.

Methamphetamine's Effects

Methamphetamine-related emergency room visits, admissions to publicly funded treatment facilities, and deaths have increased significantly. In 2011, 102,961 individuals visited emergency rooms because of methamphetamines. This is a significant increase compared to previous years where in 2007, almost 70,000 emergency room visits were attributed to methamphetamines.[98] More than half of these visits involve methamphetamine use with another drug and one-third are due to the presence of two or more drugs.[99] In more than half of the cases, patients are treated and released.

The abuse of methamphetamines is not limited to any one group of people; however, one group that

methamphetamines More potent forms of amphetamine

speed A stimulant drug; another name for methamphetamine

"speed freaks" People who use methamphetamines over a period of time

has been especially affected is Native Americans. On some Indian reservations, methamphetamine abuse rates have reached 30%.[100] Methamphetamine abuse by Native Americans are three times as high compared with White Americans.[101] Native American reservations are in remote areas, making it very difficult to police.[102] It is relevant to note that about one-half of all treatment admissions for methamphetamine abuse were referred by the criminal justice system.

Many users take methamphetamines in conjunction with other drugs such as cocaine and marijuana. Methamphetamines are the drug of choice for many young people because of the relatively low cost, and the high can last up to 14 hours. Methamphetamines produce many adverse effects, including slurred speech, loss of appetite, excitement, increased blood pressure and heart rate, irregular heartbeat, a pounding heart sensation, severe chest pain, hot flashes, excessive perspiration, anxiety, tremors, confusion, insomnia, convulsions, memory loss, violent behavior, elevated body temperature, paranoia, auditory hallucinations, and death. Recent research shows that methamphetamines can cause irreversible damage to blood vessels in the brain.[103]

In the late 1970s, **ice** entered the drug scene. Named for its clear crystal form, ice is also called **crystal meth** and **crank**. Ice has been produced largely in Far Eastern countries, primarily Korea, Taiwan, and the Philippines, and transported to the United States, most commonly into Hawaii.

The increase in the amount of ice available can be attributed to the proliferation of clandestine laboratories. Ice can be manufactured from chemicals purchased legally from chemical supply stores.

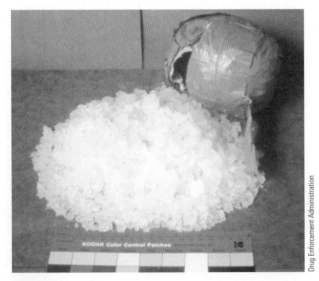

Drug Enforcement Administration

■ "Ice," so named because of its appearance, is a smokable form of methamphetamine.

Ice can be injected or smoked. When it is smoked, the user feels profound emotional and physical arousal in a few seconds. Ice is often used compulsively, and users do not eat or rest for days. The dangers from ice possibly exceed those of other stimulants because its effects last 12 or more hours. (In contrast, the effects from crack last several minutes.) Ice poses numerous problems: Users are less resistant to illness. The liver, kidneys, and lungs are especially vulnerable. Babies born to pregnant women who have taken ice tend to be asocial and incapable of bonding. Ice causes psychological dependence and withdrawal symptoms including anxiety, intense depression, fatigue, insomnia, paranoia, and delusions.

Ritalin and Adderall

Stimulants have been used to treat children's behavioral problems since 1937. The most prescribed drugs for **attention deficit hyperactivity disorder (ADHD)** are **Ritalin** (methylphenidate) and Adderall. ADHD usually begins in childhood and is characterized by developmentally inappropriate hyperactivity, impulsivity, and inattention. Changes in the criteria and their interpretation have broadened, allowing more individuals to be diagnosed with ADHD. Between 2011 and 2013, almost 10% of all children were diagnosed with ADHD.[104] ADHD is the number-one identified childhood psychiatric disorder in the United States.[105] Because diagnosis of ADHD is imprecise, some parents and physicians are questioning whether Ritalin is overprescribed. In the United Kingdom, per capita use of Ritalin is one-tenth the amount used in the United States. Guidelines from their National Institute for Health and Care provide guidance for when these drugs should be used and suggest they should be used as a last resort. However, in recent years, they have seen an increase in prescription medication use for the treatment of ADHD, which doubled from 2004 to 2010.[106]

The number of children treated with Ritalin is unprecedented. Americans consume more than 80% of the world's Ritalin.[107] The increase in the diagnosis of ADHD is partly attributable to heightened public awareness and changes in educational policy in which schools are obliged to identify children with the disorder. Children with ADHD have a higher risk for substance abuse disorders later in life. However, studies are now showing that when children are treated early with stimulant medication, their risk of a later substance abuse disorder goes down.[108,109]

Ritalin has a good safety record with school-aged children. Children on Ritalin are at no greater cardiovascular risk than children not on Ritalin.[110]

Misuse of Prescription Medication in College

With estimates between 4% and 28% of all college students having used a non-prescription stimulant medication during their academic career, it is not surprising this has become a public health concern in the United States.[1] Most college students who report using no-prescription stimulant medication do so to improve academic performance.[2] One study found a relationship among college students using non-prescription stimulant medication and alcohol use and abuse.[3] Other studies found the following characteristics associated with nonmedical use of prescription stimulants:[4]

- Excessive drinking and other drug use
- Lower GPA
- Psychiatric distress or depressed mood
- Skipping classes
- Affiliation with a Greek organization

While most college students who use nonmedical prescription stimulants cite academic performance behind the motivation for using the drug, studies show use of nonmedical prescription stimulants is associated with lower GPAs.[5] The use of these drugs by college students may be compensatory behavior for not attending class and having an overly active social life.

Sources:

1. R. M. Ward, B.B. Oswald, and M. Galante, "Prescription stimulant misuse, alcohol abuse, and disordered eating among college students", *Journal of Alcohol & Drug Education,* 60, no.1 (2016): 59-80.
2. Ibid
3. Ibid.
4. Center on Youth Adult Health and Development, "Nonmedical use of prescription stimulants", *University of Maryland-Public Health.* Accessed on February 20, 2017 from http://webcache.googleusercontent.com/search?q=cache:vpGlinSvup4J:medicineabuseproject.org/assets/documents/NPSFactSheet.pdf+&cd=19&hl=en&ct=clnk&gl=us.
5. Ibid.

Compared with amphetamines and cocaine, Ritalin is milder and causes fewer side effects. Because the high from Ritalin is brief, it is not as likely as cocaine to be abused. The typical dose is 10 to 30 mg in the morning and at midday.

Using Ritalin to treat children exhibiting ADHD is paradoxical. Logically, if a child is hyperactive, Ritalin should increase activity. Instead, the drug helps moderate a child's activity level. A low dosage of Ritalin helps children's cognitive processing, whereas a high dosage helps children with severe ADHD. Ritalin and other stimulants enhance the functioning of the reticular activating system, which helps children focus attention and filter out extraneous stimuli. It is estimated that Ritalin and other stimulants are effective with 70 to 80% of children with ADHD.[111]

Many adverse effects have been associated with Ritalin. These include insomnia, weight loss, headaches, irritability, nausea, and dizziness. Research into whether Ritalin affects a child's growth is

ice Crystals of methamphetamine that are smoked, inhaled, or injected

crystal meth A variation of methamphetamine; one example is ice

crank A term for methamphetamines

attention deficit hyperactivity disorder (ADHD) A condition in which the individual is hyperactive and easily distracted, which inhibits learning

Ritalin A mild stimulant used to treat attention deficit/hyperactivity disorder (ADHD)

inconclusive. Although some studies report weight gain, one current study indicated no significant change in height or body mass index.[112] Ritalin does not cause physical dependency in children, although psychological dependence is possible. A rare problem is facial tics. If tics appear, they tend to subside once the person stops taking Ritalin.

Caffeine

Caffeine is the world's most frequently consumed stimulant. In the United States, about 90% of people drink caffeinated beverages with 80% of adults consuming caffeine everday.[113] Many people get their stimulation through tea, which contains caffeine and **theophylline**, a stimulant from the same chemical family as caffeine. Theophylline is less potent than caffeine, but the caffeine content is greater in some types of tea than in some coffees. Theophylline acts as a bronchodilator and is effective for treating asthma. Used since the 1970s, theophylline is a safe drug that actually increases the growth rate of asthmatic children and does not interfere with sleep.

Products containing caffeine extend beyond beverages to gum, mints, beer, candy, sunflower seeds, and soap.[114] Caffeine is found in many over-the-counter and prescription medicines and chocolate. Because caffeine is so ubiquitous, many children are receiving it unknowingly. Many experts recommend that children under age 6 avoid caffeinated beverages altogether.[115] A glass of chocolate milk has about 5 mg of caffeine. A stimulant in chocolate, **theobromine**, is related chemically to caffeine but is less powerful. Theobromine is more plentiful in cocoa than in caffeine.

Because millions of people consume caffeine, they may not want to believe that the legal substances they are consuming have psychological, pharmacological, and physiological properties similar to those of illegal drugs. The difference is a matter of degree. Caffeine is milder than amphetamines and cocaine. The amount of caffeine in various soft drinks is shown in Table 11.1.

High-Energy Caffeinated Beverages

Increasingly, beverage companies are trying to boost the sale of soft drinks by adding more caffeine to new products. From 2004 to 2009, sales of energy drinks increased 240%.[116] In 2016, sales have leveled off for

TABLE 11.1 Caffeine Content in Selected Soft Drinks and Energy Drinks

Drink	Company	Milligrams of Caffeine in 12 oz.
Soft Drinks		
JOLT	Wet Planet	72
Mountain Dew Code Red	PepsiCo	55
Mountain Dew	PepsiCo	55
Mello Yello	Coca-Cola	51
Diet Coke	Coca-Cola	45
Dr Pepper	Cadbury	41
Pepsi-Cola	PepsiCo	38
Energy Drinks		
Redline Power Rush	Vital Pharmaceuticals	1,680
JOLT Endurance Shot	Wet Planet	900
Cocaine Energy Drink	Redux Beverages	400
Blow (Energy Drink Mix)	Kingpin Concepts	360
Monster	Monster Beverage	120
Red Bull	Red Bull	116

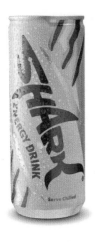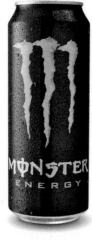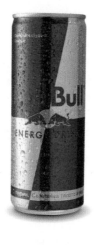

Chones/Shutterstock.com

While unregulated by the FDA, they recommend no more than 72 mg of caffeine per 12 ounces. Many energy drinks exceed that limit.

energy drinks.[117] The FDA does not regulate caffeine in food and drinks. However, its guidelines suggest that a safe level of caffeine is 72 mg per 12 ounces. Many beverages such as Red Bull, Monster, and Rock Star exceed that level.

Of emergency room visits for persons aged 12 and older, 10% of them were related to energy drinks.[118] The number of emergency room visits due to energy drinks doubled between 2007 and 2011.[119] To counter the sedating effects of alcohol, some individuals alternate with these high-energy drinks when drinking alcohol. Individuals who consume high-energy drinks and alcohol are more likely to drink alcohol more heavily than those individuals who do not drink high-energy drinks, and they are also at greater risk for becoming alcohol dependent.[120] Drinkers who consume energy drinks with alcohol are three times more likely to binge drink and are twice as likely to report being taken advantage of sexually or taking advantage of someone else sexually.[121]

Pharmacology

Although most people who use caffeine do so orally, it can be administered rectally or by injection. Like that of other drugs, the onset of its actions occurs quickly when it is injected. Caffeine acts as an antagonist to receptors for the inhibitory neurotransmitter **adenosine**. Therefore the action of caffeine as a stimulant arises from its inhibitory effect. Caffeine obstructs adenosine's inhibition of brain cells, heightening alertness and mood.

When two negative numbers are multiplied together, the product is positive. This is exactly how caffeine works. By reducing inhibition, the effect is stimulation. Peak effects from caffeine occur 30 to 45 minutes after consumption. One study found that college students are able to maintain more attention during a 75-minute lecture if they consume caffeine an hour prior to the lecture.[122] A more recent study found similar caffeine injection in the morning improved explicit memory but not implicit memory.[123] This same study showed no improvements in memory from caffeine intake during afternoon hours. Caffeine can prevent automobile accidents by keeping drivers alert and awake.[124]

Caffeine use by well-conditioned athletes has been found to improve their endurance on a short-term basis. Olympic athletes that are most likely to consume caffeine before or during competition are triathletes, cyclists, and rowers.[125] One study found the preexercise ingestion of 3 mg of caffeine increased performance among Brazilian Jiu jitsu athletes by improving dynamic and isotonic muscular force and endurance strength.[126] A moderate amount of caffeine improves cycling endurance, although there is no additional benefit when caffeine levels are significantly increased.[127]

Extreme caffeine intake, however, has been linked to a low blood sugar condition called **hypoglycemia**. Excessive sweating, feelings of tiredness, fainting, and weakness are characteristics of low blood sugar. Caffeine is metabolized by liver enzymes. The kidneys excrete almost all the caffeine ingested, but tiny amounts are eliminated through saliva, feces, semen, and breast milk. Women should be cautioned that oral contraceptives and pregnancy slow the metabolism and excretion of caffeine.

Properties and Risks

Caffeine is a member of the **xanthine** family. Xanthines are stimulants that improve work capacity, alertness, and motor performance while curbing fatigue. Caffeine may delay the progression of Alzheimer's disease.[128] Another benefit is that caffeine widens air passages in the lungs, enabling asthmatics to breathe easier and deeper. There is some evidence to suggest that moderate amounts of caffeine may reduce the risk of type 2 diabetes in younger

theophylline A stimulant found in tea; in the same chemical family as caffeine

theobromine A stimulant found in chocolate; chemically related to caffeine

adenosine A neurotransmitter for which caffeine acts as an antagonist

hypoglycemia A condition of low levels of sugar in the blood

xanthine A type of stimulant; caffeine is an example

and middle-aged women.[129] Caffeine has been associated with lower mortality rates from cardiovascular diseases, but the mechanism to which these benefits is seen is not well known as the same benefit has been seen among those who consume decaffeinated coffees.[130] A recent study discovered caffeine was inversely related to telomere length.[131] Individuals who have shorter telomere lengths have an increased risk of early death compared to those with longer telomeres. Furthermore, telomere length can be used as a predictive factor for years of healthy life.[132]

If caffeine is taken on an empty stomach, it releases stomach acids and digestive enzymes, causing an upset stomach. Caffeine increases the need to urinate and can cause dehydration.[133] Both caffeinated and decaffeinated drinks produce a laxative effect. Other effects include nervousness, anxiety, insomnia, heartburn, and symptoms of premenstrual syndrome. Although caffeine can improve motor performance, it adversely affects motor coordination.

Moderate caffeine consumption has not been shown to be deleterious to individuals with known or suspected arrhythmias.[134] Caffeine increases blood pressure within the first hour after ingestion and will remain slightly higher for up to 3 hours.[135]

Some women report breast pain symptoms improve when caffeine is eliminated from their diet. However, no research has shown caffeine impacts breast cysts or benign breast disease.[136] Furthermore, the American Cancer Institute states that there is no association between fibrocystic breast disease and caffeine. Studies conducted in the 1990s found no conclusive evidence linking breast cancer to caffeine. Recent studies confirm that caffeine does not increase the risk for breast cancer.[137] Caffeinated coffee decreases the likelihood of cancer of the oral cavity and pharynx,[138] endometrial cancer in postmenopausal women,[139] and prostate cancer.[140]

Effects of Caffeine

The effects of caffeine on wakefulness, coordination, and mood vary considerably among individuals. At moderate levels, caffeine increases blood pressure, body temperature, blood sugar levels, metabolism, urination, and hand tremors, and decreases appetite and coordination. In large amounts, it causes nausea, diarrhea, shaking, headache, and nervousness. At its worst, caffeine can cause convulsions, respiratory failure, and, if one drinks 70 to 100 cups of coffee, death.

Because caffeine stimulates the cortex of the brain, thought processes quickly improve, becoming more efficient, albeit temporarily. Memory improves and reaction time decreases. Other benefits include easing of asthma, relieving of painful bouts

of gallstones, and weight loss. Heavy caffeine use also affects the developing fetus, because caffeine crosses the placenta easily. In numerous studies, women who used moderate amounts—three cups of coffee daily—were *not* likely to have miscarriages or have any fetal abnormalities. One study found an association between caffeine intake during pregnancy and low birth weight. This study found a 3% increase in low birth rates for every additional 100 mg of caffeine ingested (1 cup of coffee or 2 cups of tea).[141] Another prospective study found that in-utero exposure to caffeine is associated with an 87% increase in childhood obesity.[142] Infants can receive caffeine through breast milk. Children nursed by mothers who drink caffeinated beverages appear more nervous or agitated. The effects of caffeine are greater in newborns and infants because they cannot metabolize and eliminate caffeine as readily as adults.

Caffeine users seem to need the drug to achieve alertness and to eliminate withdrawal symptoms, which appear in people who consume two and a half cups of coffee or more daily. Withdrawal symptoms become apparent about 12 to 16 hours after the last caffeine intake. Headache is the most commonly reported withdrawal symptom. Others include depression, lethargy, lower energy level, sleepiness/drowsiness, and irritability.

Decaffeinated Coffee

Because of the adverse publicity surrounding caffeine use, many people are drinking decaffeinated coffee, in which the caffeine has been displaced from the coffee bean using a hot water solution. The caffeine then is taken out of the water with the aid of an organic solvent. The National Cancer Institute identified the original solvent, trichloroethylene, as potentially carcinogenic. Subsequently, methylene chloride, a substance used in paint remover, was substituted. Methylene chloride also might contribute to cancer. A survey conducted by *Consumer Reports* found that decaffeinated coffee has some degree of caffeine. In six different locations where decaffeinated coffee was purchased, levels of caffeine varied from 5 to 32 mg per 10 to 12 ounces.[143] About 100 mg is considered normal in a typical cup of coffee.

Caffeinism

Dependency on caffeine is called **caffeinism**. More than one-half of moderate coffee drinkers who stop drinking it experience moderate to severe headaches. Most caffeine users acknowledge that they are dependent on it and that they have difficulty stopping. Caffeinism is marked by irritability, depression, and insomnia. Headaches and morning lethargy are the most common withdrawal symptoms. These symptoms tend to last for 3 or 4 days.[144] Despite the fact that caffeine cessation may result in withdrawal symptoms, some people contend that it is not addictive and should not be used in the same sentence as cocaine or heroin addiction.[145] Literature regarding caffeine use disorder is incomplete as well as the best methods to treat caffeine use disorder.[146] More addiction

professionals do not believe caffeine dependence should be included in the DSM.[147] About one-fourth of users experience withdrawal symptoms when they discontinue drinking it.[148]

Summary

Stimulant drugs increase activity levels and alter mood. Cocaine is the most commonly used illegal stimulant. Derived from the coca plant, cocaine is a colorless, crystalline powder after it is refined. It was included in many over-the-counter products until the Harrison Narcotic Act was passed in 1914.

A variation, freebase, appeared in the 1960s. The popularity of cocaine rose in the 1970s, accompanied by an increase in cocaine-related deaths. In the 1980s, the more affordable crack cocaine emerged. Its effects are short-lived but profound.

When it is smoked, cocaine can cause nasal, pulmonary, and cardiovascular problems and even death. Psychological effects include mood swings, distortions, and delusions. Users report feeling confident, in control, and exhilarated.

Cocaine abstinence has three phases: (1) the *crash*, marked by intense craving and deep depression; (2) *withdrawal*, when depression moderates but the person is incapable of feeling normal pleasure; and (3) *extinction*, when depression and craving subside but may reappear. Although cocaine withdrawal is unlikely to be fatal, using the drug itself can have tragic consequences because it can produce an irregular heartbeat or heart attack.

Cocaine use during pregnancy may result in poorer birth outcomes including low birthweight babies and premature delivery. Studies suggest children who were exposed to cocaine prenatally have negative effects in attention, language, and behavior.

Amphetamines, another type of stimulant, have been used to treat asthma, narcolepsy, fatigue, and hyperactivity and to promote weight loss. A stronger methamphetamine, crystal meth, or ice, is smoked and takes effect in a few seconds.

Beginning in the 1940s, amphetamines and methamphetamines, also known as speed, were a problem in the United States. As weight-reducing agents, amphetamines have limited success because people eat for reasons other than hunger and users develop tolerance.

Attention deficit hyperactivity disorder (ADHD) is the number one identified psychiatric disorder in children in the United States. Stimulants are used with children who have ADHD with a 70 to 80% effective rate. They work by stimulating the reticular activating system, which helps children focus. A drawback is that they might inhibit growth.

Medically unsupervised use of amphetamines can lead to mania, aggressiveness, paranoia, and violent behavior. Fatal overdoses are not likely, but people have died from their behaviors while they are taking amphetamines. Whether the psychotic-like effects that amphetamines produce are the result of the drugs or sleep deprivation is not clear.

Methamphetamines entered the drug scene in the 1980s. Their effects can last 12 hours or more, and their use has been linked to liver, kidney, and lung damage. Babies born to women who took methamphetamines while pregnant show signs of being asocial and incapable of bonding.

Caffeine, a member of the xanthine family, is the most widely used drug in the United States. Theophylline and theobromine, found in tea and chocolate, respectively, also part are of the xanthine family. Both are less potent than caffeine. Its peak effects appear 15 to 45 minutes after ingestion. Side effects are upset stomach, excessive urination, heartburn, anxiety, insomnia, and symptoms of premenstrual syndrome.

At moderate doses caffeine is considered safe, but at extremely high doses, caffeine can be fatal. Heavy caffeine use during pregnancy has been related to complications at birth and higher rates of miscarriage. Daily caffeine use of 600 mg for 6 to 15 days can lead to caffeinism. Cessation of caffeine use produces withdrawal symptoms including headaches, low energy levels, depression, drowsiness, and irritability. Many people have switched to decaffeinated beverages. The process of decaffeination, however, utilizes organic solvents that may be carcinogenic.

Thinking Critically

1. Consider the current crack and cocaine laws. Do you feel crack cocaine should hold a higher penalty compared to powder cocaine? Do you feel the laws contribute to racial disparities regarding jail time? Defend your answer.

2. Cocaine use can be reduced by reducing the amount of cocaine entering the country or by reducing demand for the drug. Do you favor putting more tax dollars into stopping drugs from coming into the United States or into persuading people not to take drugs? What about drug treatment?

3. Society is concerned with child abuse. Do you consider cocaine use during pregnancy to be a form of child abuse? If so, do you also consider alcohol or tobacco use during pregnancy as a form of abuse? Should pregnant women who use cocaine during pregnancy be prosecuted? Should pregnant women who use tobacco or alcohol during pregnancy be prosecuted? Defend your answer.

4. Although caffeine is a psychoactive drug, it usually is not viewed as such. The World Anti-Doping Agency has had various views regarding caffeine and athletes. It was a banned substance until 2004. Should Olympic athletes be allowed to use caffeine, or should there be restrictions on its use?

5. Energy drinks containing high amounts of caffeine have grown in popularity. The consequences of drinking these drinks, especially when used in conjunction with alcohol, can be harmful. Should age limits be imposed on purchasing energy drinks? Should there be restrictions on the levels of caffeine in energy and other drinks? Defend your answer.

12

Marijuana

Chapter Objectives

After completing this chapter, the reader should be able to:

- Explain the history of marijuana in the United States
- Describe the different species of marijuana and the forms in which they are taken
- Explain the extent of marijuana use and explain the risk and protective factors associated with its use
- Compare and contrast different methods of administration of marijuana
- Describe the process of vaping and how it is different from smoking marijuana
- Synthesize the types of dependence associated with marijuana use
- Assess behavioral, psychological, and cognitive effects of marijuana use
- Summarize the effects of marijuana on various systems in the body
- Argue whether marijuana contributes to mental illness
- Describe the medical conditions for which marijuana is prescribed
- Create an argument for and against the legalization of marijuana

Marijuana remains classified as a schedule I drug even though an increasing number of states allow its use for medicinal and recreational use.

Creative Family/Shutterstock.com

FACT OR FICTION?

1. The word *canvas* is derived from the word *cannabis,* and many famous paintings are on marijuana fibers.

2. The use of marijuana by high school students has increased in the last 5 years while alcohol consumption has decreased.

3. Marijuana does not cause dependence.

4. Marijuana arrests accounted for over one-half of all drug abuse arrests.

5. Marijuana is harmless.

6. At one time, marijuana seeds were put into birdseed.

7. The early Colonial settlers planted marijuana because they recognized its medicinal value.

8. The federal government owns a farm in Mississippi where it grows marijuana to be used for research purposes.

9. Public opinion polls reveal that the majority of Americans favor legalizing marijuana.

10. The federal government allows the medical use of marijuana only to treat the side effects of chemotherapy on cancer patients.

Turn the page to check your answers

Marijuana, or **cannabis**, is one of the world's oldest known drugs. The medicinal value of marijuana was described by the ancient Chinese, Greeks, Persians, Romans, East Indians, and Assyrians. Marijuana was used to regulate muscle spasms, lessen pain, and combat indigestion. Marijuana is also an important part of early US history. Physicians used it to treat migraine headaches and as an anticonvulsant. In the late 1800s, marijuana was used to treat menstrual cramps, labor pains, spastic conditions, and insomnia.

The early settlers in Jamestown, Virginia, planted marijuana for its fiber, which was used for making rope. Called **hemp**, it was a prominent crop during the Civil War and during World War II. Today, the plant is used in more than 25,000 industries including agriculture, textiles, recycling, and furniture.[1] The original hemp plants were cultivated in the United States for rope and contained low levels of THC, seldom exceeding 1%. The commercial growing of hemp was forbidden by the Drug Enforcement Administration until 2014 when President Obama signed the Agriculture Act of 2014 (aka Farm Bill), which allows universities and state departments of agriculture to grow or cultivate help for limited purposes.[2] In 2015, a group of US senators introduced the Industrial Hemp Farming Act of 2015 to allow farmers to produce and cultivate hemp.

Not until the 20th century was marijuana used for its euphoric effect. Marijuana was used in the early 1900s by Mexican farm workers and Caribbean dockworkers. After coming to the United States, many of these immigrants lived in the Southwest. New Orleans was a central site for marijuana distribution because of its location on the Mississippi River. Marijuana use spread quickly. People living in the North and East started smoking it during the 1920s due, in part, to alcohol prohibition.

As more people smoked marijuana, articles appeared in magazines and newspapers denigrating its effects. It was linked to crime and violence, especially in Blacks and Mexican Americans. The film *Reefer Madness* depicted marijuana use as causing the moral decay of young people, brain damage, and mental illness. Despite the American Medical Association's support of the medicinal use of marijuana, politicians and the general public presented marijuana as a heinous drug. Marijuana use was restricted, even for medical purposes, and it was banned altogether after the Marijuana Tax Act was enacted in 1937.

Characteristics

Derived from the hemp plant, the most common strain of marijuana in the United States is *Cannabis sativa*. There are over 480 natural compounds in cannabis, with about 66 being identified as **cannabinoids**.[3]

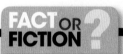

1. **FACT** The word *canvas* comes from *cannabis* and many famous paintings were done on fibers made from marijuana.

2. **FICTION** The fact is—Marijuana use has decreased from 25% in 2011 to 22.6% in 2015. Alcohol use also decreased from 45.3% in 2011 to 36.7% in 2015.

3. **FICTION** The fact is—One-fourth of adolescents who use marijuana meet the criteria for marijuana abuse or dependency and withdrawal symptoms do occur when heavy use ceases.

4. **FACT** Marijuana accounted for over half of all drug related arrests in 2015.

5. **FICTION** The fact is—Marijuana a negative impact on the respiratory, circulatory, nervous, and reproductive systems.

6. **FACT** Even after marijuana was made illegal in 1937, birdseed manufacturers were allowed to include marijuana seeds in birdseed.

7. **FICTION** The fact is—Marijuana was not used for medicinal purposes in the United States until the early 1990s.

8. **FACT** The federal government grows marijuana on a well-guarded farm in Mississippi.

9. **FACT** Almost 60% of Americans in 2016 favor making marijuana legal.

10. **FICTION** The fact is—The federal government does not allow marijuana to be used for any medical purpose.

TABLE 12.1 Types of Cannabinoids

Cannabigerols (CBG)
Cannabichromenes (CBC)
Cannabidiols (CBD)
Tetrahydrocannabinols (THC)
Cannabinol (CBN) and Cannabinodiol (CBDL)

Source: Alcohol & Drug Abuse Institute, "Learn about Marijuana: Science-based information for the public", Updated June 2013. Accessed on February 25, 2017 from http://learnaboutmarijuanawa.org/factsheets/cannabinoids.htm.

Cannabinoids are chemical compounds unique to the cannabis plant. See Table 12.1 for a list of cannabinoids found in cannabis plants. The primary mood-altering, psychoactive agent in marijuana is **delta-9-tetrahydrocannabinol**, or THC. Several factors influence THC levels: the plant's sex, soil and climate conditions, the part of the plant that is used, and how the plant is harvested, prepared, and stored.

Another cannabinoid that has been getting much attention recently is cannabidiol, or CBD. Cannabis resin contains up to 40% of CBD, making it the most abundant cannabinoid in the plant.[4] Although not psychoactive, it provides antianxiety effects, which may reduce the intensity of THC. The potential therapeutic effects from CBD include antiseizure effects, antiinflammatory effects, and analgesic effects.[5] More on the medicinal applications of marijuana will be presented later in the chapter.

Cannabinol (CBN) is the byproduct of THC. When THC is exposed to oxygen and heat, it breaks down creating CBN. CBN is only mildly psychoactive. Some of the benefits of CBN include antiinflammatory properties and as an immunosuppressant.[6] It has also been shown to reduce intraocular pressure in the eye and can be used to treat glaucoma.[7]

More recently it has been shown to produce sedative effects. Steep Hill Labs showed it can produce similar effects as diazepam.[8]

One carcinogenic compound in marijuana smoke and tobacco smoke is **benzopyrene**. Marijuana smoke contains 70% more benzopyrene and 50% more tar than tobacco smoke, and marijuana releases five times as much tar into the lungs as cigarettes.[9] This is noteworthy because marijuana smokers keep the smoke in their lungs for an extended time, inhale more deeply, and take in more smoke.

Species and Forms of Marijuana

The following are among the several species of cannabis plants:

1. *Cannabis sativa*, the most widespread, used primarily to make rope. George Washington's Mount Vernon farm grew it for that purpose. *Cannabis sativa* has a tall, woody stem and can reach a height of 20 feet.
2. *Cannabis indica*, from India originally, is grown for its psychoactive properties. This species grows to a height of only 3 to 4 feet.
3. *Cannabis ruderalis*, found mainly in northern Europe and parts of Asia, is marked by a short growing season and low potency.

Marijuana comes in a variety of forms. The marijuana plant can be separated into **ganja, sinsemilla, and bhang**. Ganja and sinsemilla are made from the top leaves and flowers of the female cannabis plant. Sinsemilla, meaning "without seeds," is derived from the unfertilized female cannabis plant and contains greater amounts of THC. Unfertilized female plants

Ganja and sinsemilla are made from the top leaves and flowers of the marijuana plant.

Michael Nosek/Shutterstock.com

cannabis A genus of plant that is also known as marijuana

hemp Marijuana plant that may be used to make rope, clothing, and paper

delta-9-tetrahydrocannabinol (THC) The psychoactive agent in marijuana

cannabinoids Chemicals found in marijuana plants

benzopyrene Carcinogenic compound found in marijuana and tobacco

ganja Top leaves and flowers of the cannabis plant

sinsemilla Seedless marijuana; derived from unfertilized female cannabis plants

bhang Lower leaves, stems, and seeds of the cannabis plant

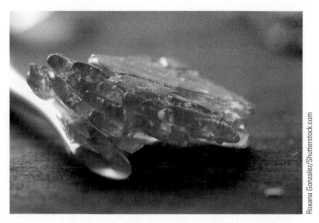

■ "Dabbing," a relatively new practice, can contain upwards of 80% THC.

produce higher amounts of THC because they do not have to expend energy toward reproduction. **Bhang** consists of the lower leaves, stems, and seeds of the cannabis plant and contains less THC compared to sinsemilla and ganja. It is a paste that is created by grinding the leaves of the plant. It is popular in India, especially during Holi, a Hindu festival of color and spring.[10]

Kief is a powder that can be sifted from the leaves and flowers of the cannabis plant. Kief can be pressed into cakes called **hashish.** Hashish, taken from the resin of the cannabis plant, is usually smoked in a pipe, though it can be eaten or vaporized ("vaped"). **Hash oil** is produced by a solvent extraction. Legally, it is produced by using carbon dioxide and ethanol to extract the oil. However, illegal producers have been using butane, a cheaper but much more explosive option.[11] Even in states where hash oil is legal, the production of "do it yourself" hash oil is illegal due to the dozens of cases of home explosions and fires linked to producing it at home.[12] A new practice, known as "dabbing," is becoming more popular in the United States. Also known as cannabis oil, shatter, and wax extract, dabbing is the inhalation of hash oil, some of which can contain upwards of 80% THC.[13]

THC levels of marijuana smoked in the United States have been rising. In the 1970s the average THC content was less than 1%. In the 1990s it ranged from 3 to 4% and today it is about 13%.[14] While the THC content is on the rise, CBD content has been declining. This cannabinoid is being studied for its therapeutic properties, which places people who rely on the CBD content of marijuana for its therapeutic benefits at a disadvantage.[15] One of the reasons there are lower levels today of CBD is because this compound does not produce any of the psychoactive properties associated with marijuana. Contaminants have also been rising. Many labs have found contaminants such as fungi, butane, and microbial growth.[16]

Points of Origin

Because the cannabis plant is resilient, it can be grown almost anywhere. Since laws regarding marijuana have been changing, marijuana production has become a home-grown product. Some estimate that between 60% and 70% of all marijuana in the United States is grown in California.[17] There has been growing concern regarding marijuana being grown in California and the damage it causes to the environment. The cannabis plant requires a lot of water to grow and thrive and California struggles with drought regularly. While winemakers have strict regulations in regards to water usage for grapes (which also require a lot of water to grow), illegal cannabis growers do not follow regulations and often divert water supply to their illegally grown crop.[18] Marijuana being smuggled in from Mexico is declining, many say from the legalized status of marijuana in many states. In 2009, over 3.5 million pounds of marijuana were seized at the southwest border, compared to 2015, where just a little over 1.5 million pounds were seized.[19] Marijuana growers in Mexico have seen a dramatic drop in the price of marijuana. In 1910, they could receive between 60 and 90 dollars per pound of marijuana compared to today where they receive between 30 and 40 dollars a pound.[20]

CONSIDER This

As marijuana's status in the United States continues to change, one of the results has been in higher amounts of THC in both illegal and legal marijuana. The result often being lower amounts of CBD, which is the cannabinoid some say is responsible for the many therapeutic benefits achieved from marijuana. Many now say CBD is the more therapeutic cannabinoid, more so than THC. The problem is CBD does not cause the "high" associated with marijuana and many feel products with more CBD and less THC would not sell as well as higher THC products.

Source: T. Coughlin-Boque, "Want to relax? Don't let them talk you into high-THC weed", *The Stranger,* (April 13, 2016). Accessed on February 26, 2017 from http://www.thestranger.com/feature/2016/04/13/23950787/want-to-relax-dont-let-them-talk-you-into-high-thc-weed.

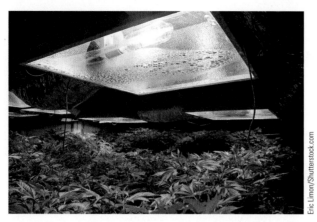

Indoor marijuana cultivation requires an extraordinary amount of energy; representing one-fifth of the cost associated with growing it.

Indoor Cultivation

The indoor cultivation of marijuana has escalated in recent years. There are several reasons for this development. First, it is easier to avoid eradication. Secondly, indoor cultivation has allowed for production of marijuana with a higher THC content. Also, the profits of indoor cultivation are higher because marijuana plants can be harvested four to six times per year.

There have been some concern regarding power usage for indoor cultivation as indoor cultivation requires 24-hour lighting, heating, ventilation, and air conditioning. It is estimated that indoor cultivation of marijuana accounts for 1% of total electricity use in the United States.[21] Furthermore, electricity represents 20% of the cost associated with growing marijuana indoors. Currently, states like Oregon and Colorado have no regulations regarding energy use for legal indoor marijuana cultivation.[22]

Extent of Use

Worldwide, marijuana is the fourth most commonly used drug, surpassed by nicotine, caffeine, and alcohol. Marijuana is the most commonly used illegal drug in the United States.[23] In 2016, 0.7% of 8th graders reported daily use, compared to 2.5% of 10th graders and 6.0% of 12th graders.[24] Furthermore, almost 40% of 12th graders report having used marijuana over the past 12 months. Since the mid-2000s, the perceived risk associated with marijuana has been on the decline. Couple this with a little over 80% of 12th graders reporting that marijuana is readily available, it is no surprise that it continues to be one of the most popular illicit drugs in the United States and

around the world.[25] In 2015, an estimated 22.2 million Americans aged 12 or older were current marijuana users.[26] Almost 10% of Americans aged 12 or older were past month users. The United States, Canada, Nigeria, and Australia rank highest on the percentage of people who smoke marijuana.[27]

Researchers have found correlations among grades, truancy, religious commitment, and marijuana use, the most important reasons that students significantly increased their use of marijuana relate to a reduced perception of risk and less disapproval of its use.[28] Many people fear the recreational medicinal legalization of marijuana will increase use by reducing people's disapproval of its use and risks. In a recent study comparing use and perceived risk among 8th, 10th, and 12th graders, researchers found an increase in perceived harmfulness of marijuana after the enactment of a state medical marijuana law. This study also found a decrease in marijuana use among 8th graders in states that have a medical marijuana law on the books.[29] However, another study found marijuana use increased and perceived harm decreased among 8th and 10th graders in Washington State after the enactment of a recreational marijuana law.[30] Perhaps the message in states that allow medicine marijuana compared to those that allow recreational marijuana are different regarding perceived risk.

There may be an association between parents with cannabis use disorder and their children. One study found children have higher risk for cannabis use disorder if they have parents who use hard drugs, have a cannabis use disorder, and/or antisocial personality disorder.[31] Marijuana use is also associated with cigarette use. One study looked at smoking prevalence rates among 8th and 4 years later administered a survey to determine marijuana use. They found marijuana use and cigarette use to be correlated. When 8th graders reported higher levels of cigarette use, it accurately predicted marijuana use 4 years later. The reverse of this also proves true; when cigarette use decreases among 8th graders, 4 years later, marijuana use also experienced a decline.[32]

Marijuana use is associated with alcohol and cigarette use. The Center on Addiction and Substance Abuse has reported that 12-year-olds who drank alcohol and smoked cigarettes within 30 days of a

kief resin of cannabis that contains trichomes

hashish A potent form of marijuana taken from resin of the cannabis plant

hash oil Substance made by separating resin from the cannabis plant by boiling the plant in alcohol; it has a very high THC content

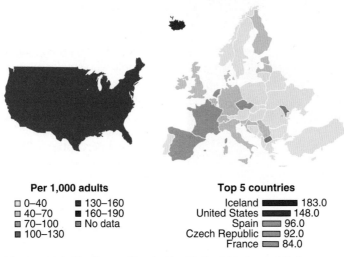

Per 1,000 adults

- □ 0–40
- ■ 40–70
- ■ 70–100
- ■ 100–130
- ■ 130–160
- ■ 160–190
- ▨ No data

Top 5 countries

Iceland	183.0
United States	148.0
Spain	96.0
Czech Republic	92.0
France	84.0

Figure 12.1 Marijuana Use in the United States Is Higher Compared to European Nations

survey were 30 times more likely to use marijuana than young people who did not use alcohol or cigarettes. One study found marijuana use among high school students had no effect on disapproval ratings for cocaine, crack, or heroin, suggesting marijuana use may not be associated with lower disapproval ratings for harder drugs.[33]

Many people worry that teenagers will have more access to marijuana in states that allow medicinal and recreational marijuana. However, the data does not appear to support an increase in marijuana use among teenagers in states that allow some form of marijuana.[34] Most teenagers acquire marijuana from a friend, regardless of whether the teenagers live in states where it is legal or not.[35]

Becoming a parent was the most important social variable leading to marijuana cessation in one study.[36] Moreover, people who used marijuana for social reasons rather than to alter their mood were more likely to quit using marijuana. Individuals who started using marijuana early in life were less likely to stop using it than those who started using it later. Also, continued marijuana use was greater among people who used other illicit drugs as well.

Pharmacology of Marijuana

Methods of Administration

The three common routes of administration for marijuana are through the lungs, oral, and through the skin. Marijuana can be smoked or ingested. Most users in the United States smoke it, but ingestion is becoming more common. Marijuana cannot be injected because the resin from the cannabis plant does not dissolve in water.

Lungs

The two ways marijuana is taken to enter the lungs are through smoking and vaping. This method has a rapid onset, but the duration tends to be shorter.[37] If it is smoked, it takes effect more quickly than if it is ingested. Factors influencing the effects of marijuana include dosage, THC content, depth of inhalation, interval between puffs, and length of time it is held in one's lungs. Pipes, joints, water pipes, and **blunts** are used to smoke marijuana. Blunts are cigars where some or all of the tobacco has been removed and marijuana added in its place. Blunts are more common among youth, males, and African Americans.[38] One of the problems associated with blunts is the dose of nicotine that is included in the smoke, which may lead to nicotine addiction. Even when all the tobacco is taken out of the cigar and replaced with marijuana, there are still quantifiable levels of nicotine in the wrapper.[39] Inhaled marijuana is metabolized quickly in the body. Studies show the effects from smoked marijuana last on average 2.5 hours.[40]

Vaping is a process where extract from the cannabis flower is heated at a lower temperature creating a gas or vapor that is then inhaled. It works the same in the body as smoking, but may better allow the person to control the dose. In a survey conducted among current cannabis users, only 8% reported using vaping to smoke the drug, but they also reported vaping as the most important harm-reduction strategy.[41]

Children and Edibles

Children love sweets and often find it difficult to keep their hands off of brownies and candies. However, in states that allow medicinal or recreational marijuana, these sweets may not be what they seem. Since 2014, Colorado has seen an increase of 150% of children exposed to marijuana through edibles. Symptoms for marijuana exposure in children include lethargy, vomiting, or agitation. While the numbers of children exposed to marijuana are still low, 163 documented cases between 2009 and 2015, they are still cause for concern. In 2015, Colorado required marijuana products to be sold in childproof packaging to help reduce the number of children exposed to marijuana.

Questions to Ponder

1. Many marijuana edibles come in forms that are appealing to children (i.e., gummy bears, candies, brownies, etc.), do you feel these types of products should be discontinued due to increase in children who are accidently exposed to edible marijuana?

2. Should parents whose children have been exposed to edible marijuana be charged with a crime? Defend your position.

Source: J. Hoffman, "Study finds sharp increase in marijuana exposure among Colorado children", *New York Times,* (July 25, 2015). Accessed on March 1, 2017 from https://www.nytimes.com/2016/07/26/health/marijuana-edibles-are-getting-into-colorado-childrens-hands-study-says.html?_r=0.

Furthermore, vaping is most common the United States and Canada, which have lower levels of tobacco use. Some argue the method of vaping marijuana may reduce tobacco use among marijuana users.[42]

Oral

Marijuana can be taken orally in the form on edibles, capsules, or oils. Cannabis is infused in oil, butter, or some other edible fat, which is then used in cooking. Some now believe the effects of ingesting marijuana are stronger compared to smoking it. Ingested marijuana goes through a first-pass metabolism, which causes a chemical change and loss to the molecular structure of the drug. When THC is ingested, it gets metabolized by the liver and delta-9 THC is converted to 11-hydroxy-THC. This new molecule passes the blood–brain barrier more rapidly and has a stronger psychedelic effect compared to smoked THC.[43] Ingesting cannabis takes on average 30 to 60 minutes for users to feel the effects of the drug and the duration of the effects last longer at 4 to 6 hours.[44] Stomach contents also influence the effect of marijuana. People who consume marijuana orally are more likely to feel nausea and discomfort than those who smoke it.

Skin

Transdermal patches contain THC and CBD and are applied directly to the skin. The drug is absorbed through the skin to enter the circulatory system. Some advantages of transdermal marijuana is the dose is more controllable and the effects are gradual and consistent.[45] Similar to edible marijuana, it can take up to an hour to take effect and can last up to 6 to 8 hours.[46]

Tolerance

Animal studies show that tolerance to the physiological effects of marijuana develops, but there is dispute regarding whether humans develop pharmacological, or physical, tolerance. In studies proving pharmacological tolerance, it was more likely to develop among daily users. One indication of tolerance is that heavy users are still capable of doing cognitive tasks.[47]

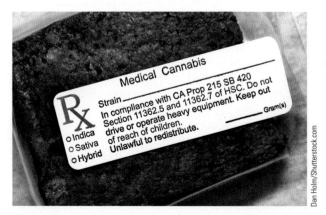

Dan Holm/Shutterstock.com

Ingesting THC takes longer to take an effect but lasts longer.

blunt A marijuana-containing cigar; to create a blunt, tobacco is removed from a regular cigar and marijuana is inserted

One study compared neurocognitive performance between heavy users (those who used cannabis more than four times a week) and occasional users (those who used cannabis less than two times a week). Researchers gave a high dose of THC to both groups and tested them on performance tasks. Occasional users showed impairments on all performance tasks while heavy users only showed impairment on one performance task.[48] This suggest heavy users develop some type of tolerance for the drug, although whether tolerance was developed through physical adaptations to the presence of the drug or behavioral adaptations was not determined.[49] Many users claim they get high from decreasing doses, though no evidence of **reverse tolerance** exists. If a person gets high more easily with subsequent use, the setting and familiarity might be factors. Euphoria, then, could result from expectations or previous experience. In short, because of previous experience with marijuana, users are able to adjust and respond to its effects. Frequent users also experience less loss of memory, coordination, and concentration.

Physical Dependence

One study of twins found that if one twin started smoking marijuana before age 17, the other twin was also more likely to initiate marijuana use by that age. This leads researchers to conclude that marijuana use may be heritable.[50] Although most experts agree that physical dependence on marijuana does *not* occur, whether marijuana causes physical dependency might depend on how dependency is defined. One study reports that one-fourth of adolescents who use marijuana frequently meet the criteria for marijuana abuse or dependency.[51]

Columbia University drug expert Denise Kandel maintains that young people may develop physical dependency because they are more sensitive to marijuana. One argument against marijuana causing physical dependency is that its use drops dramatically as people age. Half of all cannabis users went into remission 6 years after considering themselves dependent on the drug.[52] Conversely, a German study reported that individuals who smoked marijuana at least five times a week were likely to be marijuana smokers ten years later.[53] This suggests that either they did not want to stop smoking marijuana or had difficulty trying to stop.

The National Institutes for Health estimate that nearly 2.5% of adults experienced marijuana use disorder in the year 2015 and nearly 6.5% of adults have experienced marijuana use disorder in their lifetime.[54] It is estimated that 30% of current marijuana users have some degree of marijuana use disorder.[55] Marijuana use disorder is associated with the presence

WITHDRAWAL SYMPTOMS ASSOCIATED WITH MARIJUANA

- Nausea
- Vomiting
- Perspiration
- Irritability
- Runny nose
- Restlessness
- Diarrhea
- Lack of appetite
- Insomnia
- Hot flashes

of withdrawal symptoms and a difficulty in abstaining from the drug. The brain adapts to the presence of marijuana by reducing production and sensitivity to endocannabinoid neurotransmitters. Studies estimate that 9% of marijuana smokers will become dependent on the drug. This estimate increases to 17% if marijuana use is initiated during adolescence.[56] Research suggests nearly 35% of frequent cannabis users (who don't use other drugs) will experience withdrawal symptoms when abstaining from the drug.[57] Withdrawal symptoms include irritability, anxiety, appetite loss, and sleep disturbance. Peak withdrawal symptoms are likely to occur within the first 4 days of abstinence, while sleep disturbance may persist for a longer period of time.[58] Some studies suggest women experience greater withdrawal symptoms compared to men and tend to be less successful in treatment trials for the cessation of marijuana.[59]

Psychological Dependence

Most drug experts think marijuana can result in psychological dependence. Most people who smoke marijuana are occasional users, few of whom become compulsive users. If dependency develops, it is more likely to be motivated by psychosocial than by physiological factors. The drug itself does not necessarily lead to increased use. The perceived need for the drug is believed to be responsible for compulsive use and dependency.

Effects of Marijuana Use

The amount of marijuana that could be fatal has not been established; thus, the margin of safety between effective and lethal doses is wide. Nevertheless, in

Marijuana on College Campuses

Approximately 35% of college students have smoked marijuana in the past year. A recent study found negative academic consequences due to the direct and indirect effects of marijuana. Marijuana users are more likely to skip classes and have lower first-semester GPA compared to non-users. While skipping classes has been associated with lower grades, research suggests marijuana contributes to more classes skipped, thus negatively impacting GPA. Marijuana use by college students may result in poorer academic outcomes and prove to be a barrier to academic achievement at the collegiate level.

Questions to ponder

Given that marijuana use is negatively associated with college academic performance, should colleges drug test entering freshman? Defend your position.

Source: A.M. Arria, K.M. Caldeira, B.A. Bugbee, K.B. Vincent, and K.E. O'Grady, "The academic consequences of marijuana use during college", *Psychology of Addictive Behaviors,* 29, no.3 (2015): 564–575.

recent years, the number of marijuana users seen in emergency rooms has increased, along with the number of users seeking treatment. During the first year marijuana became legal in Colorado, emergency room visits doubled involving marijuana using tourists.[60] However, emergency room visits for Colorado residents did not change. Of those marijuana-related emergency room visits, there were three groups of people: those who have underlying medical conditions in which marijuana can exacerbate those symptoms; those who are directly affected by the drug (i.e., motor vehicle accidents); and those who get heavily intoxicated and become scared.[61] Thus far, there has been one death associated with edible marijuana in Colorado.[62] In 2014, a college student exceeded the recommended dose by six times and after consuming marijuana jumped from a hotel balcony.[63]

Behavioral Effects

Marijuana use has been associated with poor educational outcomes. A study conducted in Australia and New Zealand found that adolescents who use marijuana regularly are less likely to finish high school or obtain a high school diploma.[64] Also, one study of adolescents who smoked marijuana at least once a week reported that these adolescents thought about killing themselves three times more often than nonusers, felt more lonely and unloved, were six times more likely to run away from home, were six times more likely to cut classes or skip school, and were five times more likely to steal.

Among adults, heavy marijuana use has shown to have a negative impact on work/life. One study followed heavy marijuana users from adolescence to adulthood and discovered this group had lower income, greater welfare dependence, unemployment, criminal behaviour, and lower life satisfaction compared to the control group.[65, 66] Marijuana use may also impact work by contributing to workplace injuries and accidents.[67]

More than 10 million Americans have reported to driving under the influence of illicit drugs.[68] Although determining the specific effects of THC at varying levels is imprecise, driving ability is clearly affected by the presence of THC in the bloodstream. Marijuana impairs perceptual and motor skills and the ability to stay awake—skills necessary for driving a car or motorcycle. Research studies have shown that the use of marijuana while driving increases lane weaving and contributes to poor reaction time.[69] One study looked at marijuana users who resided in Colorado and Washington (where marijuana is legal) to determine the prevalence among users who admitted to drugged driving. They found that 43% of users admitted to driving under the influence of marijuana during the past year, while almost 24% admitted to driving under the influence of marijuana at least five times over the past year.[70] There have been mixed

reverse tolerance A drug user's experiencing the desired effects from lesser amounts of the same drug

results on the effects of THC on automobile crashes. One study found those who were under the influence of THC were 1.83 times more likely to be involved in a crash, while another study found no correlation between THC and automobile crashes.[71] Between 1999 and 2009, 44,000 people in the United States died from single-vehicle crashes. One-fourth of the victims tested positive for an illegal drug. Twenty-two percent of that sample tested positive for marijuana.[72] Marijuana interferes with concentration and the ability to adjust for wind conditions and maintaining a steady speed. Teenagers who smoke marijuana and drive cars are more than twice as likely to be involved in an automobile accident as when they do not smoke. The risk associated with marijuana use and alcohol is greater for the combination of drugs than either drug alone.[73]

Psychological Effects

Many variables influence the psychological effects of marijuana. Marijuana increases the release of dopamine, a neurotransmitter involved in the experience of euphoria. Therefore, most users report euphoria, as well as relaxation, often followed by sleepiness. Others say they develop insight.

The frequency of and motivations for marijuana use affect its psychological effects. One study found that adolescents who used marijuana experimentally were not as well adjusted as those who abstained from marijuana use. Some middle-school students use marijuana in an effort to be more popular.[74] This is unfortunate, as one study indicated that marijuana users who started using before age 14 were more likely to exhibit psychosis.[75]

One study compared psychosocial outcomes between alcohol and marijuana among high school seniors in the United States. They found marijuana was associated with poorer relationships with teachers or supervisors and resulted in less energy and interest.[76] However, when comparing alcohol and

marijuana users, marijuana users were more likely to report no adverse effects from the drug.

In the publication *The Link Between Marijuana and Mental Illness*, the federal government identified numerous studies supporting the connection between marijuana and mental illness.[77] These studies link marijuana use to increased risk for psychiatric disorders, depression, anxiety, and substance use disorders.[78] However, the strongest link between marijuana and psychiatric disorders are among those users who have a preexisting or other vulnerability for these problems.[79] One study found adults with depression or a serious psychological distress were at higher risk of lifetime use of marijuana, past year use of marijuana, and frequent marijuana use.[80] Adults in this study were more likely to have a higher number of quit attempts and were less successful at marijuana cessation.[81] Another study noted that marijuana use predicted an increase in depressive symptoms and a decrease in fun-seeking behavior.[82] This study also showed female marijuana users had increased anxiety symptoms.

Psychological effects are subject to interpretation. What one person may view as desirable or euphoric may be undesirable or dysphoric to another. Although using marijuana to deal with interpersonal dilemmas, stress, and other problems may seem desirable to the user, many mental health experts view this as an inadequate long-term solution to personal problems. Despite the possible connection to interpersonal problems, some researchers maintain that strict enforcement of marijuana is unwarranted.[83]

Perceptual Effects

Many people report feeling more introspective and sensitive to external stimuli when they are using marijuana. Others claim they are more artistically creative, although objective research does not support this. Marijuana alters perceptions of time and space. Mood changes are marked by anxiety, sadness, laughter, and paranoia. Some people experience panic reactions, which tend to be temporary and often are triggered by a feeling of not being in control. Others use marijuana to cope with social anxiety. Some individuals who suffer from posttraumatic stress use marijuana to cope with their negative mood states.[84] An estimated 30% of veterans who served in Iraq and Afghanistan suffer from PTSD. Marijuana may aid veterans by reducing symptoms associated with PTSD including anxiety, flashbacks, and depression. One study found patients who smoked marijuana saw a 75% reduction in symptoms.[85]

Determining how much perceptual change is attributable to marijuana itself and how much to one's beliefs about its effects is difficult. This point is illustrated in the classic study in which marijuana users were given regular tobacco cigarettes or marijuana cigarettes but did not know which they were given. In a study conducted in the 1970s, marijuana smokers reported being just as high after smoking a regular cigarette as they were after smoking a cigarette with marijuana.[86]

Participants in one study were given Marinol, a prescription drug consisting of capsules containing THC (given to chemotherapy patients to reduce nausea). About half of the subjects said they were drowsy, and one in six said they felt anxiety. Almost as many subjects receiving a placebo reported feeling drowsy, and nearly one in four said they experienced anxiety.[87] In contrast to subjects receiving Marinol, a higher percentage receiving the placebo reported feeling anxiety.

Cognitive Effects

One area that has shown negative effects on cognition is marijuana use during adolescence. During adolescence, the prefrontal and parietal cortex of the brain undergo major changes and much growth and development in those areas occur during this time. Using marijuana during this period of growth may have significant impact on the development of the brain.[88] Some studies have shown that marijuana use during adolescent and young adult years (15 to 25 years of age) is associated with cognitive deficits.[89] See Table 12.2 on the relationship between marijuana use and grades earned. Furthermore, studies also suggest marijuana use during adolescence and young adulthood has shown a decrease in attention span and verbal memory and has been

associated with lower IQs.[90] Studies involving brain imaging have conflicting results. One study conducted on adolescents who regularly use marijuana showed altered connectivity in the brain and in specific regions involved in executive functions. Another study found no structural damage to the brain region among adolescents who use marijuana.[91]

One reported cognitive effect of marijuana is impairment of working memory, although research on this effect is inconsistent. One study found working memory decreased with acute marijuana use and increased with tobacco use. When marijuana was used with tobacco, there were no effects on working memory.[92] Many scientists agree that temporary cognitive effects occur, but they do not agree on whether any effects are permanent. However, one study looked at people in their 20s, who were heavy marijuana smokers during their late teens. At the time of the study, the participants had abstained from marijuana for the past 2 years. Results from this study found changes in the brain structures related to working memory. Participants also performed poorly on memory tasks indicating that heavy marijuana use during adolescence may contribute to long-term effects, particularly in the brain.[93]

It is not known whether these cognitive deficits are permanent or temporary after a person abstains from marijuana. One study compared brain images of three adolescent groups: The first group had used marijuana in the past week, the second group had not used marijuana for the last 27 to 60 days, and the third group were nonusers. Results from this study indicate that recent marijuana use may impact how spatial working memory functions are performed in the brain and change the neural networks associated with that area of the brain. Additionally, the study showed improvement among the sustained abstinent users, which suggest the brain heals itself after abstinence.[94] In adults, verbal learning deficits disappear after 28 days of abstinence[95] while deficits are

TABLE 12.2 Percentage of High School Students Who Use Marijuana by Types of Grades Earned

Marijuana Use	A's	B's	C's	D's/F's
Ever used marijuana	21	37	50	66
Current marijuana use	10	19	30	48
Tried marijuana for the first time before age 13	3	5	12	24
Used marijuana on school property	2	3	6	17

Source: U.S. Department of Health and Human Services. "Alcohol and other drug use and academic achievement", Centers for Disease Control and Prevention. Accessed on March 7, 2017 from https://www.cdc.gov/healthyyouth/health_and_academics/pdf/alcohol_other_drug.pdf.

still observed in memory, executive functioning, and motor impairments after 28 days of abstinence.[96]

Amotivational Syndrome

Heavy marijuana users reportedly are unable to concentrate and are unmotivated, apathetic, lacking ambition, and not achievement oriented. This describes the **amotivational syndrome**. Does marijuana smoking bring about the amotivational syndrome, or are people who frequently smoke marijuana less motivated to start with? One study found THC negatively impacted high-effort choices. This study also found CBD in conjunction with THC reduced these effects.[97] However, marijuana and cigarette users have higher rates of depression, which may have influenced the results of this study as depression and amotivational syndrome share characteristics. There are still arguments among scientists regarding the existence of amotivational syndrome. Additionally, most people who use marijuana do not develop amotivational syndrome.[98] In their review of numerous studies, however, Lynskey and Hall reported that research on marijuana use and amotivational syndrome is inconclusive.[99]

The amotivational syndrome is more likely to develop in adolescents than in older people. Older marijuana smokers might view its use in a different context than younger users. For example, a college student might engage in many activities during the course of a day—attend classes, exercise, go to the library, watch a movie, study, and smoke a joint. Thus marijuana may be one small part of that person's day. In contrast, a high school student who smokes marijuana might place more importance on associated factors such as where to smoke, with whom to smoke, and when to smoke. If marijuana assumes an integral role in one's life, the amotivational syndrome is more likely to be present.

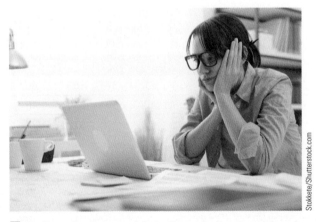

Stokkete/Shutterstock.com

■ Marijuana is often associated with amotivational syndrome; however, research in this area is not conclusive.

Physical Effects

Marijuana affects the body in many ways. A common experience is an increase in appetite. Marijuana acts on the respiratory, cardiovascular, immune, and reproductive systems, as well as on the brain. Some effects are temporary, some can be life-threatening, and others are insignificant.

Short-term effects include increased pulse rate, dilation of the pupils, reddened eyes, and dryness of the mouth and throat. Marijuana poses a greater risk to young people, pregnant and nursing women, and people with cardiovascular problems.

Oral and Gastrointestinal

Marijuana users consistently report an increase in appetite when they smoke, although no one component of marijuana has been identified as an appetite stimulant. The media has portrayed marijuana use with increased appetite, known as the "munchies." Recent studies do not support an increased appetite among marijuana users. One way to measure appetite is to look at weight gain or MBI among marijuana users as one would assume if a drug increases appetite it would also increase weight gain. Studies have been done and have shown no relationships between heightened BMI and marijuana use.[100] Other studies have confirmed these results with one showing marijuana users (both male and female) have significantly lower BMIs compared to nonusers.[101] Marijuana has been associated with an increased risk in periodontal disease. One study looked at over 1000 people in New Zealand to determine if a relationship exists between smoking marijuana and gum disease. This study found that over 50% of marijuana users had gum disease compared to only 13.5% of nonusers.[102] A similar study conducted in the United States confirmed these results showing a significant increase in periodontal disease among frequent users of cannabis.[103]

Emergency room in states where marijuana is legal are seeing an upsurge of cannabinoid hyperemesis syndrome (CHS),[104] an illness characterized by nausea and vomiting. See Table 12.3 for features associated with CHS. This syndrome, while rare, is seen among heavy and long-term marijuana users. CHS will enter remission when users abstain from marijuana use.[105]

The Respiratory System

The THC in marijuana has been used to treat asthma because THC acts as a bronchodilator. Despite this benefit, long-term smoking of marijuana is harmful to the lungs because the smoke contains many respiratory irritants and carcinogens. Daily marijuana smokers who do not use tobacco have more sick days and visits to doctors for respiratory problems than people

TABLE 12.3 Features of Cannabinoid Hyperemesis Syndrome

Current, heavy cannabis use
Abdominal pain, epigastric or periumbilical
Recurrent episodes of severe nausea and intractable vomiting
Compulsive bathing with symptom relief
Resolution of symptoms with cannabis cessation
Failure of standard antiemetics to resolve nausea and vomiting

Source: C. King and A. Holmes, "Cannabinoid Hyperemesis syndrome", *CMAJ*, 187, no.5 (2015): 355.

who do not smoke at all. The harm to the respiratory system occurs regardless of whether one smokes marijuana in cigarette form or with a water pipe or hookah.[106]

Because chronic marijuana smokers also tend to be chronic cigarette smokers, ascertaining how much lung damage is from marijuana and how much is from tobacco smoking is difficult. The evidence is contradictory. One study found that people who use both marijuana and tobacco had an increased risk for respiratory systems including wheezing and chronic airflow limitation.[107] Additionally, the use of both marijuana and tobacco created an increased risk for chronic obstructive pulmonary disease, while the use of marijuana alone did not seem to be a risk factor.

Marijuana has not been proven definitively to cause lung cancer; however, daily marijuana smokers show damage to the cells lining the airways similar to that seen in cigarette smokers who develop lung cancer. The potential for marijuana smokers to develop lung disease is a concern because marijuana contains 20 times as much ammonia and 5 times as much hydrogen cyanide as tobacco smoke.[108] Smoking marijuana is associated with chronic bronchitis symptoms and large airway inflammation among heavy users.[109] While there are currently no studies that show a direct relationship between marijuana and lung cancer, scientists agree there is biological plausibility of the link between marijuana and lung cancer.[110]

Some airway obstruction in the lungs might be reversed after a significant reduction or abstinence from smoking marijuana. One study found users who reduce or abstain from marijuana after frequent use experienced reductions in the prevalence of coughing, sputum, and wheezing.[111]

The Cardiovascular System

Marijuana dilates the peripheral blood vessels, manifested by bloodshot eyes and warm ears. Research regarding the impact of marijuana on the cardiovascular system have produced mixed results. Marijuana cigarettes cause increases in heart rate, blood pressure, and forearm blood flow.[112] Smoking marijuana has been associated with triggering myocardial infarctions (MI) and young male patients. Furthermore, smoking marijuana shows an increase in risk for MI for 60 minutes after smoking and a small increase in annual risk of MI.[113] Conversely, a recent study found no association between smoking marijuana and incidence of cardiovascular disease for both recent and cumulative effects of smoking marijuana.[114]

The Immune System

A properly functioning immune system is essential to ward off infections. Smoking marijuana can suppress the body's immune system, which may explain why recreational users of marijuana get sick more often.[115] Marijuana may also increase immune cells called myeloid-derived suppressor cells, which suppress the immune system. The increase of these myeloid-derived suppressor cells may decrease the effectiveness of cancer treatment.[116] Conversely, while the immunomodulatory effects are not fully understood, CBD may reduce the inflammatory response of the immune system, making it useful for those suffering from autoimmune diseases.[117]

The Reproductive System

Some users claim that marijuana heightens the sexual experience, and other users claim it makes them less interested in sex. Perhaps people who find marijuana sexually enhancing are predisposed to that effect. Nothing inherent in marijuana justifies its reputation as an aphrodisiac. Feelings of euphoria and increased awareness of stimuli, however, might make a person feel more sexual. In one study measuring the impact of marijuana on sexual health, daily marijuana users were more likely to have a greater number of sexual partners and having experienced an STI (for women only).[118] This study also found frequent marijuana users (men only) reported inability to reach orgasm, reaching orgasm too slowly, and reaching orgasm too quickly. No sexual problems in women were identified.[119] Another study found similar effects in men and erectile function.[120]

Marijuana has a negative effect on male sexuality because it decreases sperm count. One study looked at healthy men (ages 18 to 28) to determine the impact of marijuana on sexual health. It was determined that regular marijuana smoking is associated with lower sperm concentration, which may reduce the sperm's ability to fertilize an egg.[121] However, this same study found

amotivational syndrome A condition characterized by apathy, an inability to concentrate, and little achievement orientation

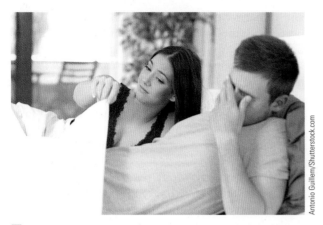

Marijuana has shown to have negative effects on the male reproductive system.

marijuana smokers have higher levels of testosterone compared to nonusers. The effects of marijuana on testosterone levels may be short-term as one study found no differences in testosterone levels between men who have ever used marijuana and those who have never used marijuana.[122] However, the same study found men who were current users of marijuana have higher levels of testosterone compared to past users and nonusers. But some research indicates that marijuana may help men experiencing erectile dysfunction.[123]

Marijuana may also affect a woman's reproductive system by reducing fertility. Careful control of the endocannabinoid system is required to reproduce and marijuana use may disturb this balance, reducing fertility in women.[124] Women who use marijuana have slightly more menstrual cycles without ovulation.[125] While use of marijuana has not been connected to an increase in miscarriages in humans, it has been associated with an increase in miscarriages in animal studies.[126] THC easily crosses the placenta to reach the fetus. It is also present in breastmilk. See Table 12.4

TABLE 12.4 Impact of Marijuana Use During Pregnancy

Age of Offspring	Effects of Prenatal Exposure to Marijuana
18-22-week-old fetus	Changes in development of brain. In male fetuses, abnormal function of the amygdala
6-year-olds	Decreased ability to understand concepts in listening and reading
10-year-olds	More impulsive and less ability to focus their attention
Age 14	Lower scores in reading, math, and spelling

Source: C.S. Louis, "Pregnant women turn to marijuana, perhaps harming infants", *New York Times,* (February 2, 2017). Accessed on March 3, 2017 from https://www.nytimes.com/2017/02/02 /health/marijuana-and-pregnancy.html.

on the impact of marijuana use during pregnancy. Use of marijuana by pregnant women can harm brain development and cognition in the fetus and may contribute to low birth weight.[127] Regardless, the American Academy of Pediatrics and the American College of Obstetricians and Gynecologists advise against prenatal use of cannabis.[128]

The Brain

It is not entirely clear how marijuana interacts with the brain. Although some past studies reported that marijuana causes serious brain damage, many of these studies were seriously flawed. Subsequent research employing more sophisticated technology has contradicted those findings. Because many marijuana smokers use other drugs, determining the precise effects of marijuana on the brain is difficult. Nonetheless, it does appear that chronic marijuana users experience cognitive deficits.[129] Cognitive impairments have been found in rats exposed to THC and structural and functional changes in the hippocampus have been observed. Smoking marijuana reduces acetylcholine in the **hippocampus**, the portion of the brain that affects memory. This relationship among marijuana, acetylcholine, and the hippocampus explains how memory is impaired.[130] The activity of the neurotransmitters norepinephrine and dopamine alters the mood, and marijuana affects these as well.

Anticholinergic drugs such as marijuana are believed to be related to schizophrenia, and schizophrenia is more likely to show up in heavy users than in nonusers. Some studies have shown that marijuana use during adolescence can increase a person's risk of later developing schizophrenia.[131] One study found the use of marijuana doubles the risk of schizophrenia and psychosis.[132]

Medical Applications

In the late 1800s, marijuana was used medically to treat convulsions, chronic cough, sleeplessness, gastrointestinal disorders, gonorrhea, and pain. With passage of the Marijuana Tax Act in 1937, physicians in the United States had to stop prescribing preparations made from cannabis, though many of them had cut back already because cannabis was unsuitable for injection and took a long time to take effect when taken orally, and other more effective drugs were available. Also, THC levels in cannabis preparations were not uniform.

After the popularity of recreational marijuana increased in the 1960s, interest in its therapeutic applications likewise surged. Recently, marijuana has been used to treat glaucoma, asthma, nausea and vomiting during cancer chemotherapy, and pain associated with multiple sclerosis.[133] A recent study found that the number of accidental opioid deaths were reduced in states where medicinal marijuana is legal.[134] There is also a safe addiction margin for cannabis with lower risks compared to anxiolytics, alcohol, cocaine, heroin, and tobacco.[135] It also has been used to alleviate withdrawal symptoms related to barbiturates, narcotics, and alcohol.

Glaucoma

Glaucoma, caused by pressure building up behind the eye, is a leading cause of blindness in the United States, afflicting 3 million Americans.[136] Although marijuana does not cure blindness, it can reduce the risk by reducing pressure behind the eye. However, the effectiveness of marijuana is limiting as it only lasts 3 to 4 hours, which means one would have to use marijuana six to eight times a day.[137] Furthermore, there has been speculation about whether marijuana may make glaucoma worse by reducing blood pressure in eye and reducing blood supply to the optic nerve.[138] Many supporters of the use of marijuana as a treatment for glaucoma cite a study that was conducted in the 1970s when treatment for glaucoma was limited.[139]

THC eye drops were developed in 1981. THC is fat soluble and it has not yet been possible to develop an eye drop that is effective.[140] Because marijuana affects heart rate and blood pressure and causes psychological problems in some patients, its widespread use for glaucoma treatment is unlikely. Moreover, other drugs are more effective for treating glaucoma.

Nausea and Vomiting

Marijuana is an effective **antiemetic** drug to counteract the nausea and vomiting that frequently

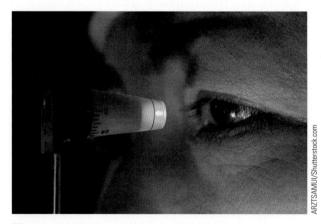

◼ Once thought to be an effective treatment for glaucoma, marijuana only temporary reduces pressure in the eye. Other treatments have been found to be more effective.

accompany chemotherapy to treat cancer.[141] In a study conducted on rats, low doses of combined THC and CBD and of each on their own were able to reduce acute nausea.[142] Mindset contributes to the effectiveness of marijuana in patients. Those who are uncomfortable taking the drug because of the negative connotations surrounding it might also have difficulty benefiting from it. These people might profit more from medications such as Marinol (THC formulated in sesame oil) or Cesamet (a synthetic cannabinoid), because they do not resemble marijuana.

First marketed in 1986, Marinol was projected to reduce the demand for prescriptive marijuana. Marinol comes in capsule form and produces fewer side effects than marijuana; however, it takes longer to act than smoked marijuana does. Marinol has been approved for nausea associated with chemotherapy treatment only after other treatments have proven to be unsuccessful.[143] Like other oral drugs, Marinol can take over 30 minutes to provide therapeutic effects; this may be problematic when treating nausea and vomiting. Synthetic marijuana has shown promise in treating headaches,[144] posttraumatic stress disorder,[145] and marijuana dependence.[146]

Debate continues to swirl around whether Marinol or marijuana is more effective for reducing nausea and vomiting. The reduction in nausea and vomiting could be the result of chemicals other than THC in marijuana. Also, some individuals complain that Marinol is more expensive (some insurances do not cover it) than marijuana and produces some undesirable side effects.[147]

Asthma

An estimated 34 million Americans are affected by asthma. One study of children with asthma indicated that about one-fourth will use some type of alternative treatment at some point.[148] The THC in marijuana is helpful in expanding lung capacity because it dilates the bronchial tubes. Paradoxically, whether smoke goes into the lungs from a marijuana cigarette or a regular tobacco cigarette, lung capacity decreases. Many of the studies looking at asthma and marijuana were conducted in the 1970s with little evidence to suggest marijuana is effective in the treatment of asthma.[149] Because of these limitations and the availability of other bronchodilators that are more effective and do not produce as many side effects, marijuana is not the drug of choice for treating asthma.

hippocampus Part of the brain involved with memory; altered by marijuana

antiemetic A drug that reduces nausea and vomiting; an example is marijuana

Epilepsy

Epilepsy is a seizure disorder and the fourth most common neurological disorder in the United States.[150] It is characterized by uncontrollable seizures and may cause other health problems. Recent studies suggest CBD may be an effective treatment for treatment-resistant epilepsy.[151] In a retrospective study on children and adolescents who were given oral cannabis for seizure control, almost 60% reported improvements.[152] Adverse reactions include increased seizures in (13%) and fatigue (12%). Showing promising results, a study in Canada among adult patients suffering from epilepsy who used marijuana, found 99% perceived seizure improvement, 98% perceived sleep improvement, and 88% perceived a reduction in antiepileptic drug side effects.[153]

Autoimmune Diseases

Almost 50 million Americans suffer from an autoimmune disorder.[154] Autoimmune disorders result from excessive inflammation and affect mainly women (three-fourths of all autoimmune diseases occur in women).[155] The body's immune system begins to attack itself because it cannot distinguish between foreign agents and the body's internal agents. Examples of autoimmune diseases include rheumatoid arthritis, celiac disease, fibromyalgia, and inflammatory bowel disease. One study found THC to be helpful in regulating the immune system, which may be useful in helping those who suffer from an autoimmune disease.[156] Cannabis's antiinflammatory properties may also help alleviate or reduce symptoms associated with autoimmune diseases.

Additional Medical Uses

Marijuana stimulates the appetite. This may be beneficial for people with AIDS and those receiving chemotherapy. When receiving chemotherapy, many people lose weight because their appetite diminishes. Marijuana can help these people regain their appetite and put on needed weight. One Australian study reported that nearly 60% of men and women living with HIV/AIDS used marijuana. Although many used the drug recreationally, over 40% believed it helped with their condition.[157]

Marijuana may help with noncancer chronic pain. In a review of controlled trials, researchers found statistical improvement in pain relief using THC.[158] However, scientists caution that more research needs to be completed to determine long-term effects of THC for the management of pain.

Marijuana has been recommended for partially or completely paralyzed individuals because it acts as a muscle relaxant and relieves pain more safely than narcotics.[159] Marijuana alleviates muscle spasms and tremors; consequently, it may prove to be beneficial to people with multiple sclerosis. One study looked at a THC/CBD oromucosal spray in patients with multiple sclerosis and found patients improved in spasticity symptoms related to sleep quality.[160]

Marijuana is recommended for epilepsy, insomnia, rheumatoid arthritis, and chronic pain conditions. Anecdotal evidence suggests that it helps people with bipolar disorders. Finally, marijuana might be beneficial in treating premenstrual syndrome and menstrual cramps. In the late 1800s, Queen Victoria used marijuana for these purposes.

Decriminalization and Legalization

In 1972, the Presidential Commission on Marijuana and Drug Abuse recommended the decriminalization of marijuana. Between 1973 and 1978, 11 states (Oregon being the first) decriminalized marijuana, making possession a minor offense punishable by a

---

CASE STUDY: Charlotte's Web

Perhaps the most well-known case regarding marijuana and epilepsy is Charlette Figi. Charlotte experienced her first seizure at 3 months and was diagnosed with Dravet Syndrome, a rare and severe form of epilepsy. At one point, she was on seven different medications, but the seizures continued. She was five years old when hospitals told her there was nothing more that can be done. She was experiencing over 300 grand mal seizures a week and lost the ability to eat, talk, and walk. At this point, the family decided to apply for a medical marijuana card. She was the youngest patient ever to apply for the card.

They tried her out on a strain that contained a high amount of CBD and low amounts of THC. Results were positive, for the first time in years, she went 7 days without having seizures. At age 6, she is now only having seizures a few times a month and only during her sleep. She has retained the ability to eat and is now riding a bicycle. Speech is also slowly coming back.

Source: S. Young, "Marijuana stops child's severe seizures", *CNN*, (August 7, 2013). Accessed on March 4, 2017 from http://www.cnn.com/2013/08/07/health/charlotte-child -medical-marijuana/.

$100 fine. Marijuana was illegal in every state except Alaska, where up to 4 ounces could be grown. In 1990, however, voters in Alaska approved recriminalizing marijuana. In 1998, the Oregon legislature introduced a referendum to recriminalize marijuana. It appeared on the November 2000 ballot, but by a 2-to-1 margin, the voters defeated the measure. In 2008, Michigan became the 13th state to approve the medical use of marijuana, while Massachusetts became the 13th state to reduce the possession of marijuana to a misdemeanor.[161] However, in a case in California, it was ruled that employers are allowed to fire a worker who tests positive for marijuana, even if it is given for medical reasons.[162] Furthermore, employers in California have the right not to hire someone if they tested positive for marijuana during a drug screening; even if the person has a prescription for the drug.[163] See Table 12.5 for information on states that allow recreational marijuana use.

Perhaps no drug has generated as much discussion regarding decriminalization and legalization as marijuana. Many people believe it is a *relatively* safe drug, although few people are in favor of anyone smoking marijuana before flying an airplane or operating a motor vehicle or heavy equipment. Concern has been voiced that relaxing marijuana laws would give young people the impression that using marijuana is acceptable.

Another argument against marijuana is that it is a gateway drug, leading to the use of more dangerous drugs. How valid is this **steppingstone theory**? Most people who have taken heroin, cocaine, and other illegal drugs have smoked marijuana. Yet, most marijuana smokers do not proceed to use other drugs. Those marijuana smokers who proceed to other drugs start their use at earlier ages and smoke more frequently. The pharmacological properties of marijuana have not been proved to increase the desire to progress to other drugs. Thus other factors are implicated if other drugs are used. One study found that the increase in the use of hard drugs after using marijuana is greatly overstated for people born since the beginning of the 1970s.[164] Alcohol and cigarettes are better predictors of involvement with illegal drugs.

To illustrate, probably most heroin users have consumed soft drinks. Yet soft drinks are not seen as steppingstone drugs. If a marijuana user progresses to other drugs, factors such as availability and desire may also be relevant.

Many marijuana proponents do not contend that the drug is harmless, only that marijuana laws present a greater danger to the public. Which is the greater problem—marijuana or laws against marijuana? One group that lobbies for a change in marijuana laws is the National Organization for the Reform of Marijuana Laws (NORML). NORML contends that the quality of marijuana would be controlled more effectively if it were legal. Marijuana has medical benefits, and legalization would allow people who would benefit from it to obtain it more easily. The opposing argument is that if marijuana could be easily obtained for medical reasons, what might start out as medical use could become personal, recreational use.

When the legalization of marijuana is debated, marijuana inevitably is compared to tobacco and alcohol. It is argued that marijuana wreaks less havoc on families and society than tobacco and alcohol do. Tobacco is connected more definitively to heart disease and lung cancer than marijuana is. The links between marijuana and heart disease and between marijuana and lung cancer have not been established. Nonetheless, if marijuana were as readily available as alcohol and tobacco, usage rates might rival those of alcohol and tobacco, and problems with marijuana conceivably could become commensurate with those of alcohol and tobacco.

TABLE 12.5 States with Recreational Legal Marijuana (as of 2017)

State	Status
Alaska	Adults 21 and over can use, possess, and transport up to an ounce of marijuana for recreational use.
California	Can use and carry up to an ounce of marijuana without a prescription.
Colorado	Legalized recreational marijuana (There are more marijuana dispensaries than Starbucks and McDonalds)
Maine	Right to possess 2.5 ounces of marijuana (retail stores will open in 2018).
Nevada	Legal to possess up to 1 ounce of marijuana (2018 retail launch)
Oregon	Grow up to 4 plants at home, legal to give edibles as a gift.
Washington	Legal to carry up to 1 ounce of marijuana. To be eligible for a grower's license, must require the drug for medicinal purposes.
Washington, DC	People may possess up to 2 ounces of pot and may gift up to 1 ounce.

Source: M. Robinson, "It's 2017: Here's where you can legally smoke weed", *Business Insider,* (January 8, 2017). Accessed on March 4, 2017 from http://www.businessinsider.com /where-can-you-legally-smoke-weed-2017-1.

steppingstone theory Hypothesis holding that use of soft drugs such as marijuana and alcohol leads to use of harder drugs such as heroin and cocaine

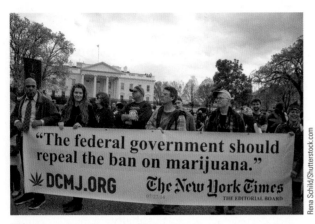

On April 2, 2016 hundreds of Americans protested the federal ban on marijuana in Washington, D.C.

In 2011, the Dutch government reversed its tolerance policies regarding marijuana. It reclassified marijuana so that it is now comparable to cocaine and ecstasy.[165] The Dutch government had taken a pragmatic approach, believing that if it had better control over marijuana use, the risks would be reduced. It is estimated that 13% of Dutch high school students have used marijuana, compared to 28% of American high school students.[166] One of the reasons for the crackdown in the Netherlands was to decrease the amount of "pot tourists" visiting the area to have access to marijuana.[167] While the new laws have reduced this problem, another problem took its place: street dealers are back. In contrast to The Netherlands, a number of European countries such as Belgium, Britain, and Luxembourg have adopted less stringent views on marijuana use.

Legalization of Marijuana for Medical Uses

Whether marijuana should be legal for medical purposes is hotly debated. One argument in favor of it is that marijuana has a long history of medical use and is reasonably safe. Opponents of medical marijuana use believe that if marijuana were available for medical use, its nonmedical use would increase dramatically. In a study looking at the impact of medical marijuana laws on recreational drug use, it was found that among adults aged 21 and older, in states that had medicinal marijuana laws, there was an increase in marijuana use and frequency of use.[168] Furthermore, among those ages 12 to 20 years old, a small increase in marijuana use was observed.

The federal government maintains that most evidence showing that marijuana works is anecdotal and is not based on solid scientific research. It has, however, begun to fund research into the efficacy of medicinal uses of marijuana. At the same time, some scientists maintain that the federal government is hindering research into marijuana's medicinal benefits by making it difficult to receive permission to conduct these studies. One concern is that medical marijuana may be illegally diverted. There is evidence that adolescents in treatment for substance abuse have received marijuana from others who obtained it for medical purposes.[169]

In November 1996, California voters passed Proposition 215, eliminating state penalties for medical uses of marijuana. Despite passage of Proposition 215, federal law takes precedence over state law, and the vast majority of politicians at the national level oppose making marijuana medically legal. In June 2001, Nevada state lawmakers approved marijuana use for seriously ill individuals. In the month preceding this approval, however, the US Supreme Court reaffirmed its stance opposing medicinal use of marijuana.

Initiatives to legalize marijuana for medical purposes were on the ballots of numerous states and the District of Columbia. In every instance except in Missouri, voters approved allowing doctors to prescribe marijuana to treat terminal or debilitating illnesses. In Alaska, 58% of voters approved the initiative; in Washington State, 59% of voters approved it; in Oregon, 55%; and in Nevada, 59%. Twenty-eight states, including the District of Columbia, have passed medical marijuana laws.[170]

The National Academies of Sciences, Engineering and Medicine (formally known at the Institute of Medicine) published a report in January 2017 regarding research on cannabis and cannabinoids.[171] The conclusions regarding its therapeutic effects were as follows.[172]

There is conclusive or substantial evidence that cannabis or cannaninoids are effective for:

- Treatment of chronic pain in adults
- Antiemetics in the treatment of chemotherapy-induced nausea and vomiting (oral)
- Improving patient reported multiple scherosis spasticity stumptoms (oral)

There is moderate evidence that cannabis or cannabinoids are effective for:

- Improving short-term sleep outcomes in individuals with sleep disturbance associated with obstructive sleep apnea syndrome, fibromyalgia, chronic pain, and multiple sclerosis

There is limited evidence that cannabis or cannabinoids are effective for:

- Increasing appetite and decreasing weight loss associated with HIV/AIDS

- Improving clinician-measured multiple sclerosis spasticity symptoms
- Improving symptoms of Tourette syndrome
- Improving anxiety symptoms in individuals with social anxiety disorders
- Improving symptoms of posttraumatic stress disorder

There is limited evidence of a statistical association between cannabinoids and

- Better outcomes (mortality, disability) after a traumatic brain injury

There is limited evidence that cannabis or cannabinoids are ineffective for:

- Improving symptoms associated with dementia
- Improving intraocular pressure associate with glaucoma
- Reducing depressive symptoms in individuals with chronic pain or multiple sclerosis

In 1988, Francis Young, the chief administrative law judge for the Drug Enforcement Agency (DEA), recommended that the DEA change marijuana from schedule I to schedule II to give support to medical patients who would benefit from it. The DEA refused to accept the recommendation because it questioned the medical value of marijuana. Ironically, morphine and cocaine, drugs with stronger psychoactive effects, are currently used in medicine. In April 2006, the US Food and Drug Administration (FDA) reaffirmed its position that marijuana should remain a Schedule I drug, asserting that marijuana has a high potential for abuse, has no currently accepted medical use in treatment in the United States, and has a lack of accepted safety for use under medical supervision.[173] However, the FDA supports research into the medical use of marijuana.[174] It is unclear what approach President Donald Trump will take on the federal government's stance on marijuana.

As more states legalize medical marijuana, there has been a shift of opinion from other organizations. The American Medical Association used to oppose marijuana, but now call for more controlled studies of marijuana and cannabinoids and urge the National Institutes of Health to review the schedule I status of marijuana.[175] While not endorsing marijuana for medicinal use, it is recognizing the need for more research. The National Multiple Sclerosis society supports the right of patients to work with their doctors to access marijuana for treatment.[176] The American Academy of Ophthalmology does not support the use of marijuana to treat glaucoma.[177] As mentioned earlier in this chapter, marijuana only provides a temporary reduction in intraocular pressure. The American College of Physicians, the nation's largest organization of internal medicine doctors, calls for the use of medical marijuana.[178] In fact, more doctors are supporting legalization of medical marijuana.[179] A group of over 50 doctors and Joycelyn Elders (former US Surgeon General) formed a national organization (Doctors for Cannabis Regulation), which endorses the legalization of marijuana for adult recreational use.[180]

The debate over whether marijuana should be medically legal raises several interesting questions:[181]

- If physicians believe marijuana could be beneficial, do they have a moral obligation to inform their patients of this possibility?
- Should physicians be prosecuted if they recommend marijuana use to their patients?
- What constitutes a legitimate medical use?
- Is improving the quality of mental health a legitimate medical use for marijuana?

Cost

Drug reform advocate and executive director of the *Drug Policy Alliance* (DPA) Ethan Nadelmann contends that treating drug offenders is much cheaper than incarcerating them.[182] Moreover, legalizing marijuana and other drugs would stem the rise in violence and criminal activity.[183] The DPA believes three principles relate to drug policy:[184]

- Freedom— People should not be punished for what they put in their body, only for crimes that hurt others.
- Responsibility— People and government should be held responsible for the harmful consequences of their actions.
- Compassion— When people struggle with drug abuse, compassion is more effective than punishment.

In the United States, almost 1.5 million people are arrested each year on nonviolent drug charges. In 2015, almost 650,000 were arrested for a marijuana law violation with 89% of those charged with possession only.[185] Over half (858,408) of these arrests were for a marijuana law violation.[186] In contrast, only 30% of drug-related arrests in 1990 were for a marijuana violation. Interestingly, the increase in arrest rates has had no impact on marijuana's rate of use.[187]

Crime and Violence

The reputation of marijuana as a cause of violence dates back to Hassan, an Arabian politico who lived during the Middle Ages, and his cult, who purportedly used hashish in preparation for aggressive acts against others. Still, whether Hassan and his followers actually consumed hashish is unclear. The 1930s film

Reefer Madness also depicted marijuana as a drug that caused users to become violent.

What effect would legalization of marijuana have on aggression and crime? No one can say for sure. Legalization might result in one set of problems replacing another. The incidence of criminal and violent behavior might go down, whereas interpersonal and intrapersonal problems might escalate. One historical precedent is alcohol prohibition. When alcohol was legally prohibited, alcohol-related arrests dropped by half, but the law laid the groundwork for organized crime, which took over the manufacture and distribution of alcohol.

An argument for legalization is that it would remove much of the profit motive.[188] Initial evidence from Colorado suggests a reduction in crime after the legalization of marijuana. The city of Denver saw a decrease in violence and property crime in 2014.[189] Additionally, traffic fatalities went down in 2014 by 3%, which was one area that people felt would increase as a result of drugged driving.

Summary

Marijuana has an extensive history. It was medically important in many countries and was economically essential to the United States in its infancy for the hemp used in making rope. Not until the 1900s was marijuana used for recreational reasons. Stories of marijuana causing mental illness, violent behavior, and immorality eventually resulted in the Marijuana Tax Act of 1937 being passed.

Marijuana comes from the *Cannabis sativa* plant and contains over natural compounds, of which 66 are cannabinoids. The primary psychoactive agent is delta-9-tetrahydrocannabinol (THC). Other cannabinoids, such as CBD and CBN, are being researched to determine therapeutic benefits. Levels of THC are affected by the plant's sex, the part of the plant used, soil and climate conditions, and how the plant is stored.

Marijuana works more quickly when it is smoked than when it is ingested. THC reaches the brain within seconds after smoking, peak effects occur in about one-half hour, and the high lasts several hours. THC levels, intervals between puffs, and depth and length of inhalation influence the effects of marijuana. Behavioral and psychological tolerance seems to occur in humans, but reverse tolerance—in which users achieve the desired effects with decreasing dosages—has not been proved.

The psychological effects of marijuana vary among users. It can affect mood, sensitivity to external stimuli, and perception of time and space. Marijuana use has been shown to have negative cognitive effects on adolescents who use the drug. This may be attributed to the disruption of brain growth during adolescence and young adulthood.

Much of the research on the long-term effects of marijuana use has been poorly conducted. Evidence regarding the respiratory system, however, is clear. Marijuana smoke damages lung tissue and impairs lung function. Also, marijuana smoke contains carcinogenic chemicals. Marijuana has not been shown to cause heart attacks in people with a healthy heart, but it could precipitate heart conditions in people who already have coronary heart disease. In males, sperm production, sperm structure, and sperm motility are affected adversely. Women who smoke marijuana might not ovulate.

Marijuana has been used to treat asthma, glaucoma, and multiple sclerosis. Its use in treating glaucoma has declined because other drugs have proved to be more effective. Because THC expands lung capacity, it formerly was used for asthma, although its benefit was limited. Marijuana seems to be effective in alleviating the nausea and vomiting associated with chemotherapy. Twenty-eight states have passed referenda approving the use of marijuana for medical purposes, although federal law overrides the state laws.

Many people consider marijuana a relatively safe drug and believe that problems stem from its illegal status. Proponents of legalization argue that it would allow for more control over the distribution and use of the drug, that marijuana causes less physical harm than alcohol and tobacco, and that treating marijuana users is cheaper than incarcerating them. Opponents argue that liberalizing marijuana laws would trigger an increase in personal use, leading to increased cost of treatment programs. These people believe illegality prevents many people from using a drug that may result in negative long-term consequences.

Thinking Critically

1. Cannabinoids, other than THC, are being researched to determine their therapeutic effects. Previous research regarding the medicinal benefits of marijuana solely focused on THC, but current research is including other cannabinoids to determine their therapeutic effects. Furthermore, the THC content seems to be rising in marijuana products, perhaps at the detriment of other cannabinoids. How much credence to previous research should be given?

2. Former Presidents Clinton and Obama publicly acknowledged to using marijuana in their youth. Yet, marijuana remained as a schedule I drug during and after their presidency. What message are they giving to the public regarding marijuana? Do you think public opinion of those presidents would change if they admitted to using harder drugs such as cocaine and heroin? Defend your answer.

3. Do you feel marijuana use leads to heavier drug use? Is marijuana a "stepping stone" to harder drugs? Justify your answer.

4. Because marijuana may result in babies with lower birth weight, smoking marijuana during pregnancy is unwise. If birth difficulties were proven to be caused by marijuana use, would it affect your decision to smoke or not smoke marijuana during pregnancy? Should pregnant women who smoke marijuana be penalized in some way? If so, how?

5. Whether marijuana should be used in the treatment of medical problems is the topic of an ongoing debate. Should the decision to use marijuana for medical purposes be made by government officials or by medical personnel?

6. One argument for legalizing drugs is that the black market in drugs would be reduced. Do you think legalization would reduce the black market? Would you be more tempted to try drugs if you could get them legally? Would the cost of obtaining marijuana affect your decision to use or not to use it? How does legality affect use?

13

Hallucinogens

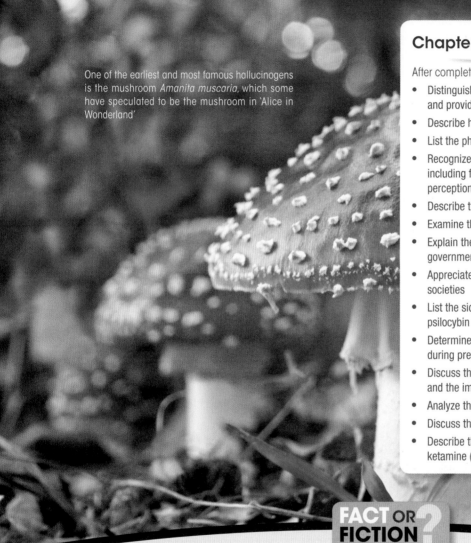

One of the earliest and most famous hallucinogens is the mushroom *Amanita muscaria*, which some have speculated to be the mushroom in 'Alice in Wonderland'

specnaz/Shutterstock.com

Chapter Objectives

After completing this chapter, the reader should be able to:

- Distinguish between classic and dissociative hallucinogens and provide examples of each
- Describe human use of hallucinogens throughout history
- List the physiological and psychological effects of LSD
- Recognize the potential long-term effects of hallucinogens including flashbacks and hallucinogen-induced persistent perception disorder
- Describe the events that led to the popularization of LSD
- Examine the relationship between LSD and mental health
- Explain the experiments with LSD conducted by the US government
- Appreciate the role hallucinogens have played in native societies
- List the side effects associated with mescaline and psilocybin
- Determine the impact of various hallucinogenic drugs during pregnancy
- Discuss the legal status of anticholinergic hallucinogens and the impact on usage
- Analyze the potential medical benefits of hallucinogens
- Discuss the trends related to emergence of salvinorin A
- Describe the physiological and psychological effects of ketamine (special K) and PCP

FACT OR FICTION?

1. Hallucinogens act as stimulants on the central nervous system.
2. Besides the U.S. military, the Russian military is also believed to have experimented with hallucinogens.
3. Hallucinogens are not addictive.
4. Hallucinogens are perfectly safe.
5. At twice its normal dosage, LSD is fatal.
6. At one time, hallucinogenic drugs were associated with witchcraft and sorcery.
7. The psychological effects of psilocybin are more powerful than the psychological effects of LSD.
8. Jimsonweed, which can result in poisoning, is illegal throughout the United States.
9. LSD and other hallucinogens may cause a psychotic disorder.
10. Albert Hofmann, who was responsible for developing LSD, died from an LSD overdose soon after developing the drug.

Turn the page to check your answers

E ver since the beginning of time, humans have sought ways to alter their consciousness. Through trial and error, certain plants were identified as having mind-altering properties. In early times, over 6,000 plants were capable of altering conciousness.[1] Today about 150 plants are used for hallucinogenic purposes. Although it is not a plant, lysergic acid diethylamide (LSD) is one of the most potent hallucinogens. Scientific interest in hallucinogenic drugs increased after World War II. The availability of mind-altering drugs was (and still is) vast.

Terminology

Terms referring to **hallucinogens** can be confusing because many terms have been used to describe drugs with hallucinogenic characteristics. The word *hallucinogen* refers to drugs that cause profound distortions in a person's perception of reality.[2] In other words, these are chemicals that alter thoughts, feelings, and perceptions. Many of these chemicals result in hallucinations only when they are taken in large quantities. Some drugs classified as hallucinogens produce no hallucinations; conversely, some drugs not classified as hallucinogens can induce hallucinations.

Lewis Lewin, a German pharmacologist in the early 1900s, called hallucinogens **phantasticants**

TERMS DESCRIBING HALLUCINOGENS

- **phantasticants**: Drugs having stimulating and inebriating properties
- **psychedelic**: Mind-manifesting
- **psychotomimetic**: Psychotic-like
- **psychotogenic**: Psychosis-generating

because of their "stimulating and inebriating properties" and their importance to research and science.[3] During the era of tie-dyed shirts, antiwar protests, flower power, Woodstock, acid rock, and political activism, the term **psychedelic**, or "mind-manifesting," was in vogue. Coined by British psychiatrist Humphrey Osmond in 1956, the word referred to the mind-altering properties of naturally occurring hallucinogenic plant substances.[4]

Because hallucinogens reportedly produced psychotic-like symptoms, they also were called **psychotomimetic**. *Psychoto* means "psychosis," and *mimetic* translates to "acting-like." Another term used to describe hallucinogens is **psychotogenic**, meaning "psychosis-generating." Current research is examining the role of LSD and other drugs as a cause of schizophrenia.[5] During closely monitored research involving hallucinogens, subjects rarely experience adverse reactions.[6]

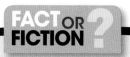

1. **FICTION** The fact is—Hallucinogens do not increase or decrease central nervous system activity.

2. **FACT** Although the evidence is not conclusive, it appears as though the Russian military gave hallucinogens to prisoners.

3. **FICTION** The fact is—While LSD is not physically addictive, it has been shown to be psychologically addictive.

4. **FICTION** The fact is—Some hallucinogens can make you physically ill and can be poisonous.

5. **FICTION** The fact is—Although one may die from behaviors while under the influence of LSD, one does not die from the pharmacological effects of LSD.

6. **FACT** Numerous hallucinogenic drugs have been applied to the practices of witchcraft and sorcery.

7. **FICTION** The fact is—LSD's psychological effects are more potent than the psychological effects of psilocybin.

8. **FICTION** The fact is—Currently, jimsonweed is illegal in several states, but the U.S. government has not declared jimsonweed illegal.

9. **FACT**

10. **FICTION** The fact is—Albert Hofmann died at age 102, from natural causes.

The Origin of Hallucinogens

Almost all drugs that have hallucinogenic properties are derived from plants. Two exceptions are LSD and methylenedioxymethamphetamine (MDMA), which are produced synthetically. Swiss chemist Albert Hofmann developed LSD as a possible headache remedy in 1938 and discovered its hallucinogenic capabilities accidentally 5 years later. The following passage is the chemist's description of his own initial experience with LSD.

> Last Friday, April 16, 1943, I was forced to interrupt my work in the laboratory in the middle of the afternoon and proceed home, being affected by a remarkable restlessness, combined with a slight dizziness. At home I lay down and sank into a not unpleasant intoxicated-like condition, characterized by an extremely stimulated imagination. In a dreamlike state, with eyes closed (I found the daylight to be unpleasantly glaring), I perceived an uninterrupted stream of fantastic pictures, extraordinary shapes with intense, kaleidoscopic play of colors. After some two hours this condition faded away.[7]

The Search for Hallucinogens

Human's early search for mind-altering drugs was described by Schultes and Hofmann's book *The Botany and Chemistry of Hallucinogens*:

> Agents that cause visual, auditory, tactile, taste and other hallucinations or that induce artificial psychoses have been undoubtedly used since earliest human experimentation with the vegetal environment.[8]

These drugs were thought to be consumed primarily for their psychic, not their physical, effects. People took them to escape their everyday existence to commune with a higher order.

Psychic, sacred, and medicinal powers were attributed to hallucinogens. Hallucinogens change awareness of reality. They alter perceptions of time, spirituality, and the universe, helping people transcend boundaries of time and space. Mind-altering drugs were central in many Eastern religions, where they were used to achieve religious revelations. Hallucinogenic drugs were used throughout Central and South America as well as by the ancient Greeks and Romans. More recently, methods of altering one's concepts of time and space involve activities that do not use drugs—such as music, chanting, meditation, and computer games.

Amanita muscaria

One of the earliest and most common hallucinogens is the mushroom ***Amanita muscaria***, also called

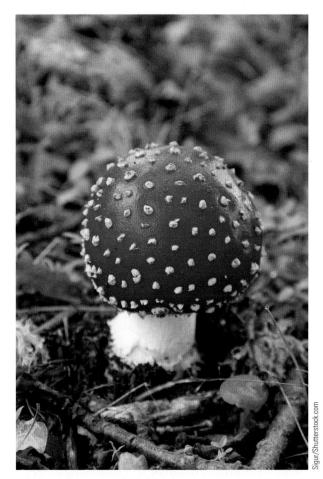

Sigur/Shutterstock.com

The *Amanita muscaria* is poisonous; although deaths are rare, they can occur.

fly agaric. It has been used in parts of Europe as an insecticide. It was crushed in milk, which would attract flies and kill them.[9] In India 3,500 years ago, the *Rig Veda*, an ancient Hindu book, contained an

---

hallucinogens A class of drugs that induce perceived distortions in time and space

phantasticants A term used to describe hallucinogenic drugs

psychedelic A term used to describe hallucinogenic drugs; means "mind-manifesting"

psychotomimetic Refers to drugs that produce psychotic-like symptoms

psychotogenic Refers to drugs that generate psychosis

Amanita muscaria One of the oldest and most common hallucinogens; derived from the fly agaric mushroom

fly agaric Another name for the hallucinogenic mushroom *Amanita muscaria*

Christmas time brings about traditions that are celebrated around the world. Those who practice it bring in trees to decorate and place presents under. On Christmas Eve, Santa rides in a sleigh pulled by flying reindeer and visits children all over the world to leave them presents while they are sleeping.

According to one theory, Santa's story may be traced back to shamans in the Siberian and Artic regions who used *Amanita muscaria*, in their religious rituals. As the story goes, shamans would collect *Amanita muscaria*, to give as gifts on winter solstice. Because these regions experience heavy snow fall, doors to homes were blocked, so the shamans would place the gifts in the openings of roofs, which were there as an alternative entrance to homes during the winter months. Similarly, Santa also enters homes through openings in the roof. Christmas trees, or pine trees, are brought in the home where presents (usually white and red wrapped) are left under the branches. In Artic regions, the *Amanita muscaria* are found under birch and conifer trees. Santa, who is dressed in red with a white edging, is said to represent the colors of the mushroom which are red with white spots. And what about flying reindeer? Reindeer in the Artic region are common, and perhaps they are flying due to the psychedelic trip experienced when taking *Amanita muscaria*.

Source: D. Main, "Magic Mushrooms may explain Santa & his flying reindeer", *Live Science*, (December 20, 2012). Accessed on March 8, 2017 from http://www.livescience.com/25731-magic-mushrooms-santa-claus.html.

elaborate description of a drug called **soma**. Soma, which was highly praised and used in religious ceremonies, was actually *Amanita muscaria*. The active parts of this drug inhibit the part of the brain responsible for instilling fear into a person.[10] Some believe the Viking warriors ingested this drug to make them feel more fierce.[11] When traveling through Siberia, Europeans noticed villagers ingesting these mushrooms. Within an hour, the villagers would twitch, tremble, feel happy, hallucinate, dance, and then fall into a deep sleep.

Other effects of *Amanita muscaria* include lower heart rate, elevated blood pressure, constriction of pupils of the eye, and excessive perspiration and salivation. This mushroom grows throughout the United States, and can be lethal.[12] A unique characteristic of *Amanita muscaria* is that it passes through the body and into the urine unchanged. Hence, it can be used more than once.

Saint Anthony's Fire

A plant with hallucinogenic properties that was used by ancient Greeks in religious rituals is a fungus of the genus *Claviceps*, which grows on certain cereals, especially rye. One species implicated in deadly epidemics in Europe and elsewhere was *Claviceps purpurea*, the ergot of rye.[13] Reports of ergot poisoning—**ergotism**—killing thousands of people surfaced during the Middle Ages.[14] Ergotism is marked by hallucinations, convulsions, epileptic symptoms, and delirium; gangrene leading to occasional loss of nose, ears, fingers, toes, and feet; and possible death.

Pregnant women would miscarry after ingesting this poisonous fungus.

The epidemic was called the "holy fire," because people had burning sensations in their hands and feet. To end the epidemic, people went on pilgrimages to the shrine of Saint Anthony, the patron saint of fire, epilepsy, and infection. The epidemics, which came to be known as **St. Anthony's fire**, ended with a change in diet that excluded rye. Incidents of ergotism have been reported as recently as 1953.

Ergot poisoning might have played a role in allegations of witchcraft in colonial New England. Young girls who appeared to be suffering from a witch's *spell* may have ingested the ergot fungus. The inability to explain the source of the girls' odd behavior led to accusations of witchcraft in Salem in the 1690s. It was from this fungus that Albert Hofmann extracted LSD in 1938.

Review of Major Hallucinogens

Hallucinogens are often placed into two categories: classic hallucinogens and dissociative drugs.[15] See Table 13.1 for examples from each category of hallucinogens.

The number of hallucinogenic drugs is quite extensive. People go to considerable lengths to find new ways to alter their consciousness. For example, some people in the United States, Canada, Australia, and South and Central America engage in "toad

TABLE 13.1 Examples of Hallucinogens

Classic Hallucinogens	Dissociative Hallucinogens
• LSD	• PCP
• Psilocybin	• Ketamine
• Peyote	• DXM
• DMT	• *Salvia divinorum*
• Ayahausca	

Source: National Institute on Drug Abuse, "Hallucinogens and Dissociative drugs", Updated February 2015. Accessed on March 8, 2017 from https://www.drugabuse.gov/publications /research-reports/hallucinogens-dissociative-drugs /what-are-dissociative-drugs.

licking," an activity in which they orally ingest glandular secretions or smoke the dried skin of the **bufo** toad. Prior research into the hallucinogenic effects of licking the bufo toad and other toads indicated that it had little effect. Furthermore, many toads excrete a toxin through their skin, which has been attributed to pet deaths. Nevertheless, aphrodisiac-like effects have been attributed to the bufo toad.[16]

In this section, we will review the better-known hallucinogens, with emphasis on their psychological and physiological effects. Notwithstanding the scarcity of clinical research into the effects of hallucinogens on humans, a review of the studies resulted in little evidence of long-term neuropsychological deficits.[17] However, two conditions have been associated with repeated use: hallucinogen-persisting disorder (HPPD) and persistent psychosis. It is worth noting these lasting conditions are more likely to occur in people with a history of psychological problems.[18] The research, however, has not been conducted over a long period of time. Also, people who use hallucinogens tend to use other drugs as well, confounding the research results. Most of the research on humans took place before the mid-1960s, when Congress prohibited the public use and sale of LSD, peyote, mescaline, and similar drugs due to its adoption as a recreational drug.[19]

Classic Hallucinogens
LSD

Of all known hallucinogens, none is more powerful than LSD. Whereas dosages of most drugs are measured in milligrams, or one-thousandth of a gram, dosages of LSD are measured in micrograms, or one-millionth of a gram. LSD produces profound effects on perception and mood.

Tolerance develops rapidly. Thus, people cannot experience the effects of LSD if they have taken it within the previous 3 or 4 days, which is the time needed for tolerance of the drug to dissipate.[20] Withdrawal symptoms do not occur and most users can easily abstain from the drug without any ill effects.[21] Also, cross-tolerance between LSD and other hallucinogens occurs.[22] LSD, which is consumed orally, is absorbed through the gastrointestinal tract, metabolized by the liver, and quickly excreted. LSD has no taste, color, or odor.

LSD is taken differently today than when it was first introduced. In the 1960s, it came in the form of a cube or tablet. Today it consists of microdots, or diluted drops, that typically are placed on blotter paper and licked. Its effects begin within an hour. Behavioral effects last 6 to 8 hours, but LSD has a half-life of only 3 hours. Hence, the effects last longer than the drug is active. LSD is detectable in urine up to 72 hours after ingestion. Despite adverse publicity, no fatal overdoses have been documented. People have died as a result of their behavior while on LSD, such as jumping out of windows, but not from its pharmacological effects.

Since 1997, the use of LSD and other hallucinogens by secondary school students has declined, although rates of use have slowly increased since the mid-2000s when use was at its lowest.[23] In 2016, annual prevalence rates for 8th, 10th, and 12th graders were 0.8%, 2.1%, and 3.0%, respectively.[24] The US Department of Defense in 2008 decided to cease testing service members for LSD because so few were testing positive, suggesting a low rate of use in this population as well.[25] In 2008, the Department of Defense decided to cease testing service members for LSD due to the low rate of LSD use among service members. Over a 3-year time period, only four tests came back positive for LSD, out of over 2 million samples.[26] Periodic screening for LSD may still take place to determine prevalence of the drug.

LSD operates on the neurotransmitter serotonin in the brain, but little is known about its precise actions. Serotonin plays a role in sensory perception and mood. As potent as LSD is its physiological effects, which begin about 20 minutes after ingestion,

---

soma An Indian drink used in ritualistic ways

ergotism A condition resulting from ingesting a fungus that grows on grains; marked by muscle tremors, burning, mania, delirium, hallucinations, and eventual gangrene

St. Anthony's fire Burning sensations caused by ergot poisoning; people during the Middle Ages would visit the shrine of St. Anthony in an attempt to cure it
Timothy Leary helped to popularize the use of LSD
A powerful hallucinogen derived from a fungus

bufo A type of toad that produces a hallucinogenic secretion

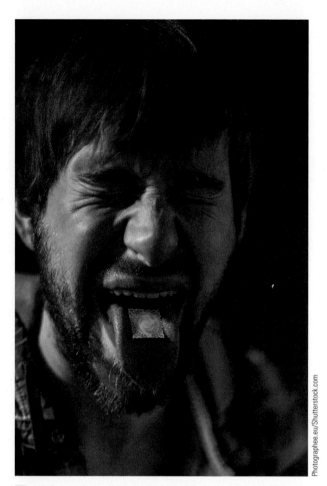
Photographee.eu/Shutterstock.com

LSD is usually consumed orally. Diluted drops are placed on blotter paper, which is then placed on the tongue.

PHYSIOLOGICAL EFFECTS OF LSD

- Dilation of pupils
- Increased blood pressure
- Dry mouth
- Increased salivation
- Twitching
- Dizziness
- Rapid heartbeat
- Slight tremors
- Higher body temperature
- Fatigue
- Muscle weakness
- Numbness
- Nausea
- Uterine contractions

Source: National Institute on Drug Abuse, "Hallucinogens and Dissociative Drugs", Updated February 2015. Accessed on March 7, 2017 from https://www.drugabuse.gov/publications /research-reports/hallucinogens-dissociative-drugs /what-are-hallucinogens.

are rather mild and brief. See the side box on the physiological effects of LSD. Because LSD can stimulate uterine contractions, pregnant women should avoid it.

Although LSD causes chromosome damage, it is just one of the many drugs, including aspirin, that do so. On closer examination, study subjects who have taken LSD have been found to have taken amphetamines, tranquilizers, or heroin at the same time. Thus, it is not possible to attribute LSD use to chromosonal damage as other drugs could have caused this damage. The same is true with studies claiming that women taking LSD gave birth to highly deformed babies and had a higher rate of miscarriage and premature delivery. These women were likely to have used other drugs as well and generally had poorer prenatal care. It is more likely that .the behavioral effects of pregnant women who use LSD lead to poorer birth outcomes, not the drug itself.[27] Furthermore, studies have been inconclusive regarding prior LSD use and birth outcomes. This does not suggest that LSD is safe but that there is not definitive proof that it is harmful.

The most significant effects of LSD are psychological, not physiological. By their nature, psychological effects are subject to interpretation. Although LSD is known to alter mood and perception, the extent to which these changes occur depends on the user's mental state, the environment in which the drug is used, previous experiences with the drug, and dosage.

Psychological changes take effect about 40 minutes after ingestion. The LSD trip consists of the following five distinct phases:[28]

Level 1: Users will experience mild visual effects.
Level 2: Users will experience mild visual effects and an increase in abstract and creative thought.
Level 3: Users may see wrapping patterns and kaleidoscopic imagery. Intermingling of sense may occur.
Level 4: Users may experience strong visual patterns, intense visions, and a perception of time.
Level 5: Considered the epicenter of the psychedelic state. Users may experience complete immersion in visions and synesthesia.

Synesthesia, the blending of senses in which the person hears or tastes colors and sees sounds, is one outcome of LSD. Depersonalization and

POSSIBLE PSYCHOLOGICAL EFFECTS OF LSD

- Time distortion
- Ego disintegration
- Depression
- Fear
- Mood swings
- Panic
- Blending of senses
- Flashbacks

disorientation are other effects. Body image may be distorted, or the user might have feelings of becoming one with the floor or whatever he or she is sitting or lying on. A user may conjure repressed memories or have a psychotic reaction lasting weeks or months. Others say that they experience mystical or religious encounters.

Although some people find changes in perception and sensation desirable, others find these changes frightening. Fear or panic can lead to a "bad trip." A person having a bad trip must be reassured that the effects are temporary and that he or she will not be left alone. A helpful person should *not* restrain this person physically. A bad trip is more likely to occur with inexperienced users and people with preexisting psychological problems. The set and setting of drug use may contribute to a bad trip. When medical intervention is necessary, major tranquilizers are administered in order to calm a person down so medical personnel are able to monitor and stabilize any physical conditions.

Another phenomenon associated with LSD is a **flashback** in which the person reexperiences the effects of LSD days, weeks, or even months after last using it. There is no consensus on how often flashbacks occur. What causes flashbacks has not been determined conclusively, but they might be precipitated by stress or fatigue. Some studies have found flashbacks to be less likely to occur among people who took LSD in a therapeutic or research setting rather than in a recreational setting.[29] However, in a recent study of 400 patients who were treated with LSD between 1960 and 1974 for a variety of psychological ailments, many suffered from severe side effects resulting from LSD use.[30] Out of the initial 400 patients, there was one homicide, two suicides, and four suicide attempts. Additionally, out of 154 cases, two-thirds reported experiencing flashbacks. The symptoms of flashbacks are similar to the active effects of the drug. While unpredictable, some

conditions have been thought to increase the chance of experiencing flashbacks including heavy or frequent LSD use, marijuana use, alcohol use, fatigue, stress, existing mental illness, and use of certain drugs such as antidepressants.[31] When flashbacks occur frequently and interfere with a person's life, it is known as **hallucinogen-induced persistent perception disorder (HPPD)**. While scientists are unsure what causes flashbacks, some theories include:[32]

- Brain may be damaged by LSD use
- Function of the brain has been changed by LSD use
- LSD or some other hallucinogen may be stored in the brain and released again later on

LSD and Mental Health

In 1953, the US Food and Drug Administration (FDA) approved a request by the Sandoz Pharmaceutical Company to register LSD as a new drug for investigative purposes. One of the first uses of LSD was to study mental illness, especially schizophrenia. Because LSD causes hallucinations, and people with schizophrenia hallucinate, the researchers believed that studying the effects of LSD on the brain would be helpful. Patients under the influence of LSD would serve as models for studying schizophrenia. This line of research was abandoned because people who were given LSD did not have the disordered thinking pattern found in schizophrenics, and LSD produces visual hallucinations, whereas schizophrenics have auditory hallucinations. Furthermore, in people with a preexisting risk of mental illness, LSD may induce real psychosis.[33] However, in a large population study of over 100,000 adults in the United States, there was no link between psychedelic use (LSD, psilocybin, or mescaline) and mental health problems later on.[34] This study also found no link between lifetime use of psychedelics and psychological distress, mental health treatment, suicidal thoughts, suicidal plans, suicidal attempts, depression, and anxiety.

Many psychiatrists gave their patients LSD and other hallucinogens to help them develop personal insight and to recall forgotten or repressed experiences.

synesthesia The hallucinogenic blending of senses (e.g., seeing sounds and hearing color)

flashback A phenomenon in which a person reexperiences the effects of LSD days, weeks, or months after it was last used

hallucinogen-induced persistent perception disorder (HPPD) Flashbacks that continue and interfere with daily life

Initial results were promising. Some patients credited LSD with giving them peace of mind after taking it during therapy. Patients who took LSD were less defensive, responded more effectively to their counselors, and exhibited positive emotional responses. In one study conducted on 12 people who suffer from anxiety, results indicate positive results from only two sessions of LSD-assisted psychotherapy.[35]

LSD was given to terminally ill cancer patients to help them cope with the specter of death and to other patients to alleviate stress and psychosomatic illnesses. Studies in the 1960s reported that LSD helped terminally ill patients adjust to their impending death and enabled them to be more responsive to their families.[36] A more recent study found that hallucinogens improve the mood of patients with a life-threatening disease. This study found significant improvements in anxiety related to the life-threatening disease and an improvement in their quality of life.[37] LSD was also used in the treatment of autism from 1959 to 1974, although the research was inconclusive.[38] In addition, LSD was used to treat heroin addiction, sexual deviance, sexual dysfunction, and alcoholism. Despite the early studies demonstrating that LSD was helpful in treating alcoholism, research was halted after the US government made it illegal. In a retrospective analysis of studies involving alcoholism and the use of LSD, it was found that LSD helped people overcome alcohol addiction.[39]

By 1965, an estimated 40,000 patients in psychotherapy had received LSD.[40] Despite indications that LSD could benefit individuals in psychotherapy and terminally ill patients, its use was discontinued because of negative publicity. In the mid-1960s, the number of research projects examining the therapeutic uses of LSD dropped from more than 70 to 6.[41] The political climate and potential risks deterred psychiatrists from using LSD in therapy, and Sandoz Pharmaceutical Company ended its production of LSD.

Presently, LSD is a schedule I drug and has no accepted medical use. However, there is still research regarding the effects of LSD. In a recent study, scientists used brain imaging to get a picture of what is going on in the brain when a person takes LSD. Results indicate an increase in connectivity among regions in the brain, especially in areas contributing to visual processing.[42] In the presence of LSD, the brain networks that deal with vision, hearing, attention, and movement become more connected with each other. This research may lead to further studies investigating using LSD as a treatment for depression and other mental health disorders.[43] The basis for using hallucinogens to study mental illness is that the drugs may help an individual to lose control of typical thought patterns, essentially reworking the brain patterns seen in depression and addiction.[44]

MICRODOSING AND HAPPINESS CASE STUDY

Author Ayelet Waldman suffered from severe depression that began to overwhelm her during perimenopause. She felt it was destroying her marriage and other relationships in her life. That is when she began researching ways to treat her depression and came across the idea of microdosing on LSD. Feeling at the end of her line, she decided to try this technique. Microdosing involves taking such small amounts of LSD so they do not produce any adverse effects.

In her book, *A Really Good Day*, she chronicles her experience as she microdoses on LSD each day for one month. She felt LSD allowed her to better control her emotions and take time to really think about how she is feeling. Ayelet described the experience as extreme mindfulness and felt LSD helped her focus her mind.

She did quit using the drug after a month, partly due because she didn't want to continue committing a crime due to microdosing LSD. Purchasing the drug on the black market is dangerous because of the lack of control to what a person is actually receiving.

Questions to Ponder

Ayelet admits to microdosing on LSD for an entire month. During this time, she cared for her children and went to work every day. Do you think the company she works for should enact some type of punishment for her admitting to showing up to work under the influence of LSD? What about notions of child abuse; as she was caring for her children during this time as well? What about the law? Should she be prosecuted for LSD use?

Source: "Is microdosing LSD the shortcut to happiness?", *Shape*, (January 16, 2017). Accessed on March 9, 2017 from http://www.shape .com/lifestyle/mind-and-body/microdosing-lsd-shortcut-happiness.

LSD and Creativity

Because LSD affects perception strongly, some people, especially artists, believe it enhances creativity. A limitation in determining whether LSD has such effects is that creativity is subjective and thus difficult to measure (one person's scribbling may be another person's masterpiece). In an article written by neuropharmacologist and psychologist David Nutt, he explains that "capturing the elusive elements of a creative act is like trying to weigh a pound of leaping mice."[45]

Objectively, LSD does not seem to improve creativity, although artists who take it largely seem to enjoy its effects. Although LSD will not make a good artist a great artist, it might make that artist more capable of expanding his or her creativity. Artists believe that the perceptual changes from LSD have a profound, positive effect, creating a sense of confusion and disorganization that they view as desirable.[46] In another study, though, many artists believed that their drawing skills vastly diminished while they were under the influence of LSD.[47] Two recent studies reported that LSD was able to evoke an emotional response to music. One of these studies found LSD could enhance music-evoked emotions in a positive way.[48] The second study found LSD changes the parahippocampal connectivity, resulting in enhanced meaningful thoughts, emotions, and imagery.[49] Music has been used in therapeutic settings to help patients find deeper emotions. The results from these studies may encourage the use of music and LSD in therapeutic settings.[50] Steve Jobs, of Apple, said he became more creative after using LSD.[51]

The US Experience

LSD did not reach the United States until 1949, when it was used initially to study mental illness, then later used by psychotherapists with their patients, by musicians and artists to enhance their creativity, and by government officials to determine its effectiveness as a mind-control agent.

Later, the drug was woven into certain segments of society. The nonmedical, unregulated use of LSD and the illicit use that followed caused much concern. We will look first at mental health uses and the related study of LSD, then its use to enhance creativity, and finally the governmental interventions and impact on the culture.

LSD and Government Experiments

Research on LSD and other hallucinogens was conducted at the Edgewood Arsenal in Maryland in the early 1950s. Mind-control experiments by the Russians and Chinese prompted the US Central Intelligence Agency (CIA) and other agencies to conduct their own experiments to assess whether LSD could control the mind and serve as a truth serum. The CIA gave LSD to about 1,500 military personnel.[52] These experiments were not always performed on willing participants, and sometimes the results were tragic.

One unfortunate incident involved a government scientist named Frank Olson. In 1953, the CIA gave LSD to Olson without his knowledge. He experienced a psychotic response and was transported from Maryland to New York City to be hospitalized. The evening before he was to be hospitalized, Olson jumped to his death from a hotel's 10th-story window. The circumstances of Olson's death were not disclosed until 1975, whereupon his family was awarded $750,000.[53] (Similarly, the British government agreed to compensate many of its servicemen who were given LSD without their consent in the 1950s.[54])

In another project, prostitutes in San Francisco were given LSD unknowingly to evaluate the drug's effect on their sexual activities and experiences and on their patrons. The prostitutes and their customers were watched through a two-way mirror.[55] The CIA was looking to determine if LSD could be used as a truth serum. Results from this study found LSD and the act of sex did not influence the talkability of the male subjects. However, it was determined during the postcoital period that subjects were more willing to engage in conversation.

LSD and the US Culture

Beginning in the early 1960s, hallucinogens became more integrated into American society. Nonmedical interest in LSD was not spurred simply by the desire to achieve euphoria; people took drugs such as LSD as a means of dealing with society and its inherent problems. In his book *LSD: My Problem Child*, Albert Hofmann stated that the appeal of the drug stemmed from

> materialism, alienation from nature through industrialization and increasing urbanization, lack of satisfaction in professional employment in a mechanized, lifeless working world, ennui and purposelessness in a wealthy, saturated society, and lack of a religious, nurturing, and meaningful philosophical foundation of life.[56]

As a result of research by Timothy Leary at Harvard University, interest in hallucinogens grew. While vacationing in Mexico, Leary and some colleagues took "magic mushrooms" and found the experience enlightening. After this experience, Leary and his associate Richard Alpert studied the

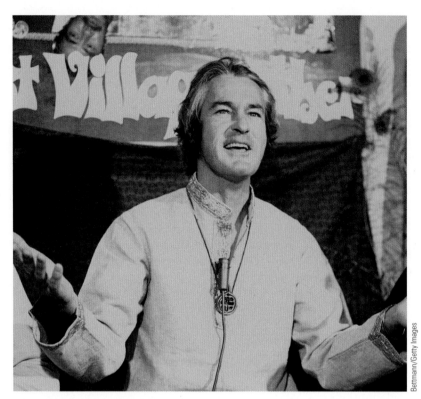

Timothy Leary helped to popularize the use of LSD in the early 1960s.

psychological effects of **psilocybin**, a hallucinogenic mushroom, on humans. They later examined the effects of LSD on humans.

Leary and Alpert believed that LSD and other hallucinogens were psychologically and spiritually beneficial. They gave these drugs to convicts reentering society, to students, and to theologians. Some people thought their research lost its scientific objectivity, and the two subsequently were fired from Harvard. Leary went on to form the League of Spiritual Discovery, whose acronym is LSD.

Around the time Leary was involved with LSD, a young writer on the West Coast named Ken Kesey was also experimenting with LSD. As a graduate student at Stanford University, Kesey participated in research at a nearby hospital in which he was paid to take various hallucinogens. At the same time, Kesey was working at a mental hospital. During the time he was participating in the research and working at the mental hospital, Kesey wrote the critically acclaimed book *One Flew over the Cuckoo's Nest*. He and a group of friends, the "Merry Pranksters," traveled around the United States promoting drugs such as LSD and marijuana.

As the popularity of LSD grew, so did the negative publicity. LSD was linked to chromosome damage, brain damage, insanity, suicide, homicide, and other acts of violence. By the end of the 1960s, interest in LSD had waned. In 1965, LSD became an illegal drug.

Peyote

Peyote is a hallucinogen the Aztec Indians used for religious rituals. The Spanish conquerors, however, condemned it for its "satanic trickery." Peyote comes from the *Lophophora williamsii* cactus. This small, spineless cactus, measuring about 3 inches in diameter, is found in Mexico and Texas. Its psychoactive agent, **mescaline**, is named after the Mescalero Apaches. Users dry the crown of the cactus, suck it, and swallow. Chemically, mescaline produces effects similar to those of norepinephrine.[57] An increase in norepinephrine causes excitation and increased motor activity whereas a decrease in norepinephrine causes depression.

The dried cactus is known as a "mescal button." Preparation of mescal buttons is difficult because of their foul odor, and ingesting them is unpleasant because of the rancorous taste. Users initially experience nausea, vomiting, and diarrhea, which often deter continued use. In small doses, mescaline produces euphoria. In larger doses, it generates striking hallucinations involving intense colors, tastes, and feelings.

Compared with LSD, peyote is less intense and more manageable. Peyote intoxication consists of the following two stages:

1. Contentment and sensitivity
2. Great calm, muscular sluggishness, and a shift of attention from external stimuli to introspection and meditation

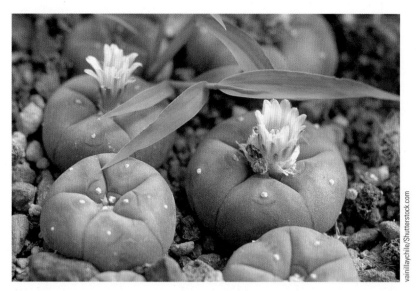

The peyote cactus is found in Mexico and Texas and has played an important role in Native religions.

Mescaline may be beneficial in treating addiction, depression, and anxiety. Some scientists had promising results when they gave peyote to alcoholics.[58] Peyote may be beneficial in treating cluster headaches. This type of headache usually occurs around the same time and in the same spot on a regular basis.[59]

Peyote takes effect within 30 to 90 minutes and stays in the body about 10 hours, although the hallucinations last only 2 hours.[60] Peyote is eliminated from the body primarily in the urine. Physiological effects include dilation of the pupils, a rise in body temperature, and increases in blood pressure and heart rate. Fatalities from its use have not been documented, although a person could die from behaviors while taking the drug. Some experts believe that peyote may cause paranoid schizophrenia, however, it is suggested this occurs in persons who were previously diagnosed as mentally ill.[61] In a 12-year period, the California Poison Control System encountered 31 instances in which individuals had adverse reactions.[62]

Mescaline is similar to LSD in that tolerance forms quickly, but physical dependence does not occur. There is cross-tolerance between mescaline and LSD. Synthetic mescaline can be made into a liquid, capsule, or tablet and is more palatable than natural mescaline, but synthesizing mescaline is difficult. What is sold on the streets as mescaline is commonly another drug, such as LSD.

In the early 1800s, the Apaches, Kiowas, and Commanches chewed mescal buttons and incorporated their use into their religious practices. Until 1990, members of the Native American Church, comprised of several North American Indian tribes, used peyote legally in the United States for spiritual reasons. Church members considered the use of peyote a sacrament, and recreational or social use was not permitted. This community also believed that the spiritual use of peyote could foster health, respect, and a sense of community.[63]

Peyote has been used as part of religious rituals among Native Americans for thousands of years. Legal use of peyote in the United States has had a turbulent history. In 1991, the US Supreme Court ruled that individual states could forbid peyote use for religious purposes. The Smith opinion, written by Justice Scalia found that, "There being no contention that Oregon's drug law represents an attempt to regulate religious beliefs, the communication of religious beliefs, or the raising of one's children."[64] In 1994, President Clinton signed into law an exempt of peyote from federal-and state-controlled substance laws for those using it for religious purposes.[65] Furthermore, in 2004, the Utah Supreme Court ruled that members of the Native American Church could use peyote without being prosecuted.[66]

Psilocybin

A drug that seems to be making a resurgence in the United States is magic mushrooms or "shrooms." The Aztecs called mushrooms containing psilocybin **teonanacatl**, which translates into "God's flesh."[56]

psilocybin A hallucinogen found in certain mushrooms in Central America

peyote A cactus containing the hallucinogen mescaline

mescaline A psychoactive agent or hallucinogen that is derived from the peyote cactus

teonanacatl Aztec word describing the psilocybe mushroom

Peyote has been used in American Indian ceremonies for at least 5,700 years. Its use among American Indians has had much conflict over the past 150 years, finally resulting in the American Indian Religious Freedom Act of 1994, which explicitly permits peyote use for religious and ceremonial purposes.

Since the pass of the American Indian Religious Freedom act of 1994, there has been an increase in peyote use among American Indians, however, there has not been an increase in the illicit recreational use of the drug by non-Indians. Additionally, the passage of this act resulted in an feeling of less repression among American Indians by being able to practice their religion without fear of being prosecuted for peyote use.

Source: B. Prue, "Prevalence of reported peyote use 1985–2010: Effects of the American Indian Religious Freedom Act of 1994", *The American Journal on Addiction*, 23 (2014): 156–161.

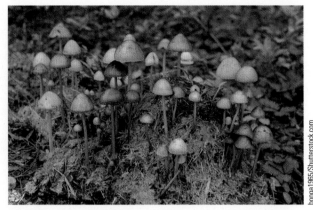

Psilocybin is being studied to determine the therapeutic benefits of the drug on depression for terminally ill patients.

This drug was spiritually significant to the Aztecs, but the Spaniards tried to squelch the religious use of mushrooms after overtaking the natives.

Several species of mushrooms containing psilocybin grow in parts of the United States, Mexico, and Europe. In 1958, Albert Hofmann isolated the psychoactive ingredient. In the early 1960s, psilocybin use increased on many college campuses, but its popularity waned when LSD became more prominent.

Psilocybin is similar chemically to LSD, although its effects are shorter and are not as intense. Psilocybin can be consumed orally in the form of dried mushrooms, by drinking a beverage containing the mushrooms, or in tablet form. Also, it can be ground up and added to foods. After psilocybin is ingested, a stomach enzyme converts it into **psilocin**.

Psilocybin is more potent than mescaline but less toxic. As with mescaline and LSD, no fatal overdoses from psilocybin have been recorded. A person can die from ingesting other types of mushrooms, though, and it is easy to mistake a poisonous mushroom for psilocybin.

In small doses (4 mg), psilocybin brings about feelings of euphoria and relaxation. Higher doses distort perceptions of time and space, and the user is distracted more easily and is open to suggestion. The hallucinations produced by psilocybin are both visual and auditory. Psilocybin also interferes with the ability to concentrate. Like peyote, psilocybin has an unpleasant taste. Psilocybin dilates the pupils and raises body temperature, pulse rate, and blood pressure. Involuntary movement of arms and legs and muscle relaxation may follow use. The drug is capable of producing an array of emotional responses, ranging from uncontrolled laughter to depression. The user experiences hallucinogenic effects within 30 minutes, which last 3 to 8 hours.

Psilocybin appears to slow brain activity, which may be beneficial in treating depression.[67] In a study at Johns Hopkins University on the effects of the hallucinogen psilocybin, individuals given this drug rated their experience very positively. Although some participants experienced anxiety, others claimed they had a mystical-type experience.[68] Following up on the results to the John Hopkins study, researchers looked at adults who reported using psilocybin in the past to determine outcomes from its use. Results from

POTENTIAL EFFECTS OF PSILOCYBIN

- Euphoria
- Easily distracted
- Difficulty concentrating
- Elevated body temperature
- Pulse rate increases
- Wide range of emotions
- Involuntary movement of limbs
- Relaxation
- Open to suggestion
- Pupils dilate
- Blood pressure increases
- Muscle relaxation
- Hallucinations

Going away to college is a time that provides a sense of freedom for students. As with other illicit drugs, college students tend to use hallucinogens more frequently compared to their non-college attending peers.

In a recent study, almost 30% of college students sampled admitted to using psilocybin. Many students cited the top reasons for using the drug were feelings of curiosity, to achieve a mystical experience, and introspection. Those who used the drug believed there were no addictive properties for psilocybin and did not believe the drug negatively impacted grades, mental or physical health. However, this study showed a high correlation between those who used psilocybin and other drugs such as ecstasy, opiates, non-prescribed prescription drugs, and LSD.

Source: R.M. Hallock, A.Dean, Z.A. Knecht, J. Spencer, and E.C. Taverna, "A survey of hallucinogenic mushroom use, factors related to usage, and perceptions of use among college students", *Drug and Alcohol Dependence*, 130, no.1–3. (2013): 245–248.

this study found all participants maintained insights gained through the experience with psilocybin after discontinuing use of the drug.[69] Other studies have looked at the therapeutic use of psilocybin for treatment of anxiety and depression. One study looked at people who were suffering from life-threatening cancer to determine the impact of psilocybin on depression and anxiety. Results from this study suggest high-dose psilocybin greatly increases symptoms associated with depression and anxiety as rated by clinicians and self-rated measures by patients.[70] A similar study confirmed these results showing significant long-term improvement in depression and anxiety 6 months after administering a single, moderate dose of psilocybin along with psychotherapy in patients suffering from life-threatening cancer.[71] Other research is being done to determine the extent of therapeutic benefits for psilocybin. One study found psilocybin to be effective in smoking cessation. Results from this study found that almost 70% of participants remained tobacco abstinent at a 12-month follow-up after using psilocybin and cognitive behavioral therapy. Additionally, almost 90% of the participants rated their psilocybin experiences as being among the five most personally meaningful and spiritual experiences of their lives.[72]

Anticholinergic Hallucinogens

Plants containing **anticholinergic hallucinogens** include belladonna, datura, henbane, and mandrake. These drugs belong to the potato and tomato families and have a long, rich history involving sorcery and witchcraft. The effects of henbane are similar to those of the mandrake root. They have been used as medicines, poisons, and beauty aids. Besides producing hallucinations, these drugs can be highly toxic in large doses. In the 1970s, anticholinergic drugs were found in many over-the-counter (OTC) preparations including Sominex, Contac, Donnagel (for diarrhea), Travel-Eze (for motion sickness), and Endotussin (cough syrup). Since the 1980s, anticholinergic drugs have been removed from OTC medications.

Belladonna

"Beautiful lady" in Italian, **belladonna** was used to increase the size of the pupils and produce a glassy effect on the eyes, which was considered desirable. Also known as **deadly nightshade**, it may have been used during the Middle Ages in witches' brews and satanic rituals. It consists of bluish black, soft berries called "love apples," because belladonna was believed to be an aphrodisiac. This plant is found in parts of Europe, North Africa, and Asia.

psilocin The psychoactive ingredient in the psilocybe mushroom

anticholinergic hallucinogens Substances found in datura and in *Amanita muscaria* mushrooms; interfere with the action of acetylcholine to produce hallucinations

belladonna (deadly nightshade) A potent hallucinogen found in Europe, North Africa, and Asia; member of the tomato and potato family

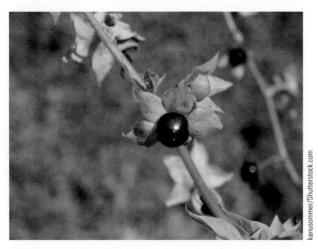

While beautiful, the Belladonna berry is toxic and can be fatal.

Belladonna is toxic and eating a small quantity of its leaves or berries can be fatal.[73] Some believe the berries from the Belladonna are the poison used in Shakespear's play "Romeo and Juliet."[74] Despite its toxic nature, the chemicals atropine and scopolamine, derived from belladonna, are still used today and have important medical properties. Both of these chemicals are used to dilate eyes during an eye exam and atropine has been used as an antidote for insecticides and chemical warfare agents.[75]

Reportedly, belladonna makes people feel like they are flying, which explains its association with witches and broomsticks. The sensation of flying probably is derived from the irregular heartbeat and drowsiness that accompany its use. In addition to its potent hallucinogenic properties, belladonna can be extremely toxic. Consuming slightly more than a dozen berries can be fatal.

Datura

One species of **datura** plant, *Datura stramonium*, is known as **locoweed** or **Jamestown weed (jimsonweed)**. American Indians used this species in many rituals. In one peculiar use, it was thought that a person under the influence of datura would have a vision in which the person who stole an object would be revealed and the location of the object would be identified.

Also, datura was used as a rite of passage from childhood to adulthood. Algonquin Indians gave it to adolescent boys, who hallucinated for several days without recollecting the experience later.

Indications are that datura was used in China, Greece, India, and Africa. The Chinese used it for medical purposes, and in India it was included in love potions. Datura was used to treat asthma, epilepsy, delirium tremens, rheumatism, and menstrual pains. Because its side effects are potentially harmful and noxious, it is seldom used recreationally. Allegedly,

in Haiti, datura is one ingredient of zombie powder, a substance that is supposed to induce a zombie-like state. Datura holds special magical and religious significance to North American and Central American Indians.

Because jimsonweed is readily available and inexpensive, its recreational use is increasing.[76] The percentage of all anticholinergic plant poisonings due to intentional exposure has increased from 22 to 44% over the past several years.[77] Jimsonweed can cause extreme delirium, making a person unable to distinguish between reality and fantasy. Physical effects of jimsonweed poisoning include dry mouth, burning thirst, dry skin, constipation, amnesia, dilated eyes in which bright lights are painful, inability to focus the eyes, rapid pulse, elevated blood pressure, and difficulty urinating.[78] Symptoms appear within 30 to 60 minutes after ingestion or smoking and may last for 24 to 48 hours. The effects can be as severe as coma and death.

Mandrake

Because the root of the **mandrake** plant resembles a human body, it has been valued for its medicinal and supernatural properties and had a reputation as an aphrodisiac. The word *mandrake* means "potent male." This powerful and toxic plant grows in southern Europe, North Africa, western Asia, and the Himalayas.

Like belladonna, mandrake belongs to the nightshade family. In ancient Egypt, the mandrake plant and the water lily were used for inducing trances and in healing rituals. In Europe during the Middle Ages, its use was associated with witchcraft, sorcery, and superstition. Europeans feared and respected the mandrake. Its effects include mental confusion, increased heart rate, dilation of the pupils, dry mouth, hallucinations, and amnesia.

MANDRAKE: AN INTERESTING HISTORY

The mandrake, made popular in the late 1990s from the novel, and later movie, *Harry Potter and the Chamber of Secrets*, has been around since before the bible and has a place in Greek mythology. In the Bible (Book of Genesis) the mandrake root helped Rachel conceive Jacob. In Greek mytholody, Circe and Aphrodite use it as an aphrodisiac.

Source: A. Calabrese, "The history and uses of the magical mandrake, according to modern witches", *Atlas Obscura*, (January 12, 2016).

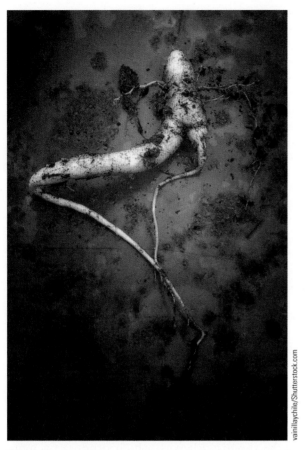

Literature and folklore contain explicit directions for harvesting up the mandrake root which has been thought to "scream" when pulled out.

Two psychoactive drugs found in mandrake and other anticholinergic hallucinogens are **scopolamine** and **atropine**. In small doses, these drugs induce euphoria, feelings of sedation, disorientation, slurred speech, silly behavior, confusion, fatigue, and dreamless sleep. Other effects are vomiting, malaise, and excessive perspiration and salivation. In large amounts, mandrake can cause coma and death. Psychological and physical dependence on both drugs is uncommon.

Scopolamine formerly was given to women during childbirth. Because it causes amnesia, the medical profession thought that women would not remember labor pains. Scopolamine is used in rats to induce memory loss in order to study new treatments for Alzheimer's disease.[79] Women given scopolamine, however, often had hallucinations or delirium, so this practice was discontinued. Scopolamine has also been used to treat motion sickness. Recent studies suggest scopolamine may be used to treat major depressive disorder in a subpopulation of patients.[80] One study highlighted the potential use of scopolamine as palliative medicine for end-of-life patients

with Parkinson's.[81] Atropine is used to dilate the pupils and reduce lung congestion (especially during surgery) and is an antidote for poisoning from some insecticides.

Scopolamine has been used for unscrupulous motives. Purportedly, prostitutes would slip it into the drink of a client, who then would fall into a stupor. The victim would be robbed and would have difficulty recalling what had happened.

Nutmeg and Mace

The Arabs introduced nutmeg into Europe as a medicine in the first century. It was used to treat heart disease, tuberculosis, digestive problems, kidney troubles, asthma, and fever. Though nutmeg is used without effect in food preparations, it can induce visual and auditory hallucinations if consumed in large quantities. It distorts time and space and creates a sense of detachment from reality.

Nutmeg is made from the seeds of the Myristica tree, and mace comes from the fruit of the same tree. Nutmeg and mace are chemically similar to mescaline. Nutmeg is chewed or snuffed with tobacco. **Myristicin**, found in nutmeg and mace, is capable of producing effects when one to two teaspoons are consumed, but it takes 2 to 5 hours before the effects are felt. Nutmeg and mace are not taken for hallucinogenic reasons because their unpleasant side effects include nausea, severe headache, vomiting, tachycardia, and sensory distortion, followed by an extremely noxious hangover.

Nutmeg and mace have been shown to contain food preservative properties as well as antibacterial qualities.[82] In higher doses, they can slow the growth of some common human pathogenic bacteria strains.[83] Due to their antibacterial and

---

datura A hallucinogen used for sacred purposes in ancient China, Greece, India, and Africa

locoweed Another term for jimsonweed

Jamestown weed (jimsonweed) A hallucinogen derived from the datura plant; also known as locoweed

mandrake A hallucinogen derived from the nightshade family; used during the Middle Ages in connection with witchcraft and sorcery

scopolamine A psychoactive agent found in mandrake and other anticholinergic hallucinogens

atropine A psychoactive agent found in mandrake and other anticholinergic hallucinogens

myristicin Substance found in nutmeg and mace; chemically similar to mescaline and capable of producing hallucinations

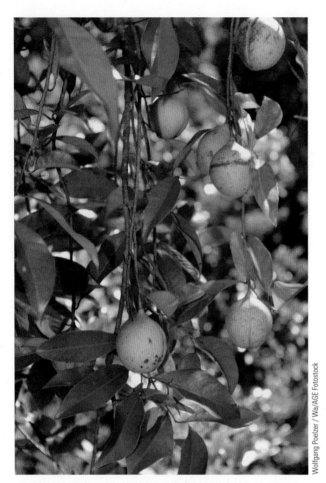

Nutmeg (the seed from the fruit of the *Myristica fragrans* tree) and mace (the lacy membrane around the seed) contain small amounts of chemicals that may produce hallucinations.

antiinflammatory properties, nutmeg and mace may help treat periodontal disease along with traditional treatment.

Dissociative Hallucinogens

Dissociative hallucinogens also distort sounds and sights, but they also produce profound feelings of detachment.

Salvinorin A

A relatively new hallucinogen is salvinorin A. Derived from the sage family, this drug has been used in traditional spiritual practices by Mazatec Indians in Oaxaca, Mexico, to produce mystical or hallucinogenic experiences.[84] The drug, known sometimes as Salvia, is nicknamed Sally-D, Magic Mint, and Diviner's Sage. Salvinorin A is not considered a controlled substance by the US Federal government, although some states have placed this substance on their own drug schedule and have banned its use.[85] Salvinorin A is illegal in Denmark, Australia, Belgium, and Italy. In 2016, the Canadian government made salvinorin A a schedule IV drug under the Controlled Drugs and Substance Act. While it is illegal to transport or possess for the purpose of transportation, production, and trafficking, simple possession is not prohibited. [86]

Information about salvinorin A is spreading. There are a number of YouTube videos showing young people on the drug.[87] It is believed that an increasing number of young people are discovering this drug through the Internet and smoke shops. They are frequently marketed as "legal highs" and are among the top 30 most common products in recreational drug use in Europe.[88] Lifetime prevalence for use of salvia is similar to lifetime prevalence of hallucinogens, with about 1.5% Americans aged 12 to 17 and a little over 5% of adults aged 18 to 24 admitting to lifetime use.[89]

There are several ways to use salvia. Mazatec Indians prepared a water-based rink from the ground leaves. Some users chew the laves, which allows salvinorin A to be directly absorbed in the mucus membrane inside the mouth. Users also smoke the dried leaves, which produces a more intense experience.[90] When smoked, salvinorin A produces a psychoactive effect that has been shown to begin within a minute and to last up to 15 minutes.[91] However, when smoked, it produces a dissociative state similar to the effects of ketamine.[92] Like other hallucinogens, salvinorin A alters human consciousness and perception.[93] According to some individuals, its potency rivals that of LSD.[94] While no deaths have been recorded regarding use of salvinorin A, there have been a few cases where users were hospitalized due to negative effects including psychosis, paranoia, and psychomotor agitation. However, in these cases there were either preexisting mental conditions present, or use of other drugs.[95] There have been little research regarding the potential therapeutic effects of salvia. In one case study involving rats, it was shown this drug may have antidepressant and anxiolytic effects.[96] However, in high doses in rats, it was associated with cognitive impairment. It is speculated that the study of salvinorin A may be beneficial in the treatment of cocaine dependence as use of salvia has been shown to reduce cocaine-seeking behavior in rats.[97] In a recent study, it was discovered that naltrexone, the drug used to treat heroin overdoses, can reduce the effects of salvinorin A, suggesting this drug works on the brain similar to heroin and other opioids.[98]

Dimethyltryptamine

Dimethyltryptamine (DMT) is derived from the leaves, bark, and seeds of various plants grown in South and Central America that contain that substance. It is classified as a schedule I drug. DMT, which is found in the psychoactive beverage called ayahuasca, has been used for spiritual purposes in these regions in order to communicate with the spirits to cure illness.[99] Natives using DMT would snort or blow it into each other's noses.

DMT was first synthesized in 1931. During the 1960s, DMT was called the "businessman's LSD," presumably because of the segment of the population that used it. The hallucinogenic effects last 1 to 2 hours. In a large global study, researchers found almost 9% of adults sampled had used DMT in their lifetime, most often smoked.[100] Euphoria and behavioral stimulation are associated with DMT. The drug may result in a psychotic episode, although long-term psychosis is not likely to occur when the drug is used on an occasional basis.[101] Unlike other hallucinogens, tolerance to DMT does not develop. DMT significantly raises blood pressure. It may have properties that reduce inflammation in the body.[102]

Phencyclidine Hydrochloride

Phencyclidine hydrochloride (PCP) is sometimes classified as a hallucinogen because it is capable of producing hallucinations, although the hallucinations differ from those produced by LSD. When it was developed in the 1950s, it was used as a surgical anesthetic. PCP is still used as a veterinary anesthetic outside the United States. Production of PCP in the United States became illegal in 1978.

Classifying PCP is complicated because it generates anesthetic, hallucinogenic, stimulating, or depressing effects depending on the dosage and method of administration. Some drug experts describe PCP as a **dissociative anesthetic** that causes the person to feel separated from reality.

Early Use

PCP has many nicknames, including angel dust, dust, rocket fuel, trank, and crystal. It was distributed on the West Coast in the early 1960s under the name PeaCe Pill. By the late 1960s, it was sold on the East Coast under the name "hog." When PCP first appeared in San Francisco, it was relatively popular, but its appeal declined because it induced bizarre, violent behavior.

Marketed under the name Sernyl, PCP was used originally as an anesthetic for humans. It was considered desirable for surgery because patients remained awake yet were unable to recall their experiences because of the amnesia that PCP produced. Moreover, it had no adverse effect on blood circulation, heart rate, or respiration. However, it was discontinued by 1965 because of undesirable effects including agitation, delirium, and disorientation. Once the effects wore off, patients became unmanageable, confused, and disassociated from nearby surroundings. PCP later was used in veterinary medicine but has been largely replaced by similar drugs such as ketamine.

In the 1960s, when PCP was initially used on the street, it was distributed in tablet or capsule form, but it can also be injected, snorted, or smoked. When PCP was smoked, it was mixed with marijuana, tobacco, or vegetable matter. Because absorption is rapid, the effects of PCP are experienced quickly. The acute effects last 4 to 6 hours, but the user may be in a state of confusion for 8 to 24 hours. Neither tolerance nor physical dependence results, and no physical withdrawal symptoms are apparent after the person stops using the drug.

Illegal Use

Despite the unpredictable and behaviorally disruptive effects of PCP, its illegal use escalated toward the end of the 1960s and into the 1970s. Contributing to this increase was its low cost. In 1979, nearly 13% of high school seniors had tried PCP. By 1996, about 4% of seniors had tried it; in 2016, 1.3% of seniors had tried PCP.[104]

PCP frequently is used in place of other drugs such as LSD, THC, mescaline, or amphetamines. Many users view it as a desirable substitute for LSD, and it sometimes is mixed with marijuana to augment its effects. "Killer joints" and "sherms" refer to cigarettes containing PCP and marijuana.

Because PCP has a reputation for making users violent and incredibly strong, police and hospital personnel are wary of people who are using it. Media accounts have reported average-sized people breaking handcuffs, simultaneously wrestling several police officers, and being shot repeatedly before succumbing. Yet, nothing in PCP increases one's strength. Considering the fact that users are disoriented, paranoid (often the basis for violent behavior), and anesthetized, one can imagine the person failing to respond to restraints that would prevent the behavior.

dimethyltryptamine (DMT) A hallucinogen in which effects last 1 to 2 hours

phencyclidine hydrochloride (PCP) Originally developed as an anesthetic for humans and, later, animals; also called "angel dust"

dissociative anesthetic Substance that alters the perception of pain without loss of consciousness

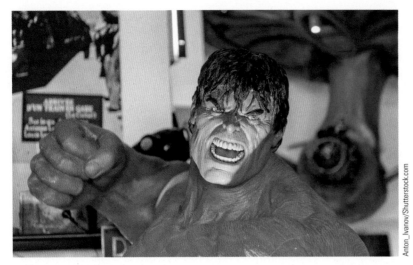

An inaccurate depiction of PCP by media shows it giving a person "super-human" strength.

Effects

In small doses, PCP brings about feelings of relaxation, warmth, euphoria, and numbness; however, it interferes with concentration, distorts body image, and creates a sense of depersonalization. With increasing dosage, the user experiences confusion, poor coordination, nystagmus (irregular movement of the eyes), agitation, and impaired reaction time. With high doses, muscular rigidity, blank staring, and excessive salivation may occur. Users may have sudden mood swings and engage in repetitive actions.

There is a slight increase in heart rate, blood pressure, respiration, and body temperature. In the extreme, PCP can bring about coma, seizures, and death. Dosage levels of 10 to 25 mg can be life-threatening. The synergistic effect of PCP when combined with other depressants such as alcohol and barbiturates increases its potency. Death from PCP is caused by overdose, suicide while under the influence, or behavior either during intoxication or during withdrawal.[104]

PCP can produce psychotic-like effects similar to those of schizophrenia. PCP psychosis is marked

---

EFFECTS OF PHENCYCLIDINE HYDROCHLORIDE (PCP)

Small Dosage

- Feelings of warmth
- Relaxation
- Poor concentration
- Depersonalization
- Nystagmus
- Agitation
- Muscle rigidity
- Sudden mood swings
- Faster heart rate
- Elevated blood pressure
- Euphoria
- Numbness
- Distorted body image
- Confusion
- Poor coordination
- Slow reaction time
- Excessive salivation
- Repetitive behavior
- Respiration
- Higher body temperature

Large Dosage

- Anorexia
- Violent behavior
- Restlessness
- Suicide
- Seizures
- Paranoia
- Insomnia
- Amnesia
- Depression
- Coma
- Death

by restlessness, memory problems, inability to eat or sleep, paranoia, and physical aggressiveness. It has been reported that recovery from PCP-induced psychosis may take 4 to 6 weeks, although later research shows that recovery may take longer.[105] PCP has been linked to suicide, drownings, and self-inflicted injuries. In recent years, treatment specialists have found that synthetic compounds called dopamine D_3 receptor agonists may help treat PCP abusers.[106] There is also research aimed at developing a vaccine to prevent PCP abuse, although none has made it past phase II trials.[107]

Ketamine

Ketamine is used in veterinary medicine in place of PCP and is a schedule III drug. It is not uncommon for ketamine to be diverted from veterinarians' offices and medical supply offices.[108] It is effective for pain management in humans.[109] Nonmedical use of ketamine, also known as special K, K, and vitamin K, is increasing. Like PCP, ketamine is considered a dissociative anesthetic, with the user feeling separated from reality. Also, ketamine is capable of producing confusion, hallucinations, delirium, excitement, irrational behavior, muscle rigidity, tremors, respiratory depression, irregular heartbeat, loss of appetite, skin

ketamine A drug very similar to PCP

rashes, nausea, and cardiac arrest. Studies with animals demonstrate that ketamine and PCP cause significant damage to the developing fetus. Ketamine has been associated with ulcers and bladder pain, kidney problems, stomach pain, depression, and poor memory.[110] Ketamine can be injected, snorted, or ingested. Its effects begin within 5 to 10 minutes and last up to an hour. Like Rohypnol and gamma-hydroxybutyrate (GHB), ketamine has been used as a date-rape drug. In combination with alcohol, it induces vomiting. Many users have reported the effects of the drug as intense and dissociative. Like cocaine, ketamine does not produce a physiological withdrawal syndrome, but some users become dependent on ketamine by demonstrating a craving for the drug.[111] In a clinical setting, ketamine is currently being administered to reduce the craving for heroin among addicts. Preliminary research also indicates that ketamine may be effective for treating treatment-resistant depression.[112]

Summary

Hallucinogens—plants and synthetic materials, capable of producing hallucinations—also have been called phantasticants, psychedelic, psychomimetic, and psychotropic. These drugs have been used for psychic purposes, to transcend boundaries of time and space, to escape from daily pressures, to communicate with a higher order, for medical reasons, and for recreation. They are generally separated into two categories: classic and dissociative.

The FDA approved lysergic acid diethylamide (LSD) for medical use in 1953. It was used to study schizophrenia but without success. LSD also was given to alcoholics, psychiatric and terminally ill patients, and sexual deviants. Despite promising results, adverse publicity and unfounded fears that it caused brain damage brought an end to its use.

On the East Coast in the 1960s, Timothy Leary popularized hallucinogens. He studied the effects of hallucinogens on personality and later formed the League of Spiritual Discovery. On the West Coast, writer Ken Kesey and his followers promoted LSD experimentation. Negative publicity caused its use to decline, and LSD was made illegal in 1965. In the last several years, LSD use by high school seniors has declined further.

LSD is an extremely potent drug, capable of altering consciousness for 6 to 8 hours, though the physiological effects are short and moderate. LSD has a significant effect on mood, perception, and time. LSD is odorless, colorless, and tasteless. Tolerance develops rapidly, but its use is nonfatal unless the person engages in fatal behaviors while under the drug's influence.

Mescaline is the psychoactive ingredient in the peyote cactus and has been used for thousands of years by Native cultures. Although its effects range from euphoria to intense hallucinations lasting up to 2 hours, peyote has unpleasant side effects related to its foul odor and taste. The physiological effects are modest.

A hallucinogen gaining in popularity is psilocybin. The mushrooms that contain psylocybin are chemically similar to LSD, but their effects are shorter and less intense. Psilocybin is more powerful than mescaline. Scientists are researching the therapeutic benefits of psilocybin, and it has been shown to be beneficial in treating depression among terminally ill patients. Additionally, some research shows that psilocybin may be effective in reducing alcohol abuse.

Examples of anticholinergic hallucinogens are belladonna, datura, henbane, and mandrake. They are associated with use in sorcery and witchcraft. Belladonna, also called deadly nightshade, gives users a feeling of flying and was used to enhance beauty. Datura, better known as locoweed, was significant in North American and Central American Indian cultures and was given to boys during rites of passage into adulthood, among other rituals. Mandrake, containing scopolamine and atropine, is said to hold special powers as an aphrodisiac. It induces euphoria, confusion, and sleep.

Another hallucinogen, dimethyltryptamine (DMT), is derived from plants grown in South America and Central America. It has its origins in spiritual uses. DMT was popular briefly in the United States in the 1960s. Called the "businessman's LSD," its effects lasted just 1 to 2 hours.

Phencyclidine hydrochloride (PCP) can be classified as a hallucinogen, a stimulant, or a depressant because of its varying properties. PCP first was used as a human anesthetic during surgery but this was stopped as a result of undesirable effects. It later was used as an animal tranquilizer. Paranoia, amnesia, restlessness, and thoughts of suicide sometimes accompany PCP use. In high doses, it can be fatal.

Ketamine, popularly known as special K, has replaced PCP as an animal tranquilizer. Its effects are similar to those of PCP. Reportedly, ketamine has been used as a date rape drug.

Thinking Critically

1. Currently, LSD is listed as a schedule I drug. This means that it cannot be used for medical purposes under any circumstances. Would you support experimental use of LSD in psychotherapy? For other medical conditions? Why or why not?
2. Because LSD is nonfatal, some people consider it safe. Because it produces a powerful effect on the mind, others deem it dangerous. On what basis would you judge a drug safe or dangerous? Should one look at only the physical effects of a drug, or are the psychological effects just as important? Explain.
3. There is some research supporting the therapeutic benefits of LSD and psilocybin for helping terminally ill patients deal with depression and anxiety. Examine the potential benefits and consequences for using these drugs as therapeutic agents.

14

Over-the-Counter Drugs

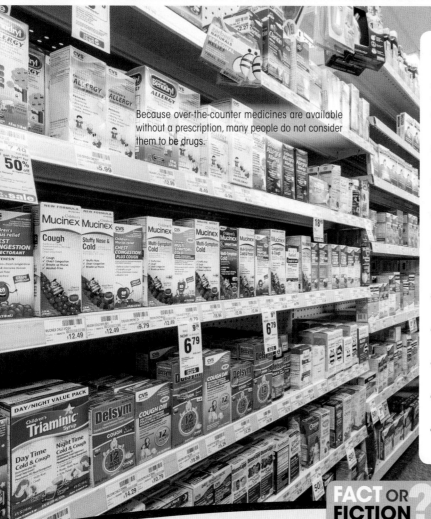

Because over-the-counter medicines are available without a prescription, many people do not consider them to be drugs.

Chapter Objective

After completing this chapter, the reader should be able to:

- Discuss the impact of the Food, Drug, and Cosmetic Act of 1938
- Differentiate between the OTC drugs in Category I, Category II, and Category III
- Argue the benefits of generic drugs over brand-name drugs
- Access the benefits and side effects of OTC analgesic drugs
- Examine how herbal drugs are regulated and how these regulation protocols are different compared to prescription drugs
- Create an argument for and against changing prescription drugs to OTC drugs
- Explain how antitussive cough suppressants and expectorants differ
- List the major ingredient in OTC sleep aids and discuss the effectiveness of these drugs
- Identify the drawbacks related to various types of antacids
- Evaluate the effectiveness and side effects of weight-reducing medications

FACT OR FICTION?

1. About 1 in 20 high school students have taken cough medicines in the previous year to get high.

2. A "child-resistant" container is a container that 80% of 5-year-olds need more than 5 minutes to open.

3. OTC drugs are completely safe.

4. For preventing a heart attack, a baby aspirin is just as effective as an adult aspirin.

5. Acetaminophen accounts for more emergency room visits than aspirin.

6. OTC are not habit forming.

7. Natural supplements are always a safer choice.

8. Brand name medications work better than their generic equivalents.

9. For many people, drinking warm milk at bedtime allows them to go to sleep more easily.

10. Because of the media's attention on obesity, children today are less obese than they were 20 years ago.

Turn the page to check your answers

Billions of dollars are spent each year on over-the-counter (OTC) drugs in the United States and abroad. In 2015, almost 70% of Americans took dietary supplements.[1] People typically perceive OTC drugs as being relatively harmless. OTC drugs are readily accessible; moreover, a number of drugs are being switched from prescription to OTC. For example, the morning-after pill, an emergency contraception, went from being a prescribed drug to an OTC drug.[2] Some people may reason that if a drug does not require a prescription to be purchased, it can't be that harmful. A 2015 survey indicated that 1 out of every 12 Americans do not follow directions regarding prescription medicine.[3] A *Consumer Reports* survey found that 31% of respondents indicated that they did not follow the directions for nonprescription drugs very carefully.[4]

The perception that nonprescription drugs are completely safe can have grave consequences. Not only can one become euphoric from OTC drugs, but some drugs are known to cause hallucinations.[5] The abuse of OTC medicines is most common among teens.[6] The most common OTC drug abused is dextromethorphan (DXM). It is estimated that 1 in 10 teens have abused DXM.[7] Because it contains 30 mg of DXM, the drug of choice is Coricidin HBP.[8] The federal agency that regulates OTC drugs is the US Food and Drug Administration (FDA), which has been in existence for more than 100 years.[9] In 2004, the FDA implemented regulations requiring that more information be included on labels of OTC drugs.[10] Because discussions of drugs often focus on illegal drugs, the potentially adverse effects of OTC drugs, as well as alcohol and tobacco, tend to be overlooked. Abuse of OTC drugs by teenagers is increasing, especially abuse of decongestants, antihistamines, cough suppressants, and laxatives.

One can easily understand how the use of OTC drugs has become ingrained in our society. Advertisements try to convince consumers of their need for drugs. The message is that no one has to feel pain or discomfort. Regardless of the problem, some type of medication is always available to remedy it. Advertisers prefer the term *medication* to *drug* because the former implies that the product is helpful and the latter implies that it is harmful. The FDA oversees ads for prescription drugs while the Federal Trade Commission oversees ads for OTC drugs.[11]

Over-the-Counter Drug Market

For many years, OTC drugs were unregulated. People could get **patent medicines**—another term for OTC drugs—from traveling side shows or from a local pharmacist or physician. The contents of these drugs were not regulated. The Pure Food and Drug Act, passed in 1906, changed that. This law stipulated that ingredients ranging from alcohol (the most common ingredient), to opium, to cocaine, to almost anything had to be listed on labels. Despite the Pure Food and Drug Act, problems persisted. Eventually, the Food, Drug, and Cosmetic Act was enacted.

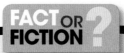

1. **FACT** According to data from the federal government, over 5% of 10th- and 12th-grade students took cough medicine to get high.

2. **FACT** Child-resistant containers are containers that most 5-year-olds should not be able to open within 5 minutes, although many 5-year-olds open the containers in less than 5 minutes.

3. **FICTION** The fact is—OTC medicines are responsible for many emergency room visits due to adverse effects and combining different medications. Each year, over 7,500 deaths occur from non-steroidal anti-inflammatory drugs (aspirin, ibuprofen, naproxen, ketoprofen).

4. **FACT** A baby aspirin is as effective as an adult aspirin, without the potential for as many side effects.

5. **FACT** Acetaminophen accounts for about four times more emergency room visits than aspirin.

6. **FICTION** The fact is—More than 6 million people reported using cough and cold medicine to get high.

7. **FICTION** The fact is—Supplements are not regulated in the same way as drugs - many contain contaminants and other substances that are not listed on the label. In addition, many produce adverse effects when combined with other medication.

8. **FICTION** The fact is—Generic medications have the same active ingredient as brand name medications and are just as effective.

9. **FACT** Warm milk produces a chemical that makes falling asleep easier.

10. **FICTION** The fact is—It is estimated that obesity is three times more common for children today than it was 20 years ago.

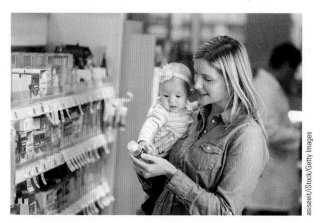

Children are more at risk than adults for adverse reactions to over-the-counter drugs.

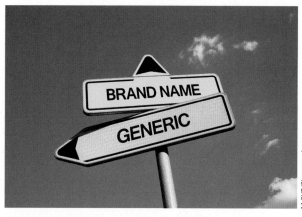

Generic drugs are a less expensive option and contain the same active ingredients as brand name drugs

Regulating Over-the-Counter Drugs

The Food, Drug, and Cosmetic Act, passed in 1938, required that prescription drugs be proved safe and effective before being marketed. This act, however, applied only to prescribed drugs. Not until the Kefauver-Harris Amendment in 1962 did *nonprescription* drugs have to be proved safe and effective. The law stipulated that all OTC drugs had to be proven safe and effective. This task was enormous because more than 300,000 OTC preparations were on the market already.

To simplify its task, the FDA evaluated ingredients in OTC drugs rather than examining each product. The FDA identified 26 classes of OTC products and had advisory panels review the active ingredients in these classes. Existing OTC drugs could remain on the market until they were tested, a process that took many years. The FDA presented its findings in 1985. Among the 348 new drugs from the largest 25 drug companies in the United States, the FDA found that 3% made important contributions to existing therapies, 13% made modest contributions, and 84% made little or no potential contribution.[12]

In 2007, the FDA proposed a new category for drugs called "behind-the-counter" (BTC) drugs. BTC drugs are nonprescription drugs that consumers have to ask for after consultation with their pharmacist. This resulted from the Combat Methamphetamine Epidemic Act of 2005, whose purpose was to reduce the production of illicit methamphetamines.[13] Drugs that are regulated under this Act contain pseudoephedrine, ephedrine, and phenylpropanolamine, which are commonly found in cough and cold medicines. Under this Act, the following restrictions were created:[14]

- Limits on the amount of drug an individual can purchase

- Individuals must present photo identification to get the drug
- Requires retailers to keep a logbook on customers who make these purchases for at least 2 years

BTC drugs were prescribed drugs previously. This new category for drugs improves access to drugs for people who lack health insurance or adequate prescription drug coverage because they do not have to pay to see a physician before obtaining these drugs.[15]

Generic Versus Brand-Name Drugs

Generic drugs are copies of brand-name drugs and have the same dosage, safety, strength, and quality. They are also similar in how they are administered and in their intended use. The FDA requires that all drugs, whether they are generic or brand-name drugs, be safe and effective. One advantage of generic drugs over brand-name drugs is that they cost less.

Although generic drugs contain the same ingredients as brand-name drugs, they appear different. Trademark laws in the United States require that generic drugs not look exactly like brand-name drugs. Although generic drugs are less expensive than brand-name drugs, not every brand-name drug has a generic equivalent.[16] Generic drugs are 80 to 85% less expensive than name-brand drugs. In the past. a number of physicians surveryed had concerns.[17] However, in recent years, physicians' attitudes have been changing with one survey showing the majority of physicians support FDA process for generic drugs.[18]

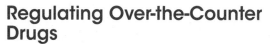

patent medicines A synonym for over-the-counter drugs

Categories of Over-the-Counter Drugs

The FDA devised a three-tier system for categorizing OTC drugs.

Category I:
  a. "generally recognized as safe" (GRAS)
  b. "generally recognized as effective" (GRAE)
  c. "generally recognized as honestly labeled" (GRAHL)

Category II: Not generally recognized as safe or effective or is improperly labeled; these drugs are supposed to be removed from the shelves within 6 months unless the manufacturer demonstrates that the drug should be Category I; if research in regard to a drug's safety and effectiveness is insufficient, the drug is included in Category III.

Category III: Cannot be sold; if a drug manufacturer contests the FDA's decision, the manufacturer can request a formal hearing.

Besides reviewing OTC drugs, the FDA looks at many prescription drugs to assess their safety and effectiveness. In several instances, the FDA has ruled that a prescription drug can be marketed as an OTC drug because it is relatively safe and effective. These prescription drugs have been reformulated to be less potent. Hence, the difference between many OTC and prescription drugs is the amount of active ingredient.

Another difference between prescribed and OTC drugs is that many chemicals in prescription drugs are not available for use in OTC drugs. Prescription drugs that have been switched to OTC drugs include ibuprofen (an analgesic drug sold as Nuprin, Advil, and Motrin), Dramamine (used for motion sickness), Actifed (a decongestant), Dimetapp (a cold medicine), levonorgestrel (Plan B), and orlistat (alli). Moving drugs to an OTC classification is cost effective for consumers. Even among those with health insurance, cost savings derive from no longer having to go to a doctor to get the prescription, travel time, and time off work.[19]

Herbal Drugs

A largely unregulated segment of the marketplace is that of herbal drugs. Part of the problem with regulating these products is that it is unclear whether they should be classified as drugs, foods, or herbs. The Dietary Supplement Health and Education Act of 1994 was created to define and regulate dietary supplements. Included under this act are vitamins, minerals, herbs, and other botanicals.[20]

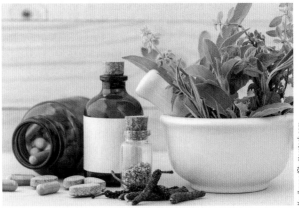

Many people equate the terms "herbal" and "natural" as safe alternatives to traditional medicine. Many of these supplements contain contaminants that can cause adverse effects.

Kerdkanno/Shutterstock.com

While regulated by the FDA, they differ from the way drugs are regulated. Marketers of these products are held accountable for branding products, as adulterated or misbranded products are not allowed. Additionally, these products must comply with the Current Good Manufacturing Process of the FDA, which provides practices required for product manufacturing including quality control, recordkeeping, and cleanliness of manufacturing facilities.[21] Thus, if there are numerous complaints regarding a herbal drug, it can be removed from the market.

The use of herbal drugs in China, India, Rome, Greece, Egypt, and Syria dates back to 500 years ago. Today, the use of herbal dietary supplements has been increasing each year, up 6.8% in 2014 totalling over 6 billion in US sales.[22] One-third of Americans use herbal drugs. While herbal drugs have evolved from fringe drugs to mainstream drugs, research into the safety and effectiveness of these drugs is still lacking.[23] In 2011, the European Union banned hundreds of herbal remedies, although other herbal remedies can be sold if they are licensed. Licenses are given if the products meet safety, quality, and manufacturing standards and provide information on possible side effects.[24]

Some herbal remedies can interfere with the effectiveness of conventional drugs. For example, St John's Wort, used for depression, may reduce the effectiveness of the birth control pill, while ginseng is not suitable for diabetics, and garlic may interfere with HIV medication.[25] There is also concern that herbal drugs will be used for euphoric or hallucinogenic purposes.[26] Table 14.1 lists selected herbal drugs and their intended uses.

Analgesics

The vast majority of Americans reported using an OTC pain reliever within the past year. Advertisements constantly remind us that pain relievers are indispensable. We are told that we do not have to live with minor aches and pains that affect our daily lives. The message is clear: Pain and discomfort are nuisances that we do not have to tolerate. Despite their benefits, all analgesic drugs have adverse side effects.[27]

The two basic types of **analgesics** are internal and external:

1. *External analgesics*, such as Ben-Gay and Absorbine, are applied to the skin for sore muscles. Their benefit is more psychological than physical.
2. *Internal analgesics* are taken into the body. Most analgesics are internal. Aspirin is the drug used most commonly. Americans ingest more than 10,000 *tons* of aspirin each year, which equates to 80 million aspirin or aspirin-containing tablets consumed every day.

At one time, aspirin dominated the analgesic market. Now, competitive analgesic products include

analgesics Drugs that relieve pain

TABLE 14.1 Commonly Used Herbal Supplements

Herb	Common Uses	Cautions
Chamomile	Used for GI complaints	Can cause toxicity of calcium channel blockers and antihyperlipidemics Has an additive effect when taken with alcohol or sedatives
Ginkgo	Used to improve circulation impaired by vascular disease Used to improve cognition and memory	Can increase bleeding in individuals already taking aspirin or warfarin
Melatonin	May help reestablish proper circadian rhythm	Should be taken in the early evening Can cause some stomach upset
St. John's wort	Used as an antidepressant Used as an antiviral	Can cause photosensitivity
Echinacea	Enhances the immune system Can be used as a sun protectant	Immunosuppression can occur with usage of more than eight weeks (immunocompromised individuals should not use)
Ginseng	Used for energy	Contraindicated in individuals with blood-clotting disorders Will increase blood pressure Can reduce the effectiveness of antihypertensive agents
Glucosamine	Stimulates the biosynthesis of a cartilage-building compound May also reduce inflammation	May exacerbate diabetes
Goldenseal	Used for High blood pressure Poor appetite Infections Menstrual problems Minor sciatic pain Muscle spasms Eye wash	Contraindicated in heart patients Should not be used with ear infections
Valarian	Used for its sedative action	Should not be used in children Should not be used in individuals with altered hepatic (liver) function
Kava	Used for anxiety, psychosis, and depression	Interacts with Levodopa, sedatives, central nervous system depressants, and barbiturates
Ginger	Used for motion sickness/stomach disorders	Multiple known drug interactions Can increase bleeding in individuals already taking aspirin or warfarin

acetaminophen, ibuprofen, naproxen sodium, and ketoprofen. These products effectively alleviate moderate pain, though they differ in other respects. Like aspirin, they have adverse side effects. From 2006 to 2010, over 400,000 people went to the emergency room for problems related to acetaminophen. Over 45% were admitted and less than 1% of the patients died. Women represented 65% of the cases and more than half of the cases involved intentional self-harm.[28]

Aspirin

Aspirin is one of the best documented medicines in the world. It is the most frequently used and least expensive drug of all times.[29] **Acetylsalicylic acid**, the active agent in aspirin, is similar to a chemical found in the bark of willow trees. Using willow bark for pain

and fever was common among the ancient Greeks and American Indians. At one time, people in pain were given salicylic acid, but it resulted in stomach upset and nausea. By 1897, chemist Felix Hoffman of Bayer Laboratories had developed a compound combining salicylic acid and acetyl acid to help treat his father's arthritis.[30] This new compound, called aspirin, caused less stomach distress than salicylic acid. Aspirin is a pain-reliever, fever reducer, and has anti-inflammatory properties. Additionally, it has antiplatelet properties that decrease platelet formation and inhibit the formation of blood clots, which may benefit circulation. Aspirin works best for dull, constant pain but is ineffective for sharp pain. Aspirin is nonaddicting; it does not alter consciousness, and the senses of the user remain intact.

When a cell in the human body is injured, hormone-like chemicals called **prostaglandins** are activated. High levels of prostaglandins can cause headaches, inflammation, fever, blood clots, and menstrual cramps. These chemicals can also affect the reproductive, circulatory, and digestive systems. Aspirin inhibits the synthesis and release of prostaglandins, thereby reducing moderate pain by affecting the body's pain receptors and ameliorating inflammation and fever.

Because aspirin reduces inflammation, it is especially helpful in relieving symptoms of rheumatoid arthritis. In 2013, almost 25% of the US adult population suffered from arthritis.[31]

Aspirin acts as an **antipyretic**, or fever-reducing drug. It works on the hypothalamus, which dilates peripheral blood vessels. This increases respiration and blood flow, and the body cools down as a result. Antipyretic action is not always advantageous. Although a fever causes discomfort, it can be helpful because an elevation in body temperature destroys many bacteria and viruses. Thus, the fever-reducing effect of aspirin can be counterproductive. If the body temperature is normal, aspirin does not lower it.

Among the significant benefits attributed to aspirin is prevention of heart attacks and strokes. The American Heart Association recommends low doses of aspirin (81 mg) for people at risk for heart attacks and heart attack survivors.[32] One study found that taking low-dose aspirin cut the risk of major cardiovascular events by more than 20%.[33] It is now considered to be a primary prevention tool in the prevention of cardiovascular disease among women.[34]

There are additional benefits to regular aspirin use. It has been shown that 100 mg of aspirin every other day reduces the risk of adult-onset asthma.[35] However, there are some among the asthma population who cannot tolerate aspirin. Aspirin intolerant asthma refers to a group of asthmatics whose condition becomes worse after taking aspirin. It is estimated to affect up to 20% of the asthmatic population.[37] Similarly, aspirin may exacerbate other respiratory conditions, a condition known as nonsteroidal anti-inflammatory drug-exacerbated respiratory disease.[38]

Among diabetics, aspirin use reduces the risk of retinopathy, the leading cause of blindness among people aged 20 to 65,[39] and is recommended as a primary and secondary prevention strategy for those with diabetes and higher risk of cardiovascular disease.[40] Another benefit of aspirin and other analgesic drugs is a reduction in cataracts. However, there is a relationship between regular aspirin use and aging macular disorder, a vision disorder.[41] Aspirin has also shown to reduce the risk in a number of cancers.[42] The US Preventive Services Task Force recommends low-dose aspirin to reduce the risk for colorectal cancer among adults aged 50 to 70.[43] However, many elderly people who take aspirin also drink alcohol—and this combination is particularly harmful because it may result in internal hemorrhaging and prolonged bleeding.[44] The risk of internal bleeding increases when aspirin is used with other anticoagulant drugs such as warfarin.[45] Even at low dosage levels, aspirin can result in kidney damage for many elderly people.[46] A British study noted that the administration of low doses of aspirin for 5 or more years resulted in a 34% decline in deaths from all types of cancers.[47]

People who are allergic to aspirin develop rashes, weakness, stomach pain, breathing problems, wheezing, and asthma-like attacks that can be fatal. In other people, aspirin causes nausea, vomiting, blood loss, and iron-deficiency anemia. With as few as two to three aspirins, a person can bleed twice as long as normal. Patients having surgery and women in the late stages of pregnancy are advised not to take aspirin. Taking aspirin during pregnancy has been linked to postpartum hemorrhaging, prolonged labor, and higher perinatal mortality.

People with bleeding disorders, especially hemophilia and gastrointestinal problems, are cautioned not to use aspirin. Aspirin also aggravates peptic ulcers.[48] To reduce stomach irritation, some people use buffered aspirin, though it does not diminish the irritation. The purpose of making buffered aspirin is to increase sales. To minimize irritation, taking a full glass of water with aspirin helps.

Other problems related to extensive aspirin use include hepatitis, bone-marrow depression, and kidney damage. Most overdoses are seen in children. In children younger than age 5, aspirin is one of the leading causes of death by accidental poisoning. Symptoms of aspirin toxicity include perspiration, dizziness, hyperventilation, headache, thirst, ringing in the ears, and hearing loss. Unfortunately, 25% of Americans who use OTC pain drugs exceed the recommended dosage.[49]

Aspirin inhibits **interferon**, a natural substance in the body that helps ward off viruses. Hence, it results in people being more susceptible to viruses, including colds.

Children with chicken pox or flu-like symptoms should not be given aspirin because of the slight risk of developing Reye's syndrome. This serious

acetylsalicylic acid The agent in aspirin that relieves pain

prostaglandins Chemicals in the body that produce pain and inflammation; aspirin alters their synthesis

antipyretic Having fever-reducing properties

interferon A natural substance in the body that wards off viral infections

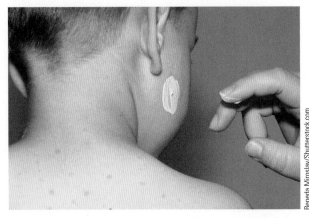

Children with chicken-pox or flu-like symptoms should never be given aspirin without first consulting a doctor. It can cause Reye's syndrome, a serious, but rare condition.

condition is marked by severe personality changes, vomiting, disorientation, lethargy, and death in up to one-fourth of patients. Reye's syndrome does not occur with other analgesic drugs. Although aspirin is approved for use in children ages 2 and up, it should not be used without first consulting a doctor.[50]

Acetaminophen

Because of concerns about the side effects of aspirin, many people have switched to other analgesics. One popular alternative is acetaminophen, a byproduct of **phenacetin**. Phenacetin was distributed widely in the 1940s and 1950s in combination with aspirin and caffeine. After a review, however, the FDA recommended that phenacetin use be limited to 10 days. Eventually, it was banned altogether in the United States because it was linked to kidney problems as well as heart disease, hypertension, and cancer.

First marketed in 1955, acetaminophen is used to reduce pain and fever. Since that time, its popularity has grown immensely. OTC products with acetaminophen include Tylenol, Datril, Anacin-3, and Panadol. Acetaminophen is believed to interfere with the synthesis of prostaglandins. However, it is not a safe alternative to aspirin. According to one research group, out of every 1,000 men who take acetaminophen for arthritis, 715 will improve, 4 will go to a hospital with a bleeding ulcer, and 12 will have a heart attack.[51] The most common cause of acute liver failure in the United States and United Kingdom is from

acetaminophen.[52] Unintentional use and chronic overdose of acetaminophen account for 50% of all acute liver diseases.[53] The recommended daily dose is 4 g of acetaminophen. Among those who exceeed the recommended limit of acetaminophen, one study discovered it was due to redosing too soon, exceeding the one-time dose, and combining a prescription medicine containing acetaminophen and an OTC containing the same drug.[54]

Signs of overdose, which might not appear for up to 48 hours, include stomach pain, fatigue, diarrhea, nausea, and vomiting. Children have died, usually from liver failure, after taking only a few Extra Strength Tylenol tablets. More cases of liver toxicity have occurred after people consumed two to three times the suggested dose within a 24- to 48-hour period.[55] Also, combining acetaminophen and alcohol is especially dangerous to the liver. In addition to these detrimental effects, one study of 51,529 male health professionals found that using acetaminophen four to five times a week increased the risk of hypertension.[56]

On the other hand, two advantages of acetaminophen over aspirin are that

1. it causes less stomach irritation and
2. it does not prolong bleeding time.

Acetaminophen is one of the only pain relievers doctors recommend for pregnant women.[57] However, recent studies suggest an increase in the risk for ADHD symptoms, autism, and asthma in children born to mothers who took acetaminophen while pregnant.[58] Although experts are divided on the issue, they agree that untreated pain or fever also carries risk for the baby and mother. Thus, it is a better alternative for people who are allergic to aspirin or who are pregnant. In a large Danish cohort study of over 60,000 children, it was found there was an increased risk of autism with hyperkinetic (movement) disorders

ADVANTAGES AND DISADVANTAGES OF ACETAMINOPHEN

Advantages

- Lessens pain
- Reduces fever
- Irritates stomach less than aspirin
- Does not prolong bleeding

Disadvantages

- Is ineffective for inflammation
- Can cause liver damage
- Can cause diarrhea, nausea, and vomiting
- May increase risk of hypertension
- Can cause death

ADVANTAGES AND DISADVANTAGES OF IBUPROFEN

Advantages

- Reduces pain
- Lessens inflammation
- Produces less stomach upset
- May reduce risk of breast cancer and Alzheimer's disease

Disadvantages

- Prolongs bleeding time
- Can cause allergic reaction
- Has numerous side effects
- May increase risk of peptic ulcers and enlarged prostate
- Can cause death

among children whose mothers used acetaminophen while pregnant.[59] Another study found an increased risk of ADHD symptoms of children whose mothers took acetaminophen during pregnancy.[60]

Arthritis sufferers do not receive the same anti-inflammation benefit from acetaminophen as from aspirin. Another disadvantage is that the analgesic benefit of acetaminophen is delayed if it is taken with or shortly after eating high-carbohydrate foods. In a study of individuals with tension-type headaches and dental pain, acetaminophen, with codeine included, was less effective than aspirin.[61] It is difficult to avoid acetaminophen because it is found in at least 100 other medications.[62]

Ibuprofen

Another OTC drug that reduces moderate pain and inflammation is ibuprofen. It is sold under the names Advil and Motrin.[63] It is a more potent pain reliever than aspirin and acetaminophen. When it was introduced, ibuprofen could be obtained only by prescription. In 1984, it was approved for OTC sale. Ibuprofen is less likely than aspirin to cause stomach upset, but it does prolong bleeding time. Doctors advise against using alcohol while taking ibuprofen because the combination increases the risk of stomach problems. Taking ibuprofen with food or milk helps to relieve upset stomach and mild heartburn.

If you have any of the following conditions, it is recommended you speak to a doctor before taking ibuprofen:[64]

- stomach ulcer
- inflammatory bowel disorder

- asthma
- pregnancy, trying to get pregnant, or breastfeeding
- high blood pressure
- blood-clotting problems
- high blood sugar or cholesterol levels

Unlike acetaminophen, ibuprofen reduces inflammation. Thus it is recommended for relieving symptoms of rheumatoid arthritis. People who are allergic to aspirin, however, might also be allergic to ibuprofen. In a meta-analysis of current publications, researchers found ibuprofen was preferred among patients who suffered from acute pain, osteoarthritis, acute pain, and migraines.[65] As with aspirin and acetaminophen, individuals taking ibuprofen are cautioned against exceeding recommended dosages. Ibuprofen can impede concentration and cause drowsiness and thus it is not a good idea to operate equipment after taking it.

Possible side effects from ibuprofen include vomiting, loss of hearing, nausea, elevated blood pressure, diarrhea, visual disturbances, heartburn, and congestive heart failure for people with impaired cardiac function. Its use has been linked to cataracts and death from liver failure. Ibuprofen has been shown to cause an increased risk of stroke and heart attacks among people with heart disease, and can cause stomach or intestinal bleeding.[66] These risks increase

phenacetin An alternative to aspirin now linked to kidney problems; its sale is prohibited

if ibuprofen is taken for an extended period of time, an individual is in poor health, or an individual consumes three of more alcoholic drinks a day.[67] On a positive note, ibuprofen may reduce the risk of breast cancer in women.[68] Another positive finding is that ibuprofen, as well as aspirin, might reduce the risk of developing Alzheimer's disease.[69]

Naproxen Sodium and Ketoprofen

Two other entries into the OTC analgesic market are **naproxen sodium** and **ketoprofen**. Aleve is a popular brand of naproxen sodium, and Orudis KT and Actron are brands containing ketoprofen. Naproxen sodium is comparable to ibuprofen in effectiveness, and its analgesic effects last up to 12 hours. Ketoprofen is as effective as ibuprofen, and it produces results in about 30 minutes. Like aspirin, acetaminophen, and ibuprofen, naproxen sodium and ketoprofen reduce fever, and like aspirin and ibuprofen, it also reduces inflammation.

One advantage of naproxen sodium is its long-term pain relief. One study reported that among people who took the drug for moderate and severe headaches, 52% experienced significant pain relief when the drug was first used and 90% experienced pain relief after 3 months.[70] In a separate study of 3,000 migraine sufferers, those who were given naproxen sodium were more likely to experience relief than those individuals given placebos.[71] The majority of people taking naproxen sodium do not encounter adverse side effects, although some patients experience gastrointestinal bleeding.[72] Naproxen sodium can sometimes cause bloating and dizziness.

Doctors advise consumers not to drink alcohol while taking these drugs. Both drugs work best for muscle pain, arthritis, and menstrual pain. One study found that there is minimal risk cardiovascular risk for those taking OTC doses of naproxen.[73] In 2003, a ketoprofen patch was approved for use as treatment for joint pain.[74] Ketoprofen has been shown to be more effective than acetaminophen for reducing fever in children.[75] Asthmatics and people who are allergic to aspirin should not take these drugs.

Cold and Allergy Drugs

OTC drugs sold to treat colds and allergies do not cure these conditions.[76] In 2015, the incidence of colds and flu was down almost 11%.[77] This may be attributed to warmer winter seasons, as warmer tempuratures impact how many people experience colds, which leads to fewer cough and cold OTC sales.[78]

What these drugs do is relieve symptoms of colds and allergies. This could be counterproductive in the long run, however. Colds are self-limiting conditions that go away notwithstanding treatment. Many people overcome colds (and other ailments) more quickly

---

ON CAMPUS

North Carolina has seen an upward trend among college students using cough syrup to get high. Sometimes called Skittles or Triple-C, students are using cough syrup containing DXM to get high. It is often mixed with soda or marijuana and can have devastating effects. At high doses, the effects of DXM are similar to the effects from PCP.

Effects of DXM include dizziness, impaired physical coordination, rapid heartbeat, confusion, and disorientation. Abuse of DXM can lead to liver damage and death. There is additional risks, such as respiratory failure, when mixing the cough syrup with alcohol, another depressant.

Questions to Ponder

What role should college health centers play in preventing the abuse of cough syrup?

Source: D. Wilson, "NC Parents shocked to learn children are abusing over-the-counter drug", *ABC13*, (November 5, 2014). Accessed on March 14, 2017 from *http://abc13.com/health/parents-shocked-kids-are-abusing-over-the-counter-drug/382140/*.

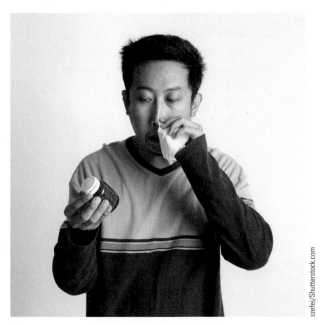

Cough and cold medicines do not cure the disease, they only provide treatment for the symptoms.

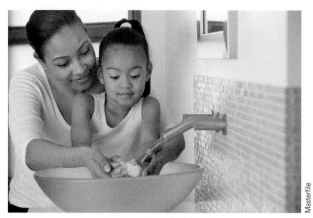

Washing the hands is one of the most effective means of preventing colds and other infectious diseases.

when physicians prescribe medications, even if the medications are **placebos**. A familiar adage says "A cold will end in a week with aspirin or in 7 days without anything."

The common cold has no cure. One problem with finding a cure is that a cold is far from "common" and is actually a complex condition. In addition, cough and cold remedies for children can be hazardous. One study involving 63 emergency rooms, dating from 2004 to 2005, found that 7,091 children under age 12 received treatment for adverse reactions to cough and cold medicines. The majority of children seen were between ages 2 and 5.[79] In 2008, the labels on cough and cold medicines were updated with warning that these medicines are not appropriate for children under 4 years old. As a result of this change, there were fewer emergency room visits from adverse reactions to cough and cold medicines for children.[80] The following discussion examines the types of drugs that comprise the cold and allergy market.

Antihistamines

When allergens are present, the body releases chemicals called **histamines**. Histamines protect the body from diseases by releasing antibodies that attack antigens (foreign bodies), viruses, bacteria, and chemicals in the body. In doing so, they produce runny nose and eyes, sneezing, congestion, nausea, and itching. One study found that antihistamines were effective for relieving itching[81] and for nasal inflammation.[82] One study found that using antihistamines alone does not

provide meaningful relief from the common cold, but researchers did find that combining antihistamines with other OTC (decongestants, analgesics, etc.) has small to moderate effects on the common cold.[83] Second-generation antihistamines, which do not cause drowsiness, are more effective than older antihistamines and also improve seasonal allergy symptoms.[84]

Antihistamines interfere with the release of histamines and thereby provide symptomatic relief from allergies. One study found that 85% people who used second-generation antihistamines were satisfied with the efficacy of the drug.[85] Besides treating allergies of the nose and eyes, second-generation antihistamines are effective for treating skin allergies.[86] They are also more effective than placebos for relieving headaches.[87] They do not cure colds. In fact, one study found that antihistamines may actually prolong ear infections in children,[88] and are not recommended for children experiencing ear infections.[89]

Antihistamines are found in cough syrups, hay fever and motion sickness preparations, and decongestants such as Contac, Dimetapp, Sudafed, and Triaminic. Antihistamines in Benadryl and similar allergy relievers make people drowsy and thereby affect driving ability. Antihistamine medications often contain alcohol, which contributes to drowsiness. Antihistamines also can produce dry mouth, nose, and throat; weakness; and constipation. An allergic

naproxen sodium An over-the-counter analgesic

ketoprofen An over-the-counter analgesic

placebos Inert substances that do not have a physical effect but may produce psychological and associated physiological reactions

histamines Chemicals that are released by the body in response to the presence of allergens

reaction to antihistamines can cause blurred vision, dizziness, nervousness, headaches, hives, and an inability to urinate. While various studies on the use of antihistamines during pregnancy show no harm to the fetus, there have been animal studies done that suggest antihistamines have a teratogenic effect. Thus, none of the antihistamines have been declared safe by the FDA to take during pregnancy.[90]

Cough Medicines

A cough can be productive—meaning that it produces secretions—or nonproductive. Nonproductive coughs irritate the throat. Drugs that suppress or prevent coughing are called **antitussives**. These cough suppressants act on the medulla, the brain's cough center. One study of children given antitussive cough medicines reported that 46 to 56% had satisfactory responses.[91] Efficacy regarding cough and cold medicine has not been established in children, and some recommend not giving these drugs to children altogether.[92]

Two antitussive drugs are codeine and dextromethorphan:

- **Codeine** provides relief within 15 to 30 minutes, and the effects last 4 to 6 hours after ingestion. One interesting study, however, found that chocolate was more effective than codeine in suppressing coughs.[93] Although codeine-based cough syrups do not require a prescription, their sale is regulated. Codeine causes dependency, but the risk is low compared with that for morphine. In 2007, the FDA issued a warning for nursing mothers who take codeine because there was a report of an infant who died after having been breastfed by its mother who took codeine. Cough medicines with codeine are associated with a higher frequency of adverse effects and toxicity in children.[94]
- **Dextromethorphan (Delsym)** is nonnarcotic and does not produce dependency, although it induces drowsiness, nausea, and dizziness. In recent years, DXM has become popular among

CHOCOLATE VS. CODEINE

A few studies have shown that dark chocolate is more effective in treating coughs compared to codeine. Evidently there is an alkaloid in cocoa that is better at reducing coughs than codeine. This is especially true if experiencing a tickle or hacking cough as chocolate's texture is better at coating the throat and protecting the nerve endings that trigger the cough.

So, next time you experience coughing, try a bar of chocolate!

Source: Purewow, "When it comes to coughs, chocolate is more effective than codeine", *Food and Wine*, (January 22, 2016). Accessed on March 16, 2017 from http://www.foodandwine .com/fwx/food/when-it-comes-coughs-chocolate-more-effective -codeine.

young people as a mind-altering substance because it is easy to obtain, the negative effects are not widely known, and it is socially approved. The inappropriate use of DXM is also referred to as "robo-tripping."[95]

- Dextromethorphan, also known as DXM, can be lethal. In 2010, an advisory panel for the FDA met to discuss whether DXM should be listed as a controlled substance but the panel voted against this measure.[96] At recommended doses, DXM is safe; however, at 10 times the recommended dose, it produces hallucinations.[97]
- DXM is chemically related to PCP and ketamine. Young people who use DXM often use alcohol and illegal drugs in conjunction with it. DXM contributes to injuries and fatalities because one's judgment is impaired. When used with Ecstasy, DXM can cause hyperthermia.[98]

A productive cough helps respiration by removing mucous secretions and foreign matter from the lower respiratory tract. Cough syrups that increase mucous secretions, making a cough productive, are called **expectorants**. The most common expectorant, guaifenesin, is found in Nortussin, Anti-Tuss, and Robitussin. If large amounts are consumed, expectorants produce drowsiness, nausea, and vomiting.

At least 80% of cough and cold remedies are unnecessary.[99] Studies have cast doubt on the efficacy of codeine. Moreover, codeine produces a number of adverse effects including irritated stomach, tiredness, gastric hemorrhage, and renal impairment.[100] Sucking on hard candies can be just as effective in increasing mucous secretions and relieving throat irritation.

SIDE EFFECTS OF ANTIHISTAMINES

- Dizziness
- Weakness
- Nervousness
- Poor concentration
- Headache
- Drowsiness
- Blurred vision
- Difficulty urinating
- Constipation
- Hives
- Dry mouth, nose, and throat

Decongestants

Decongestants constrict blood vessels of the nasal passages, improve air flow, and obstruct secretions that go to the back of the throat. Although decongestants are effective, they do have drawbacks. Some produce a **rebound effect**, in which the congestion becomes worse than it was originally. Increasing the intake of decongestants exacerbates the rebound effect. Dependency on decongestants is possible. Instructions in nasal spray packages indicate that they should not be used for more than three consecutive days.

Because antihistamines in decongestants shrink swollen nasal passages and relieve sinus headaches, they alleviate allergies. One decongestant is **pseudoephedrine**, the active ingredient in the OTC decongestant Sudafed. Side effects of pseudoephedrine include dry mouth, anxiety, dizziness, tremors, tachycardia, vomiting, nausea, headache, difficulty urinating, and insomnia.

Antacids

As a result of eating habits and lifestyle, stomach-related problems are prevalent. The so-called good life has wreaked havoc on our sedentary bodies. Advertisers constantly remind us that upset stomach, acid indigestion, heartburn, constipation, and diarrhea are annoyances that are easily remedied by using their products. In response, US residents spent more than 2.19 billion dollars on antacids in 2015.[101] What causes the stomach to be irritated in the first place? The culprit is **hydrochloric acid**, which aids in digestion but also aggravates the stomach's lining. It is estimated that almost 60% of adults suffer from indigestion or heartburn each given year.[102] Antacids curtail stomach acidity[103] but have many side effects. Therefore, the FDA established guidelines for antacids: They should not be used for more than 2 weeks at a time, and if a problem persists for more than 2 weeks, the user should consult a physician. Some antacids have high sodium levels, which can cause either constipation or diarrhea.

Liquid antacids are more effective than tablets. A tablet should be taken with a full glass of water. Effervescent tablets should be dissolved completely. Also, aspirin and antacids should not be taken at the same time because this combination can increase stomach upset. Although antacids are relatively safe, one concern is that they could mask symptoms of more serious underlying problems.[104] Also, some antacids impair calcium absorption, resulting in an increase in broken bones for people as they age.[105] In addition, antacids may interfere with the function of certain antibiotics.[106]

Sodium Bicarbonate

A popular antacid used to neutralize excess stomach acid is Alka-Seltzer. A primary ingredient in Alka-Seltzer is **sodium bicarbonate**, otherwise known as baking soda. People with high blood pressure have to monitor their sodium intake. Because sodium bicarbonate can raise blood pressure, people with hypertension should know which antacids contain it. Side effects related to sodium bicarbonate are belching and flatulence. Although neither of these effects is fatal, they can be uncomfortable and embarrassing.

Calcium Carbonate

Some people with acid indigestion have switched to **calcium carbonate** because it is free of sodium. Two popular OTC drugs containing calcium carbonate are Rolaids and Tums. The benefits of calcium carbonate are temporary. In the long run, it creates more problems than it solves because it produces a rebound effect in which stomach acidity actually increases after the drug's effects wear off. Constipation can result from the use of calcium carbonate. Also, it is contraindicated for people who have severe kidney disease. On the other hand, one benefit is that it is rich in calcium.

Salts of Magnesium and Aluminium

Other ingredients frequently found in antacid medications are salts of magnesium and salts of aluminium. These counteract each other: Salts of magnesium

antitussives Drugs that act as cough suppressants

codeine A mild narcotic that suppresses coughing; a derivative of opium

dextromethorphan (Delsym) An over-the-counter nonnarcotic drug found in cough preparations

expectorants Cough medicines that make a cough productive by increasing mucous secretions

decongestants Substances used to relieve congestion

rebound effect The side effects produced by a drug that make a condition worse than it was originally; for example, sinuses become more congested by nasal sprays

pseudoephedrine A nasal decongestant

hydrochloric acid Acid in the stomach that can ease digestion and irritate the stomach lining

sodium bicarbonate Baking soda; an ingredient in antacids designed to neutralize excess acid in the stomach

calcium carbonate An antacid designed to relieve acid indigestion

TABLE 14.2 Drawbacks of Various Types of Antacids

Antacid	Side Effects
Sodium bicarbonate	Increased blood pressure Belching Gas
Calcium carbonate	Rebound effect Constipation Kidney damage
Salts of magnesium/salts of aluminium	Bowel irritation Vomiting Abdominal cramps

cause constipation, and salts of aluminium bring about diarrhea. People with intestinal disorders such as irritable bowel syndrome are cautioned against using these products.

To relieve diarrhea, some people use products such as Kaopectate, a mixture of kaolin and pectate, which decreases the fluid content in the stool. Antidiarrheal drugs can cause abdominal cramps, nausea, and vomiting, as well as dependence. An old standby to relieve constipation is castor oil, which stimulates contractions of the smooth muscles of the intestine. Table 14.2 identifies the disadvantages of various types of antacids.

H2 Blockers and PPIs

Newer remedies include histamine (H2) blockers and proton pump inhibitors (PPIs). Both types of drugs effectively treat heartburn, although they may produce side effects such as diarrhea, constipation, and headache. In less severe cases of heartburn, H2 blockers are effective. Examples of H2 blockers are Tagamet HB and Zantac. The American College of Gastroenterology recommends PPIs because they are more effective. Some studies indicate PPI increases the risk of hip, spine, and any-site fracture.[107] There has also been some recent research that suggests the use of PPIs has been associated with an increased risk of ischemic strokes.[108] To make matters worse, many users do not adhere to taking PPIs.[109] Examples of PPIs include the OTC drug Prilosec and the prescription drug Nexium.

Sleep Aids and Sedatives

Stress, tension, and anxiety are epidemic in contemporary society, and many people depend on OTC drugs for relief. Insomnia affects more than one-third of adults within any given year.[110] In addition, women are twice as likely to suffer from insomnia compared to men, and the risk of insomnia increases as one ages. Insomnia results in irritability, restlessness, ineffectiveness at work, lethargy, and moodiness. To overcome insomnia, some individuals take an OTC medication or sedative. The primary ingredient in many OTC sedatives and sleep aids is some type of antihistamine.[111]

Antihistamines produce drowsiness, and the sedating effects of antihistamines increase greatly in conjunction with alcohol. Therefore, taking alcohol and antihistamines at the same time is not prudent. Also, a person should not drive an automobile or engage in potentially hazardous activities while taking antihistamines. In addition, anyone who is planning to take an allergy skin test should not take antihistamines.

The benefits of antihistamines as sedatives and sleep agents are limited. Nytol, Sominex, and Sleep-Eze are advertised as OTC sleep aids, and Compoz is advertised as an OTC sedative. These products are essentially the same.

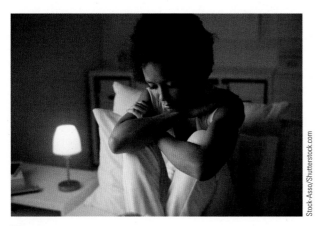

■ About one in three Americans suffer from insomnia in a given year.

Over-the-Counter Stimulants

Just as some people have difficulty going to sleep, others have trouble staying awake. To combat fatigue and drowsiness, OTC stimulants have been designed to help people stay awake and alert. The primary ingredient in these drugs is caffeine.

Although some people use OTC stimulants in an attempt to reverse alcohol intoxication, the stimulants do not work. Giving caffeine to an intoxicated person results in a wide-awake drunk. OTC stimulants such as Vivarin and No Doz are common on many campuses. Since March 1989, the only drug that has been allowed in OTC stimulants is caffeine.

The popularity of energy drinks, in which caffeine is a primary ingredient, has exploded in recent years. Sales of energy drinks having been soaring and it is now the second sales performer in the drinks market (water is still number 1).[112] In 2012, an inhalable form of caffeine appeared on the market. While with coffee it takes about 20 minutes before the effects of caffeine are experienced, the effects of inhaled caffeine are felt almost instantly. Inhaling caffeine produces quicker effects compared to digesting caffeine.[113] Some are concerned that young people who drink alcohol may take energy drinks or inhalable caffeine in the belief that caffeine will make the effects of alcohol dissipate more quickly. In 2012, the FDA sent a warning letter to the company stating false advertisement; the company had marketed the product as being both an inhaled and ingested product.[114]

The amount of caffeine in a recommended dose of OTC stimulants is equal to two to three cups of coffee. Labels on the packages of OTC stimulants caution consumers against taking other caffeine-containing beverages—such as tea, coffee, and soft drinks—at the same time.

One consequence of excessive caffeine consumption is **caffeinism**, a condition marked by nervousness, anxiety, tachycardia, sweating, and panic in some instances. As reported in Chapter 2, "look-alike" and "sound-alike" stimulants are promoted through mail-order advertisements. These typically include nothing more than caffeine.

Weight-Loss Aids

Many people are obsessed with dieting. In the United States, an estimated $30 billion annually is spent on dietary supplements, books, foods, and related services.[115] Books on dieting are among the top sellers year after year. Magazines are replete with articles on weight loss. Many Internet Web sites promote herbal weight-loss supplements. However, despite the disclaimer statements posted on each of these Web sites, only a few mention potential drug interactions or adverse reactions.[116]

Society constantly reminds us that "thin is in" and help is available for anyone who wants to achieve that desired state. Too often, thinness is equated with attractiveness. Television shows and other media have popular actors and actresses leading viewers through aerobic exercises. Advertisements for health clubs abound in the media.

Ironically, most of the people leading the aerobic activities and appearing in the health club advertisements are thin in the first place and do not need weight-loss products. And, the same magazines that feature articles about how to lose weight include articles with recipes that would kill any diet. Many companies tout their products as helping with (in some cases guaranteeing) the loss of excess pounds with little effort. If all else fails, fat can be suctioned out through liposuction.

One drug used for weight loss is ephedrine (ephedra). Ephedra is a Chinese herb that was used to treat asthma. When combined with other stimulants such as caffeine, ephedrine can be fatal.[117] Because of its toxic effects, it has been banned in many countries.[118] Metabolite, a popular weight-loss product, contains this dangerous combination of ephedra and caffeine. Metabolite was responsible for 18 heart attacks, 26 strokes, 43 seizures, and 5 deaths between 1997 and 2002.[119] The FDA banned the sale of ephedrine in April 2004.[120]

Orlistat

One of the more effective weight-loss drugs is orlistat, also known as **alli**. It is the only FDA-approved weight-loss product available to adults without a

caffeinism Excessive caffeine consumption resulting in caffeine dependency

alli A weight-loss drug that blocks the absorption of fat

Moving from RX to OTC

Many support initiatives to move prescription drugs to over-the-counter drugs. They argue OTC drugs are more accessible to consumers since a prescription and doctor's visit is not necessary to purchase these drugs; thus removing some of the barriers to obtaining these drugs.

On the other hand, some content moving prescription drugs to OTC classes negatively impacts consumers while reducing healthcare costs for the government and health insurance companies. By taking the doctor's visit out of the equation, health insurance costs go down because they do not have to pay for a doctor's visit. Additionally, while many health insurance companies cover prescription drug costs, they do not cover OTC medicines; thus placing the burden on the consumer to pay for these drugs.

Questions to Ponder

Does the movement from RX to OTC reduce/increase barriers to access?

Socioeconomic status (SES) can be used as a health marker, as those with lowers SES generally have poorer health outcomes compared to those with higher SES. How does the movement from RX to OTC impact the health disparity gap?

prescription. Until June 2007, orlistat was available only by prescription. The prescribed version of this drug is known as Xenical. The only difference between alli and Xenical is that alli comes in 60 mg capsules and Xenical comes in 120 mg capsules.

Orlistat works by blocking the absorption of about 25% of the fat in the foods that people consume. Orlistat, especially in conjunction with counseling, effectively helps obese individuals to lose weight.[121] However, there is pressure on the FDA to ban Orlistat because of concerns regarding its safety. Orlistat has been linked to acute pancreatitis, liver damage, and kidney damage.[122]

Phenylpropanolamine and Benzocaine

At one time, the FDA permitted OTC sales of **phenylpropanolamine (PPA)**, caffeine, and **benzocaine** for purposes of weight loss. It is believed that stimulants such as caffeine suppress appetite, but no long-term research is available to support this hypothesis. PPA is a frequently used appetite suppressant, and is structurally similar to amphetamines but does not produce euphoria unless it is taken in large doses. PPA seems to affect appetite over a short time, but long-term effectiveness has not been demonstrated. Despite concerns regarding the safety and effectiveness of PPA, an FDA advisory panel approved it as a supplement for weight reduction for up to 12 weeks.

Side effects of PPA include headache, rapid heartbeat, anxiety, higher blood sugar levels, nausea, insomnia, and hypertension. It is contraindicated for clinically depressed and hypertensive individuals. The most commonly encountered problems with PPA are psychotic episodes, seizures, and stroke. In 2000, the FDA issued a strong warning against the use of PPA, stating that PPA may be responsible for 200 to 500 hemorrhagic strokes (bleeding in the brain) each year in US adults younger than age 50.[123] In response, many manufacturers have voluntarily removed PPA from their products. An example of a product that used to include PPA (but no longer does) is Dexatrim. Because it acts as a decongestant, PPA also is found in OTC cold and allergy preparations.[124]

Another purported weight-reducing drug is **benzocaine**, a topical anesthetic that is put into chewing gum and candy. When one eats candies or chews gum containing benzocaine, the tongue and palate become numb. As numbness sets in, the desire for food diminishes. The effectiveness of benzocaine as an appetite suppressant has not been determined, although it might work under the same principle that one does not usually feel like eating after visiting the dentist and receiving an anesthetic!

Being a Smart Consumer

Because of the escalating costs of health care, many people are turning to self-care and self-medication. Visiting the doctor every time a minor ache or ailment arises is time-consuming and costly. At the same time, many advertisements for OTC drugs make claims about their benefits. Consumers must look at these

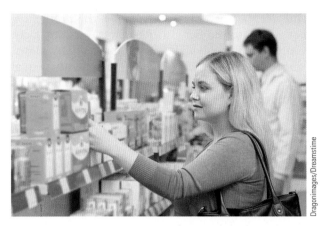

Become a health-wise consumer by reading labels and following directions.

Dragonimages/Dreamstime

phenylpropanolamine (PPA) A decongestant also used as an appetite suppressant

benzocaine A topical anesthetic put into candies or chewing gum to diminish appetite

mended dosage, warnings, and date of expiration. Being a prudent consumer requires reading labels.

Another concern regarding self-medication is that OTC drugs often provide relief of symptoms only. Ameliorating the symptoms of an illness can encourage the ill person to minimize the seriousness of the illness or disregard its cause. This is potentially hazardous because the person might not seek additional or more appropriate treatment. *Relieving the symptoms of an illness is not the same as curing the illness.* Furthermore, some OTC drugs—such as stimulants, nasal sprays, sedatives, eye drops, cough syrups, and laxatives—can result in dependency. In short, consumers should not assume that OTC drugs are harmless.

advertisements carefully because, though advertisers legally cannot make false claims, they may give inaccurate impressions.

Information on labels of OTC medicines includes a list of active ingredients, directions for use, recom-

Summary

The over-the-counter (OTC) drug market is a multibillion-dollar business. People are taking health care into their own hands, and advertisers are trying to convince consumers of the need for their products. Consumers are told that a product is available to address almost every problem. Just because nonprescribed drugs are readily accessible, this is no guarantee that they are safe and effective. A growing problem is the lack of regulation of herbal drugs.

The first attempt to regulate OTC drugs came with the Pure Food and Drug Act of 1906, but persistent problems led to enactment of the Food, Drug, and Cosmetic Act in 1938. This law stipulated that prescribed drugs had to be proven safe and effective. By 1962, the legislation was expanded to include OTC drugs. An FDA advisory panel reviewed the active ingredients in OTC drugs and, based on its findings, drugs were placed into one of three categories, relating to their OTC status.

Among the most commonly used OTC drugs are analgesics. External analgesics are used for muscle soreness. Internal analgesics reduce dull, constant pain.

The active agent in aspirin is acetylsalicylic acid, which alleviates pain, fever, and inflammation. Aspirin can help prevent heart attacks and strokes. However, it prolongs internal bleeding, and some people are allergic to it.

Aspirin is a leading cause of accidental poisoning deaths in children younger than 5 years of age. Aspirin use is not advised in children up to age 18 with chicken pox or flu-like symptoms because of an increased risk, though slight, of Reye's syndrome, a potentially deadly disease.

Alternatives to aspirin are acetaminophen, ibuprofen, naproxen sodium, and ketoprofen. Acetaminophen reduces pain and fever but does not alleviate inflammation; thus, it is not recommended for arthritis. Although many people switched from aspirin to acetaminophen because it causes less stomach upset and does not prolong bleeding time, it is not safer. Acetaminophen has been implicated in a number of liver-related problems. More people have gone to hospital emergency rooms from acetaminophen use than from aspirin use, and it accounts for more deaths than aspirin.

Ibuprofen lessens inflammation and pain. Although it extends bleeding time, it causes less stomach upset than aspirin. Ibuprofen use can be fatal in certain circumstances. Both naproxen sodium and ketoprofen are alternatives for reducing fever and inflammation. Naproxen sodium is as effective as ibuprofen, and its effects last up to 12 hours. Ketoprofen works as well as ibuprofen and produces results in about 30 minutes.

Cold and allergy medications provide symptomatic relief but do not cure colds and allergies. Their primary agents are antihistamines. A common side effect is drowsiness.

Because of our typical eating habits and lifestyles, stomach-related disorders are prevalent. Many stomach problems are caused by excessive hydrochloric acid, which aggravates the stomach lining. Antacids are ingested to neutralize stomach acidity. Two types of antacids are sodium bicarbonate and calcium carbonate.

Stress, anxiety, tension, and sleeplessness affect millions of people, and many products are available to address these concerns. Antihistamines, which induce drowsiness, are prominent in many OTC sedatives and sleep agents. For some people, the problem is not going to sleep but rather staying awake and alert. Caffeine is the only OTC stimulant the FDA allows. The amount of caffeine in OTC stimulants is equal to that in two or three cups of coffee. Too much caffeine causes nervousness and anxiety.

With the availability of OTC products and the desire to assume more responsibility for our own health care, people have to be wise consumers. Most OTC products relieve symptoms but do not offer cures. Therefore, consumers might think their health is improving when they actually are getting worse. People would be wise to become more informed about drugs. Being a smart consumer, at a minimum, means reading labels and following directions.

Thinking Critically

1. Although pain is a common experience, individuals have different thresholds. Some people reach for a pain reliever almost instantly when they feel discomfort. Others resist any type of medication as long as they can. How would you describe your threshold level? How soon after getting a headache do you take medicine for it?
2. The incidence of Reye's syndrome after aspirin use is very low. Should warnings regarding Reye's syndrome be included on aspirin containers? Why or why not?
3. Though many people realize that cold remedies do not cure colds, they continue to buy them. Studies suggest their efficacy is minimal at best. Given that research is lacking about the effectiveness of cough and cold medicines, why do you believe they are so popular?
4. Since the 1970s, the size of women shown in advertisements has gone down. In the 1950s Marilyn Monroe, the icon of sexiness, was a size 14. Today, she would be considered a plus-size model. As the media shows smaller and thinner women as the image of beauty, the percentage of obesity and overweight women continue to rise, increasing the gap between media's portrayal of beauty and the average woman. Given societal pressures on being thin, it is no surprise OTC diet aids are so popular. Many of these aids only produce minimal and temporary results. How should the effectiveness of these aids be studied and marketed?

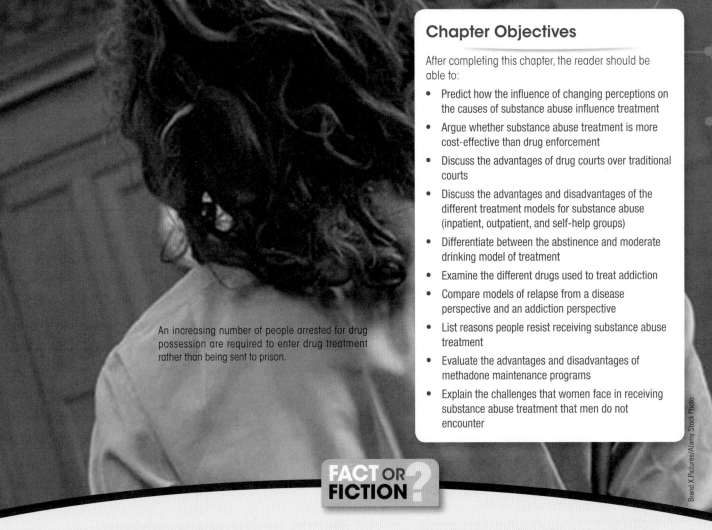

15

Substance Abuse Treatment

Chapter Objectives

After completing this chapter, the reader should be able to:

- Predict how the influence of changing perceptions on the causes of substance abuse influence treatment
- Argue whether substance abuse treatment is more cost-effective than drug enforcement
- Discuss the advantages of drug courts over traditional courts
- Discuss the advantages and disadvantages of the different treatment models for substance abuse (inpatient, outpatient, and self-help groups)
- Differentiate between the abstinence and moderate drinking model of treatment
- Examine the different drugs used to treat addiction
- Compare models of relapse from a disease perspective and an addiction perspective
- List reasons people resist receiving substance abuse treatment
- Evaluate the advantages and disadvantages of methadone maintenance programs
- Explain the challenges that women face in receiving substance abuse treatment that men do not encounter

An increasing number of people arrested for drug possession are required to enter drug treatment rather than being sent to prison.

Brand X Pictures/Alamy Stock Photo

FACT OR FICTION?

1. The most common reason for not receiving drug abuse treatment is the stigma associated with receiving treatment.

2. A person has to want drug treatment in order for it to be effective.

3. In the early 1900s, drug addiction was viewed as a public health problem rather than as a legal problem.

4. Adults in the United States are more likely to seek treatment for marijuana than for any other drug.

5. Although twice as many men as women enter drug treatment, the number of adolescent boys is nearly the same as the number of adolescent girls.

6. Drug addicts who enter into drug abuse treatment voluntarily have higher success rates than drug addicts who are required to go into treatment.

7. Less than 5% of people dependent on alcohol can stop on their own without any type of formal program.

8. More adolescents are in drug treatment for marijuana than for any other drug.

9. A relapse means treatment was not successful.

10. Drug and alcohol rehabilitation can cure addiction.

Turn the page to check your answers

The economic cost of illicit drug abuse for society amounts to $700 billion annually.[1] In 2015, an estimated 21.7 million persons aged 12 or older needed substance abuse treatment. Of these, only 10% of those who needed substance abuse treatment services received treatment.[2] The vast majority of all admissions to state substance abuse agencies can be attributed to five drugs: alcohol (36%), opiates (30%), marijuana/hashish (15%), cocaine (5%), and methamphetamines/amphetamines (9%).[3] Socially, economically, and interpersonally, drug abuse is expensive. The federal government has allocated $14 billion for drug-abuse treatment for 2017, which represents 46% of the Drug Control spending budget.[4] The need to prevent substance abuse is indisputable, and treatment is essential for people who require it. The majority of Americans view drug abuse as a serious problem in the United States and two-thirds of Americans would like to see drug offenders in programs that focus on rehabilitation, not jail.[5] Additionally, more than half of Americans believe mandatory minimum sentences should be eliminated.

Underlying Causes of Drug Abuse

A national study found that people in treatment for substance abuse had problems that extended beyond drug abuse. Compared with the general population, they were disadvantaged in education and employment.[6] Proportionately, people in treatment were more likely to be male, Caucasian, aged 25 to 45, and unemployed or out of the workforce, and have less than a high school education.[7] One group of concern are veterans, who experience higher rates of abuse compared to nonveterans. One study found 60% of homeless veterans suffered from a substance abuse disorder, of which half of those had an alcohol and drug abuse disorder.[8] Another group that is concerning is the elderly, where substance abuse has been rising. A growing number of elderly are at risk for hazardous drinking, prescription misuse, and illicit use and abuse.[9] This group is particularly at risk because they generally have more medical conditions, with multiple prescriptions, making substance abuse difficult to diagnose. Approximately 26% of all substance abusers in treatment are aged 45 or older.[10] By 2030, the number of Americans aged 65 and older is expected to be twice what it was in 2000.[11] Substance abuse services for the elderly are likewise expected to increase.

How effective is treatment? What type of treatment is best? Also, the goals of a treatment program differ, depending on whether drug abuse is seen as a medical problem, as a breakdown in society, or as a personality weakness. If the cause of drug abuse is medical, some type of drug therapy might be in order. If the cause is social, the abuser might be taught how to deal with society. If the cause is seen as a personality defect, therapy would consist of restructuring the abuser's personality.

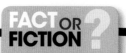

1. **FICTION** The fact is—Although many people perceive a stigma to receiving drug abuse treatment, the most common reason was that abusers were not ready to stop using the drug.

2. **FICTION** The fact is—Treatment has a positive impact on the patient regardless of their desire to receive treatment.

3. **FACT** Drug addiction was originally seen as a public health or medical problem. It was not until drugs were made illegal that addiction was viewed as a legal problem.

4. **FICTION** The fact is—Alcohol accounts for the highest percentage of individuals seeking substance abuse treatment.

5. **FACT** According to data from the federal government, the numbers of adolescent males and females entering drug treatment are very comparable.

6. **FICTION** The fact is—Individuals who enter treatment voluntarily leave more quickly. The longer one stays in treatment, the more effective it is.

7. **FICTION** The fact is—As many as one-third of alcoholics stop their abusive drinking without any formal treatment program.

8. **FACT** More than half of juveniles in drug treatment are there because of problems with marijuana.

9. **FICTION** The fact is—Relapse is a normal part of recovery and can be seen as helpful tool to indicate a need to restart or adjust treatment.

10. **FICTION** The fact is—There is no cure for addiction. Addiction is a chronic disease that may enter remission, but will never be cured.

THE LINK BETWEEN EDUCATION, DRUGS, AND CRIME

While most Americans favor treatment over incarceration for drug offenders, the budget for state and local corrections continues to rise, while the budget for education remains stagnant. State and local spending on corrections has increased by almost 90%, while spending on higher education remains flat since 1990.

There is an association between education and incarceration. As educational attainment increases, incarceration rates decrease. Currently, two-thirds of state prison inmates have not completed high school. Black men ages 20 to 24, who do not have a high school diploma or equivalent, have a greater chance of being incarcerated than employed. Additionally, some researchers say for every 10% increase in high school graduation rates, a 9% decrease is seen in criminal arrest rates.

The budget increase on prisons reflects a problem that is not being addressed. To reduce incarceration rates, the focus needs to remain on prevention through educational attainment. This will help reduce drug dependency, especially among young, Black men, where more than half of them did not use hard drugs until after being sent to jail.

Questions to Ponder

What is the relationship between education and incarceration? Why does it exist?

If the budget allotment were reversed, and states and local government spent more on education, how could the money be spent to achieve the greatest impact?

Some say the focus on incarceration, rather than preventative efforts, creates greater racial disparities. Create an argument either supporting or negating this statement.

Source: Press Office, "Report: Increase in spending on corrections far outpace education", U.S. Department of Education, (2016). Accessed on March 17, 2017 from https://www.ed.gov/news/press-releases /report-increases-spending-corrections-far-outpace-education.

How substance abuse treatment is funded reflects society's view of the cause of substance abuse. Should tax dollars be used to treat people who could have prevented their substance abuse by not starting to use the substance? On the other hand, if substance abuse is the result of heredity, people have no control over their abuse of a substance. As mentioned earlier, public opinion regarding drug offenders is changing, with most Americans favoring treatment compared to incarceration. While prevention is often thought of the best approach, only 5% of the National Drug Control budget for 2017 was allocated to prevention.[12] Though the immediate problem for many people might be the drugs themselves, most professionals believe treatment must address the underlying causes of drug abuse, which could include poverty, inadequate health care, hunger, ethnic discrimination, and an inefficient educational system.

Should drug abusers receive treatment or incarceration, and is misuse of a substance a cause or a result of their behavior? Of prison inmates who had used heroin, methadone, cocaine, PCP, or LSD, half did not use these drugs until *after* their first arrest. Treatment is much less costly than incarceration. The annual cost of treatment for one person is $4,700, while the annual cost for incarcerating that same individual is $24,000.[13] Half of all state prisoners are drug dependent, with only 10% of them receiving substance abuse treatment. Researchers estimate that if just 40% of drug-dependent prison inmates received treatment, it would save the taxpayers $12.9 billion.[14] If substance abusers are viewed as deviant, they are blamed for their drug use. On the other hand, if substance abusers are seen as ill, they are not blamed for their drug use.

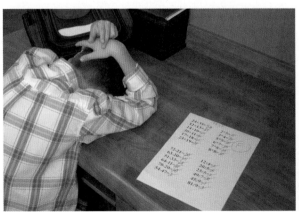

kilukilu/Shutterstock.com

▨ There is a relationship between educational achievement, incarceration, and substance use and abuse; lower educational attainment increases the risk of the latter.

Drug Courts

One avenue for helping substance abusers is through drug courts. Because there is a strong relationship between substance abuse and criminal behavior, there is a need for the criminal justice system and substance abuse treatment programs to work with each other to curtail this problem. Almost 10 years ago, a report was published by the Office of National Drug Control Policy addressing policies and programs that would reduce drug use. According to the publication *What Works: Effective Public Health Responses to Drug Use*:

> For nonviolent drug offenders whose underlying problem is substance use, drug treatment courts combine the power of the justice system with effective treatment services to break the cycle of criminal behavior, alcohol and drug use, child abuse and neglect, and incarceration.[15]

Although the first drug court was established in 1989, there are currently over 3,000 problem-solving courts in the United States.[16] The purpose of these courts is to reduce crime by offering drug treatment programs to be completed instead of prison sentences. If a treatment program is successfully completed, offenders do not have to serve time in jail. The benefits of drug courts are supported by research. Fewer people are rearrested and convicted. One study found that for every $1 invested in drug court, taxpayers save $3 in criminal justice costs.[17] A study in Washington State indicated that drug courts saved $4,767 per person in terms of reduced crime and taxpayer expenses. On average, drug courts reduce recidivism rates by 10 to 15%.[18] Other studies have found reductions in recidivism to last at least 3 years following drug court. One study even found that 75% of drug court graduates remained arrest-free for at least 2 years after leaving the program.[19] According to the US Government Accountability Office (GAO), "drug court participants who completed their program had re-arrest rates 12 to 58 percentage points below those of the comparison group."[20] One downside is that the more intensive one's criminal background, the less likely that treatment will be effective.[21] One study found participants were more likely to be terminated from drug court if they did not have a high school diploma upon entering, did not have a job or were a student, had more positive drug tests, and had a criminal history.[22] However, even among this group, drug courts have better recidivism rates compared to probation alone. Unfortunately, even with studies highlighting the benefits of drug courts, funding has been limited. One of the greatest frustrations among those who advocate for drug courts is the lack of resources including money, access to residential and outpatient treatment programs, and mental health treatment.[23]

Profile of the Drug Abuser

Most people in drug treatment are males. For those who seek drug treatment services, 5% are between the ages of 12 and 17, 34% are between the ages 18 and 29, 35% are between the ages 30 and 44, and 26% are over the age of 45.[24] Of those who enter treatment, 62% are White, 18% are Black, and 13% are Hispanic, with the rest having other racial/ethnic identity.[25] Almost 40% of those in treatment are unemployed and almost 30% of those aged 18 and over had not completed high school or attained a General Education Development. A substantial portion of drug-abusing patients have mental health problems, especially depression, psychotic and mood disorders, and antisocial personality disorders. Almost 42% of those with a substance abuse disorder also suffer from a mental illness.[26] Moreover, as many as 30 to 40% of the homeless population consists of substance abusers.

Most people in treatment use more than one drug.[27] Polydrug use seems to be dictated by drug availability rather than by a desire for the effects from a particular drug. To be drug-dependent does not mean necessarily that a person uses drugs daily. To support their behavior, drug abusers often resort to selling drugs, theft, and prostitution. People in treatment are more likely to be unemployed and to have a low family income, and are less likely to be college graduates. Table 15.1 shows admission rates to drug treatment based on employment status and education.

History of Treatment

Using drugs to treat drug abuse was common in early treatment programs. To help abusers overcome their dependency on opiates, Freud experimented with cocaine as a substitute. Opium was also used to treat alcohol problems. When drug abuse treatment was initiated in the United States, therapy focused primarily on addiction to opiates. Until the Harrison Act of 1914, treatment was administered by private doctors who addressed opiate addiction as a medical problem.

The US Public Health Service established two hospitals to serve the growing number of addicts in federal prisons. The first hospital was opened in Lexington, Kentucky, in 1935 and the second in Fort Worth, Texas, in 1938. Besides treating drug addicts

TABLE 15.1 Admissions to Treatment by Primary Substance of Abuse, According to Employment Status (Ages 16 and Over) and Education (Ages 18 and Over): TEDS 2014

Employment status and detailed not in labor force	All Admissions aged 16+	Alcohol Only	Alcohol With Secondary Drug	Heroin	Other Opiates	Smoked Cocaine	Other Route	Marijuana/ Hashish	Methamphetamine/ Amphetamines	Tranquilizers	Sedatives	Hallucinogens	PCP	Inhalants	Other/None Specified
Total admissions aged 16 and older	1,584,465	326,407	255,326	357,123	132,110	57,466	29,921	223,632	142,952	14,990	2,800	1,792	4,905	737	34,304
Employment status															
Employed	23.9	35.3	25.2	15.0	24.1	11.5	24.3	27.4	18.4	16.1	15.2	18.7	17.3	20.8	24.5
Full time	16.1	26.6	17.1	9.3	16.0	7.0	16.7	16.3	11.3	10.1	10.2	10.5	10.2	12.9	16.3
Part time	7.8	8.7	8.1	5.6	8.0	4.5	7.6	11.1	7.1	6.0	5.0	8.2	7.1	7.9	8.3
Unemployed	39.2	34.7	37.2	42.5	44.7	38.3	38.2	36.0	45.3	39.4	31.4	40.5	46.1	39.7	38.4
Not in labor force (see detail below)	36.9	30.0	37.6	42.5	31.3	50.2	37.5	36.7	36.3	44.5	53.4	40.8	36.6	39.5	37.1
Total	100.0	100.0	100.0	100.0	100.0	100.0	100.0	100.0	100.0	100.0	100.0	100.0	100.0	100.0	100.0
No. of admissions	1,561,385	323,069	253,489	353,597	130,801	57,059	29,657	222,219	142,287	14,829	2,771	1,764	4,835	731	24,277
Detailed not in labor force[1]															
Total admissions aged 16 and older and not in labor force	576,264	96,771	95,349	150,406	40,905	28,667	11,127	81,546	51,635	6,593	1,480	720	1,769	289	9,007
Disabled/Retired	24.9	30.2	32.0	16.9	30.4	26.2	26.2	16.3	25.5	24.0	22.7	17.9	16.1	25.0	31.1
Student	9.0	4.8	5.4	2.3	4.7	1.3	3.5	37.9	6.1	5.8	4.5	21.9	2.9	13.5	15.6
Inmate of institution	6.0	4.0	5.2	5.1	5.8	5.7	9.0	7.2	16.0	3.5	3.8	14.9	17.1	11.5	7.7
Homemaker	3.1	3.7	2.2	1.3	8.1	1.8	2.6	3.2	6.1	4.4	4.4	1.2	2.4	1.9	6.2
Retired	3.1	9.4	2.5	1.5	2.1	1.8	2.0	0.7	0.6	2.5	44.0	0.5	1.6	1.2	3.1
Other	53.8	47.9	52.7	72.8	48.8	53.4	56.7	34.7	45.6	59.8	20.6	43.7	59.9	46.9	36.3
Total	100.0	100.0	100.0	100.0	100.0	100.0	100.0	100.0	100.0	100.0	100.0	100.0	100.0	100.0	100.0
No. of admissions	478,352	85,549	84,854	127,074	35,129	24,349	10,358	68,170	24,310	6,225	1,327	659	1,540	260	8,548

[1]*Detailed not in labor force* is a Supplemental Data Set item. Individual Supplemental Data Set items are reported at each state's option.

Notes: Based on administrative data reported to TEDS by all reporting states and jurisdictions. Percentages are based on all admissions with known and valid values. Admissions for which values were not collected, unknown, or missing are excluded from the percentage base (denominator).

Source: Center for Behavioral Health statistics and Quality, Substance Abuse and Mental Health Services Administration, Treatment Episode Data Set (TEDS). Data received through 02.01.16.

who were prisoners, the hospitals treated voluntary patients. The goals of treatment were to gradually withdraw opiates from the addict, offer a drug-free environment, and provide psychotherapy. Originally, the recommended length of stay was 6 months, but later it was reduced to 4 months.

This treatment was considered ineffective. The **relapse** rate of people released in the 1940s through the early 1960s ranged between 87% and 96%.[28] Relapse usually occurred within 6 to 12 months after patients left treatment. Based on the high relapse rate of opiate addicts, this addiction was thought to be incurable; however, the high relapse rate occurred among patients who left the hospitals before completing treatment.

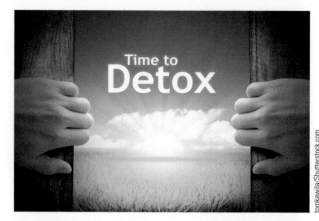

Detoxification from drugs is the first step in a treatment program.

Current Treatment Options

In the 1960s, drug abuse treatment services expanded greatly. One type of program was the therapeutic community, a residential facility staffed by former drug addicts. The emphasis in these communities is on restructuring the addict's personality and maintaining an abstinent lifestyle.

Methadone maintenance programs, initiated in the 1960s, are outpatient programs in which opiate addicts receive methadone daily. Methadone eliminates the withdrawal symptoms from opiates and prevents addicts from getting high. Before entering treatment, addicts go through **detoxification**, a medically supervised program to withdraw gradually from the drugs on which they are physically dependent. This can be done in either an inpatient or outpatient setting.

In essence, detoxification allows the body to adjust to the absence of drugs. According to the Center for Substance Abuse Treatment, three immediate goals of detoxification are:

1. To provide safe withdrawal from drugs
2. To provide withdrawal that is humane and protects the person's dignity
3. To prepare the person for ongoing treatment

Methadone, naltrexone, or buprenorphine is used in lieu of heroin to enable the addict to function normally, not just to alleviate withdrawal symptoms. Moreover, treatment programs address psychological and behavioral factors that contributed to drug addiction in the first place. Drug abusers can be treated in short-term or long-term residential facilities. Long-term residential programs are geared to individuals with severe dependency problems. Furthermore, there are outpatient treatment programs,

individualized counseling, and group counseling programs. These will be highlighted in the following sections.

Successful treatment programs approach drug treatment from a comprehensive view; not just focusing on the behavior, but also the reasons behind the drug abuse. See Figure 15.1 regarding a comprehensive approach to substance abuse treatment. The best programs include a combination of therapies and other services to meet the needs of the patient, considering individual characteristics (gender, race, ethnic background, parenting, housing, etc.) that has contributed to the drug-dependence behavior.[29] In July 2016, President Obama signed into law the Comprehensive Addiction and Recovery Act (CARA) to combat opioid drug abuse. This law favors the comprehensive view for drug treatment, specifically in the areas of prevention, treatment, recovery, law enforcement, criminal justice reform, and overdose reversal.[30]

Sometimes, drugs other than methadone are used to help an addict who is in withdrawal, because abuse of multiple drugs has become the norm. Drugs such as methadone will not help an opiate addict who also abuses cocaine or alcohol. Determining which drug or drugs to use in treatment is difficult because of these variables. Self-help programs are growing in popularity. These programs are based on the principles of Alcoholics Anonymous. These will be discussed later in the chapter.

Substance abuse dependence is a chronic disease, to which there are no quick fixes or treatment options. Like chronic diseases, addiction is heritable (runs in families), influenced by environmental conditions and behavior, and responds differently to different treatment options. Like a disease, relapse may occur even in the best situations. See Figure 15.2 for relapse rates for addiction and other chronic diseases.

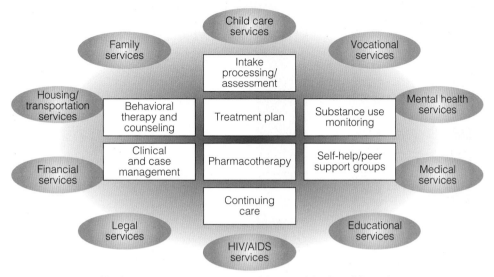

Components of Comprehensive Drug Abuse Treatment

The best treatment programs provide a combination of therapies and other services to meet the needs of the individual patient.

Figure 15.1 Components of a Comprehensive Drug Treatment Program

Source: National Institute on Drug Abuse, "Components of comprehensive drug abuse treatment". Accessed on March 19, 2017 from https://www.drugabuse.gov/publications/principles-drug-addiction-treatment-research-based-guide-third-edition/frequently-sked-questions/what-drug-addiction-treatment.

SUMMARY OF CARA

- Expand prevention and educational efforts—particularly aimed at teens, parents and other caretakers, and aging populations—to prevent the abuse of methamphetamines, opioids and heroin, and to promote treatment and recovery.

- Expand the availability of naloxone to law enforcement agencies and other first responders to help in the reversal of overdoses to save lives.

- Expand resources to identify and treat incarcerated individuals suffering from addiction disorders promptly by collaborating with criminal justice stakeholders and by providing evidence-based treatment.

- Expand disposal sites for unwanted prescription medications to keep them out of the hands of our children and adolescents.

- Launch an evidence-based opioid and heroin treatment and intervention program to expand best practices throughout the country.

- Launch a medication assisted treatment and intervention demonstration program.

- Strengthen prescription drug monitoring programs to help states monitor and track prescription drug diversion and to help at-risk individuals access services.

Source: CADCA, "Policy priorities". Accessed on March 19, 2017 from http://www.cadca.org/comprehensive-addiction-and-recovery-act-cara.

Treatment Programs

The range of treatment programs available complicates the decision as to which treatment program to choose. Treatment programs have different philosophies and practices and different degrees of effectiveness. Because effectiveness means different things to different people, assessing the effectiveness of a treatment program is not easy. To some, effectiveness means

relapse Failure to maintain a course of action, such as returning to drug abuse after initiating a treatment program

methadone maintenance program A type of therapy used in the treatment of heroin addiction

detoxification Eliminating drugs from the body; usually the initial step in treatment of alcohol and other drugs

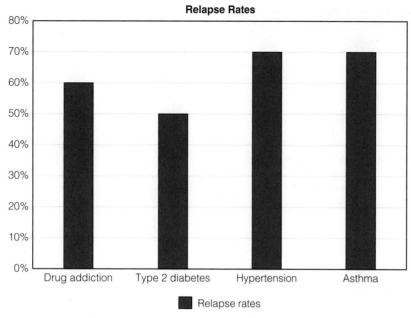

Figure 15.2 Relapse Rates for Addiction and Diseases

Source: National Institute on Drug Abuse, "Addiction is a chronic disease". Accessed on March 23, 2017 from https://archives.drugabuse.gov/about/welcome/aboutdrugabuse /chronicdisease/.

PRINCIPLES OF AN EFFECTIVE TREATMENT PROGRAM

The following principles were identified by the *National Institute on Drug Abuse,* as guidelines to look for in a treatment program:

- People need to have quick access to treatment
- Staying in treatment long enough is critical
- Medications are often an important part of treatment
- Treatment plans must be reviewed often and modified to fit the patient's changing needs
- Treatment should address other mental disorders
- Medically assisted detoxification is only the first state of treatment
- Drug use during treatment must be monitored

Source: National Institute on Drug Abuse, "Treatment approaches for drug addiction", (Updated July 2016). Accessed on March 20, 2017 from https://www.drugabuse.gov/publications/drugfacts /treatment-approaches-drug-addiction.

a reduction in criminal activity or drug use. To others, nothing less than total abstinence from crime or drug use indicates effectiveness. Some require abstinence for a period of 1, 2, or 5 years to denote success. People seeking treatment often have different goals as well. In a large-scale English study, participants were asked of their goals for treatment; responses included: 71% wanted to stop using drugs altogether, 47% wanted to "sort out life," 20% wanted to "improve health," 19% wanted to "improve employment changes," and 16% wanted to "improve relationships."[31] Among this sample, only 7% believed their treatment goals would be met during their first round of treatment.

Some people go into **spontaneous remission**. They stop taking drugs without undergoing any kind of formal treatment. Some research shows most people are able to modify their behavior without any formal treatment.[32] However, success will vary depending on the nature of dependence and the severity of the disease. For example, while binge and problematic drinking tend to rise for young adults in college, these behaviors tend to reduce when they enter the workforce. In a study of 841 drug abusers spanning 25 years, it was found that spontaneous remission was the rule and not the exception.[33] However, as one author points out, most people do not spontaneously overcome addiction; instead, people actively engage in changing their behavior.[34]

TABLE 15.2 Costs and Success Rates for Treatment Programs

	Average Length of Stay (Days)	Economic Price per Treatment Episode	Success Rates
Long-term residential	71	$3,100	51% complete treatment 21% remain sober after five years
Short-term residential	31	$3,200	73% complete the program 21% remain sober after five years
Detox		$2,200	33% complete treatment 17% remain sober after 5 years
Outpatient drug-free	164	$1,200	43% complete treatment 18% remain sober after five years

Source: L. Lazzara, "Does drug rehab work? See success rates and statistics", *The Recovery Village*, (October 6, 2016). Accessed on March 19, 2017 from https://www.therecoveryvillage.com/recovery-blog/drug-rehab-success-rates/.

The forms of treatment discussed here include inpatient treatment, methadone maintenance, outpatient treatment, and self-help groups. Alcohol treatment programs are discussed separately.

Inpatient Treatment

Typically, **inpatient treatment**, or residential treatment programs, are hospital based or are in a licensed treatment facility.[35] These types can be short term or long term. Inpatient treatment programs offer 24-hour structured and intensive care, safe housing, and medical attention. Because this form of treatment is based on a hospital model, it is expensive. Only 10 to 11% of substance abusers are treated on an inpatient basis.[36] The number of inpatient treatment programs grew because of financial support from insurance companies and businesses, which now are reexamining their position on financing inpatient treatment. Inpatient treatment has been found to be no more effective than intensive outpatient treatment. Many inpatient treatment centers quote high success rates, however, it is unknown how these centers define success. Is it program completion? Remaining drug free after the program? Many fail to follow up on the success rates of patients after they have left treatment. One article states that even a 30% success rate may be overarching.[37] Therefore, the financial concerns of businesses and insurance companies might be justified as the goal of treatment programs should emphasize sustained recovery, not just immediate sobriety during the duration of stay.

Generally, inpatient treatment programs tend to be highly structured, and patients are expected to abide by regimented schedules and rules of conduct. On admission, patients are asked about their drug-taking history and are given tests to evaluate their physical and psychological status. Group therapy and drug education are stressed in many inpatient programs. Table 15.2 shows the average length of stay in various treatment programs, cost for treatment, and their respective short- and long-term success rates. Inpatient treatment programs can fall into one of the following categories:[38]

- Therapeutic communities: Highly structured. Patients remain at residence between 6 and 12 months. The entire community is involved in the helping those in recovery. Initially, these programs were run by peers in recovery, but in recent years have incorporated professional staff and medical staff onsite.[39] However, more than half of staff are in recovery themselves.
- Shorter-term residential: These programs typically focus on detoxification and provide some initial intensive counselling. It is recommended that patients should continue counseling and therapy after the initial program.
- Recovery housing: Provides short-term housing for patients following initial treatment in an inpatient treatment program. The purpose of recovery housing is to help people make the transition to an independent, drug-free life.

Outpatient Treatment

The most common form of community drug abuse treatment is **outpatient treatment**. Outpatient programs are popular because they are readily available,

spontaneous remission Cessation of drug abuse without any type of formal treatment inpatient

inpatient treatment A residential drug treatment program based on a hospital model

outpatient treatment A nonresidential drug treatment program; least expensive form of treatment

THERAPEUTIC COMMUNITIES

Therapeutic communities (TCs) focus on the whole person and lifestyle changes, not just on drug abstinence. Recovery is a gradual and long-process and relapses are viewed as opportunities for learning. TCs encourage participants to examine their own personal behavior to discover what led them to their addiction and help them become more prosocial, so when they leave the community, they are more adept at handling personal problems. As individuals progress through the program, they assume greater responsibilities, and the goal is for participants to either be employed or enrolled in school by the time they leave the TC.

Much of the "work" in TCs are through active participation through social learning, self-help groups; as all individual participation aids in their peers' recovery process. TCs recognize the need for ongoing support after they have completed the residential treatment program to help avoid relapses.

Participants who stay at TCs for at least 3 months show the greatest improvements, as measured by reduced drug use, reduced illegal activity, and improved employment outcomes. See figure below.

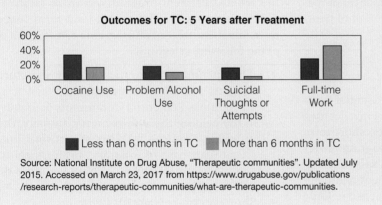

Outcomes for TC: 5 Years after Treatment

■ Less than 6 months in TC ■ More than 6 months in TC

Source: National Institute on Drug Abuse, "Therapeutic communities". Updated July 2015. Accessed on March 23, 2017 from https://www.drugabuse.gov/publications /research-reports/therapeutic-communities/what-are-therapeutic-communities.

less disruptive and stigmatizing than inpatient treatment for abusers with jobs and families, and less expensive. Treatment might involve family therapy or psychotherapy.

Outpatient treatment ranges from counseling centers to halfway houses to community centers. Many outpatient programs are identified as intensive, meaning that clients attend group therapy three times a week for 2 to 3 hours per session. Traditional outpatient programs provide social, vocational, and educational services. Outpatient therapy frequently is used after a client leaves methadone maintenance, although outpatient treatment is used in conjunction with abuse of any drug, not just narcotics. These programs use behavioral therapy in either group or individual settings.

Cognitive-Behavioral Therapy

This is a short-term, goal-oriented psychotherapy treatment. It works by changing the way people think about their problems and emotions.[40] The purpose of this type of therapy is to increase a person's coping strategies so that they can identify situations that place them at risk for relapse and plan accordingly.[41] One study, among cocaine-dependent persons, found the use of cognitive behavioral therapy, along with a methadone maintenance program, to be more effective compared to methadone maintenance alone.[42] However, improvement rates for the cognitive behavioral therapy group were only slight, with only 36% being able to achieve abstinence three or more consecutive weeks, compared to 17% for those receiving methadone alone.

Family Therapy

This is usually the first type of therapy offered to adolescents and parents who are substance abusers. It addresses not only the substance abuse issues, but includes therapy to address family conflict. This type of therapy includes the client along with a parent or cohabitating partner. The purpose of this therapy is to teach patients new skills to be used in the home

When considering incentive-based treatment programs, one would assume these would work better for those from lower socioeconomic status backgrounds, as incentives would be more meaningful for those who have less. This has not proven to be the case. One study done on cocaine-dependent individuals found contingency management treatment programs to be just as effective for those with higher socioeconomic statuses as those with lower socioeconomic statuses.[1] Income was not associated with any change in effectiveness of a contingency management treatment program.

However, the same is not true regarding race. In another study looking at cocaine-dependent persons, race was a factor for success related to contingency management programs. This study looked at success rates for Whites and African-Americans after completing a contingency management program and found rates to be higher among White participants.[2] This was especially true for those individuals who entered treatment with a cocaine-positive urine sample. Among those who entered treatment abstinent from drugs, success rates were about the same.

Sources:

1.   R. Secades-Villa, G. Garcia-Fernandez, E. Pena-Suarez, O. Garcia-Rodriquez, E. Sanchez-Hervas, and J.R. Fernandez-Hermida, "Contingency management is effective across cocaine-dependent individuals with different socioeconomic status", *Journal of Substance Abuse Treatment*, 44, no. 3 (2013): 349–354.

2.   L. Montgomery, K.M. Carroll, and N.M. Petry, "Initial abstinence status and contingency management treatment outcomes: Does race matter", *Journal of Consulting and Clinical Psychology*, 83, no. 3 (2015): 473–481.

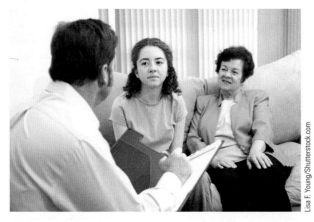

Lisa F. Young/Shutterstock.com

▨ Family therapy has been shown to be one of the most effective forms of therapy for treatment substance abuse.

environment with the goal of reducing the substance use behavior.[43] In a large European study, family therapy was shown to be effective for the reduction of cannabis use by adolescents.[44]

Motivational Enhancement Therapy (MET)

This type of therapy involves changing internal motivations for drug use and uses motivational interviewing to build a plan for change. The five elements of MET include developing and expressing empathy, acknowledging the disparity between thoughts and reality, avoiding arguments, accepting resistance as a part of the process, and supporting a recovering addict's self-efficacy.[45] MET is more effective in helping patients seek out drug treatment options. It is less effective for treatment of substance abuse disorders.[46] Thus it is a good place to start when thinking about treatment for substance abuse.

Contingency Management

This process involves giving patients rewards to reinforce positive behaviors. Sometimes known as incentive-based interventions, this type of therapy may offer vouchers or prizes for remaining drug-free.[47] Among homeless persons with substance abuse problems, transitional housing is offered if they are able to provide a drug-free specimen. Thus, if they are able to produce a urine sample free of drugs, they are able to obtain housing. A study comparing incentive-based housing found a higher number of drug-negative samples compared to homeless people who did not receive a housing initiative.[48]

Evaluations of outpatient programs reveal limited effectiveness. In a literature review conducted on substance-abusing pregnant women enrolled in outpatient clinics, there were few differences in maternal

therapeutic communities (TCs) Residential drug treatment centers that utilize confrontation techniques

outcomes, birth rates, or abstinence rates among the different outpatient programs.[49] Benefits of an outpatient treatment program include being able to live at home, continue working, and remain close to family and friends while engaging in treatment. One study found that clients who travel shorter distances to receive substance abuse treatment are more likely to complete the treatment.[50] Another study reported that outpatient treatment effectively reduces criminality while improving employment.[51] One problem is that clients attending outpatient treatment centers often go back to the environments that contributed to their drug abuse initially. Outpatient treatment can be more costly for the client than inpatient treatment because insurance programs pay less for outpatient care than for inpatient care.

Self-Help Groups

In recent years, the public has grown skeptical of the healthcare system, and many people are assuming responsibility for their own health needs. Consequently, self-help groups have proliferated as a grassroots response to perceived inadequacies within the healthcare system. Members of self-help groups are bound by a common denominator such as alcohol, gambling, food, shopping, or sex.

The largest self-help group is Alcoholics Anonymous (AA), which is based on a 12-step model and has been incorporated into many professionally sponsored treatment programs for alcoholism (see "Alcohol Treatment" section). This model has also been applied for other self-help groups including Narcotics Anonymous, Cocaine Anonymous, Gamblers Anonymous, Overeaters Anonymous, and Sexaholics Anonymous.

Not only do self-help groups offer fellowship and support, they are also used in lieu of traditional therapies or after a person stops other therapies. Self-help groups complement other types of treatment. They are seen as cost-effective for maintaining changes that clients undertake and for preventing relapse. Participants in self-help groups give and receive help for their problems. However, not everyone is well-suited for self-help groups. To benefit from them, clients have to be motivated.

Narcotics Anonymous

Narcotics Anonymous (NA) emanated from the AA program. The first meetings were held in Los Angeles in the early 1950s. In 1983, NA published its self-titled *Basic Text* book, contributing to tremendous growth of the organization with chapters in Australia, Brazil, Colombia, Germany, India, Ireland, Japan, New Zealand, United Kingdom, eastern Europe, and Africa.

NA is open to all drug addicts, regardless of the particular drug or combination of drugs being used. Membership is not restricted by social class, religion, economic status, race, ethnicity, nationality, or gender. Membership is free, although members often contribute small sums to help cover the expenses of meetings.

Critical to NA's success is the therapeutic value of addicts working with other addicts. Successes and challenges in overcoming active addiction and living drug-free, productive lives resulting from the principles contained within the 12 Steps and 12 Traditions of NA are shared by members. The principles of the NA recovery program include:

- admitting there is a problem;
- seeking help;
- engaging in thorough self-examination;
- confidential self-disclosure;
- making amends for harm done; and
- helping other drug addicts who want to recover.

NA emphasizes the practice of spiritual principles. NA itself is nonreligious, and each member is encouraged to cultivate an individual understanding—religious or not—of this "spiritual awakening." NA is not affiliated with other organizations, including other 12-step programs, treatment centers, or correctional facilities. NA does not employ professional counselors or therapists nor does it have residential facilities or clinics or vocational, legal, financial, psychiatric, or medical services.

NA's one mission is to provide a setting in which addicts can help one another stop using drugs and find a new way to live. NA encourages its members to abstain completely from all drugs including alcohol, although the use of psychiatric medication and other medically indicated drugs prescribed by a physician and taken under medical supervision is not seen as compromising a person's recovery in NA. Meetings are led by individual members while other members take part by sharing in turn about their experiences in recovering from drug addiction.

NA does not express positive or negative opinions on civil, social, medical, legal, or religious issues. In addition, it does not profess positions on addiction-related issues such as criminality, law enforcement, drug legalization or penalties, prostitution, HIV/HCV infection, or syringe programs.

NA membership is voluntary and no attendance records are kept. Thus, it is difficult to provide comprehensive information about its members. However, individuals who attend meetings three times a week are more likely to remain abstinent than those individuals who attend infrequently.[52] The following information was gathered from a survey completed by attendees (n=23,000) at the 2015 NA Convention held in Rio de Janeiro, Brazil:[53]

- Gender: male, 59%; female, 41%
- Age: 20 years old and under, 1%; 21–30 years old, 11%; 31–40 years old, 21%; 41–50 years old, 24%; 51–60 years old, 29%; over 60 years old, 14%
- Ethnicity: Caucasian, 74%; African American, 11%; Hispanic, 6%; other, 9%
- Employment status: employed full-time, 60%; employed part-time, 9%; unemployed, 11%; retired, 7%; homemakers, 4%; students, 4%
- Continuous abstinence/recovery: ranged from less than 1 year up to 40 years; 8.32 years on average

Perhaps the greatest achievement by NA attendance is improvement of quality of life. In the same survey mentioned above, the greatest area of improvement by attending NA meetings was in family relationships (92%) and social connections (88%).[54]

Alcohol Treatment

In the United States, it is estimated that 17.3 million people are heavy drinkers and 66.7 million engaged in binge drinking in the previous month.[54] Additionally, almost 6% of people aged 12 or older have an alcohol use disorder. Much debate surrounds the most effective treatment for alcoholics. Some cures for alcoholism, dating between 1860 and 1930, were most unusual. The Hay-Litchfield antidote promised to eliminate the desire for alcohol by creating feelings of disgust and nausea at the sight of alcohol; some ingredients included codfish, milk, eel skin, cow's urine, and alcohol. Another product was the White Star Secret Liquor Cure, which sold for 94 cents for a box of 30 capsules. The main ingredient in the capsules was *Erythroxylon coca*—cocaine. Other peculiar therapies included inducing convulsions and psychosurgery in which part of the brain was surgically removed.

Of the various modalities for treating alcohol abuse today, none rivals the popularity of AA. A key feature of AA is total abstinence, a view that is not universally accepted. Some treatment personnel advocate a **controlled drinking approach** in which the patient learns to drink in a nonabusive manner. Drug therapy in the form of **Antabuse (disulfiram)** has been used as well.

There have been a number of behavioral and medicinal advances in the treatment of alcoholism. Unfortunately, relapse remains high. People with

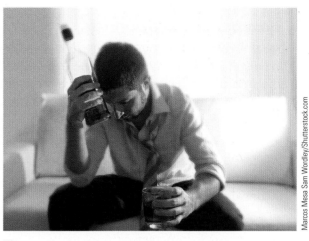

Should the goal for treating alcoholism be abstinence or moderation?

alcohol use disorder are more likely to relapse during periods of stress or when around people or places associated with past drinking.[55] In terms of long-term remission, those individuals who are most likely to succeed are female, those who initiated alcohol abuse later in life, and those who had friends who were less approving of drinking.[56] Motivation and having the support of family, therapists, self-help groups, or friends are instrumental in overcoming alcohol abuse regardless of treatment.[57]

Alcoholics Anonymous

During Prohibition, many facilities were available to help alcoholics. After Prohibition, however, these facilities closed, except for those that treated wealthy individuals. The absence of treatment for alcoholics set the stage for AA. Started in 1935 by an alcoholic surgeon (Dr. Bob) and an alcoholic stockbroker (Bill W.) helping each other achieve sobriety, AA is the oldest self-help group. At its inception, AA was not a formal treatment program.

The only requirement for membership in AA is the desire to stop drinking. AA's goals are sobriety and spiritual renewal. AA groups have been established in more than 100 countries.

AA membership consists of about twice as many males as females, although there is less disparity

---

controlled drinking approach Alcohol treatment based on behavior modification, in which the person learns to drink in a nonabusive manner

Antabuse (disulfiram) A drug that interferes with the metabolization of alcohol, making the drinker violently ill

SIGNS OF AN ALCOHOL PROBLEM

Alcohol use disorder is a medical condition when a person's alcohol use is causing harm to one or more areas in their life. If a person answers "yes" to two or more of the following questions, it may indicate problematic drinking.

- Had times when you ended up drinking **more, or longer** than you intended?

- More than once wanted to **cut down or stop drinking**, or tried to, but couldn't?

- Spent a **lot of time** drinking? Or being sick or getting over the aftereffects?

- Experienced **craving** — a strong need, or urge, to drink?

- Found that drinking — or being sick from drinking — often **interfered with taking care** of your **home** or **family**? Or caused **job** troubles? Or **school** problems?

- Continued to drink even though it was causing **trouble** with your **family** or **friends**?

- **Given up** or **cut back** on **activities** that were important or interesting to you, or gave you pleasure, in order to drink?

- More than once gotten into situations while or after drinking that **increased your chances of getting hurt** (such as driving, swimming, using machinery, walking in a dangerous area, or having unsafe sex)?

- Continued to drink even though it was making you feel **depressed or anxious** or adding to **another health problem**? Or after having had a **memory blackout**?

- Had to **drink much more** than you once did to **get the effect** you want? Or found that your **usual number** of drinks had **much less effect** than before?

- Found that when the effects of alcohol were wearing off, you **had withdrawal symptoms**, such as trouble sleeping, shakiness, irritability, anxiety, depression, restlessness, nausea, or sweating? Or sensed things that were not there?

Source: National Institute on Alcohol Abuse and Alcoholism, "Treatment for alcohol problems: Finding and getting help", (2014). Accessed on March 23, 2017 from https://pubs.niaaa.nih.gov/publications/treatment/treatment.htm.

ON CAMPUS

It is estimated that 65% of college students drink alcohol, with a large percentage drinking alcohol to excess. In addition, 40% of college students report getting drunk in a given month. Risk factors for college student alcohol consumption include being Caucasian, male, members of a Greek organization, athletes, students coping with psychological distresses, and on campuses with a high density of alcohol outlets.

Consequences for students who drink to intoxication include increase risk of injury, traffic crashes, being taking advantage of sexually, and injuring others. These risks are higher for those who drink to "get drunk." Academically, students who consume alcohol report more missed classes, falling behind in class, doing poorly on exams or papers, and receiving lower grades.

Source: A. White, and R. Hingson, "The burden of alcohol use: Excessive alcohol consumption and related consequences among college students", *Alcohol Research*, 35, no. 2 (2014): 201–218.

among younger members. AA employs no professional counselors, but some members emerge as leaders. AA is based on the premise that alcoholism is a disease over which the person has no control. Clients often participate in AA after having been discharged from other treatment programs. Additional groups, such as Alanon and Alateen, were derived from AA. Alanon is geared toward helping friends and others

12 STEPS OF ALCOHOLICS ANONYMOUS

1. We admitted we were powerless over alcohol—that our lives had become unmanageable.

2. Came to believe that a Power greater than ourselves could restore us to sanity.

3. Made a decision to turn our will and our lives over to the care of God as we understood Him.

4. Made a searching and fearless moral inventory of ourselves.

5. Admitted to God, to ourselves, and to another human being the exact nature of our wrongs.

6. Were entirely ready to have God remove all these defects of character.

7. Humbly asked Him to remove our shortcomings.

8. Made a list of all persons we had harmed, and became willing to make amends to them all.

9. Made direct amends to such people wherever possible, except when to do so would injure them or others.

10. Continued to take personal inventory and when we were wrong promptly admitted it.

11. Sought through prayer and meditation to improve our conscious contact with God as we understood Him, praying only for knowledge of His will for us and the power to carry that out.

12. Having had a spiritual awakening as the result of these steps, we tried to carry this message to alcoholics and to practice these principles in all our affairs.

The Twelve Steps are reprinted with permission of Alcoholics Anonymous World Services, Inc. ("AAWS") Permission to reprint the Twelve Steps does not mean that AAWS has reviewed or approved the contents of this publication, or that AAWS necessarily agrees with the views expressed herein. A is a program of recovery from alcoholism only—use of the Twelve Steps in connection with programs and activities which are patterned after A, but which address other problems, or in any other non-A context, does not imply otherwise.

close to the alcoholic, and Alateen assists teenage children of alcoholics.

Central to the mission of AA is its 12 steps. Among these, the person must admit to having no control over alcohol. The person is seen as powerless over alcohol and cannot overcome alcoholism until coming to this realization. Religious conviction is important. No specific religion is promoted, but the member has to believe in a higher power for help in surmounting personal shortcomings and achieving recovery.

AA promotes character traits including honesty, humility, and patience. Two other features of the 12 steps are self-examination leading to behavior change in the way members treat themselves and others. AA considers alcoholism a disease but takes a nonmedical approach regarding its treatment.

AA meetings might be open or closed. Open meetings allow partners, friends, and other interested people to attend. Closed meetings are restricted to members. During meetings, members recount their own histories of alcohol abuse, enabling others to identify with them. In this way, new members benefit from others' experiences.

Meetings provide opportunities for members to develop alcohol-free social relationships. Learning to socialize without alcohol is part of the recovery process. Also, members learn to rely on people rather than on alcohol. The social support AA members receive improves the likelihood of remaining abstinent especially when coupled with outside therapy.[58] Sponsorship is another vital component. This involves a relationship between a member who has been sober for some time and one who has not been sober as long. During times when maintaining sobriety is difficult, members can turn to their sponsors for help. The sponsor program is therapeutic for the person assuming the role of sponsor *and* for the person being sponsored. Either person can terminate the relationship.

Determining the effectiveness of AA is difficult because of the standard of anonymity for its members. Results from a 2014 membership survey state the following of its members:[59]

- 62% male
- 38% female
- 89% White
- 3% Hispanic
- 4% Black
- 1% Native American
- 1% Asian
- 1% Other

In addition, the average age of members is 50, with members attending on average 2.5 meetings a week. Of those who attend meetings, 27% remain sober less than 1 year, 24% remain sober between 1 and 5 years, 13% remain sober between 5 and 10 years, 14% remain sober between 11 and 20 years, and 22% remain sober over 20 years.[60] While difficult to gather data for those who drop out of AA, it is generally accepted that drop-out rates are high.[61] One study suggests AA may work better for those who attribute spiritual gains achieved by AA, which are also related to better outcomes.[62] However, in another study, there was no association between higher levels of spirituality and levels of sobriety.[63] Despite the obstacles in evaluating AA, research has shown that increased attendance for AA is related to short- and long-term decreases in alcohol consumption.[64] Another study found that 8 years after beginning treatment, 49% of those who had attended AA were abstinent, compared to 46% who received formal treatment. Those who attended AA in combination with formal treatment had the highest abstinence rates.[65]

Criticisms of AA include the following:

- AA treats the underlying *symptoms* of alcoholism but not its underlying causes.
- People who become dependent on AA are substituting one dependency (AA meetings) for another (alcohol).
- AA advocates that alcoholism is a disease, a position that undermines personal responsibility for behavior.
- AA ignores environmental factors that can contribute to alcoholism, such as advertising, poverty, and racism.
- AA is rigid in its beliefs.

Because AA strongly emphasizes belief in a higher power, it does not meet the needs of people who are not religious. Youth who do not engage in religious practices do not achieve very good outcomes in its 12-step program.[66] The New York State Court of Appeals ruled that prisoners cannot be required to participate in AA because of its religious orientation. Two self-help groups for alcoholics that do not refer to God or a higher power are Secular Organizations for Sobriety (SOS) and Rational Recovery (RR). SOS does not practice anonymity of its members. RR maintains that alcoholism is not a disease but, rather, a behavioral disorder that can be overcome by rational thinking. SOS and RR both believe that alcoholics should credit themselves if they abstain. They emphasize that sobriety is a matter of accepting personal responsibility, and they promote self-reliance and self-confidence in their members.

Moderate Drinking

For many alcoholics, abstinence is the only viable treatment. For others, the idea of lifetime sobriety dissuades them from stopping their abuse. A controlled drinking approach might be more suitable for them. Also called reduced-risk drinking, this approach encourages drinkers to cope with peer pressure and situations that tempt them to drink excessively.[67] The controlled drinking model is based on behavior modification. Controlled drinking is more viable if the drinker has a stable job and marriage and *no* family history of alcoholism. The longer a person has been an alcoholic, the less likely it is that he or she can return to social drinking.

One advantage of programs emphasizing controlled drinking is that more people with severe drinking problems are likely to seek help from them to reduce their alcohol use. One dilemma is determining what is "moderate." Moreover, many alcoholics justify their continued drinking by labeling it as "controlled drinking."

The controlled drinking model is contrary to the disease model. The phrase "one drink is too much and a thousand is not enough" typifies the idea that alcoholism is a disease and argues against the controlled drinking approach. The controlled drinking model also has its critics. Can alcoholics realistically learn to drink moderately? Can cigarette smokers be satisfied with two or three cigarettes a day? Furthermore, what criteria determine who can drink moderately?

For people with a liver disease, a controlled drinking approach is not recommended. Likewise, people who lack self-control and decision-making skills are not good candidates. Moreover, the greater one's alcohol dependence, the less likely one can adopt a moderate approach to drinking.[68] AA rejects the controlled drinking approach. If a person can learn to consume alcohol moderately, claims AA, he or she was not an alcoholic in the first place. Despite AA's reservations, moderate drinking programs have been adopted in Europe, Britain, Australia, and Canada. In a survey of alcohol specialists in France, almost one-half identified controlled drinking as a goal.[69]

Moderation Management (MM) was started for problem drinkers. Like other controlled drinking models, MM is based on behavioral self-management. It offers a supportive environment for those who want to come together to reduce their alcohol use and change their lifestyle. MM views alcohol abuse as a learned behavior and does not classify alcohol abuse as a disease. MM offers a "Alcohol Dependence Questionnaire" on their website to help score the severity of a person's drinking problem. For scores 20 or above, abstinence is recommended. MM works best among those who have a less severe alcohol problem. Moderation-oriented programs are common in many countries including Great Britain, Sweden, Denmark, Germany, Australia, and New Zealand.

It has been shown that many people who do not seek alcohol treatment may gravitate to a moderation model. Many of these same people eventually change their goal to abstinence.[70] Not all research supports a moderate drinking approach. One study found that a moderate drinking approach was effective initially but that it was ineffective 3 years later.[71]

Reduced-risk drinking may be most effective for those who consider themselves problem drinkers. Among problem drinkers, reduced-risk drinking and abstinence are equally effective, and success rates for either program are greater when patients can choose their treatment goals.[72]

Medications

Disulfiram (Antabuse)

Disulfiram, better known as Antabuse, is a medication that acts as an aversive agent by interacting with alcohol in such a way that the drinker becomes violently ill. It helps drinkers who do not think they can control their impulsive use of alcohol. Disulfiram interferes with the metabolism of alcohol and increases the level of acetaldehyde in the blood. Adverse reactions from disulfiram include drowsiness, fatigue, nausea, vomiting, decreased libido, anxiety, depression, a metallic taste, and headache.[73] Because of its adverse side effects and its questionable effectiveness, disulfiram is not the first pharmacological choice for treating alcoholism.[74] Generally, it is best for those with high medication compliance or when medication intake is supervised.[75]

The severity of effects of Antabuse depends on the amount of alcohol consumed. Both alcohol and disulfiram have to be present simultaneously in the body for the effects to occur. One limitation is the necessity of getting alcoholics to take the drugs. Another problem is that some alcoholics continue to drink despite disulfiram's noxious effects. Despite disulfiram's adverse effects, individuals who take disulfiram remain abstinent longer than those given placebos.[76]

Naltrexone

Naltrexone was approved by the US Food and Drug Administration (FDA) in 1994 to treat alcoholism although it is used primarily to block the effects of opiates.[77] A number of studies have found it to be beneficial for treating alcohol dependence. The FDA approved naltrexone as a treatment adjunct to reduce the risk of relapse. It does not seem to prevent alcoholics from taking just one drink, but alcoholics are less likely to binge drink while they are taking it.

Naltrexone may be most helpful after detoxification. A number of alcoholics relapse, but naltrexone reduces that number. One study looked at the effectiveness of naltrexone among young adults and found no significant differences in percent of drinking days among the ones treated with naltrexone and the placebo group.[77] However, this study did show a reduction in drinks per day among the participants who were taking naltrexone. Oral naltrexone has a modest effect on preventing relapse over three months for heavy drinking.[78]

Extended-release naltrexone has been shown to reduce alcohol use among heavy drinkers, although it has not been shown to result in abstinence.[79] Compared to a placebo, naltrexone reduced the risk of returning to heavy drinking by 17%.[80] There may be some moderators that increase the effectiveness of naltroxene including family history of alcohol problems and the Asn40Asp polymorphisms (opioid receptor gene); however, more research is needed to determine the impact of these on treatment.[81] One study found women experienced fewer cravings for alcohol compared to men on naltrexone.[82]

Besides reducing the craving for alcohol, naltrexone is a safe drug that many alcoholics find acceptable. Its side effects, which last 1 to 2 weeks, include agitation, anxiety, nausea, light-headedness, sweating, and dysphoria. In addition to its use with alcoholics, naltrexone has been tested with smokers wanting to quit. One study found naltrexone increased 12-week smoking abstinence rates and decreased smoking urge and alcohol use among heavy drinking smokers.[83] Interestingly, these decreased rates were not seen among moderate to light nondrinking smokers. Naltrexone may also helpful for those with opioid use disorder, gambling disorder, and kleptomania.[84]

Acamprosate

A third type of pharmacological drug approved by the FDA for treating alcoholism is acamprosate. Approved in 2004, this drug inhibits the craving for alcohol and food. It has been found that acamprosate helps to maintain abstinence; more so if the patient went through detoxification before medication was administered.[85] The precise mechanism by which acamprosate works is unclear; some believe it works by interacting with glutamate receptors, while others maintain its effectiveness can be attributed to calcium.[86] The drug is effective for both males and females.[87] Because acamprosate is absorbed poorly when taken orally, it is desirable that the drug be administered several times daily. Also, the drug is excreted primarily through the kidneys. Thus, it should not be used with patients who have kidney problems. Acamprosate has not been shown to be effective in treating cocaine dependence, pathological gambling, or binge-eating.[88]

Methadone Maintenance

A program of giving methadone to heroin addicts started in New York City in the early 1960s. Federal guidelines define a methadone maintenance program as any form of treatment that involves the dispensing of methadone for opiate addiction for more than 30 days. Methadone is a synthetic drug that eliminates withdrawal symptoms from opiates and prevents an opiate addict from experiencing euphoria. It is given orally and is effective for 24 hours.

Methadone is effective only for heroin and not other drugs to which a person might be addicted. To be admitted into a methadone maintenance program, addicts must have been dependent for at least 1 year. An estimated 250,000 heroin addicts are enrolled in methadone maintenance programs.[89]

Patients come for the dose of methadone daily, although many clients administer the methadone to themselves at home. The demand for methadone maintenance is high, with waiting lists up to 1 year. This is unfortunate, as heroin addicts are at high risk for mortality while waiting for treatment.[90] Many clinics offer medical, psychiatric, and vocational services. These services vary considerably from one clinic to another.

Psychotherapy in conjunction with methadone yields the best results. Having a case worker interact with a patient is more effective than merely having the patient take methadone.[91] Success rates are higher when patients come daily for methadone, as opposed to two to three times per week. Deep brain stimulation, a process in which a medical device delivers electrical impulses to parts of the brain, also has shown to be effective when used with methadone.[92] When patients attend methadone clinics, personnel counsel them about AIDS and the risks of needle-sharing. A growing problem is the number of patients with the hepatitis C virus (HCV), which, like HIV, is blood-borne. Attending methadone maintenance has been shown to reduce the risk of HCV infection and is dose related.[93]

In the United States, the average cost to support a patient taking methadone for 1 full year is almost $5,000.[94] Unfortunately, not all health insurance companies cover methadone maintenance. For those on Medicaid, one study found that 17 states do not cover methadone maintenance, thus limiting access to treatment.[95] It is cost-effective to treat opiate abusers prior to release from incarceration because those who receive methadone while incarcerated are more likely to seek treatment upon release and less likely to return to drug abuse.[96]

Methadone maintenance has been shown to:[97]

- Reduce use of illicit drugs
- Reduce criminal activity
- Reduce needle sharing behavior
- Reduce HIV infection rates
- Reduce commercial sex work
- Improvements in social health and productivity
- Improvement in health conditions
- Retention in addiction treatment
- Reduction in suicide
- Reduction in lethal overdose

The success of methadone maintenance is noteworthy because people in these programs have a history of substance abuse that is longer and more serious than is found in patients who enter outpatient centers or inpatient therapeutic communities (discussed later). Despite its effectiveness, methadone is not a panacea. Patients receiving methadone often lack emotional response.[98] A review of 15 different studies found that methadone maintenance had no effect on alcohol use.[99]

Methadone treatment does not eliminate poverty, psychological problems, homelessness, illegal drug use, or crime. One concern is whether pregnant women addicted to heroin should be placed in a methadone maintenance program. Most experts agree methadone maintenance treatment can prevent heroin withdrawal symptoms in pregnant women (which can cause the uterus to contract and bring on miscarriage or premature birth), and decrease the use of needles (which carries a high risk for infection).[100] Methadone maintenance does carry risks, which include sudden infant death syndrome, jaundice, and thrombocytosis among infants born to mothers on methadone.[101] Furthermore, infants who were born to moms who were in methadone maintenance programs will likely need treatment for methadone withdrawal. Clients are required to come for treatment daily, and critics charge that the daily routine perpetuates dependency. Clients' acceptance of methadone maintenance is widespread, and fewer people drop out of methadone maintenance than other forms of treatment. Nonetheless, methadone maintenance programs have come under criticism due to reports of fatal overdoses.[102] Each year, approximately 5,000 people die from methadone overdoses.[103]

To address concerns over the daily use of methadone, an alternative drug, **levo-alpha-acetylmethadol (LAAM)**, received FDA approval in 1993. Because of health concerns related to

LAAM, the FDA requires additional warnings on LAAM labels.[104] Methadone blocks the withdrawal symptoms of heroin for a day, but LAAM works for 3 days. In contrast to methadone, addicts given LAAM were more likely to remain in treatment and less likely to get arrested.[105] Side effects of LAAM include muscle aches, difficulty breathing, impaired circulation, dizziness, vomiting, sweating, and diarrhea. Due to side effects, its use has been discontinued in Europe.

Other drugs that block the effects of opiates are naltrexone, naloxone, clonidine, and buprenorphine. Countries including Switzerland, Australia, Germany, and the Netherlands are experimenting with giving heroin to addicts. Until 1968, the British government allowed physicians to prescribe heroin. However, this program was abandoned because many unnecessary prescriptions were being filled, increasing the number of heroin addicts. However, heroin-assisted programs do reduce the craving for illicit heroin.[106] In a study in Switzerland in which heroin addicts were given either heroin or methadone, the addicts preferred heroin because they reported fewer side effects.[107] Another study in Germany found that addicts given heroin had improved physical and mental health while in treatment.[108]

Buprenorphine is increasingly used to treat opiate dependency. The effectiveness of buprenorphine in reducing illicit opiate use appears mixed. One study found that buprenorphine was effective in reducing illicit opiate use, although its effectiveness increased as the dosage increased.[109] However, buprenorphine retains fewer participants compared to methadone when doses are flexible. This study also found methadone was superior in retaining people in treatment and suppressing illicit opioid use.[110] The drug Suboxone, which combines buprenorphine with naloxone, was used because it did not produce a high. Unfortunately, while Suboxone was effective for reducing illicit drug use, over 90% of patients in the study relapsed after stopping Suboxone use.[111] Other studies have shown that an increasing number of people are abusing or misusing buprenorphine.[112]

Some narcotic addicts say that methadone withdrawal is worse than going **cold turkey**. Several studies indicate that 70 to 80% of patients resume use of narcotics within one or two years after treatment, and between 15% and 20% continue to use cocaine intravenously. Side effects include increased perspiration, chronic constipation, sexual dysfunction, and difficulty sleeping. These effects tend to subside within the first 6 months of treatment. Concerns remain about the long-term effects of using methadone, although nothing points to any serious negative outcomes.

Treatment Issues

Funding substance abuse treatment has economic and political ramifications. Many people question the efficacy of funding treatment programs; therefore, funding is under constant public scrutiny. An important question is: What is the most effective use for the money being allocated? The treatment programs that are most cost-effective are more likely to be funded. Four pertinent issues in treating drug abuse are (1) determining whether voluntary or compulsory treatment is better, (2) matching the patients to the treatment that works best for them, (3) determining whether treatment programs designed for adults would be equally effective with adolescent substance abusers, and (4) designing programs to address the special circumstances of female addicts.

Voluntary Versus Compulsory Treatment

Many drug users enter treatment under their own volition. Others are compelled to do so; prisoners, for instance, often are required to enter treatment programs. Sometimes, a drug offender is given a choice between prison and treatment. A relevant question is whether compulsory participation is as effective as voluntary participation. Early studies of institutionalized clients in drug treatment in the Public Health Service hospitals in Lexington, KY and Fort Worth, TX showed that volunteers fared better than those required to be in treatment.[113] Other studies, however, indicate that clients who are required to receive treatment make as much progress, as measured by relapse and recidivism, as those who enter voluntarily.[114] More recent studies also show mixed results. In a systematic review on compulsory treatment versus voluntary treatment, three studies showed no outcome differences between compulsory and voluntary treatment approaches. This same study found mixed results regarding criminal recidivism.[115]

The key issue could be how long the person stays in treatment and the type of services received after initial treatment. For example, in a study on two prison cohorts who completed a drug treatment program in prison, prisoners who received aftercare, especially after being released from prison, had

levo-alpha-acetylmethadol (LAAM) An experimental drug that prevents narcotic withdrawal symptoms for about 3 days

cold turkey Elimination of a negative behavior all at once, as opposed to gradually (with or without a substitute)

significantly less likelihood of recidivism compared to the control group who received no aftercare services (44% and 15%, respectively).[116]

Matching Patients and Treatments

Because individuals have different learning styles, we can logically assume that individuals respond to different modalities for treating substance abuse. No single type of treatment applies to everyone. Many drug abusers drop out of treatment because the specific program they have attempted is poorly defined in terms of content, goals, approach, and duration. However, family therapy has been demonstrated to improve the likelihood of success for both adults and adolescents.[117]

Increasing evidence suggests that matching clients to specific treatments increases effectiveness of the treatment. For example, one study of cocaine abusers found that those with high abstract reasoning ability and low religious belief responded better to cognitive-behavioral therapy than to a 12-step approach. It has also been found that there is no significant difference in the success rate of different treatments, although "motivational interviewing," which helps patients identify reasons for change, has been found to be effective in helping those with dependency problems seek out treatment.[118]

Matching clients to treatment is not a new concept. Before one matches clients to treatment, several questions have to be addressed:

- Which treatment produces the best outcomes for a specific group or person?
- Do members of certain ethnic or socioeconomic groups respond similarly to certain types of treatment?
- Is the effectiveness of a specific program linked to age of participants?
- Do females and males differ in their responses to treatment?

Matching treatment to gender, culture, ethnicity, language, and sexual orientation improves the likelihood of positive outcomes. Patients with severe psychiatric problems and patients from lower socioeconomic backgrounds tend not to benefit from most types of treatment, especially outpatient treatment. Also, the majority of patients with co-occurring psychiatric disorders abuse more than one substance and require treatment that is able to address mental disorders along with the substance abuse disorder.[119] Individuals from supportive social and economic backgrounds and with few psychiatric problems tend to respond positively to treatment. Many professionals believe that poor matching between clients and treatment approaches accounts for poor results.

Treating Adolescent Drug Abusers

In 2014, in the United States, 5% of all substance abuse treatment admissions were between the ages 12 and 17 and the primary substance of abuse was marijuana.[120] Among adolescents admitted into treatment, the majority are male.[121] Adolescents tend to do reduce substance abuse behavior by a variety of treatment modalities; however, one study found the two most effective treatment modalities to be family therapy and mixed and group counselling.[122] Family counseling helps the adolescent and parent/caregiver work through the substance abusing behavior together and address other problems such as family communication and conflict as well as support parents/caregivers as their children struggle through treatment.[123] Group therapy has also shown to be efficacious for adolescents because it reinforces positive social interactions with peers. However, one author cautions that these group sessions may also carry a risk of conversation that glorifies drug use or using behavior.[124] Also, among adolescents in treatment for marijuana, more intensive, longer programs (3 months) are more effective than short (two session) programs.[44] One study examined the relative effectiveness of various modalities of treatment and found that group treatment was more effective and less expensive than family-based or individual treatment.[125] However, other research shows that adolescents have better treatment outcomes when parents are involved with the treatment.[126]

One encouraging finding is that there are similar success rates for all adolescents regardless of demographic or racial backgrounds and identities.[127] This suggests all treatment modalities can be used to treat adolescents. However, reductions in substance-abusing behavior were smaller for adolescents using heavier drugs (e.g., heroin and cocaine) compared to marijuana. This suggests, at least for adolescents, that marijuana dependence responds well to treatment.[128] Another study found the younger a person is when drug abuse starts, the less likely treatment will be successful.[129] Adolescents develop different patterns and problems of drug abuse than adults. Therefore, treatment programs have to be designed specifically for adolescents.

Women and Treatment

In 1974, the National Institute on Drug Abuse's Program for Women's Concerns expanded treatment options for drug-addicted women. Nevertheless, treatment programs for women are scarce. Women with substance abuse problems are more likely to have poor family relationships and psychological health than men with substance abuse problems.[130] Women receive treatment at lower rates compared to men. Even when treatment is available, many women are reluctant to enter a program because they are not ready to stop their drug use, the cost dissuades them from receiving treatment, or they feel stigmatized.

Among women entering treatment for the first time, the highest percentage were never married (44%), followed by formerly married women (37%), followed by currently married women.[132] Other studies have identified being currently married as a protective factor against substance abuse for women. Similarly, a history of divorce among women is associated with higher illicit drug use.[133] Many women seek treatment differently from men and usually seek the guidance from their general physical before seeking out treatment options. Additionally, women may be scared to seek out treatment due to being pregnant or having small children for fear of legal or judicial repercussions.[134] Women, with children at home, have the additional burden of having to fit in treatment with personal household responsibilities. According to the National Advocates for Pregnant Women, false claims about the effects of illegal drugs during pregnancy has led to the unjustified arrest of hundreds of pregnant women, with low-income and women of color being disproportionately targeted for these punitive interventions.[135] However, other women are motivated to participate in treatment in order to regain or retain custody of their children.[136]

To address prenatal drug use, the emphasis is on punishing the pregnant drug user rather than on treating her. Paradoxically, many women seek treatment to reduce drug-related harm to their children. Many treatment programs fail to recognize that

HOMICIDE CHARGES FOR DRUG USING PREGNANT WOMEN

In 1999, Regina McKnight experienced a stillbirth in South Carolina. She was an African-American woman with little education, numerous health problems, and a drug problem. As in many stillbirths, there was no obvious cause. However, when she tested positive for cocaine, the state decided her drug use was the cause of the stillbirth and charged with homicide. In 2001, she was convicted of homicide by child abuse based on her behavior during pregnancy. She was the first woman in America to be convicted of such a crime. She was sentenced to 20 years in prison, with the final 8 years being suspended.

In 2008, the Supreme Court unanimously ruled that she did not have a fair trial because her defense did not use expert testimony and also stated the prosecutor did not use sound medical or scientific information regarding the impact of cocaine use during pregnancy.

Questions to Ponder

What should be the consequences for pregnant women using drugs? Should they focus on punishment, treatment, or a combination of both? Justify your answer.

Source: D. Kasdan, "Victory in the Regina McKnight Case", *ACLU*, (May 15, 2008). Accessed on March 23, 2017 from https://www.aclu.org/blog/speakeasy/victory-regina-mcknight-case.

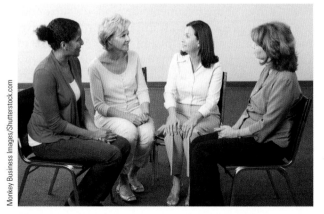

Women tend to do better in women only support groups compared to mixed gender groups.

women in treatment often have concomitant problems such as divorce, family violence, psychiatric problems, and other family members with substance abuse problems.

Women have different drug-using behaviors, and while more men use illicit drugs, women are more susceptible to craving drugs and relapses. African American and Indian/Alaska Native women are more likely to be victims of rape, physical violence, and stalking by an intimate partner in their lifetime—all are factors associated with an increased risk in substance abuse.[137] The majority of women in treatment have a history of rape, aggravated assault, or posttraumatic stress syndrome. For women who have experienced these abuses, a female-only drug abuse treatment centers may be more appropriate. Women in treatment also have significantly higher rates of eating disorders, depression, anxiety, and PTSD than women in general.[138]

Problems Associated with Treatment

Treatment poses several problems. One is retention of clients and counselors. The client dropout rate is high, with a majority of people who enter treatment dropping out within the first month. Another problem arises when people resist having treatment facilities located near their home, school, or workplace. And always problematic is the rate of relapse; a high percentage of clients return to drug use.

Client Resistance to Treatment

Access to treatment is often not enough to promote those who need help to seek it. There are many barriers that are cited for not seeking out treatment including a perception that treatment is not needed, lack of readiness to stop using the drug, cost/limited insurance and stigma associated with treatment.[139] Among older adults, one study showed the two barriers to obtaining treatment for substance use was a lack of readiness to change and cost/limited insurance concerns, while younger adults were more concerned with the stigma associated with getting treatment.[140] Gender is another factor that affects whether one seeks treatment. Twice as many men as women have alcohol-related problems, but men are four times more likely to get treatment. A double standard exists in that women are more stigmatized than men for having a problem with alcohol or other drugs.

Several factors account for the reluctance to seek treatment:

- Many treatment facilities are not readily available or accessible.
- A large percentage of clients lack insurance and cannot afford the cost of treatment.
- The policies and philosophies of some facilities deter drug abusers from pursuing help.
- For some drug abusers, the benefits of using drugs outweigh the disadvantages.
- Some clients think that legal authorities will be made aware of their drug-taking behavior if they enter treatment.

The likelihood of an individual receiving treatment improves when a family member, friend, coworker, or clergy member contacts the treatment agency for an appointment.

Community Resistance

In general, people are in favor of treatment for drug abusers but do not want drug treatment centers in their neighborhoods. Although many communities do not like treatment centers located near them,

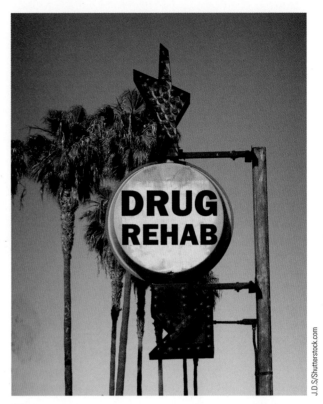

J.D.S/Shutterstock.com

■ Many people do not want a drug treatment center in their neighborhood.

one of the most important reasons people drop out of treatment is that they do not live near the treatment facility.[141] Residents living near sites designated for drug treatment are concerned about more crime, more traffic, exposure of children to bad influences, and lower property values. The **NIMBY (not in my backyard)** syndrome should prompt treatment staffs to make concerted efforts to dispel the misgivings surrounding treatment centers.

Relapse

Although no single cause accounts for relapse during or after drug abuse treatment, the person's surrounding environment plays an important role. Relapse rates range between 50% and 90%.[142] Because of financial restraints, clients receive little follow-up care once they leave treatment. Treatment centers that focus on long-term continuing care tend to have lower relapse rates.[143] Treatment clients usually return to the environments from which they came, and when confronted with high-risk situations, many of them relapse to unhealthy patterns of drug use because they lack the necessary coping skills or social support system. Also, if the drug abuser's spouse uses drugs, the likelihood of relapse increases.[144] In essence, the drug is not what causes the relapse but, rather, events associated with taking the drug.

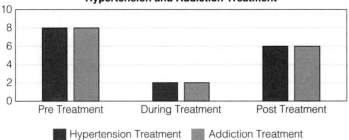

Figure 15.3 A Comparison of Relapses Among Hypertension and Addiction Treatment

Source: National Institute on Drug Abuse, "Principles of drug addiction treatment: A research-based guide (3rd Edition)". (Updated December 2012). Accessed on March 23, 2017 from https://www.drugabuse.gov/publications/principles-drug-addiction-treatment-research-based-guide-third-edition/frequently-asked-questions/how-effective-drug-addiction-treatment.

Even when a person completes drug rehabilitation successfully, the compulsion to use drugs often reappears. A former addict is conditioned to experience withdrawal symptoms even after long periods of abstinence.

Sometimes, objects trigger the desire for drugs. For example, white sugar or talcum powder might be a trigger for a former cocaine addict. Certain people, places, or odors—or even talking about drugs—could evoke the urge. Former cigarette smokers testify to the propensity for relapse. Mark Twain, a smoker, commented that it was easy to stop smoking—he'd stopped hundreds of times! An all-too-familiar scenario illustrating the paradox of using drugs against one's better judgment is related in the following:

> The patient has been through a rehabilitation program; he has returned to his job; he is reunited with his family; and he can present an apparently genuine and logical argument that he never intends to touch the drug again. And then, as one patient said recently, "I bumped into a guy that I used to do coke with, and my heart started pounding and I started shaking. Then I went on automatic pilot."[145]

Three factors contribute to relapse among alcoholics:

1. Negative emotional states such as frustration, anxiety, depression, anger, or boredom
2. Interpersonal conflicts with a spouse, family member, friend, or employer
3. Social pressure from a person or group of people

Four factors related to recovery are compulsory supervision, new relationships, a substitute dependency, and membership in an inspirational group.

Another way to look at relapse is as a natural progression of the disease and not as failure, see Figure 15.3. As with most chronic diseases, the return of

CONSIDER This

What are the goals for substance abuse treatment? Should they be to reduce or eliminate drug use? Reduce crime recidivism? Improve general health? Improve relationships? Improve employment opportunities?

There are many ways to measure success for substance abuse treatment programs. If you were asked to measure the success of a drug treatment facility, which factors would you look for? Explain how you decided which factors to include and exclude.

symptoms is likely, and signifies treatment needs to be restated or adjusted.[146] For the treatment of most chronic diseases, a reduction of symptoms is considered a success, why is it for addiction treatment, the same principles are not applied? This brings us back to the original questions presented at the beginning of this chapter, what are the goals of drug treatment? The US Surgeon General released a report in November 2016 stating the methods for treating substance use disorders should be viewed similarly to the treatment of chronic diseases; that a reduction of key symptoms and an improvement of health and functional status should be goals of treatment.[147]

NIMBY (not in my back yard) A term describing how some people feel about having a controversial facility located in their neighborhoods

Personnel Recruitment and Retention

Recruiting and retaining staff members in treatment programs are difficult because of the intense demands on the staff. According to the National Institute on Drug Abuse, treatment facilities are operating at more than 90% capacity, and personnel feel overworked because of the heavy caseloads. The quality and quantity of services in many facilities have been curtailed severely. Also, the high relapse rate of clients is discouraging. Because of these reasons, plus inadequate wages and poor working conditions, personnel often seek other employment.

The New York State Division of Substance Abuse Services found that the largest obstacles for attracting and retaining staff were inadequate fringe benefits and low wages. In a vicious cycle, low staff retention causes poor morale. Additional factors that hamper staff recruitment and retention include the following:

- Reluctance to work with drug abusers
- Undesirable locations of facilities
- Inadequate supply of applicants with professional experiences and qualifications
- Fear of contracting AIDS

Benefits of Treatment

Regardless of the type of treatment, treatment is desirable. The benefits are summed up as follows:

- Less expensive than incarceration
- Reduced use of illicit drugs
- Decline in criminal activity
- More stable employment
- Reduced transmission of AIDS

If the costs of drug abuse treatment are compared with the alternative costs of continued drug abuse, associated criminal activity, and medical treatment of AIDS, there is no question that the social benefits are worth the expense of drug abuse treatment.[148]

Not only do many people benefit from substance abuse treatment, but society benefits economically as well. Pregnant women in substance abuse treatment have healthier children than substance abusing pregnant women not in treatment.[149] One group of researchers conducted lifetime simulations to determine what impact drug treatment and aftercare prison programs would have on society. In all of their tested scenarios, they found that the societal benefits outweighed the cost of the program, with an improvement in lifetime earning potential of released inmates, decreased crime, and increased productivity.[150] More research reveals that there is a $4 to $7 reduction in the cost of drug-related crimes for every dollar spent on substance abuse treatment.[151] Despite the social,

TABLE 15.3 Drug Treatment and Criminal Activity: Percentage of Clients Engaged in Criminal Activity in 12 Months Before Versus 12 Months After Treatment Exit (N = 4,411)

	Before	After	Percentage Difference
Selling drugs	64.0	13.9	278.3
Shoplifting	63.7	11.7	281.6
Beating someone up	49.3	11.0	277.7
Arrested for any crime	48.2	17.2	64.3
Most support illegal	17.4	9	48.3

Source: National Treatment Improvement Evaluation Study (SAMHSA, 1997).

economic, and medical benefits of substance abuse treatment, a number of states have chosen to decrease spending for substance abuse in order to deal with budget deficits.[152]

A review of drug abuse research spanning 25 years concluded that intensive and appropriate drug treatment reduces both drug use and crime.[153] A comprehensive study of the benefits of treatment conducted in the 1990s, the National Treatment Improvement Evaluation Study, reported that after treatment, drug selling declined by 78%, shoplifting went down 82%, and arrests declined 64%.[154] Arrested juveniles who went through treatment were less likely to commit felonies as adults.[155] Table 15.3 shows the impact of drug treatment on crime.

Of the 4,411 people in the National Treatment Improvement Evaluation Study, drug use declined from 73% before treatment to 38% one year after treatment. Cocaine use went from 40% before treatment to 18% one year after treatment. Heroin use declined from 24% before treatment to 13% within 1 year after treatment. Other benefits included the following:[156]

- An increase in employment from 51 to 60%
- A decline in clients receiving welfare from 40 to 35%
- A drop in homelessness from 19 to 11%
- A 53% decline in substance-related medical visits
- A 56% reduction in people exchanging sex for money or drugs
- A 51% drop in people having sex with an intravenous drug user

Another area in which treatment is beneficial is in curbing AIDS. Many drug users who inject drugs share syringes. According to the Centers for Disease Control and Prevention (CDC), injected drug use is the second most frequent behavior reported by individuals with AIDS. Through its drug treatment services, the US Public Health Service initiated AIDS outreach education projects, educating clients about high-risk behaviors that lead to transmission of HIV.

Summary

Although drug abuse treatment is costly, the expense of not treating it is even greater. Most Americans support spending more money for treatment. Even though funding for drug treatment programs has increased, only a small proportion of drug abusers receive treatment. Most drug abusers are socially disadvantaged young males with histories of criminal activity and psychological problems. Drug abuse treatment reduces illicit drug use and criminal activity.

Drug courts were first established in 1989 to address the need for the criminal justice system and substance abuse treatment system to work together. The purpose of these courts is to reduce crime by offering drug treatment to offenders as a substitute to serving jail time. Benefits of drug courts include reduced recidivism, reduced crime, and cost less money compared to jail.

Substance abuse treatment falls into the three categories: inpatient, outpatient, and self-help groups. Outpatient treatment is more popular than inpatient treatment because of easier access and lower cost; it also is less disruptive and stigmatized. Self-help groups were developed in response to traditional health care that was unresponsive to meeting people's needs. Self-help groups are cost-effective and are used mainly as aftercare. Regardless of the type of treatment, people from supportive social and economic backgrounds respond best to treatment.

One of the more successful programs for treating opiate addicts is methadone maintenance. Methadone eliminates withdrawal symptoms and blocks euphoria. During treatment, clients are given medical, vocational, and psychiatric services. Two drawbacks are that clients must come daily for treatment and that methadone causes its own dependency. Drugs such as naloxone and naltrexone have been used in place of methadone because they prevent withdrawal symptoms and euphoria for a longer time. For alcohol abuse, the drug disulfiram (Antabuse) interacts with alcohol to make the drinker ill. This treatment works while the drinker is in treatment. After treatment ends, the relapse rate is high. Two other drugs approved by the FDA to treat alcoholism are naltrexone and acamprosate.

Relapse rates are high among those undergoing treatment and traditionally have been viewed a sign of failure. However, when comparing relapse rates of a chronic disease and drug dependency, the patterns are similar, suggesting relapse is a natural progression of the disease and is a signal to restart or modify treatment.

An alternative to total sobriety is a controlled or moderate drinking model, based on principles of behavior modification. This program works better for problem drinkers. The person learns to drink alcohol in a nonabusive manner. The results of moderate or controlled drinking programs are mixed.

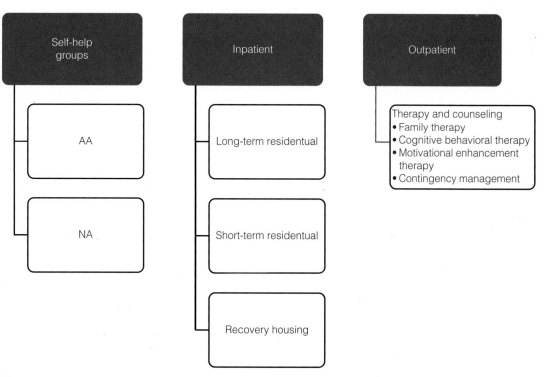

Models of Substance Abuse Treatment

Thinking Critically

1. Drug abuse can be viewed as a personality weakness, as a medical problem, or as a consequence of society. What do you think is the cause of drug abuse? Is it a flaw in personality, a medical issue, or the result of society?

2. Do you feel treating drug addiction should be viewed from the same lens as treating a chronic disease? Justify your answer.

3. Should pregnant women who use drugs be incarcerated or treated for drug addiction? Should they be treated as criminals or as sick people who require treatment? Explain your answer.

4. Methadone maintenance clinics are being met with community resistance. How would you feel about having a clinic located near you? Why?

5. Drug treatment centers are often very expensive. Research has shown mixed results in success rates for different types of centers and treatment modalities. Should success rates of treatment centers be considered when deciding how to treat an addiction? Should insurance companies be required to pay for any type of substance abuse treatment?

16

Drug Prevention and Education

Chapter Objectives

After completing this chapter, the reader should be able to:

- Evaluate the factors hindering drug prevention efforts
- Compare the advantages and disadvantages of the gateway drug theory
- Identify the principles of an effective drug prevention programs
- List the criteria identified by Shin required to be an effective drug education program
- Identify the difficulty in determining goals for prevention programs
- Examine the challenges in evaluating drug prevention programs
- Compare and contrast the levels of prevention (primary, secondary, tertiary) to the behavioral health continuum of care model
- List the characteristics of resilient children
- Identify factors that contribute to and prevent high-risk behaviors
- Examine the educational approaches to drug education

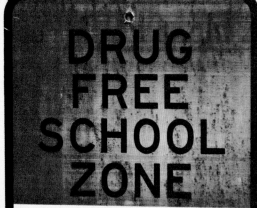

In an effort to reduce availability of drugs at school, the federal government increases penalties if caught with illicit drugs in a school zone.

DRUG FREE SCHOOL ZONE

Alcohol, Tobacco and Other Drugs Are Not Allowed Anywhere On This Campus Violators will be prosecuted

Ben Carlson/Shutterstock.com

FACT OR FICTION?

1. Short-term prevention programs are effective in reducing drugs.
2. The more a person is educated about drugs, the less likely they will be to try drugs.
3. Higher cigarette taxes result in fewer teens smoking.
4. Adolescents who attend religious services frequently are less likely to use drugs than adolescents who do not attend religious services.
5. Adolescents who identify with a minority racial status are more likely to use drugs.
6. Those who used alcohol before age 15 are five times more likely to abuse or become dependent on alcohol when compared with those people who first used alcohol at or after age 21.
7. Unsupervised children are more likely to use drugs than supervised children.
8. Teens are less likely to use illegal drugs if their parents strongly disapprove of drug use.
9. Overall, there is more drug use among youths in urban areas than in rural areas.
10. D.A.R.E., also known as Drug Abuse Resistance Education, is a very effective drug prevention program.

Turn the page to check your answers

Prevention is vital to keeping new drug users from becoming chronic, hardcore users.[1] Parents, schools, and communities have been shown to make a difference in reducing drug use by young people. For every $1 spent on school-based drug prevention, there are cost savings of $5.60 from less frequent use of drugs.[2] Efforts to prevent drug abuse started more than 200 years ago, when the first surgeon general of the United States, Dr. Benjamin Rush, initiated an educational campaign to address the detrimental effects of alcohol. At the start of the 20th century, public health workers successfully conquered tuberculosis, malaria, and smallpox. Although successful strategies to prevent drug abuse have been elusive, some signs are encouraging.

Among the reasons for persistent drug use is the fact that millions of people derive satisfaction from using drugs, particularly alcohol and tobacco. Also, many drugs provide immediate gratification, a quality that has become ingrained in American culture. The immediate impact of drugs is analogous to the immediate impact that credit cards provide, in that using credit cards is comparable to buying goods without waiting. The worry of paying for goods is delayed until the bills arrive. Moreover, Americans do not like being told what to do, as evidenced during Prohibition.

The adage "An ounce of prevention is worth a pound of cure" is trite but apropos. Various approaches have been used to stem drug abuse, raising several important questions:

- What should be the goals of drug education and prevention?
- When should drug education and prevention efforts be initiated?
- What education and prevention efforts are effective?
- Who should be responsible for drug education and prevention?

Funding Drug Prevention

In the United States, most of the funds for drug prevention come from the federal government. In the 2017 National Drug Control Budget, over $1.5 billion was allocated to drug prevention, which represents only 5% of the drug control budget.[3] Despite the success of drug education programs, the federal government allocates more money for domestic law enforcement than for drug prevention. One could argue that if more efforts and resources were placed on drug prevention, money needed for domestic law enforcement would decrease. In a survey of Americans, more than 50% believe there is not enough education for the public and students regarding drug prevention.[4] The need for drug education is reflected in the fact that

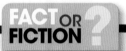

1. **FICTION** The fact is—Prevention programs should be long term, from elementary school to high school, with consistent messages throughout.

2. **FICTION** The Fact is—Early drug prevention attempts focused solely on providing information on the dangers of drug use. These were not effective programs in reducing behaviors of drug use, only knowledge about drug use.

3. **FACT** Cigarette smoking, especially among middle-class and economically disadvantaged youths, decreases significantly as cigarette taxes increase.

4. **FACT** Young people who attend religious services frequently (at least 25 times per year) have significantly lower levels of drug use.

5. **FICTION** The fact is—Positive racial identify can serve as a protective factor against alcohol, tobacco, and drugs.

6. **FACT** Sixteen percent of people who consumed alcohol by age 15 were likely to abuse or become dependent on alcohol, compared with 3% of those who used alcohol for the first time at or after age 21.

7. **FACT** Numerous studies point out that young people who are unsupervised are more likely to experiment with drugs.

8. **FACT** Teens do listen to parents and are less likely to use drugs if parents demonstrate strong disapproval of drug use.

9. **FICTION** The fact is—Although cocaine and crack are more likely to be used in urban areas, overall drug use among youths is as great or greater in rural areas.

10. **FICTION** The fact is—D.A.R.E. is a widely used drug prevention program in the United States, but it has not been proven to be effective.

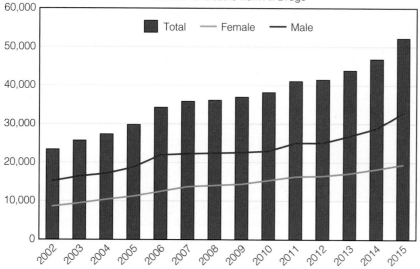

National Overdose Deaths
Number of Deaths from All Drugs

Legend: Total — Female — Male

Figure 16.1 National Overdose Deaths 2002–2015

Source: National Institute on Drug Abuse, "Overdose death rates", (Revised January 2017). Accessed on March 24, 2017 from https://www.drugabuse.gov/related-topics/trends-statistics /overdose-death-rates.

drug overdose deaths have over doubled from 2002 to 2015, with almost 60,000 people dying each year from drug overdoses.[5] See Figure 16.1.

The national agency overseeing drug prevention is the Substance Abuse and Mental Health Services Administration (SAMHSA). It is responsible for the Center for Substance Abuse Prevention (CSAP), the National Institute on Alcohol Abuse and Alcoholism (NIAAA), the National Institute on Drug Abuse (NIDA), the Office of Treatment Improvement, and the National Institute of Mental Health (NIMH). Private groups involved in drug prevention include the National Council on Alcoholism and Drug Dependence, the American Public Health Association, Mothers Against Drunk Driving (MADD), and the Center for Science in the Public Interest.

Drug Abuse Prevention

Drug prevention programs in the United States have changed significantly in the last two decades. This is not surprising, considering how society has changed. With the increasing popularity of social media, prevention efforts should be reexamined to determine the best ways to prevent drug use using current technologies. With so many changes in society, reexamining efforts designed to prevent drug abuse is certainly reasonable. Using the same approaches today that were used in the 1970s might not be appropriate.

Drug Prevention in Retrospect

The primary focus of drug prevention in the 1970s was to reduce the supply of drugs by stopping their importation, sale, and manufacture. **Interdiction** remains a popular preventive strategy but now is complemented by other measures. Logically, if drugs are not available, they cannot be abused. The problem is that the supply of drugs entering the United States can be curtailed but not stopped completely. If one drug is unavailable, people will use other drugs in its place. Thus, the absence of drugs does not diminish the public's appetite for drugs.

Beginning in the 1980s, the focus on stopping drug abuse in the United States shifted. Some drug experts began to contend that prevention should not be directed toward prosecuting drug users or halting the flow of drugs but, rather, toward the underlying factors that contribute to drug abuse. Representative Charles Rangel, chairman of the Congressional Select Committee on Narcotics Abuse and Control, proposed that prevention focus on social and economic problems that lead to drug abuse.[6] He said that until federal politicians confront issues of poor education, inadequate health care, homelessness, unemployment, and poverty, efforts to abate drug abuse will

interdiction Intervention

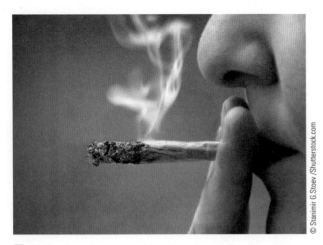

Marijuana was once considered a gateway drug; however, alcohol and tobacco use in adolescents have shown to increase the risk of harder drug use later on.

Effectiveness of Prevention Programs

Determining the effectiveness of drug prevention programs is difficult. Problems in assessing the effectiveness of prevention programs include the absence of control groups, poor data collection, groups that are too small, and inappropriate statistics.[12] Another problem has been that some prevention programs do not differentiate drug use and abuse. Should responsible drug use be a goal of prevention programs? Last, many prevention programs were not followed up on to determine how long any change in drug use persisted. The prevention's effects diminish as time goes on.[13] It is also believed that drug use during adolescence should be expected because this time of life is characterized by increased freedom and independence.[14]

A number of school-based programs reduce drug use and promote positive behaviors. A program called Communities That Care (CTC) reported that teens who participate in its support system were 25% less likely to have health problems and 33% less likely to have behavioral problems.[15] Additionally, program participants were 32% less likely to have initiated the use of alcohol and 33% less likely to imitate tobacco use.[16] Effective programs consist of a social-behavioral curriculum, parental involvement/education, peer leadership, and community-wide task force activities. Unfortunately, a number of middle schools use drug prevention programs that have not been shown to work.[17] There is an inconsistency among drug prevention programs in the United States. In a systematic review of alcohol, tobacco, and other drugs curriculum across schools in the United States, researchers discovered that two-thirds of states do not include standards and the majority of states fell below the recommended curricula and delivery benchmarks.[18] The National Institute on Drug Abuse developed principles to help prevention efforts, as follows:[19]

- Principle 1: Prevention programs should enhance protection factors and reverse of reduce risk factors.
- Principle 2: Prevention programs should address all forms of drug abuse, alone or in combination, including the underage use of legal drugs (e.g., tobacco or alcohol); the use of illegal drugs (e.g., marijuana or heroin); and the inappropriate use of legally obtained substances (e.g., inhalants), prescription medications, or over-the-counter drugs.
- Principle 3: Prevention programs should address the type of drug abuse problem in the local community, target modifiable risk factors, and strengthen identified protective factors.

fall short. Many inner-city youths turn to street-level drug sales because of high unemployment, poor educational outcomes/opportunities, violence, and poverty.[7] Some believe the focus of drug preventions should be aimed at lower socioeconomic communities to improve outcomes for families raising children. If more opportunities existed, they argue, drug dealers would be reduced.[8]

Society was concerned primarily with **hard drugs** such as heroin, LSD, cocaine, crack, and PCP. Drugs such as alcohol, tobacco, and marijuana were perceived as **soft drugs**. Although alcohol and tobacco are not desirable drugs, they are *legal*, and many honest, law-abiding, hardworking citizens smoke and drink. The **Gateway drug** theory is an idea that suggests that the use of certain soft drugs leads to the use of harder drugs.[9] "Gateway" implies that these drugs are used as an introduction to other drugs. While considered controversial, the main gateway drugs identified are alcohol, tobacco, and marijuana. Some believe that if young people do not use gateway drugs, they will not try drugs that have more serious consequences. High school students who use tobacco—whether in the form of cigarettes or smokeless tobacco—are more likely to binge drink, as well as use marijuana and cocaine, than are students who do not use tobacco. However, in a recent study, alcohol is the main culprit behind the gateway drug theory as among 12th graders, the first drug used is alcohol.[10] Inhalants and cocaine act as gateway drugs in some groups and communities. Crack is considered a gateway drug in some poor, urban centers. However, some argue the "gateway drug" hypothesis is outdated and does not consider the social, environmental, and biological factors related to drug use and abuse.[11]

- Principle 4: Preventive programs should be tailored to address risks specific to population or audience characteristics, such as age, gender, and ethnicity, to improve program effectiveness.
- Principle 5: Family-based prevention programs should enhance family bonding and relationships and include parenting skills; practice in developing, discussing, and enforcing family policies on substance abuse; and training in drug education and information.
- Principle 6: Prevention programs can be designed to intervene as early as infancy to address risk factors for drug abuse, such as aggressive behavior, poor social skills, and academic difficulties.
- Principle 7: Prevention programs for elementary school children should target improving academic and socioemotional learning to address risk factors for drug abuse, such as early aggression, academic failure, and school dropout.
- Principle 8: Prevention programs for middle or junior high and high school students should increase academic and social competence.
- Principle 9: Prevention programs aimed at general populations at key transition points, such as the transition to middle school, can produce beneficial effects even among high-risk families and children. Such interventions do not single out risk populations and therefore reduce labeling and promote bonding to school and community.
- Principle 10: Community prevention programs that combine two or more effective programs, such as family-based and school-based programs, can be more effective than a single program alone.
- Principle 11: Community prevention programs reaching populations in multiple settings—for example, school, clubs, faith-based organizations, and the media—are most effective when they present consistent, community-wide messages in each setting.
- Principle 12: When communities adapt programs to match their needs, community norms, or differing cultural requirements, they should retain core elements of the original research-based intervention.
- Principle 13: Prevention programs should be long-term with repeated interventions (i.e., booster programs) to reinforce the original prevention goals. Research shows that the benefits from middle school prevention programs diminish without follow-up programs in high school.
- Principle 14: Prevention programs should include teacher training on good classroom management practices, such as rewarding appropriate student behaviour, achievement, academic motivation, and school bonding.
- Principle 15: Prevention programs are most effective when they employ interactive techniques, such as peer discussion groups and parent role-playing, that allow for active involvement in learning about drug abuse and reinforcing skills.
- Principle 16: Research-based prevention programs can be cost-effective. Similar to earlier research, recent research shows that for each dollar invested in prevention, a savings of up to $10 in treatment for alcohol or other substance abuse can be seen.

Regarding prevention programs for school, the following components were addressed in Shin's review of effective drug education programs. Five criteria were found to be essential: (1) an adequate number of hours of curricula, over at least 3 years; (2) peer involvement; (3) an emphasis on social influences, life skills, and peer resistance; (4) a change in perceived norms; and (5) involvement of parents, peers, and the community in changing norms.[20]

Goals of Drug Prevention

When discussing drug prevention, three questions require consideration:

1. What does prevention actually mean?
2. Should the goals of drug prevention be different for a person who has never used drugs than for a person who uses drugs occasionally or daily?
3. Should drug prevention be defined as a delay in the onset of drug use, the complete elimination of drug-related problems, or a significant decline in drug use?

A major limitation of drug prevention programs is that these programs do not clearly establish the goals they are striving to achieve. When goals are identified, a broad perspective might be helpful. Rather than identifying one goal, identifying several goals might be more useful. Goals could be geared to individuals with different levels of drug involvement. Drug prevention goals for nonusers might not

hard drugs Drugs that are perceived to be dangerous, such as heroin, cocaine, and LSD

soft drugs Drugs perceived to be less harmful than hard drugs; include marijuana, tobacco, and alcohol

gateway drugs Substances that are used before use of more dangerous drugs; alcohol, marijuana, tobacco, and inhalants are considered gateway drugs

CONSIDER This

If you were a principle of a local elementary school. What type of drug prevention goals would you look for in a program? Which goals do you feel would parents want to adopt in a program? Do you think parents/teachers/students/community members would choose the same goals for a prevention program?

be the same as those for occasional or heavy users. Also, drug prevention efforts should take cultural differences into account.

The goals of drug prevention do not have to be mutually exclusive. Goals can be written to try to reduce the individual risk of drugs as well as minimize costs to society. They can also be written to try to delay the onset of drug use with the intent of preventing drug use altogether. The latter is a sound approach because the longer people delay using drugs, the less likely they will be to use drugs. The goals of drug prevention programs are often dictated by the individuals being served or by the community and according to whether the drug is legal or illegal. With alcohol, the goal could be to reduce excessive use, whereas the goal regarding illegal drugs might be complete abstinence.

Levels of Drug Prevention

According to the Health and Medicine Division of The National Academies of Science, Engineering and Medicine, the term *prevention* is reserved for interventions that take place before the initial onset

of disorder.[21] This is a simple definition. The term is confounded because of the different levels of prevention:

1. **Primary prevention:** Strives to reach people before they start using alcohol, tobacco, or other drugs. It should be initiated at a young age because most children already have tried drugs, especially alcohol, by the time they get to high school.
2. **Secondary prevention:** Attempts to minimize the potential damage resulting from drug use by targeting people who have some experience with drugs. Secondary prevention is considered an early intervention stage.
3. **Tertiary prevention:** Geared to heavy drug users and those whose patterns of drug use are well established. Basically, tertiary prevention refers to drug treatment.

Primary Prevention

Primary prevention can be aimed at reducing the demand for drugs or at curtailing the supply of drugs. Drug education is the principal approach for reducing the demand for drugs. Other strategies include mass media campaigns, community-oriented programs sponsored by service groups, drug testing, and legislation aimed at drug users. The mass media can play a significant role. According to the National Cancer Institute, a causal relationship between exposure to depictions of smoking in movies and youth smoking initiation is indicated.[22]

Secondary Prevention

Secondary prevention is geared toward those who do not use drugs abusively. Again, drug education is an important component. If people are drinking alcohol legally, the goal might not be to prevent alcohol use but, rather, to encourage them to consume alcohol in a responsible way. Some argue that "responsible use" of alcohol by young people is a contradiction because it is against the law for minors to use alcohol.

The main goals of secondary prevention are to alter drug-related attitudes and behaviors to provide alternatives to drugs and to stress a healthy lifestyle and physical fitness. As fitness improves, drug use tends to decline. Moreover, self-concept improves as fitness levels improve. There has also been some research showing that sport's participation in school may lead to reduced illicit drug use, although it may also increase alcohol use.[23]

Tertiary Prevention

Because tertiary prevention involves treatment, it is beyond the scope of educational institutions.

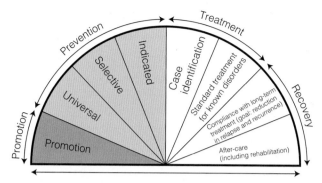

Figure 16.2 Behavioral Health Continuum of Care Model

Source: SAMHSA, "Prevention of substance abuse and mental illness", (Updated on August 9, 2016). Accessed on March 24, 2017 from https://www.samhsa.gov/prevention.

Nevertheless, schools can perform an important function by referring students who abuse drugs to appropriate facilities. In addition, schools can implement prevention programs after students have gone through intensive treatment in order to prevent them from relapsing.

Behavioral Health Continuum of Care Model

First introduced by the Health and Medicine Division of The National Academies of Science, Engineering and Medicine in 1994, the **behavioral health continuum of care** addresses the multiple ways health behaviors can be addressed.[24] The components of this model include:[25] See Figure 16. 2.

- Promotion: Strategies to create environments and conditions that support positive behavioral health.
- Prevention: Strategies delivered prior to the onset on a behavioral disorder or problem. The goal is to reduce or prevent a disorder from developing. This includes primary and secondary prevention strategies.
- Treatment: Services for people identified with a substance abuse problem. This is similar to tertiary prevention or drug treatment.
- Recovery: Services that support the ongoing effort to remain drug free.

Identifying High-Risk Youths

High-risk behavior refers not only to drug abuse but also to delinquent behavior, self-destructive behavior, dropping out of school, and unprotected intercourse.

Among adolescents, antisocial behaviors, delinquency, and illicit drug use are strongly correlated.[25] This does not mean that substance abuse directly causes delinquent behavior or that delinquency directly causes the use of alcohol and other drugs, merely that there is a relationship between the two variables. Some children succumb to the pressures of their circumstances and surroundings, and others rise above their situation. Still others inherit a propensity for drug misuse and abuse. Psychological factors also play a role. Figure 16.3 illustrates the relationship between drug use and various types of delinquent behavior.

Resilient Children

Children from high-risk backgrounds often surmount their circumstances and avoid the temptation to turn to drugs. Many children from impoverished backgrounds become healthy, competent young adults. They display **resiliency**, suggesting that they can sustain competent functioning despite the presence of major life stressors.

Resilient children have many noteworthy characteristics. They are flexible, responsive, adaptable, and active. They have positive relationships with others and maintain a sense of humor. Somehow they are able to disengage or distance themselves from dysfunctional family environments. Although they are able to see their parents' problems, resilient children view themselves as different and recognize that they have control over their environments. Resilient children do not avoid stress but, instead, learn to master it, and to use it to their advantage. Boys and girls differ in that boys tend to be more resilient in adolescence whereas girls display more resilience during early childhood. Resilient children tend to form a strong bond with at least one person (not necessarily a parent) during the first year of life. Also, children who are given responsibilities and chores become more resilient, presumably because they

primary prevention Preventing drug use before it begins

secondary prevention Early intervention to block more serious problems; halts escalation of drug use

tertiary prevention Treatment that seeks to help individuals after they have misused drugs

behavioral health continuum of care model A comprehensive approach to care that includes promotion, prevention, treatment, and recovery.

resiliency A person's ability to overcome obstacles, such as resisting drug use despite a background that increases the likelihood of drug use

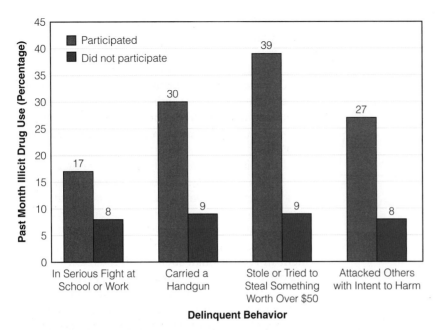

Figure 16.3 Past Month Illicit Drug Use among Youths (12–17) by Participation in Fighting and Delinquent Behavior

Source: Teens, Drugs & Violence: A Special Report, Office of National Drug Control Policy, June 2007. p. 2.

CHARACTERISTICS OF RESILIENT CHILDREN

- Responsive
- Flexible
- Form positive relationships
- Caring
- Skillful problem-solvers
- Educationally motivated
- Disengaged from dysfunctional family environments
- Active
- Adaptable
- Good sense of humor
- Empathetic
- Success oriented
- Persistent

PARENTS CAN RAISE RESILIENT CHILDREN

While some of the characteristics associated with resilient children are innate (e.g. temperament), others can be encouraged through parenting. Parents who practice the following skills can improve healthy development and prevent later substance abuse behaviors:

- Warmth
- Consistency
- Age-appropriate expectations
- Praise for accomplishments
- Consistent routines and rules

Source: National Institute on Drug Abuse, "Principles of substance abuse prevention for early childhood", (Updated March 2016). Accessed on March 24, 2017 from https://www.drugabuse.gov/publications /principles-substance-abuse-prevention-early-childhood /chapter-2-risk-protective-factors.

contribute to the family and feel important to its functioning.

At-Risk Factors

Many young people are not resilient. A number of variables predispose young people to abuse alcohol and other drugs. These variables can be broadly grouped as hereditary and familial factors, peer influence, psychosocial factors, biological factors, and community factors.

Hereditary and Familial Factors

Regardless of whether the cause is environmental or genetic, the sons of men with alcohol-related problems are more likely to have alcohol-related problems. Some risk factors for substance abuse are heritable, meaning they are passed down from parents. In a

RISK FACTORS FOR DRUG USE BY ADOLESCENTS AND CHILDREN

Individual Behavioral Factors

- Academic failure
- Early antisocial behavior
- Early drug experimentation
- Early drug use

Individual Attitudinal Factors

- Rebelliousness against authority
- Lack of commitment to school
- Attraction to deviance
- Unfavorable attitudes toward adult behavior

Individual Psychosocial Factors

- Low self-esteem
- Low self-efficacy
- Sensation seeking
- Lack of social skills

Family Factors

- Family history of drug use or antisocial behavior
- Family management problems (inadequate parenting skills)
- Parental tolerance for deviance
- Family disorganization

Community Environment Factors

- Economic and social deprivation
- Community disorganization
- Community norms favorable to deviance
- Availability of drugs
- Friends/peers who use drugs

study on nicotine addiction, a variant in the gene for the nicotine receptor is believed to double the risk of nicotine addiction among persons who carry the variant gene.[26] One Swedish study looked at siblings and twins and concluded drug abuse is highly heritable, even if the twins were raised in different environments.[27] Further, rates of alcohol, cocaine, marijuana, and tobacco dependence are greater if siblings are dependent on these drugs.[28] Sons and daughters of parents with drinking problems have poor coping skills and personality problems and are more

likely to be involved with alcohol. In addition, father involvement can serve as a protective factor against substance abuse and promote positive educational, behavioral, social, and psychological outcomes.[29] Furthermore, the attachment of males 12 to 14 years of age to their natural father in an intact family is significant as to whether young males resist abusing drugs, especially in neighborhoods where drug abuse is prevalent.[30]

Drug prevention has to address the factors contributing to drug abuse in the first place. Family factors are significantly related to delinquency and drug abuse by both boys and girls.[31] Many drug-dependent families have higher stress levels, fewer friends, more family conflict, parental depression, and less involvement in recreational, social, religious, and cultural activities. Substance-abusing parents spend half as much time with their children as nonabusing parents. Adults with a history of abuse and neglect as children are at high risk of developing substance abuse disorders. Moreover, these adults are at risk of abusing their own children.[32]

Research suggests that more emphasis should be placed on strengthening the family. Positive family influence may be protective. Parents who expect their children not to use drugs have children who are less likely to use drugs. Conversely, parents who do not agree about drug use are more likely to have children who use drugs.[33] Family structure also plays a role in drug use. Adolescents raised in single family households are at higher risk for substance use. This may be due to less intense monitoring by the single parent and having fewer resources compared to dual-parent households.[34] Additionally, there is some research to suggest that girls who are raised by fathers only are at higher risk for substance use; this same association is not seen for boys. Living with a gender-matched single matched parent may affect in reducing later drug use.[35] There is a strong relationship between family dinners and substance use.[36] In a large telephone survey conducted on over 1,000 teens ages 12 to 17, teens that reported frequent family dinners (5 to 7 a week) were more likely to have high-quality relationships with their parents.[37] When teens report positive and high-quality relationships with their parents they are less likely to have used marijuana, alcohol, and tobacco.[38]

Peer Influence

Various studies point out that the influence of peers is not consistent. For example, one study found close friends' attitudes on drugs influenced teens' substance use. Rates of substance use were increased if one's close friends had indifferent attitudes regarding substance use.[39] Conversely, rates of substance use decreased if one's close friends disapproved of substance use. This effect was greatest among White

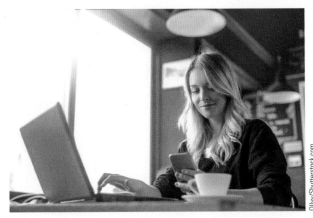

Teens who use social media for more than 2 hours a day are at higher risk for depression which can lead to substance use.

adolescents.[40] Adolescents are highly engaged in using social media to connect with friends. In a study conducted on 10th graders' use of social media, researchers found that connecting with friends on social online networks was not associated with increased risk behaviors.[41] Additionally, studies have found an increased risk between the number of hours spent on social media and psychological health. One study found that students who report to using social media for more than 2 hours a day were more likely to suffer from poor mental health, higher levels of psychological distress, and suicidal ideation,[42] all of which are risk factors for substance use. The issue might not be peer pressure as much as peer approval, as young people crave approval from their friends. Adolescents tend to choose peers with similar drinking behaviors.[43]

Psychosocial Factors

Many psychosocial factors are related to drug use by teens. Among these are rebelliousness and alienation from adults, school failure, lack of interest in school, antisocial behavior at an early age, and lack of aspirations regarding adult achievement.[44] Additional manifestations are frequent lying, indifference to

punishment, lack of empathy toward others, and a desire for immediate gratification rather than delayed gratification. Moreover, these young people are not likely to have positive bonds with adults, nor are they likely to respond to messages about the possible hazards of drugs. The more risk factors a person accumulates, the greater the risk of using a drug.

Biological Factors

Some people are genetically more predisposed than others to drug dependence. Relatedly, some individuals derive more pleasure from drugs than others. The more pleasurable the drug experience is, the more likely it is that a person will be at risk for drug dependency. It has also been noted that the more self-control one has, the less likely one is to engage in drug abuse.[45] Poor self-control, which may be due to abnormalities in the function and organization in the brain, may lead to drug abuse.[46]

Community Factors

Drug use is more prevalent in communities where people move often. Also, drug use is more common when children grow up in extreme poverty and deprivation. Drug taking is more prevalent in communities that lack stability because social support and controls regulating behaviors, including drug use, are not in place. In response to this knowledge, early-intervention programs are tied to treatment services in many communities.

Preventing High-Risk Behavior

Two factors associated with high-risk behavior—heredity and biology—cannot be changed. Other high-risk factors, however, can be modified. In this

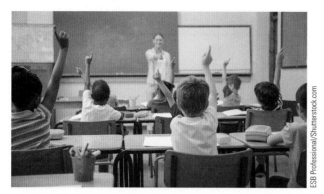

Academic achievement serves as a protective factor against drug use.

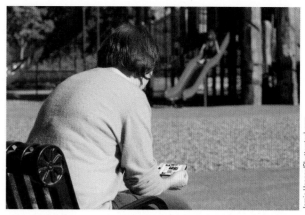

Children whose parents take a "hands-off" approach are more likely to use drugs.

section, we will explore strategies that can reduce the likelihood of individuals engaging in high-risk behaviors connected with drug use.

Education

Poor school performance and low expectations for school are strong predictors of drug use. Therefore, a good argument can be made for changes within the educational system as well as for developing more preschool programs such as Head Start. Many schools are implementing programs with emphases on team teaching, school-based planning, individual tutoring, and cooperative learning. School performance improves and high-risk behaviors are reduced particularly through *experiential* education, including community service and part-time employment.

Schools often serve as the focal point for community programs. School facilities have been used to provide health care, recreational activities, after-school programs, and counseling. School alternative programs focusing on community and recreational activities, physical activities, and job training have helped youths at risk to stay off drugs. Most illicit drug use starts during the teenage years. Thus incorporating prevention programs at school is necessary to reduce drug use. Furthermore, these programs should begin in elementary school and continue each year.

Moreover, schools that maintain high expectations for students while providing support have seen academic failure decline. The consensus among experts is that children need responsible adults who are responsive to their needs. Outside of the family, a favorite teacher may be the most important role model for helping children develop resilience.

Role of Parents

The role of parents should not be underestimated. Parental drug use greatly increases the likelihood of children's drug use. Children growing up in a household with much discord have many difficulties, although many children in families marked by a pathologic environment and poverty do *not* develop drug problems.[47] Studies on children of alcoholics show they are more likely to marry into a family with a background of alcoholism, use drugs and alcohol as adults, and are four times more likely to become alcoholics.[48] Additionally, children who grow up in homes with a substance abusing parent are more at risk for abuse and neglect.[49]

On the other hand, parents can serve as a protective factor against drug and alcohol use. Parents who have high expectations for their children foster their academic success and resilience. According to the NIAAA, "Parents can have a major impact on their children's drinking, especially during the preteen and early teen years."[50]

Adolescent drug users are more likely than non-using adolescents to perceive their parents as distant, uninvolved, mistrusting, and punitive. Thus, parents need to be more supportive of their children. In a study conducted by the National Center on Addiction and Substance Abuse (CASA), it was found that parents who take a "hands-off" approach have children who are four times more likely to use alcohol, tobacco, and illegal drugs. Confirming these results, another study found that children who rated their parents as permissive and having less maternal control were more like to use alcohol, tobacco, and marijuana.[51] Children are less likely to use drugs if they grow up in households where parents practice an authoritative parenting style and engage in high levels of parent-child communication.[52] One nationwide program for helping parents to dissuade their children from drug use is Parents' Resource Institute for Drug Education (PRIDE). Parental involvement in schools also helps to reduce their children's high-risk behaviors.

Examples of Risk Factors and Protective Factors for Drug Abuse

Risk Factors	Domain	Protective Factors
Early aggressive behavior	Individual	Self-control
Poor social skills	Individual	Positive relationships
Lack of parental supervision	Family	Parental monitoring and support
Substance abuse	Peer	Academic competence
Drug availability	School	Antidrug policies
Poverty	Community	Strong neighborhood attachment

Source: National Institute on Drug Abuse. *Drugs, Brains, and Behavior: The Science of Addiction* (Rockville, MD: National Institute on Drug Abuse, 2010).

Community Efforts

Collaboration among schools, communities, social agencies, religious organizations, businesses, and the media is vital. However, before community efforts can reduce drug use, community leaders as well as retailers, parents, and school personnel need to be ready to mobilize their efforts.[53] Spiritual/religious involvement is a particularly important protective factor against substance abuse. One study found that adolescents who identified as Agnostic had an increased risk for use of marijuana, cocaine, ecstasy, and nonmedical use of opioids and amphetamines.[54] Study also found high levels of religious attendance had protective factors against drug use, but these factors were diminished if adolescents lied in areas where they were exposed to drugs.[55]

Drug use is more prevalent in impoverished, urban neighborhoods. Neighborhoods marked by disorganization, violent crime, and illegal drug activity spawn drug use.[56] Young people growing up in disadvantaged neighborhoods face many environmental barriers. They lack amenities such as supermarkets, libraries, healthcare facilities, adequate housing, and social institutions. At the same time, they have an inordinate number of bars. Jobs have been shown to help curb drug use, yet employment opportunities for young people are in short supply. Too often the services in urban areas are fragmented because no lead agency takes charge.

According to Pentz, there are several barriers to institutionalizing community prevention efforts. These barriers are (1) community leaders' lack of perceived empowerment to continue prevention work; (2) communities' insufficient preparation for adopting programs that have been successful; (3) public resistance to spending more money on drug prevention programs after much money has already been spent on ineffective programs; and (4) the notion that every community is unique, and thus programs that are effective in one community will not necessarily work in other communities.[57]

Drug Education

Society often turns to schools to resolve social problems, whether they be teenage pregnancy, apathy, violence, racial or sexual discrimination, or drug abuse. Schools are logical places for dealing with drug problems because they have the potential to reach all children.

The Evolution in Drug Education

In the 1970s, the thrust of drug education was to provide information about the dangers of drugs, under the assumption that the more knowledge young people had about drugs, the less likely they would be to use them. Another assumption was that if young people feared drugs because of their potential harm, they would resist them. These are faulty assumptions. Knowledge does not lead to behavior change. For drug education to have any impact, emphasis has to be placed on the immediate effects of drugs. Harmful effects that take years to develop, such as emphysema and cirrhosis, have less relevance to teenagers than the effects of drugs on their breath or social standing.

The scare tactics and horror stories used in the 1970s did not prevent experimentation with drugs.[58] In some drug education programs, former addicts described how drugs ruined their lives, researchers demonstrated the effects of drugs on laboratory animals, and police warned young people about the criminal penalties for drug use. Unfortunately, these types of activities have *not* been shown to reduce drug use. Some teachers warned students that marijuana use will lead to heroin use and that once one uses heroin, one is addicted forever. Based on their own experiences, many students know this information is inaccurate or exaggerated. In addition, it has been shown that many young people are skeptical about information they are given about drugs.[59]

Values Clarification

By the mid-1970s, drug education programs were stressing **values clarification** and affective education. The focus was not on drugs but, instead, on the underlying values contributing to drug use. It was thought that improving self-esteem and interpersonal skills was essential. The belief was that, if young people were to understand and articulate their values (assuming these are life-affirming values), they would recognize the potential destructiveness of drugs.

The goal of this movement was to help students recognize their values which was then believed to help them make moral decisions based on those values. However, this approach was ineffective in changing students' behavior because drug use is often consistent with their values. Critics of this approach felt it was inappropriate for teachers, and schools, to probe in the personal lives of students and ask students to share and disclose personal feelings.[60] It tends to make assumptions that personal values and morals should naturally be against drug use; which is not always the case. Consider students who grow up in families with drug use, the values they learn at home are stronger than the ones taught at school. Another critique of the values clarification approach is that values are personal and individualized, created through life experiences, thus, there is no right or wrong value.[61] However, this approach assumed that there are right and wrong values, as "right" values would decrease drug use, while 'wrong' values would increase drug use. Moreover, some students indicated that they valued the feelings that drugs gave them and that drug use helped them to be accepted by friends. Others used values clarification as an excuse or a rationalization for using drugs. Also, some political and religious groups oppose values clarification on the basis that parents and churches, not schools, should teach values.

Alternatives Approach

One approach to drug education that was popular and that is still promoted by many drug educators is the alternatives approach. The rationale is that, for any reason for using drugs, an alternative is available to satisfy the reason. If a person takes drugs to get high, drug-free activities can provide natural highs. To relax, a person can do relaxation exercises. To cope with stress, an individual can learn stress-reducing activities. People who want to alter their consciousness can meditate. Those who have a compulsive need to take drugs can substitute a positive addiction for the negative addiction. To be effective, the alternatives must be more desirable than the drugs. While this approach seemed to be successful in increasing students' knowledge about alternatives to drug use, actual behavior change was not affected.[62]

A Change in Direction

In 1974, Robert DuPont, former director of the NIDA, reported that most students and teachers believed that drug education programs should be abolished. In the previous year, the US Special Action Office on Drug Abuse Prevention recommended a 6-month moratorium on prevention materials, prevention activities, and the implementation of prevention programs. What evolved was more emphasis on health in general and less emphasis on the pharmacology of drugs.

Current Programs

Today, drug education emphasizes developing resiliency skills, learning peer-refusal techniques, and gaining life skills. Students should be taught how to apply the knowledge they learn in the classroom to the decisions they are required to make every day. A sound drug education program teaches young people the negative effects of drugs and how to resist pressure from others to use drugs. Previously, many drug curricula were not evaluated.[63] However, from the mid-2000s to the late-2000s, there was an increase in curricula with more emphasis on evaluation.[64]

Limitations of Drug Education

Rather than dissuade students from trying drugs, many early programs stimulated curiosity, which contributed to more drug use initially, although most young people did not continue to use drugs. One way to get people to do something they should not do is to tell them they are not allowed to do it. This is analogous to the idea that forbidden fruit is sweeter.

Teachers, researchers, and drug program specialists indicate that honesty, communication, trust, and respect are the most desirable attributes of a drug education teacher. A continuing problem with drug education has been the credibility of the teacher. Some teachers distort or exaggerate the physical, psychological, and social effects of drugs. Moreover, providing false or inaccurate information can be harmful to young people.[65]

Others take a moral stance in which they preach about the evils of drugs, creating an atmosphere of distrust. Students with a drug problem will probably hesitate to talk to a teacher who moralizes, for fear of being scolded rather than helped. Teachers should not glamorize drugs, but they have to be nonjudgmental and honest. Teachers can best help a student if they neither condemn nor condone the behavior.

Many students know more (or think they know more) about drugs than their teachers. The knowledge that students have might come from their *experience* with drugs, not from their *understanding* of

> **values clarification** A teaching strategy in which individuals are asked to express and support their values

Goals of Drug Education

Drug education can have a number of possible goals. One might be to impart knowledge. This has some value, as many young people are misinformed about drugs. Presumably, if students are armed with information, they can decide for themselves whether to use drugs. This approach, however, assumes that information leads to abstinence. In reality, no link between drug knowledge and behavior has been demonstrated. When asked if a lack of knowledge was a factor in their students using drugs, teachers indicated it was not.[66]

Other goals include reducing drug abuse or dependency, preventing or delaying first-time drug use, curtailing students' drug use, and teaching responsible drug use. With young people who have experimented with or used drugs already, moderate use might be a more realistic goal. Goals for drug education are not mutually exclusive. For example, a program can delay initial drug use and also encourage drug users to explore alternatives.[67]

One-Size-Fits-All Drug Education

Drug education programs should be tailored to the students' ages and to the needs of the students and the community. Earlier in this chapter, principles from

drugs. Experience does not translate into knowledge, although some teachers who have had experience with alcohol and tobacco believe they can help their students by relating their own experiences.

Teachers do not have to have used drugs to be credible, but they do have to be informed. States such as New York require everyone receiving teacher certification to have coursework covering drugs. Because of the constant flow of new information, every teacher has to keep abreast of the field, and schools must provide staff development.

ON CAMPUS

College students drink more alcohol, and tend to get more drunk compared to their non-college attending peers. Drinking alcohol peaks during times when school is not in session, particularly during spring break. Spring break fills students with images of beaches, parties, and consuming a large amount of alcohol. However, alcohol-related consequences during spring break also increases, especially for women. Women are at an increased risk for sexual assault and rape during heavy episodic drinking periods associated with spring break.

One study incorporated components from the deviance regulation theory, which assumes people will stray from social norms to preserve a positive social image, to reduce heavy alcohol use during spring break among women. While this approach did not impact the amount of alcohol consumed by women during spring break, it did reduce the amount of alcohol-related consequences.

Questions to Ponder

- What goals should colleges set for alcohol education on campus? What type of campaigns do you think would be effective for college students?

Source: R.D. Dvorak, M.P. Kramer, B.L. Stevenson, E.M. Sargent, and T.M. Kilwein, "An application of deviance regulation theory to reduce alcohol-related problems among college women during spring break", *Psychology of Addictive Behaviors,* 31, no. 3, (2017): 295–306.

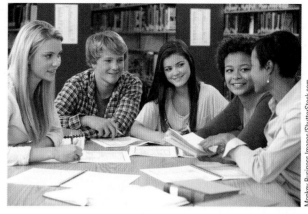

Social skills training improves relationships among teens and can impact their ability to resist drugs.

the National Institute on Drug Abuse were presented. These principles include guidelines that should be addressed in drug education. In schools, drug education programs should be customized to reflect the different cultures, backgrounds, and needs of the community.[68] For example, if a community is experiencing an increase in heroin use, education efforts at the school should address this issue. Additionally, curriculum should be age appropriate. To expect that techniques for first-grade students would be the same as those for high school seniors is unreasonable. Elementary students do not have the aptitude of high school students to think conceptually, and their decision-making and problem-solving abilities are less developed; they understand literal messages and respond to direct instruction. Prevention programs start as early as infancy. School programs should begin in elementary school and target improving academic and social-emotional learning along with drug education.[69]

In its 1989 publication *What Works: Schools Without Drugs*, the US Department of Education developed a model for drug education. The message was clear: *abstinence*. Topics for elementary students included responsible decision-making, handling feelings, and the proper use of medicines. The secondary school model emphasized the actual effects of drugs and the role of advertising.

Current Approaches to Drug Education

The primary foci of drug education today are social norms, resiliency skills, personal development, refusal skills, decision-making skills, and coping skills. Information about drugs and alternatives to drug use is included in many programs. Developing personal competence is believed to be more important than pharmacology in helping young people decide about drug use. Young people who rate high in **self-efficacy**—the belief that one is in charge of oneself—are more likely to avoid harmful patterns of drug use.

Personal and Social Skills Training

The premise of personal and social **skills training** is that drug-taking behavior is *learned* through modeling and reinforcement. Drug use results from the interplay of social and personal factors. This model is derived from Bandura's social learning theory[70] and Jessor and Jessor's problem behavior theory.[71] The skills training model is comprehensive, not limited to drugs. It teaches personal and social skills applicable to various situations. They have also been identified as useful skills needed in the workplace, thus this type of curriculum not only is effective for drug education, but helps students gain the skills needed later in life.[72] Included are skills for resisting media and interpersonal influences, problem-solving and decision-making, relieving stress and anxiety, relaxation, self-control, self-esteem, interpersonal relations, and assertiveness.

Poor social skills have been associated with an increased risk of drug abuse.[73] A study conducted in Estonia found social skill levels were related to both illicit and licit drug use among 15- to 16-year-old

self-efficacy Personal success based on one's own efforts

skills training A drug prevention program in which one learns skills to prevent drug use

students; with the effect on girls being much higher compared to boys.[74]

Drug abuse prevention programs that focus on social influences have been shown to be more effective than other prevention efforts with young adolescents.[75] Students who feel personally competent are less likely to consume alcohol.[76] In a small study conducted on female students who scored high on an addiction potential scale, the use of social skills training was evaluated against a control group to determine the impact of the training. Results from this study suggest social skills training has the potential to reduce addiction tendencies among female high school students.[77] Project Northland, a substance abuse program based in Minnesota, has been shown to reduce the use of alcohol, tobacco, and other drugs significantly. Project Northland focuses on three particular domains: *environmental factors*—aspects of the environment that support, permit, or discourage alcohol use by adolescents, including such things as influential role models, social support, specific opportunities or barriers to drink, and community norms and standards related to adolescent drinking; *intrapersonal factors*—personality characteristics and ways of thinking that increase or decrease the likelihood of an adolescent using alcohol, including an adolescent's level of knowledge about alcohol use consequences, personal values, attitudes, and self-efficacy; and *behavioral factors*—these include past alcohol, cigarette, and other drug use, intentions to drink in the future, and skills to resist offers to use alcohol.

Social Norms Approach

A drug education approach that has become more popular over the last 20 years, especially on college campuses in the United States, is the social norms approach. The premise of this approach is two-fold. On one hand, injunctive norms refer to whether the behavior is approved/disapproved by a peer group. For example, if a student feels his/her peers approve of tobacco use, that student is more likely to try

---

EXAMPLES OF SOCIAL NORMS APPROACH

- Think everyone is doing it? Guess again. 90% students at your school do not use tobacco products.

- Everyone is getting drunk? Think again. Most students at your school drink no more than three drinks when they go out to bars.

---

tobacco. On the other hand, descriptive norms refer to perceptions of how many peers engage in a certain behavior. For example, if a student perceives most of his/her classmates as smokers, that student is more likely to smoke. In one study on adolescents, altering descriptive norms regarding tobacco and marijuana use reduced those behaviors.[78] However, in a meta-analysis of descriptive norms of alcohol and college students, there were no meaningful benefits to using a social norms approach for this population.[79]

Resistance Skills Training

Young people are exposed to drugs in many situations. Perhaps they are at a party where drugs are passed around or involved romantically with a partner who encourages drug use. In **resistance skills training**, students are taught how to recognize, manage, and avoid situations that could involve drug use. Students are instructed on how to refuse drugs *effectively*, often through role-playing. The belief is that students succumb to peer pressure regarding drug use because they do not have the skills needed to refuse these pressures. Peer educators are included in many of these programs because students perceive their peers as more credible than adults. This approach has seen some success; one study among American Indian middle school students found that teaching culturally relevant communication skills, specifically resistance skills, increased students' repertoire of drug resistance skills.[80] However, whether this translates to reduced drug, alcohol, and tobacco use was not disclosed.

Resistance skills training also teaches students how to counter mass-media messages that encourage drug use, especially tobacco and alcohol. One difference between resistance skills training and personal and social skills training is that the former focuses on specific problems whereas the latter teaches general skills for coping with life.

Drug Prevention Programs

Two drug prevention programs grounded in social learning, which have met with some success, are Project ALERT and Life Skills Training (LST). Project ALERT has been shown to reduce weekly alcohol and marijuana use, at-risk drinking, and alcohol use resulting in negative consequences, as well as attitudes and perceptions conducive to drug use.[81] It is used in all 50 states with more than 1 million adolescents being exposed to this curriculum each year.[82] The goals of Project ALERT are to:[83]

- Keep low-risk nonusers from starting to use harmful substances

- Keep moderate-risk experimenters from escalating substance use
- Help high-risk users to reduce substance use

In LST, students are taught how to avoid being persuaded by others, to manage anxiety, to communicate more accurately, to be assertive, and to enhance their self-esteem. A 5 and 1/2-year study of 1,677 students found that this program significantly reduced cigarette smoking and frequency of drunkenness and marijuana use.[83] Another study confirmed these results and found the impact of LST to be long term. This study also found that LST can reduce health risk behavior as well as improve academic success.[84]

In a study of approximately 2,000 students in grades 6 through 10, teaching refusal skills resulted in significantly reduced alcohol misuse.[85] A review of smoking prevention programs found that 7th- to 9th-grade students who were taught to identify social influences promoting tobacco use and skills to resist tobacco use were less likely to smoke, and that this resistance persisted for 1 to 4 years.[86] The effectiveness of these programs, however, lessened over time. This program is also effective for young adults, as one study found an increase in drug abuse preventive behavior that remained in effect for 4 years after LST implementation, among college students.[87] One factor that strengthened the effectiveness of school-based programs was community involvement, especially by parents, youth groups, community organizations, and the mass media.

Drug Abuse Resistance Education

One popular drug education program is Drug Abuse Resistance Education (D.A.R.E.), which began as a joint program between the Los Angeles Police Department and the Los Angeles School District. Police officers go to classrooms and teach elementary students about drugs and personal safety. Students are asked to write essays critical of drug use and to publicly pledge their opposition to drug use. To illustrate its popularity, President George Bush proclaimed April 10, 2008, to be National D.A.R.E. Day.[88] On April 6, 2011, President Obama made a similar proclamation.[89]

Despite the hundreds of millions of dollars going to the D.A.R.E. program, studies of D.A.R.E.'s effectiveness are not encouraging. Over a short period, D.A.R.E. may reduce drug use, but one year after the program ends, there is no difference in drug use.[90] Suffolk County, one of the largest counties in New York, discontinued its D.A.R.E. program after 20 years because the program was found to be ineffective.[91]

In its review of numerous studies, the US General Accounting Office found that D.A.R.E. had little

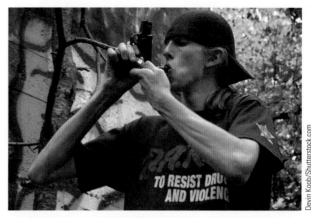

D.A.R.E., one of the most prominent drug education programs used in school, has been shown to be ineffective in reducing drug use.

impact on drug use.[92] Despite the fact that D.A.R.E. has not been shown to work, it continues to be used because it is believed that it improves the relationships between police, children, and schools.[93]

To counter some of its critics, D.A.R.E. officials developed a new curriculum for elementary and middle school students called keepin' in REAL (KiR). The new curriculum is oriented to self-awareness and management, responsible decision making, understanding others, relationship and communication skills, and handling responsibilities and challenges.[94] In a review of literature regarding this new version, researchers remained concerned in the following areas:[95]

- KiR has only been tested on a narrow audience and may not be appropriate for D.A.R.E.'s larger audience
- KiR may not be effective in reducing substance use among elementary school students
- The specific versions of KiR implemented by D.A.R.E. have yet to be tested for efficacy

Just Say No!

During the Reagan administration beginning in 1980, First Lady Nancy Reagan promoted the "Just Say No" campaign. The concept was simple: Tell young people that if someone tries to persuade or encourage them to use drugs, they should refuse the drugs and walk away. For many youngsters, this approach is adequate, but for others it is not, as some students do not recognize peer pressure or have the skills to refuse drugs.

resistance skills training Resistance skills training involves recognizing, managing, and avoiding situations that may encourage drug use.

Effectiveness of Drug Education

Although many drug education programs have increased knowledge and produced significant attitude changes, traditional drug education programs have not proved to be effective. Information alone does not alter behavior. For example, 7-year-old children are aware of the health hazards of smoking, yet many children smoke despite this knowledge. Students who most benefit from drug education may be those who least need it. In addition, many teachers do not have the skills and knowledge to teach about drugs in an effective way.[96]

Recent evaluations of current programs are very encouraging. The Safe Schools/Healthy Students (SS/HS) initiative, which provided $32.8 million to 18 states and the District of Columbia, found that 96% of school staff indicated that school safety improved, there was a 263% increase in students receiving mental health services, and more than 80% of school staff members reported that they saw decreases of alcohol and drug use among their students.[97]

Working with disadvantaged 6th-grade schoolchildren, an alcohol prevention program was effective in reducing alcohol use up to 1 month after the program, but a 1-year follow-up demonstrated no long-term benefit.[98] Another program directed at deaf students in grades 7 through 12 showed that a tobacco-related curriculum significantly affected tobacco-related practices, attitudes, and knowledge.[99] Similarly, a curriculum involving an educational cartoon and storybook for students in grades 1 to 3 demonstrated that tobacco-related knowledge has increased.[100]

Before addressing the effectiveness of current drug education programs, criteria to determine effectiveness have to be identified. Should a drug education program be judged effective if students are better informed about drugs, if they espouse negative attitudes about drugs, if their drug use declines, or if the number of drug-related problems (such as emergency room visits from drugs) goes down? Is drug education successful if students switch from illegal drugs to alcohol and tobacco?

Sometimes drug education has the opposite effect on behavior because it stimulates curiosity and drug use may go up initially. If students experiment with drugs, though, they might do so more safely. Adolescence is a time for experimentation, and a certain amount of drug use should be expected. Rather than attempting to totally eliminate drug use, some contend that educators should work toward *reducing* drug use and misuse. This harm-reduction approach recognizes that people always have and will always use drugs, but education efforts should be focused on minimizing the risks associated with drug use.[101] The research findings are contradictory, although results of programs dealing with resistance training seem to be somewhat encouraging.

To influence drug use, *social norms* have to be changed. Although schools have an important role in drug prevention, they are just one piece of the mosaic. Students are under much pressure from sources outside of school to use illegal drugs, alcohol, and tobacco. Participation by the media, parents, and the community is essential. Also, programs emphasizing personal skills and psychosocial approaches can effectively reduce the use of alcohol and other drugs.

Effective programs include the following components:[102]

- The curricula are based on an understanding of the theory and research in drug abuse prevention.

- Information is developmentally appropriate; short-term, negative social consequences are emphasized.
- The curricula emphasize social resistance skills training as part of comprehensive health education that incorporates personal and social skills training.
- The program includes normative education, in which adolescents are taught that most people do not use drugs.
- Teachers use interactive teaching techniques such as role-playing, discussions, and small-group activities.
- Teachers receive training and support.
- The amount of time devoted to drug abuse prevention is sufficient and continued.
- Programs are culturally sensitive.
- School-based programs include the family, the community, and the media.
- Evaluation is necessary to determine effectiveness.

Health Education

In the 1800s, students were taught about the dangers of alcohol, tobacco, and other drugs. Today, drug education at the secondary level typically is taught in health education classes, and its impact is encouraging. The School Health Education Evaluation showed that sequential health education from kindergarten through 12th grade had a positive effect on knowledge, attitudes, *and* behaviors. Administrative support and teacher training are important to the success of health education.

Red Ribbon Certified Schools

Since 1985, the Red Ribbon Campaign is celebrated by schools nationwide to raise awareness about the killing and destruction caused by drugs.[103] It is a yearly initiative where schools use activities and awareness programs during the last week in October. The Red Ribbon Campaign was initiated in honor of Enrique (Kiki) Camarena, a DEA enforcement agent, who was tortured and killed in Mexico. His family and friends started wearing red badges to honor Kiki's memory.[104]

The Red Ribbon Certified School program is a federally funded program designed for schools who meet certain criteria in their comprehensive drug prevention initiatives.[105] The goals for the Red Ribbon Certification initiatives include:[106]

- Produce safe, healthy drug-free kids
- Increase parental involvement in schools
- Improve academic performance
- Improve awareness and social norms around drugs and alcohol

Schools that achieve the Red Ribbon Certification show prevention plans that include a healthy school environment, use of best practices in education, high levels of parent involvement, and include year-round red ribbon activities.[107]

In a study comparing Red Ribbon certified schools against non-certified schools, significant differences were seen among Red Ribbon schools in the areas of frequency of drug use, attitudes toward drug use, academic performance, community environment, and parental attitudes toward drug use.[108]

Peer Programs

Various peer programs have been incorporated into drug prevention programs. Not all peer programs are alike. In some, peers serve as tutors; that is, older students teach younger students about drugs. In other programs, peers facilitate discussions about drugs with others of the same age, or peers counsel peers. Peer programs typically function under the auspices of adults but sometimes operate without adult supervision.

Choosing appropriate peers is paramount. Administrators and teachers might identify one student as desirable whereas students identify someone else. Unconventional but responsible peer leaders seem to be best. Besides acting as role models, peer leaders have to be able to communicate effectively.

Results from peer-oriented programs are encouraging. In five approaches—knowledge only, affective only, peer programs, knowledge plus affective, and alternatives—peer programs were the most effective with the average student; for at-risk students, alternative programs were most effective.[109] Another program demonstrated that an alcohol prevention program resulted in reduced alcohol use, although an important consideration was identifying appropriate peers.[110]

ELEMENTS OF A SUCCESSFUL PEER EDUCATION PROGRAM

- Recruitment of Peer Educators: These can be self-nominated or recruited by other peer educators.
- Training and Supervision: Peer educators need additional training and ongoing supervision to support their efforts.
- Compensation: Prizes, college credit, or other forms of compensation may help increase participation.

Source Research to Prevention, "Peer education: Rigorous evidence-usable results", (December 2010). Accessed on March 25, 2017 from http://www.jhsph.edu/research /centers-and-institutes/research-to-prevention/publications /peereducation.pdf.

Summary

Most people would agree—prevention is easier than treatment. However, preventing drug abuse has proven to be difficult millions of people derive pleasure from drugs, special interest groups hinder prevention efforts, and Americans do not like being told what to do. In the past, drug prevention was directed mainly at heroin, cocaine, and LSD. Now the attention has shifted to tobacco, alcohol, and marijuana—sometimes called gateway drugs. Rather than focus on drugs, some drug experts believe the causes underlying drug abuse—poverty, homelessness, poor education, and inadequate health care—should be addressed.

Evaluating prevention programs is difficult because the goals vary and "prevention" has no standard definition. Drug prevention occurs along a continuum of primary, secondary, and tertiary objectives.

Children from impoverished backgrounds tend to be designated as high-risk youths. Yet, many rise above their circumstances and exhibit a resiliency to high-risk behaviors. High-risk youths often grow up in households in which drugs are used, good parenting skills are lacking, and supervision is minimal. Children who are abused are at greater risk of becoming substance abusers as adults. Communities in which high-risk youths live are marked by high mobility, deprivation, population density, poverty, and disorganization. Educational programs in which students experience success, are exposed to alternative programs, and are involved in their learning have been shown to reduce high-risk behavior. Nurturing, supportive parents who give their children responsibilities are less likely to have children who use drugs. Communities can reduce drug use by providing jobs, better housing, and adequate health care.

When drug education was initiated, the emphasis was on information and scare tactics, under the incorrect assumption that knowledge and fear of the dangers of drugs would deter drug use. Drug education later promoted values clarification and affective education. These approaches were not effective, and evaluations of early drug education programs revealed that drug use actually went up, probably in part because of curiosity and the permission to explore values.

The focus today is on developing resiliency, refusal skills, decision-making ability, coping skills, and personal and social skills. Students are taught how to recognize, avoid, and manage instances that place them at risk of using drugs. Peer programs have been particularly successful in curtailing drug use.

Thinking Critically

1. If you were hired to teach at a high school and were asked to develop a drug prevention program, what goals would you strive to achieve?
2. Even though D.A.R.E. has proven to be ineffective, it is still used today. How does the commercialization of D.A.R.E. contribute to its popularity? If you were a parent of a child in a school that is considering using D.A.R.E. as a drug prevention program, would you support their decision? Why or why not?
3. Children growing up with parents who abuse drugs are more likely to use drugs than children whose parents do not abuse drugs. Should children of parents who abuse drugs be removed from their parents?
4. Some of the most effective prevention programs take a comprehensive approach to drug education that involves students, parents, and the community. If you were working at a low-income school district, how would you encourage parents to become involved in school-based programs? Consider that in low-income neighborhoods many households are run by single, working parents or in households where both parents work full-time.

GLOSSARY

Acculturation *The adaptation and acceptance of cultural and social norms of a new environment*

Acetaldehyde *Product of metabolism of alcohol by the liver; also found in tobacco smoke*

Acetylcholine (ACH) *A neurotransmitter synthesized from a molecule of choline and from acetyl CoA*

Acetylsalicylic acid *The agent in aspirin that relieves pain*

Action potential *The procedure by which the nerve impulse is sent down the axon*

Acute *Describes a condition that arises abruptly and is not long lasting*

Acute dyskinesia *Inappropriate motor movements as a side effect of antipsychotic drugs*

Adenosine *A neurotransmitter for which caffeine acts as an antagonist*

Adrenaline *A hormone secreted by the adrenal gland in the fight-flight-fright response; another name for epinephrine*

Akathesia *Jerky, uncontrollable constant motion, motor restlessness, occasional protruding tongue, and facial grimace*

Alcohol abuse *A state characterized by physical, social, intellectual, emotional, or financial problems resulting from the use of alcohol*

Alcohol dependence *Condition in which one's body requires alcohol or else withdrawal symptoms will occur; also marked by tolerance*

Alcoholism *Condition in which an individual loses control over intake of alcohol*

Alcopops *Malt, distilled alcohol-containing, or wine-containing beverages that have been flavored with fruit juices or other added ingredients; an example is Mike's Hard Lemonade*

Alli *A weight-loss drug that blocks the absorption of fat*

Amanita muscaria *One of the oldest and most common hallucinogens; derived from the fly agaric mushroom*

Amotivational syndrome *A condition characterized by apathy, an inability to concentrate, and little achievement orientation*

Amphetamines *Powerful central nervous system stimulants*

Amyl nitrite *An inhalant used to treat angina pectoris and congestive heart failure*

Anabolic steroids *Substances used to increase muscle mass; related to male sex hormones*

Analgesics *Drugs that relieve pain*

Analog *A synthetic derivative of an existing drug*

Anaphylactic shock *A condition caused by an allergic reaction to contaminants such as quinine, which are used to cut or dilute heroin*

Androstenedione *Food supplement used for muscle development*

Antabuse (disulfiram) *A drug that interferes with the metabolization of alcohol, making the drinker violently ill*

Antagonists *Drugs that occupy receptor sites and inhibit narcotic activity*

Anticholinergic hallucinogens *Substances found in datura and in*

Amanita muscaria *mushrooms; interfere with the action of acetylcholine to produce hallucinations*

Anticonvulsant *Also referred to as antiseizure durgs, these are classes of medications used to treat epileptic seizures*

Anti-emetic *A drug that reduces nausea and vomiting; an example is marijuana*

Antipyretic *Having fever-reducing properties*

Antitussives *Drugs that act as cough suppressants*

Anxiolytic *Refers to anxiety-reducing drugs*

Aphrodisiac *Any substance that increases sexual desire and performance*

Atropine *A psychoactive agent found in mandrake and other anticholinergic hallucinogens*

Attention deficithyperactivity disorder (ADHD) *A condition in which the individual is hyperactive and easily distracted, which inhibits learning*

Autonomic nervous system (ANS) *Part of the peripheral nervous system that is automatic and involuntary*

Autoreceptors *Units that alter the synthesis of neurotransmitters after they are released by the nerve cells*

Axons *Parts of the neuron that send nerve impulses away from the nerve's cell body*

Barbital *A sedative-hypnotic drug used to treat anxiety and nervousness; the original barbiturate*

Barbiturate (barbituric acid) *A member of a class of drugs that have depressant effects*

Basal ganglia *Part of the central nervous system*

Behavioral health continuum of care model *A comprehensive approach to care that includes promotion, prevention, treatment, and recovery.*

Behavioral tolerance *Adjustment or behaviors learned by an individual to compensate for the presence of drugs*

Belladonna (deadly nightshade) *A potent hallucinogen found in Europe, North Africa, and Asia; member of the tomato and potato family*

Benzedrine *An amphetamine used to treat nasal congestion and asthma*

Benzocaine *A topical anesthetic put into candies or chewing gum to diminish appetite*

Benzodiazepines *A type of minor tranquilizer; examples are Librium and Valium*

Benzopyrene *Carcinogenic compound found in marijuana and tobacco*

Bhang *Lower leaves, stems, and seeds of the cannabis plant*

Bidis *Flavored cigarettes from India that have considerably higher concentrations of nicotine than regular cigarettes*

Binge drinking *Consuming five or more drinks (men) or four (women) in a short period of time*

Biphetamine *A powerful stimulant*

Bipolar affective disorder *A mental condition characterized by alternating moods of depression and mania; formerly called manic-depression*

Blackouts *A common symptom of problem drinking; characterized by temporary memory loss*

Blood alcohol concentration (BAC)/blood alcohol level (BAL) *Percentage of alcohol in the bloodstream*

Blunt *A marijuana-containing cigar; to create a blunt, tobacco is removed from a regular cigar and marijuana is inserted*

Bradykinesia *Motor movements that are slow and limited*

Bromides *Nonbarbiturate sedatives used to treat epileptic convulsions*

Brompton's cocktail *A combination of heroin and cocaine sometimes used to treat terminally ill patients*

Bufo *A type of toad that produces a hallucinogenic secretion*

Buprenorphine *A semi-synthetic opiate that has an analgesic effect and is used to treat opioid addiction*

Butyl nitrite *An inhalant no longer used for medical purposes but found in products such as perfume and antifreeze*

BZP Similar, but much less potent, to amphetamines

Caffeine *A mild stimulant found in coffee, tea, soda pop, and chocolate*

Caffeinism *Excessive caffeine consumption resulting in caffeine dependency*

Calcium carbonate *An antacid designed to relieve acid indigestion*

Cannabinoids *Chemicals found in marijuana plants*

Cannabis *A genus of plant that is also known as marijuana*

Carbon monoxide *Gas in cigarette smoke that interferes with oxygen-carrying capacity of blood*

Catecholamines *A group of neurotransmitters that includes epinephrine, dopa-mine, and norepinephrine*

Category I drugs *Drugs determined to be safe, effective, and properly labeled*

Category II drugs *Drugs generally recognized as unsafe and ineffective or as mislabeled; must be removed from medications within 6 months after the FDA issues its final regulations*

Category III drugs *Drugs for which data are insufficient to determine general recognition of safety and effectiveness*

Central nervous system (CNS) *The brain and spinal cord*

Cerebral cortex *Part of the brain involved in intellectual functioning; affects speech, motor movement, sensory perception, hearing, vision, sensory discrimination, memory, language, reasoning, abstract reasoning, and personality*

Cerebrum *Part of the brain that contains the cerebral cortex*

Charas *A potent form of marijuana also known as hashish*

China white *A synthetic analgesic drug derived from fentanyl that mimics heroin but is considerably more potent*

Chippers *Nickname for individuals who use narcotics occasionally or on weekends*

Chloral hydrate *A nonbarbiturate sedative; also called "knockout drops" or Mickey Finns; induces sleep*

Chlorpromazine *An antipsychotic drug*

Cholinesterase *An enzyme necessary for the metabolism of acetylcholine*

Chronic drug use *The habitual use of drugs*

Circumstantial-situational drug use *Short-term drug use to contend with immediate distress or pressure*

Clove cigarettes *Cigarettes made from tobacco and cloves; contain more tar, nicotine, and carbon monoxide than commercial cigarettes*

Codeine *A mild narcotic that suppresses coughing; a derivative of opium*

Cold turkey *Elimination of a negative behavior all at once, as opposed to gradually (with or without a substitute)*

Compulsive drug use *Obsessive drug use without regard for society*

Congeners *The nonalcoholic ingredients in some forms of alcohol, such as flavoring agents or other residual substances*

Controlled drinking approach *Alcohol treatment based on behavior modification, in which the person learns to drink in a non-abusive manner*

Crack cocaine *A variation of cocaine made by heating cocaine after mixing it with baking soda and water*

Crank *A term for methamphetamines*

Creatine monohydrate *Natural substance used to increase strength and short-term speed*

Cross-tolerance *Transference of tolerance to a drug to chemically similar drugs*

Crystal meth *A variation of methamphetamine; one example is ice*

Datura *A hallucinogen used for sacred purposes in ancient China, Greece, India, and Africa*

Deadly nightshade *See belladonna*

Decongestants *Substances used to relieve congestion*

Decriminalization *The reduction or elimination of penalties for illegal activities*

Delta-9-tetrahydrocannabinol (THC) *The psychoactive agent in marijuana*

Dendrites *Parts of the neuron that allow nerve impulses to be transmitted to the nerve's cell body*

Depression *Dejection characterized by withdrawal or lack of response to stimulation*

Designer drugs *Synthetic substances that are chemically similar to existing drugs*

Desvenlafaxine (Pristiq) *an antidepressant in a group of drugs called selective serotonin and norepinephrine reuptake inhibitors (SNRIs).*

Detoxification *Eliminating drugs from the body; usually the initial step in treatment of the effects of alcohol and other drugs*

Dextromethorphan (Delsym) *An over-the-counter non-narcotic drug found in cough preparations*

Diacetylmorphine *See* heroin

Diethyl glycol *A chemical solvent*

Dimethyltryptamine (DMT) *A hallucinogen in which effects last 1 to 2 hours*

Disease *Applied when the underlying pathology is known and identified*

Disorder *Applied to a collection of symptoms*

Dissociative anesthetic *Substance that alters the perception of pain without loss of consciousness*

Distillation *A heating process that increases alcohol content*

Distilled spirits *Beverages such as whiskey, rum, gin, and vodka that are produced by boiling various solutions*

Disulfiram *See* Antabuse

Dopamine *A neurotransmitter that affects emotional, mental, and motor functions*

Dose-response curve *Graphic representation of the effects of drugs at various levels*

Drug *Any substance that alters one's ability to function emotionally, physically, intellectually, financially, or socially*

Drug abuse *The intentional and inappropriate use of a drug resulting in physical, emotional, financial, intellectual, or social consequences for the user*

Drug addiction *Continuing desire for drugs based on a physical need*

Drug dependency *Recurring desire for drugs based on a psychic or a physical need*

Drug misuse *The unintentional or inappropriate use of*

prescribed or over-the-counter drugs

Drug paraphernalia *Items that are aids to using drugs*

Dual Diagnosis *A term to describe when a person has a substance abuse problem and a mental illness simultaneously*

Duloxetine (Cymbalta) *A drug used to treat depression and peripheral neuropathy (pain, numbness, tingling, burning, or weakness in the hands or feet) that can occur with diabetes.*

Dysthymia *Mild, but long-lasting depression*

Dystonia *A type of dyskinesia marked by involuntary and inappropriate postures and muscle tones*

Ecstasy *See* MDMA

Effective dose (ED) *The amount of drug required to produce a specific response*

Electroconvulsive therapy (ECT) *Controlled administration of electric shock as a treatment for mental illness*

Elixir sulfanilamide *An antibiotic that killed more than 100 people in the 1930s*

Emasam *The levorotatory form of the monoamine oxidase inhibitor deprenyl*

Employee assistance programs (EAPs) *Company-sponsored programs to help employers deal with their employees who have problems, including drug use*

Encounter groups *A type of confrontational treatment frequently used at therapeutic communities*

Endorphins *Naturally occurring chemicals with opiate-like properties*

Enkaphalins *Endorphins found within the brain*

Environmental tobacco smoke (ETS) *Smoke in the air as a result of someone smoking*

Epinephrine *A natural chemical, also called adrenaline, involved in the fight-flight-fright syndrome*

Equanil *The first modern drug developed to relieve anxiety*

Ergogenic aids *Substances that provide an athleticadvantage, also known as performance-enhancing drugs*

Ergotism *A condition resulting from ingesting a fungus that grows on grains; marked by muscle tremors, burning, mania, delirium, hallucinations, and eventual gangrene*

Erythropoietin *Hormone that enhances cardiovascular endurance by increasing red blood cell production*

Erythroxylon coca *Coca plant from which cocaine is derived*

Ether *An inhalant dating back to the late 1700s*

Ethyl alcohol *The form of alcohol that people consume*

Eugenol *Ingredient in clove cigarettes that provides aroma and reduces coughing reflex*

Expectorants *Cough medicines that make a cough productive by increasing mucous secretions*

Experimental drug use *Infrequent drug use usually motivated by curiosity*

Extrapyramidal symptoms *Neurological symptoms characterized by difficulty walking, shuffling, and inflexible joints*

False negative *A test that is negative for drugs even though drugs are present in the urine*

False positive *A test that is positive for drugs even though no drugs are present in the urine*

Fentanyl *A synthetic narcotic that is 1,000 times more potent than heroin*

Fermentation *The process of transforming certain yeasts, carbon, hydrogen, and oxygen of sugar and water into ethyl alcohol and carbon dioxide*

Fetal benzodiazepinesyndrome *A condition of infants caused by the mother's use of benzodiazepine during pregnancy; affected children have malformed face, poor muscle tone, tremors, poor coordination, delayed mental development, and learning disabilities*

Fight-flight-fright syndrome *Psychological response of the body to stress, which prepares the individual to take action by stimulating the body's defense system*

Flashbacks *A phenomenon in which a person reexperiences the effects of LSD days, weeks, or months after it was last used*

Fly agaric *Another name for the hallucinogenic mushroom Amanita muscaria*

Fortified wines *Beverages produced by adding alcohol to slightly sweetened wines*

Freebase *A variation of cocaine in which cocaine is separated from its hydrochloride salt by heating, using a volatile chemical such as ether*

Gamma-aminobutyric acid (GABA) *An inhibitory neurotransmitter that regulates muscle tone in mammals*

Gamma-hydroxybutyrate (GHB) *A type of neurotransmitter that produces relaxation and sleepiness; one of the "date rape" drugs*

Ganja *Tops and flowers of the cannabis plant*

Gas chromatography *A drug-testing procedure that is more specific, sensitive, and expensive than the immunologic assay*

Gas chromatography/mass spectrometry *A type of drug-testing procedure that is highly sophisticated and sensitive, but time-consuming and expensive*

Gateway drugs *Substances that are used before use of more dangerous drugs; alcohol, marijuana, tobacco, and inhalants are considered gateway drugs*

Halcion *A drug used to induce sleep*

Hallucinogens *A class of drugs that induce perceived distortions in time and space*

Hallucinogen-induced persistent perception disorder (HPPD) *Flashbacks that continue and interfere with daily life.*

Hard drugs *Drugs that are perceived to be dangerous, such as heroin, cocaine, and LSD*

Harm reduction *A series of practical interventions that respond to the needs of drug users and the community where they live in an effort to reduce the harm caused by illicit drug use*

Hash oil *Substance made by separating resin from the cannabis plant by boiling the plant in alcohol; it has a very high THC content*

Hashish *A potent form of marijuana taken from resin of the cannabis plant*

Hemp *Marijuana plant that may be used to make rope, clothing, and paper*

Heroin (diacetylmorphine) *A potent drug that is a derivative of opium*

Hippocampus *Part of the brain involved with memory; altered by marijuana*

Histamines *Chemicals that are released by the body in response to the presence of allergens*

Homeostasis *A condition in which the body's systems are in balance*

Human growth hormones *Hormones that stimulate protein synthesis; used by athletes to enhance performance*

Hydrochloric acid *Acid in the stomach that can ease digestion and irritate the stomach lining*

Hypnotic *Also referred to as sleeping pills, these are classes of medications used to induce sleep*

Hypoglycemia *A condition of low levels of sugar in the blood*

Hypothalamus *Gland situated near the base of the brain; maintains homeostasis; affects stress, aggressiveness, heart rate, hunger, thirst, consciousness, body temperature, blood pressure, and sexual behavior*

Hypoxia *A lack of oxygen within body tissues. Hypoxia can lead to brain damage resulting from an inadequate supply of oxygen to the brain*

Ibogaine *A hallucinogen that is used to treat cocaine dependence*

Ice *Crystals of methamphetamine that are smoked, inhaled, or injected*

Illicit drugs use *Illegal drug use*

Immunoassay *A drug-testing procedure that tests for metabolites of drugs*

Inhalants *Drugs that are inhaled or "sniffed"*

Inpatient treatment *A residential drug treatment program based on a hospital model*

Intensified drug use *Taking drugs on a steady, long-term basis to relieve a persistent problem or stressful situation*

Interdiction *Prohibition and enforcement*

Interferon *A natural substance in the body that wards off viral infections*

Iproniazid *A monoamine oxidase inhibitor*

Isobutyl *One type of nitrite that is used to treat angina pain; also causes vasodilation, flushing, and warmth*

Jamestown weed (jimsonweed) *Any hallucinogen derived from the Datura plant; also known as "locoweed"*

Ketamine *A drug very similar to PCP*

Ketoprofen *An over-the-counter analgesic*

Kief *resin of cannabis that contains trichomes*

Kola nut *A part of a plant originally used in Coca-Cola*

Laudanum *A drug derived from opium*

Lethal dose (LD) *The amount of a drug required to result in death*

Lethal hyponatraemia *Fatal water overdose from taking in too much water*

Levo-alpha-acetylmethadol (LAAM) *An experimental drug that prevents narcotic withdrawal symptoms for about 3 days*

Limbic system *Part of the central nervous system that plays a key role in memory and emotion*

Lithium *A psychotherapeutic drug used to treat symptoms associated with mania*

Locoweed *Another term for jimsonweed*

Look-alike drugs *Substances that appear similar to illegal or pharmaceutical drugs*

LSD (lysergic acid diethylamide) *A powerful hallucinogen derived from a fungus*

Mainstream smoke *Smoke exhaled by a smoker*

Major tranquilizers *Antipsychotic drugs*

Mandrake *A hallucinogen derived from the nightshade family; used during the Middle Ages in connection with witchcraft and sorcery*

Mania *A mood disorder characterized by inappropriate elation, an irrepressible mood, and extreme cheerfulness*

Margin of safety *The difference between a beneficial level and a harmful level of a drug*

MDA *A hallucinogen that is structurally similar to amphetamines*

MDMA (methylenedioxymethamphetamine) *A synthetic hallucinogen related to amphetamines; also called Ecstasy*

Medial forebrain bundle (MFB) *Serves as a communication route between the limbic system and the brain stem; affects pleasure and reward*

Medical model *The premise that a pathogen is responsible for a person's illness or disease*

Medulla oblongata *One of two structures constituting the brain stem; helps control respiration, blood pressure, heart rate, and other vital functions*

Mental illness *A condition caused by a mood disorder or by disorganized thinking*

Meperidine *A synthetic derivative of morphine*

Meprobamate *A minor tranquilizer marketed under the trade names of Miltown and Equanil; also used for treating psychosomatic conditions*

Mescaline *A psychoactive agent, or hallucinogen, derived from the peyote cactus*

Methadone *A drug given to heroin addicts to block withdrawal effects and euphoria*

Methadone maintenance program *A type of therapy used in the treatment of heroin addiction*

Methamphetamine *A more potent form of amphetamine*

Methaqualone *A sedative-hypnotic drug that relieves tension and anxiety without barbiturate-like after effects*

Methyl alcohol *Wood alcohol; not fit for human consumption*

Midbrain *Part of the brain stem that connects the larger structures of the brain to the spinal cord*

Miltown *Brand name for meprobamate*

Minor tranquilizer *Drug used primarily to relieve anxiety*

Monoamine oxidase inhibitor (MAO) *An antidepressant drug used for acute anxiety, obsessive-compulsive behavior, and phobias*

Mood disorder *A form of psychosis that affects the person's emotions; can be depression or mania*

Morphine *An analgesic drug derived from opium; used medically as a painkiller*

MPPP *A synthetic drug that is similar to meperidine*

Myristicin *Substance found in nutmeg and mace; chemically similar to mescaline and capable of producing hallucinations*

Naltrexone *A narcotic antagonist that blocks the reinforcing effects of narcotics*

Naproxen sodium *An over-the-counter analgesic*

Narcolepsy *Condition in which the person involuntarily falls asleep; commonly called sleeping sickness*

Narcotic *An opium-based central nervous system depressant used to relieve pain and diarrhea*

Negative reinforcement *Relief or avoidance of pain achieved by a behavior, motivating one to repeat the behavior*

Neuroleptics *The European term for antipsychotic drugs*

Neurons *Messengers in the brain that transmit information via chemical and electrical processes*

Neurosis *A long-term disorder featuring the symptoms of anxiety and/or exaggerated behavior dedicated to avoiding anxious feelings*

Neurotransmitter *A chemical substance manufactured in vesicles of the brain*

Nicotine *Psychoactive component in tobacco responsible for stimulation and tobacco dependence*

NIMBY (not in my back yard) *A term describing how some people feel about having a controversial facility located in their neighborhoods*

Nitrous oxide *An inhalant also known as laughing gas*

Norepinephrine *A neurotransmitter that may help regulate appetite and reduce fatigue*

Normalization *A term used by the Dutch for the practice of not prosecuting users of soft drugs such as marijuana*

Opiate *A class of drugs derived from opium*

Opioid *A family of drugs with characteristics similar to those of opium*

Opium *The plant from which narcotics are derived*

Outpatient treatment *A nonresidential drug treatment program; least expensive form of treatment*

Paraldehyde *A nonbarbiturate sedative-hypnotic drug used with severely disturbed mental patients*

Parasympathetic nervous system *Branch of the autonomic nervous system that includes acetylcholine and alters heart rate and intestinal activity*

Parasympathomimetics *Drugs that mimic actions of the parasympathetic system, which allows the body to rest during states of emergency*

Parenteral drug use *Drug administration by injection*

Parkinsonism *A form of acute dyskinesia marked by tremors, weakness in the extremities, and muscle rigidity*

Passive smoke *Tobacco smoke present in the air from someone else's smoking and inhaled by others*

Patent medicines *A synonym for over-the-counter drugs*

Pathogen *Any organism that produces disease*

Pentothal *See thiopental*

Peptides *Substances linking amino acids; include endorphins, which are naturally occurring chemicals with opiate-like properties*

Peripheral nervous system (PNS) *Consists of the autonomic and somatic nervous systems*

Periventricular system *Part of the central nervous system implicated with punishment or avoidance behavior*

Peyote *A cactus containing the hallucinogen mescaline*

Phantasticants *A term used to describe hallucinogenic drugs*

Pharmacological tolerance *Adjustment or compensation of the body to the presence of a given drug*

Pharmacology *The professional discipline that studies the relationships and interactions between living organisms and substances within them*

Phenacetin *An alternative to aspirin now linked to kidney problems; its sale is prohibited*

Phencyclidine hydrochloride (PCP) *Originally developed as an anesthetic for humans and, later, animals; also called "angel dust"*

Phenobarbital *Second barbiturate developed; produces relaxation and relieves anxiety*

Phenylpropanolamine (PPA) *A decongestant also used as an appetite suppressant*

Pituitary gland *The "master gland"; responsible for controlling many bodily functions by secretion of hormones*

Placebo *An inert substance that does not have a physical effect but may produce psychological and associated physiological reactions*

Polydipsia *Frequent and excessive consumption of water*

Polyuria *Frequent urination*

Pons *One of two structures constituting the brain stem, connecting the medulla with the brain stem*

Positive reinforcement *Pleasurable sensations associated with a behavior, motivating one to repeat the behavior*

Potency *A drug's ability to produce an effect relative to other drugs; the less that is needed to produce a response, the more potent the drug*

PPA *See phenylpropanolamine*

Primary prevention *Preventing drug use before it begins*

Primary reinforcers *Stimuli that reduce physiological needs or are inherently pleasurable*

Proof *Amount of alcohol in a beverage expressed as twice the percentage of the alcohol content*

Propoxyphene hydrochloride *A mild narcotic that has the potential to cause dependence*

Proprietary drugs *Drugs that can be purchased without a prescription; over-the--counter drugs*

Prostaglandins *Chemicals in the body that produce pain and inflammation; aspirin alters their synthesis*

Protective factor *Reduces a person's risk for drug use behavior*

Prozac (fluoxetine) *An antidepressant drug*

Pseudoephedrine *A nasal decongestant*

Psilocin *The psychoactive ingredient in the psylocybe mushroom*

Psilocybin *A hallucinogen found in certain mushrooms in Central America*

Psyche *Refers to the mind*

Psychedelic *A term used to describe hallucinogenic drugs; means "mind-manifesting"*

Psychoactive drug *Any substance that has the capability of altering mood, perception, or behavior*

Psychoanalysis *A form of talk therapy based on Freudian principles*

Psychosis *A severe mental condition marked by loss of contact with reality*

Psychotogenic *Refers to drugs that generate psychosis*

Psychotomimetic *Refers to drugs that produce psychotic-like symptoms*

Purity *Quality of a substance; state of noncontamination of a drug*

Quaalude *Brand name for methaqualone*

Rapid eye movement (REM) *A stage during sleep that is needed for the sleep to be restful*

Rapid smoking *Aversive smoking-cessation technique in which one smokes rapidly to exceed tolerance and becomes ill*

Rebound effect *The side effects produced by a drug that make a condition worse than it was originally; e.g., sinuses become more congested by nasal sprays*

Rebound insomnia *A side effect of sleeping pills in which falling asleep becomes more difficult rather than less difficult*

Recidivism *Relapse*

Reinforcers *Stimuli or events that lead to certain behaviors being repeated*

Relapse *Failure to maintain a course of action, such as returning to drug abuse after initiating a treatment program*

Resiliency *A person's ability to overcome obstacles, such as resisting drug use despite a background that increases the likelihood of drug use*

Resistance skills training *Instruction in which students are taught to recognize, manage, and elude situations involving drugs; includes dealing with peer pressure and media messages*

Risk factor *Increases a person's risk for drug use behavior*

Reticular activating system (RAS) *Part of the central nervous system; affects sleep, attention, and arousal*

Reuptake *A process by which a chemical is reabsorbed into the cell from which it was discharged*

Reverse tolerance *A drug user's experiencing of the desired effects from lesser amounts of the same drug*

Ritalin *A mild stimulant used to treat attention deficit/hyperactivity disorder (ADHD)*

Rohypnol *A powerful depressant; one of the "date rape" drugs*

Roid rage *Uncontrollable violence associated with use of anabolic steroids*

Salvinorin A *A hallucinogen that alters perception and consciousness; effects last less than one hour*

Schizophrenia *A type of functional psychosis; literally, "split mind"*

Scopolamine *A psychoactive agent found in mandrake and other anticholinergic hallucinogens*

Secondary prevention *Early intervention to block more serious problems; halts escalation of drug use*

Secondary reinforcers *Stimuli that signal the increased probability of obtaining primary reinforcers*

Sedative-hypnotic *Class of drugs that produce relaxing to sleep-inducing effects depending on dosage*

Selective serotonin reuptake inhibitors (SSRIs) *A class of antidepressant medications that increase the concentration of the chemical, serotonin, in the brain*

Selegeline (Ensam) *the levorotatory form of the monoamine oxidase inhibitor deprenyl*

Self-efficacy *Personal success based on one's own efforts*

Serotonin *An inhibitory neurotransmitter located in the upper brain stem; plays a role in regulating sensory perception, eating, pain, sleep, and body temperature*

Serotonin and norepinephrine reuptake inhibitors (SNRIs) *A class of antidepressant medications that inhibit both the reuptake of serotonin and norepinephrine*

Set *The psychological state, personality, and expectations of an individual while using drugs*

Setting *The physical and social environment in which drugs are used*

Shooting gallery *A place to buy and inject drugs*

Sidestream smoke *Smoke that comes from the burning end of a cigarette, pipe, or cigar*

Sinsemilla *Seedless marijuana; derived from unfertilized female cannabis plants*

Skills training *A drug prevention program in which one learns skills to prevent drug use*

Snuff *A form of smokeless tobacco*

Social-recreational drug use *Taking drugs in a social environment to share pleasurable experiences among friends*

Sodium bicarbonate *Baking soda; an ingredient in antacids designed to neutralize excess acid in the stomach*

Soft drugs *Drugs perceived to be less harmful than hard drugs; include marijuana, tobacco, and alcohol*

Soldier's disease *A name given to morphine dependency during the Civil War*

Soma *1. From the Greek; literally means "body" 2. An Indian drink used in ritualistic ways.*

Somatic nervous system *Part of the nervous system that controls movement of the skeletal muscles*

Sound-alike drugs *Substances with names that sound similar to those of illegal or prescription drugs*

Speed *A stimulant drug; another name for methamphetamine*

Speedball *Injectable combination of heroin and cocaine*

"Speed freak" *Someone who uses methamphetamines over a period of time*

Spontaneous remission *Cessation of drug abuse without any type of formal treatment*

St. Anthony's fire *Burning sensations caused by ergot poisoning; people during the Middle Ages would visit the shrine of St. Anthony in an attempt to cure it*

Stacking *Ingesting or injecting several steroids at the same time*

Stepping stone theory *Hypothesis holding that use of soft drugs such as marijuana and alcohol leads to use of harder drugs such as heroin and cocaine*

Sympathetic nervous system *A branch of the autonomic nervous system that releases adrenaline*

Sympathomimetic effects *An increase of blood to the brain and muscle, allowing the body to flee or fight*

Sympathomimetics *Drugs that mimic actions of the sympathetic nervous system, which is involved with fight-flight-fright activity*

Symptoms *An observable or stated behavior*

Synthetic cannabinoids *Related to chemicals found in the marijuana plant*

Synthetic cathinones *Related to the stimulant in the khat plant related to the stimulant in the khat plant*

Synapse *The space between an axon and a dendrite*

Synergistic effect *An enhanced, unpredictable effect caused by combining two or more substances*

Synesthesia *The hallucinogenic blending of senses (e.g., seeing sounds and hearing color)*

Synthetic drugs *Drugs that are synthesized by chemicals to mimic illicit drugs*

T lymphocytes *Type of white blood cells that help in fighting infections*

Tachycardia *Faster than normal heart rate*

Tar *A carcinogenic component of tobacco*

Tardive dyskinesia *A side effect of antipsychotic drugs marked by involuntary repetitive facial movements and involuntary movement of the trunk and limbs*

Temperance *Moderate alcohol use, rather than abstinence*

Temperance movement *A social trend that developed in the United States in the 1800s when groups sought to reduce alcohol use*

Teonanacatl *Aztec word describing the psylocybe mushroom*

Teratogenic *Refers to substances that cause harm to the fetus*

Tertiary prevention *Treatment that seeks to help individuals after they have misused drugs*

Tetrahydrogestrinone (THG) *A designer drug, closely related to the banned anabolic steroids gestrinone and trenbolone*

Thalidomide *A sedative that was found in the 1960s to cause birth defects including missing or malformed limbs*

THC *See delta-9-tetrahydrocannabinol*

Theobromine *A stimulant found in chocolate; chemically related to caffeine*

Theophylline *A stimulant found in tea; in the same chemical family as caffeine*

Therapeutic community (TC) *A residential drug treatment center that utilizes confrontation techniques*

Therapeutic window *The amount of drug needed for therapeutic purposes*

Thin-layer chromatography *A simple, inexpensive, urine-based drug test*

Thiopental (pentothal) *A barbiturate that is used as a general anesthetic*

Thorazine *Major tranquilizer used to treat psychosis*

Threshold dose *The smallest amount of a drug required to produce an effect*

Tinnitus *A condition marked by constant ringing in the ears*

Toluene *The psychoactive agent in glue*

Toxicity *A drug's ability to disturb or nullify homeostasis*

Transdermal method *Administration of drugs by applying them on the surface of the skin*

Tricyclic antidepressants *Drugs that effectively remove the symptoms of acute depression*

Tryptophan *An amino acid that affects serotonin levels, allowing one to fall asleep more easily*

Tyramine *An amino acid that interacts with monoamine oxidase inhibitors to cause very high levels of hypertension*

Unipolar depression *A mental disorder marked by alternating periods of depression and normalcy*

Valium *(diazepam) A minor tranquilizer*

Values clarification *A teaching strategy in which individuals are asked to express and support their values*

Venlafaxine (Effexor XR) *An antidepressant drug that acts by inhibiting the reuptake of serotonin and norepinephrine by neurons*

Veronal *Brand name for barbital*

Vesicles *Saclike structure at the end of the axon*

Wellbutrin *An antidepressant drug that is used to help people stop smoking*

Whiskey Rebellion *A protest by farmers in southwestern Pennsylvania against a tax on whiskey*

Withdrawal symptoms *Physical signs that appear when drug use is stopped*

Xanthine *A type of stimulant of which caffeine is one*

INDEX